INTRODUCTORY

Mental Health Nursing

Cynthia A. Kincheloe, MSN, BSN, ADN, RN

Reusable Medical Equipment (RME) Coordinator
Albuquerque, New Mexico
Past Nursing Chair and Educator
National American University
Albuquerque, New Mexico

T0178851

FIFTH EDITION

Wolters Kluwer

Philadelphia • Baltimore • New York • London
Buenos Aires • Hong Kong • Sydney • Tokyo

Vice President, Nursing Segment: Julie K. Stegman
Manager, Nursing Education and Practice Content: Jamie Blum
Senior Acquisitions Editor: Jodi Rhomberg
Development Editor: Phoebe Jordan-Reilly
Editorial Coordinator: Venugopal Loganathan
Editorial Assistant: Devika Kishore
Production Project Manager: Frances Gunning
Marketing Manager: Wendy Mears
Manager, Graphic Arts & Design: Stephen Druding
Art Director: Jennifer Clements
Manufacturing Coordinator: Margie Orzech
Prepress Vendor: Aptara, Inc.

5th Edition

Library of Congress Cataloging-in-Publication Data

Names: Kincheloe, Cynthia A., author. | Womble, Donna M. Introductory
   mental health nursing
Title: Introductory mental health nursing / Cynthia A. Kincheloe.
Description: Fifth edition. | Philadelphia, PA : Wolters Kluwer, [2024] |
   Preceded by Introductory mental health nursing / Donna M. Womble, Cynthia A. Kincheloe. Fourth edition. 2020. | Includes
   bibliographical references and index. | Summary: "Created specifically for LPN/LVN students, Introductory Mental Health
   Nursing, 5th Edition, instills the comprehensive understanding and clinical confidence for success in today's evolving mental
   health nursing practice. This approachable, easy-to-use text prepares students for the clinical challenges ahead by providing a
   summarized overview of the theories integral to current treatment modalities accompanied by integrated study exercises that
   stimulate critical thinking and clinical reasoning. Unit I presents a picture of mental health and mental illness including an
   expanded emphasis on cultural, ethnic, and religious influences. Building upon those concepts, Unit II discusses the delivery of
   mental health care, moving from early views to current issues. Unit III explores the nursing process and how it relates to mental
   health, followed by a detailed breakdown of specific psychiatric disorders in Unit IV and disorders related to age and development
   in Unit V. This 5th Edition is extensively updated throughout, delivering the current information and clinical preparation essential
   to your students' success in class, on their exams, and beyond." —Provided by publisher.
Identifiers: LCCN 2023026509 (print) | LCCN 2023026510 (ebook) |
   ISBN 9781975211240 (paperback) | ISBN 9781975211264 (epub)
Subjects: MESH: Mental Disorders–nursing | Psychiatric Nursing | BISAC:
   MEDICAL / Mental Health
Classification: LCC RC440 (print) | LCC RC440 (ebook) | NLM WY 160 | DDC
   616.89/0231–dc23/eng/20230706
LC record available at https://lccn.loc.gov/2023026509
LC ebook record available at https://lccn.loc.gov/2023026510

To the points on my compass that help guide me:
Jay, Deanna, Kathryn, Kinley, Deloris, Mary, Paula,
Jean, and Sally.

—Cynthia

Preface

New to This Edition

- NEW! Cultural Considerations boxes familiarize you with cultural, ethnic, and religious considerations that may affect care.
- NEW! Test Yourself recall exercises throughout each chapter help you identify areas you have mastered and areas requiring further review.
- UPDATED and redesigned Nursing Process sections in all chapters on specific disorders clarify each step in the nursing process.
  - NEW! Two Nursing Care Focus subsections were added to each Nursing Process section with examples of goals, implementations, and evaluations of outcomes to help you understand how the nursing process can be applied to the care of mental health clients.
- UPDATED! Language reviewed and revised for inclusive terminology that strengthens your clinical communication.
- REVISED and IMPROVED Case Studies:
  - NEW! Each case study now includes a picture of the client to help you immerse yourself in the scenario and focus on client care.
  - UPDATED! Case Studies have been added so all chapters have a minimum of two per chapter.
- STREAMLINED Appendices, including two NEW Appendices:
  - Sample Patient Health Questionnaire-9 (PHQ-9)
  - Sample Abnormal Involuntary Movement Scale (AIMS)
- UPDATED! Key Terms in each chapter with a REVISED Glossary in the back of the book for a quick review of all Key Terms and definitions included in the text.
- UPDATED! Student Worksheet in every chapter with new and revised questions to test your understanding.
- NEW! Chapter 17 has been heavily revised and renamed from "Sexual Disorders" to "Mental Health Issues Related to Gender Identity and Sexuality," broadening the focus to discuss mental health concerns of people with a range of sexual and gender identities. Content in this chapter has been updated with the latest terminology, discussion of historical social discrimination, and a tool to help nurses self-assess beliefs that may influence care.

A Note From the Author

I am excited to present the fifth edition of this textbook. It is my mission to continue to update and streamline the basic principles and foundations of mental health nursing for the LPN/LVN student. As mental health is a component of the whole client, it is essential for every nurse to have a basic understanding of the essential information presented in this text to provide holistic nursing care to a variety of clients in a variety of settings. Awareness has been made to keep the focus of the text on the nursing model of care. It is my intent that the fifth edition of this textbook will continue to help students better understand mental health and its presence and impact in the nursing care of all clients.

LPN/LVN student nurses do not always have the opportunity for in-depth inpatient psychiatric unit experience, but they will encounter mental health concerns and issues in a variety of health care settings as both students and graduates. To help supplement their learning experience, case studies are included in every chapter to help the student tie the content to potential situations they may encounter. I have attempted to discuss different practice settings and functional roles of the LPN/LVN.

This book presents mental health and illness by first establishing the essential groundwork related to this subject. Unit I presents an overview of mental health concepts including cultural, ethnic, and religious influences. A basic understanding of how mental health is viewed and approached is essential for caring for clients from multicultural and diverse backgrounds. Factors that affect mental health are also discussed in this unit. Stress, anxiety, grief, and loss are discussed along with variations of human responses to these factors. The delivery of mental health care, including historical views, is presented. The section on outpatient and community mental health details information on services offered in various settings. The various practice settings for mental health care are included to provide an all-encompassing picture of how mental health is a common encounter for the nurse in every health care setting. Legal and ethical considerations, including client rights and nursing accountability, are addressed. The unit concludes with an overview of various theories of personality and psychological development to help provide a foundation for understanding human behavior.

In Unit II, the treatment process is discussed, beginning with an introduction to the treatment team, holistic and different approaches to treatment, and the client's role. The various types of psychotherapy are presented along with an overview of psychotropic medications used in the treatment of mental illness. The importance of establishing a therapeutic relationship between the nurse and the client is described. Difficult client situations, including the impact of anger, violence, bullying, and abuse are discussed. The subjects of crisis and suicide prevention are presented including client risk factors, exhibited behaviors, nursing interventions, and nursing care.

Unit III looks at the fundamental nursing roles in mental health nursing. This unit begins with a discussion of therapeutic communication. Techniques that facilitate communication and interactions with the mental health client, as well as what can hinder them, are discussed. A detailed discussion of the nursing process, including specifics to mental health nursing, is provided. Application of the nursing process in relation to mental health is included as part of the chapter case studies.

Unit IV deals with specific mental health disorders. The different disorders are discussed in terms of symptoms exhibited, risk factors, populations seen in, and treatments for the disorder. Medications, including action and therapeutic use, are incorporated into the discussion of treatment. Current research and references are used to substantiate the information presented and are also included in the end-of-chapter bibliography. Nursing care of the client with a mental illness specific to the chapter topic is described in the Nursing Process section.

Unit V examines disorders that have diagnostic criteria or are influenced by age. The first chapter in the unit is on disorders specific to the child and adolescent, and those that are commonly first diagnosed in childhood or adolescence. The final chapter addresses issues and types of mental disorders seen in older adults.

To help supplement the content, there are several features throughout every chapter to aid the LPN/LVN student's understanding. Opening each chapter are chapter objectives, which are written concisely and purposefully to guide learning outcomes. They are also intended to provide an outline for the student as they read the chapter. Key terms are boldfaced in the manuscript to provide easy access to their meaning. In addition, the key terms are listed in the glossary for easy reference. Enhanced features for content understanding are presented multiple times throughout every chapter in the form of specialty call-out boxes. Thought-provoking questions are presented to encourage critical thinking in the "Mind Jogger" boxes. Important information is summarized or added in "Just the Facts" boxes. A new feature has been added, the "Test Yourself" box, which helps to break up the chapter and provides an opportunity for students to quiz themselves on the information presented. Boxes and tables are located throughout the chapter to give the student a summary of information in an easily viewed and compressed format. A minimum of two case studies are integrated into each chapter to provide opportunities for reflection and content application. Last, another new feature, the "Cultural Considerations" box, has been added at the end of each chapter to provide multicultural information related to a topic in the chapter.

Each chapter is followed by a study guide, or worksheet, with various methods of appraising the student's recall of the content presented. This component is designed for the student to practice deductive thinking and reasoning. Questions are written so that the answers are easily discernible after reading the chapter. Terminology and key terms are reinforced through completion and matching exercises. Multiple-choice questions are written using an NCLEX item-writing format to help prepare the LPN/LVN student for entry-level testing. Included are questions that ask the student to select all answers that are applicable. An answer key is provided for all worksheets at the end of the textbook. A supporting bibliography for content is provided at the end of each chapter that includes internet addresses to references as applicable.

Building Clinical Judgment Skills

Nursing students are required to obtain nursing knowledge and apply foundational nursing processes to practice effective clinical judgment. Being able to apply clinical judgment in practice is critical for patient safety and optimizing outcomes. The content provided in this text includes features such as Case Studies; Nursing Process Sections; and Mind Jogger, Test Yourself, and Just the Facts boxes that strengthen students' clinical judgment skills by giving them opportunities to apply knowledge and practice critical thinking. In addition, accompanying products CoursePoint and Lippincott NCLEX-PN PassPoint provide an adaptive experience that allows students to build confidence by answering questions like those found on the Next Generation NCLEX (NGN) examination.

Inclusive Language

A note about the language used in this book: Wolters Kluwer recognizes that people have a diverse range of identities, and we are committed to using inclusive and nonbiased language in our content. In line with the principles of nursing, we strive not to define people by their diagnoses, but to recognize their personhood first and foremost, using as much as possible the language diverse groups use to define themselves, and including only information that is relevant to nursing care.

We strive to better address the unique perspectives, complex challenges, and lived experiences of diverse populations traditionally underrepresented in health literature. When describing or referencing populations discussed in research studies, we will adhere to the identities presented in those studies to maintain fidelity to the evidence presented by the study investigators. We follow best practices of language set forth by the *Publication Manual of the American Psychological Association, 7th edition* but acknowledge that language evolves rapidly, and we will update the language used in future editions of this book as necessary.

A Comprehensive Package for Teaching and Learning

Ancillary Package

To further facilitate teaching and learning, a carefully designed ancillary package has been developed to assist faculty and students.

Instructor Resources

Tools to assist you with teaching your course are available upon adoption of this book on thePoint® at http://thepoint.lww.com/Kincheloe5e

- A **Test Generator** features National Council Licensure Exam (NCLEX)-style questions mapped to chapter learning objectives.
- **PowerPoint Presentations** provide an easy way to integrate the textbook with your students' classroom experience; multiple-choice and true/false questions are included to promote class participation.
- A sample **Syllabus** is provided to use in your course.
- An **Image Bank** lets you use the photographs and illustrations from this textbook in your course materials.
- An **ebook** serves as a handy resource.
- Access to all **Student Resources** is provided so that you can understand the student experience and use these resources in your course as well.

Student Resources

An exciting set of free learning resources is available on thePoint® to help students review and apply vital concepts in mental health nursing. Multimedia engines have been optimized so that students can access many of these resources on mobile devices. Students can access all these resources at http://thepoint.lww.com/Kincheloe5e using the codes printed in the front of their textbooks.

- **Journal Articles** offer access to current research relevant to each chapter and available in Wolters Kluwer journals to familiarize students with nursing literature.
- **Videos** reinforce topics from the textbook and appeal to visual and auditory learners.

A Comprehensive, Digital, Integrated Course Solution: Lippincott® CoursePoint

Lippincott® CoursePoint is an integrated, digital curriculum solution for nursing education that provides an other-course knowledge and be prepared for practice. The time-tested, easy-to-use and trusted solution includes engaging learning tools, case studies, and in-depth reporting to meet students where they are in their learning, combined with the most trusted nursing education content on the market to help prepare students for practice. This easy-to-use digital learning solution of *Lippincott® CoursePoint*, combined with unmatched support, gives instructors and students everything they need for course and curriculum success!

Lippincott® CoursePoint includes:

- Engaging course content provides a variety of learning tools to engage students of all learning styles.

- Adaptive and personalized learning helps students learn the critical thinking and clinical judgment skills needed to help them become practice-ready nurses.
- Unparalleled reporting provides in-depth dashboards with several data points to track student progress and help identify strengths and weaknesses.
- Unmatched support includes training coaches, product trainers, and nursing education consultants to help educators and students implement CoursePoint with ease.

Acknowledgments

First, I want to thank Donna Womble for her willingness to pass the text on to me and entrusting me with this revision and future editions.

The development and final product of this textbook would not be possible without the support of many individuals and the immense assistance of the editorial and production team. There are several dedicated individuals at Wolters Kluwer Health that I would like to recognize. Without their help and guidance, this text would not be possible.

My heartfelt thanks to Jodi Rhomberg, Senior Acquisitions Editor, for her encouragement and support during this revision. I am grateful for Staci Wolfson, Manager of Content Editing. Thank you for your encouraging words and especially for your guidance and input with Chapter 17. I am thankful for Jonathan Joyce, Senior Acquisitions Editor for his encouragement to start this revision and willingness to hear and accept my ideas for this revision. Thank you to Alex Kapitan for your review and input on Chapter 17.

Last, but most importantly, my sincerest and deepest gratitude to Phoebe Jordan-Reilly, Development Editor. Phoebe, your skills amaze me and I am so fortunate to have been able to work with you on this text! I am grateful for ALL of your support including a critical eye to detail, extra guidance on current standards and terminology, research to support a weak statement to make it stronger, awkward sentence rephrasing, and an awareness of sensitive items. Your input on Chapter 17 is greatly appreciated. In addition to your outstanding skills you have been a major source of moral support and encouragement throughout this process. Your kindness on a personal level also shows what a wonderful person you are. Thank you doesn't begin to express my appreciation for all you did for me and this text.

As important as the production and editorial team is, this revision would not exist without the love, support, and encouragement from my family and friends. Jay, your love and humor has helped keep me on track. You center me. Deanna and Kathryn, you both are amazing and talented women with the kindest hearts for others. Your encouragement and interest in this book has been a source of inspiration. Mary, I am so blessed to call you my best friend. Your support has kept me in balance and helped me in the toughest moments. Kinley, you are a blessing and help me have fun even in everyday moments! Mom, your faith and strength are a guide to follow. Paula, your professionalism, skills, and wisdom model what a nurse is. Your friendship is a gift. Sally, you led me in the beginning and continue to teach me. I treasure our friendship. Jean, not only an outstanding mental health nurse but a strong mentor and a trusted friend. I'd be lost without all of you and am thankful you are all part of my compass. Thank you for believing in, and encouraging, me during this extensive revision. All of this wouldn't be possible without faith in my Savior Jesus.

I close by restating what Donna so eloquently stated in the 4th edition, and what I also heartfully believe and acknowledge: "I am thankful most of all to my Heavenly Father for blessing me with the ability to give back to others what experience has taught me. My hope and prayer is that the students who read and study this textbook will continue to offer knowledgeable and compassionate care to those who search for the balance of mental health and those who encounter the challenges of mental illness along life's path."

Contents

Unit V   Age-Specific Disorders and Issues

Appendices

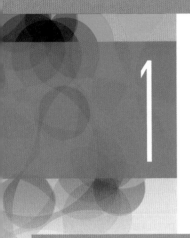

Unit I | Introduction to Mental Health and Mental Illness

1 Mental Health and Mental Illness

LEARNING OBJECTIVES

After learning the content in this chapter, the student will be able to:

1. Describe the nature of mental health and mental illness.
2. Describe factors that influence mental health.
3. Describe how culture affects the perception of mental health.
4. Differentiate between adaptive and maladaptive coping strategies.
5. Define stress and its relationship to anxiety.
6. Identify factors that contribute to stress and anxiety.
7. Differentiate between the four levels of anxiety.
8. Identify and describe different types of grief.
9. Describe grief as a process.
10. Describe the different stages of grief.
11. Discuss ways to assist individuals to cope with the grieving process.

KEY TERMS

adaptation
adaptive coping
anticipatory grief
anxiety
bereavement
conventional grief
cultural identity
distress
dysfunctional grief
eustress
external stressors
"fight-or-flight" response
grief
internal stressors
job-related burnout
loss
maladaptive coping
mental health
mental illness
palliative coping
reframing
stress
stress reaction
unresolved grief
visualization

Defining Mental Health and Mental Illness

We exist in a society composed of many different types of people. Although genetics provides a blueprint for the physical body, the human mind is unique in that it contains a combination of thoughts, perceptions, memories, emotions, will, and reasoning. Each of these is developed as the individual grows, thinks, feels, and reacts to the world around them. The individual interprets, and interacts with, their own thoughts in a private way, with the ability to communicate them to others as they choose. The well-being of this aspect of the body may be referred to as the state, or health, of the mind. While the terms "mental health" and "mental illness" sound similar, they are actually two different concepts.

Mental Health

Many large bodies (e.g., Centers for Disease Control and Prevention, World Health Organization, American Psychiatric Association, and National Alliance on Mental Illness) have defined mental health. While their definitions vary slightly, **mental health** involves the components of emotional, psychological, and social well-being; the balance between the individual's cognitive, behavioral, and emotional states; and the individual's ability to handle stress and adversity, relate to others, emote (express) their feelings, and make healthy choices.

There are many factors that influence an individual's mental health. These include socio-economic, biologic, and environmental factors. In addition, mental health is affected by the individual's ability to realize their own abilities; to work productively (examples of work can include, but are not limited to, attending school, holding a job, or tending a family); contribute to their community or family; and to enjoy life. It is important to understand that mental health is *not* characterized by the absence of a mental illness.

Mental health impacts the way an individual sees their surroundings, how they think, and the decisions they make. How the individual feels about themselves and those around them has an influence on how they cope with life and meeting the expectations it creates. The ability to act independently, directed by inner values and strengths, to face life with assurance and hope, and seek a meaningful balance between work, play, and love produces satisfying relationships with others. Further evidence of mental health is seen in the ability to function well alone or with others, to make sound judgments and accept responsibility for the outcomes, to love and be loved, and to adapt when faced with adversity.

Mental Illness

Definitions of mental illness, like mental health, vary slightly depending upon the focus of the organization defining it. In **mental illness**, the individual demonstrates a change in one or more of the following: emotions (sometimes referred to as mood), thinking, or behavior. These changes are accompanied by problems relating to others in personal, work, or social relationships or an inability to perform activities of daily living (ADLs).

In the individual with mental illness, interpersonal relationships are often stressed or ineffective as mental distress impacts the emotional stability and coping efforts of the individual. Thinking is often distorted as misconceptions and thinking errors take the place of rational and realistic processing. The distress experienced in the mind sets in motion the behavioral patterns characteristic of the various mental disorders. Box 1.1 lists some warning signs that might indicate a mental illness. Since medical issues can present with symptoms similar to those of a mental condition, the client who presents for medical or mental health treatment should have data collected for both possibilities.

BOX 1.1

Warning Signs of a Mental Health Issue

- Changes in eating or sleeping routines
- Feelings of hopelessness or like nothing matters
- Increase in drinking or illegal drug use
- Withdrawing from close family and/or friends and/or activities
- Hyper or reckless activity
- Hearing voices that others do not hear
- Thoughts of self-harm, or harming others
- Neglecting activities of daily living (eating, bathing, dressing, work, or caring for dependents)
- Change in thinking that include illogical ideas or magical thinking (e.g., believing that one can control the behavior of a television character)

Adapted from Parekh, R. (2018). *Warning Signs of Mental Illness.* American Psychiatric Association. https://www.psychiatry.org/patients-families/warning-signs-of-mental-illness

TABLE 1.1	Comparison of Mental Health and Medical Conditions	
Mental Health Condition(s)	**Symptoms**	**Medical Condition(s)**
Anxiety	Sweating, headaches, tremors	Hyperthyroidism, Pheochromocytoma
Depression	Lethargy, increased sleeping, weight gain, difficulty concentrating	Hypothyroidism
Schizophrenia, Bipolar	Psychosis	Systemic lupus erythematosus

Chapter 2 also details medical issues that have major psychological effects.

Table 1.1 lists some common mental health conditions that have similar symptoms to medical conditions.

Causes and descriptions of mental disorders vary. Reasons for these variances include, but are not limited to, the organization's focus of treatment, the individual's response to medications or treatment, and the culture of the individual or the health care professional.

Often the terms "mental illness" and "mental disorders" are used interchangeably. For the purpose of this textbook, "mental disorder" will refer to a specific, or group of similar, conditions while "mental illness" will encompass a broader issue or a global discussion of disorders.

Impact and Incidence of Mental Illness

Mental illness is seen in all cultures, socioeconomic levels, and genders. The National Institute of Mental Health (NIMH) estimates that in 2019 there were 51.5 million adults in the United States that have some form of a mental condition that ranges from mild to severe. This is roughly 20.6% of the population (close to 1 in 5 adults). This number does not include individuals with a developmental or substance use disorder. Most mental health hospitalizations are seen among individuals with a serious mental illness. Serious mental illness (SMI) is, "a mental, behavioral, or emotional disorder resulting in serious functional impairment, which substantially interferes with or limits one or more major life activities" (NIMH, 2022). The estimated number of those adults with serious mental illness in 2019 was 13.1 million, or 5.2% of the US population.

In 2019 the United States spent $225 billion on mental health services (Leonhardt, 2021). Although spending for mental health services has been increasing, there are still issues to access of care due to cost and lack of availability of services, compounded by stigma related to seeking, and receiving, mental health care.

Factors That Affect Mental Health

Mental health is achieved as the individual successfully maintains a balance between the ups and downs of everyday life. Daily there are enumerable issues encountered that require adaptation, both physically and emotionally. Stress, anxiety, grief, and loss are unavoidable issues of daily life, making it necessary for the individual to be flexible and adaptive. Faced with these challenges, their mental equilibrium may become temporarily disrupted. The ability to reestablish a stable state depends on them being able to utilize coping strategies and adapt.

Many factors influence mental health and the individual's perception of their mental health or mental illness. Cultural influences, including religion, help shape their view of what constitutes mental health, who the individual goes to for mental health advice, and acceptable treatment options. Additionally, mental health is affected by factors related to family, sleep, substance use, and exposure to trauma or violence. Coping strategies that the individual has experienced to be effective are utilized. Past experiences with stress, anxiety, grief, or loss help shape how the individual responds to the current situation.

Chapter 6 further discusses issues of anger, violence, abuse, crisis, and suicide. These all have the ability to disrupt an individual's mental state temporarily, with most individuals adapting and growing from the experience.

Cultural Heritage—Beliefs, Norms, and Values

Culture is a term that describes a common heritage and a set of social practices that are central to that group. This binding force between members of each group is often referred to as **cultural identity** and may include a common language, family structure, customs, country of origin, religious and political beliefs, food, dress or clothing, traditions, and holidays. Factors related to the group to which an individual belongs also affect how they relate to other groups. Individual behavior often, but not always, mirrors that of their group and may be altered as changes occur within the group.

With so many cultures in the world, it is not surprising that variances can be seen among the exhibition, explanation, perception, coping, and management of mental health symptoms or issues. While some individuals may respond outwardly to life situations, others may be reluctant, or discouraged, from visibly showing emotional and mental problems. This expression can be influenced by their culture. The tendency to seek help from religious or faith healers within the cultural group rather than professional providers is common. Although many families meet the challenge of a member's mental illness by seeking professional care, the stigma and shame created by a mental illness can lead some families to hide or dismiss the issue and to deal with the affected person in their own ways. Some families may simply deny that a problem exists. Others may see the symptoms as a punishment or judgment for wrongdoing.

Religious coping may include prayer, religious music, talking to God or a higher power, reading religious materials, or meditation. Some cultural beliefs conclude that mental symptoms are related to witchcraft, demon possession, or substance use and can be eliminated by traditional healing remedies or a ritual. Rituals may include the use of prayer, touch, candles, eggs, pollen, roots, herbs, or religious medals. The ritual is often provided by those seen as healers within the group and viewed by the group as an acceptable practice.

Cultural approaches remain the customary choice for some individuals to manage mental illness regardless of the availability of mental health services. Different cultures have specific syndromes that involve mental health. These syndromes are involuntary, familiar to the members, widespread in the specific culture, and treated by a healer of that culture. These conditions are referred to as culture-bound syndromes. Recognizing the client may be experiencing a culture-bound syndrome is important to provide culturally appropriate care. Also, the nurse should explore the client's meaning of the terms used (e.g., what does it mean to the client when they talk about "nerves"?). Table 1.2 lists some of these syndromes and a generalized description of each.

Religion

Religion provides routine, structure, and coping for some individuals, while for others it may be a stressor. If the client identifies a religious preference, it is important for the nurse to obtain information on what practices the client finds beneficial and if there are parts that they identify as stressors. Some individuals may not practice an organized religion but may have spiritual practices that are important to them. Religious themes are frequently seen in mental illness, especially in themes of delusions or hallucinations that are seen in psychosis. For example, a client experiencing psychosis may draw a religious symbol or write out a specific religious term repeatedly.

Family

Similar to religion, the individual's family can either be a protective factor against, or a stressor that can exacerbate, mental health issues. A strong family system can provide the individual with needed support. Conversely, if the individual has a dysfunctional or absent family, the individual will need to rely on other support systems for help.

Culture can influence the way a family views mental illness and the support they provide. In some cultures, families may view the individual with mental illness as an embarrassment or disgrace to the family name; some may even go to the extreme and disown the individual. In other cultures, the family may deny the presence of the mental illness and be unwilling to provide support but still include the individual in the family. In both cases, the individual with a mental illness will need extra support from outside the family system.

In individuals with a long history of mental illness, the family may experience caregiver burnout and may no longer be able to provide support. It is important for the nurse to be nonjudgmental when caring for a person whose family is not acting as a support system.

Sleep

Sleep is an important component of mental health. An individual who has balanced sleep and is well rested is better equipped to face daily challenges. Sleep also enhances coping mechanisms. A lack of sleep can impair the individual's ability to cope and can magnify their mental health issues. An increase or decrease in sleeping habits is seen in mental health issues such as in manic

TABLE 1.2	Common Examples of Culture-Bound Syndromes	
Syndrome	**Predominant Culture(s)**	**Description**
Amok	Malaysia Indonesia Philippines	An acute outburst of unrestrained violence, such as attempts to kill or seriously injure anyone encountered, and ends with exhaustion and amnesia.
Ataque de nervios	Latin America Mediterranean	Uncontrollable shouting, attacks of crying, trembling, heat in the chest and head, and verbal and physical aggression.
Brain fag	West Africa	Headaches, blurring or watering of eyes, difficulty grasping meaning of words, poor retention of information, and sleepiness while studying.
Dhat *Shenkui*	India China	Fear of loss of power due to loss of semen through premature ejaculation, masturbation, or from passing semen in the urine. Symptoms may include weakness, fatigue, palpitations, insomnia, guilt, or anxiety.
Hikikomori	Japan	Social withdrawal (usually longer than 6 months) and the individual exhibits a strong focus on personal interests or is apathetic with no interest in hobbies or activities.
Koro *shook yang*	Southeast Asia China	Extreme anxiety or panic that the penis will retract into the body or even may disappear.
Latah	Malaysia Indonesia	The afflicted person responds to a frightening stimulus with an exaggerated startle or jump, utters improper words, and imitates the words or movements of people nearby.
Piblokto	Some Inuit or arctic populations	Screaming, uncontrolled wild behavior, depression, insensitivity to extreme cold (such as running around in the snow naked), and echolalia.
Susto (also known as "fright sickness" or "soul loss")	Latin America	After a traumatic, or frightening, experience the individual has symptoms of nervousness, loss of appetite and strength, insomnia, listlessness when awake, depression, and introversion.
Taijin kyofusho	Japan	Excessive nervousness or fear in social situations, extreme self-consciousness, fear of contracting disease. Also an intense fear that they (or their body part or body function) will displease, embarrass, or offend others. The fear is of offending or harming other people with a focus on avoiding harm to others (rather than to oneself).
Zar	East Africa Middle East	Experience of spiritual possession, which may include dissociative episodes of laughing, hitting, singing or weeping. Apathy and withdrawal may also be seen.

Note: This is not a complete list. These are some of the more common syndromes discussed in various sources. Different cultures may have a syndrome with similar symptoms but with a different name.

Sources: Correll, C. U., Stetka, B. S., & Harsinay, A. (2018). *Culture-specific psychiatric syndromes: A review.* Medscape. https://www.medscape.com/viewarticle/901027#vp_1

Teodoro, T., & Afonso, P. (2020). Culture-bound syndromes and cultural concepts of distress in psychiatry. *Revista Portuguesa De Psiquiatria E Saúde Mental, 6*(3), 118–126. https://doi.org/10.51338/rppsm.2020.v6.i3.139

or depressive disorders. Tracking the individual's hours, and quality, of sleep is important in determining their mental health balance and the effectiveness of treatment therapies. Sleep, therefore, is an important vital sign in mental health nursing.

Substance Use

Substance use includes alcohol, medications, and illegal drug use. Individuals who use substances are at an increased risk for mental illness as the substance can cause changes to the brain's function and structure. An example of this is the individual who huffs an aerosol to get high. The aerosol physically damages the brain, leading to behavioral and cognitive changes.

Substance use is frequently seen in individuals who have an existing mental illness. Often the individual uses the substance to help cope with or lessen the symptoms of the mental illness. An example of this would be the individual with post-traumatic stress disorder (PTSD) who drinks alcohol to help forget the events that led to the post-traumatic stress disorder (PTSD). This is referred to as "self-medication."

Trauma and Violence

Exposure to trauma and violence can cause mental health issues. A child who is exposed to violence or trauma at a young age, when the brain is developing, is at risk for mental health issues. A traumatic brain injury can create mental health issues in an individual who did not previously have a mental illness. Disorders that affect the brain, such as Parkinson disease or a cerebral vascular accident (CVA, also known as a stroke), can cause mental health issues.

The Substance Abuse and Mental Health Services Administration (SAMHSA) states that trauma is "an event, series of events, or set of circumstances that is experienced by an individual as physically or emotionally harmful or life threatening and that has lasting adverse effects on the individual's functioning and mental, physical, social, emotional, or spiritual well-being" (SAMHSA, 2019).

Coping

When dealing with stress and the unpleasant situations that cause stress, the individual will need to cope to manage the emotions that arise. The ability to cope is learned from previous unpleasant experiences and by observing how others deal with similar situations (e.g., children learn to cope with situations by watching and imitating family members). Coping can be either conscious or unconscious and learned or automatic. It can also be positive or negative. For example, after a busy day at work, the individual who practices 30 minutes of yoga "to unwind" would be demonstrating positive coping while the individual who drinks heavily to "forget about work" would be demonstrating negative coping.

In most situations, the sense of control an individual feels over a particular stressor determines how they think about or perceive it. The first step in coping with a threatening situation is to assess if it really is what it seems to be. Once this has been determined, options can be reviewed to resolve the problem. The solution may be trying to deal with the situation itself or trying to control the emotional reaction that is felt in response to the stressor.

Coping Strategies

Not everyone copes the same way in a similar situation. For example, a student who feels overwhelmed by requirements of a full semester course load with a fear of failing may decide to drop one or two classes to perform better in the remaining subjects while another student with the same course load may decide to work out in the gym each day, along with budgeting time between the required subjects. Both students coped with the

similar situation in the way they felt was best for them—in other words, they used different coping strategies.

Coping strategies are the methods used to manage stress and anxiety. Coping strategies generally fall into four categories: adaptive, palliative, maladaptive, and dysfunctional. Adaptive and palliative coping strategies usually result in a positive outcome. On the other hand, maladaptive and dysfunctional strategies usually do not result in a positive outcome. Behavior is the result of the individual's perception regarding the situation and thought processes. Behavior provides a clue to the underlying motive for action.

An individual's successful management of stress or anxiety is referred to as **adaptation**. Therefore, when a rational and productive way of resolving a problem to reduce stress or anxiety is used, it is said to be **adaptive coping**. The students mentioned above both demonstrated adaptive coping skills, as they both took steps to address and successfully resolve their problems. Conversely, **palliative coping** is when the solution temporarily relieves the stress or anxiety but the problem still exists and must be dealt with again at a later time. Examples of palliative coping would be when a drama student feels anxiety as time for a performance approaches and asks a classmate to review the script to refocus on the lines. A second student who feels anxious about the performance goes jogging with music to relieve the anxiety and increase their mental alertness to remember the lines. For both students, the stressor of performing their lines still exists but the stress of learning the lines has been temporarily relieved.

If unsuccessful attempts are made to decrease the anxiety without attempting to solve the problem, the strategies are described as **maladaptive coping** and the stress or anxiety remains. For example, the drama student might decide to ignore the anxiety and go to a movie the afternoon before the performance and rapidly look over the lines immediately before going on stage. During the performance, they forget several lines and need to be prompted.

The individual who does not attempt to reduce the anxiety or solve the problem is considered to have dysfunctional coping. For example, another student decides to get drunk the night before the performance, fails to show up for the performance until the second act, and is replaced by their understudy.

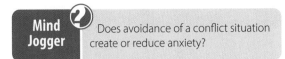

Mind Jogger ② Does avoidance of a conflict situation create or reduce anxiety?

Promoting Adaptive Coping Strategies

In managing and coping with the anxiety experienced in response to stress, it is important to accept and deal with the anxiety rather than fight it. Stress is a part of life. The individual has a choice to replace negative feelings with more positive ones. They can stand back and look realistically at the situation while functioning along with the anxiety. The outcome is rarely as bad as what is feared the most. Negative thoughts drive a perception that the worst is likely to happen. Coping strategies, whether adaptive or maladaptive, are learned by observation of those who model them in the family and social environment. When dealing with life stressors, the individual tends to use the coping skills that they know best.

Nurses play a major role in helping clients cope more effectively with anxiety. To help clients deal with their stress levels, the nurse must learn to handle their own stress. Each success the individual has in dealing with an anxiety-producing situation provides a foundation for helping to manage or control the anxiety the next time. Two examples of effective coping strategies are reframing and visualization.

Reframing is a way of restructuring thinking about a stressful event into a form that is less disturbing and over which the individual can have some control. Table 1.3 illustrates examples of how irrational beliefs can be reframed into rational thoughts. By changing the view to a more realistic expectation, the individual can pursue a solution more effectively.

Visualization involves mentally viewing a place of peaceful solitude to allow the individual a momentary reprieve from the stress (e.g., visualizing a vacation spot or pastime that brings relaxation

such as imagining oneself on the seashore listening to the sounds of water and seagulls). The reprieve provides a temporary defense of withdrawing from the anxiety, gives the individual renewed energy, and is another effective means of coping with stress.

Test Yourself
- ✔ Describe the difference between mental health and mental illness.
- ✔ How does palliative coping differ from adaptive coping?
- ✔ Name seven factors that can affect mental health.

Stress and Anxiety

Stress and anxiety can arise from any thought or issue that creates frustration or a feeling of uneasiness. Situations are seen differently by everyone with some things being stressful to one and not to another. What causes the uneasy feeling is not necessarily apparent to the person experiencing it, which adds to the tension experienced.

Defining Stress

Stress is defined as the condition that results when a threat or challenge to one's well-being requires the person to adjust or adapt to the environment. There are two kinds of stress: distress and eustress. **Distress** is a response to a threat or challenge and is harmful to one's health. This is a negative stress and demands an exhausting type of energy. **Eustress**, on the other hand, is positive and motivating, increasing one's confidence in the ability to master a challenge or stressor. This type of stress may enhance the feeling of well-being. For example, eustress is demonstrated in a football player whose stress about an upcoming football game challenges them to play better. Distress, on the other hand, might be seen in the student who is disqualified from the football team because of poor grades, resulting in a feeling of low self-worth.

TABLE 1.3	Examples of Reframing Irrational Thoughts
Irrational Belief	**Restructured Positive Thought**
I always mess things up.	Even if things didn't turn out right this time I can do it differently next time.
He never does what I want him to do.	If I want him to do something I need to communicate that to him.
She never pays any attention to me.	If I give her more attention, she might be more attentive to me.
I should have done better on the exam.	I can study harder and do better on the next one.
I can't be happy unless I am loved by the person I really care about.	If this person does not return my love, I can give my energy to finding someone better.

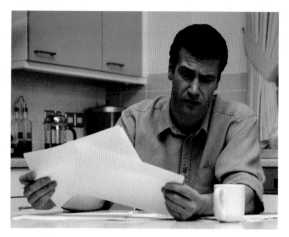

Figure 1.1 Stress is a common experience. Common sources of stress include work, family, financial problems, and world events.

Stress is further defined in terms of acute or chronic stress. Acute stress is the reaction to an immediate threat, commonly called the **"fight-or-flight" response**, occurring when there is a surge of the adrenal hormone epinephrine (also known as adrenaline) into the bloodstream. It is referred to in this way because it provides the energy or instant strength to either fight the threat or danger or run away from it. This type of response can occur in situations where there is a sense of imminent danger, such as when walking in a darkened parking lot or upon losing track of a child in a crowd. The response is usually reversed to a relaxation mode once the danger is past. Chronic stress occurs when the situation is ongoing or continuous, such as chronic illness of a family member or job-related responsibilities (Fig. 1.1).

There are common symptoms that are seen in both acute and chronic stress (Box 1.2). Common symptoms of stress generally fall into four categories: physical, mental, emotional, and behavioral. The physical response to the stressor, or the **stress reaction**, is triggered by the arousal of the autonomic nervous system.

Just the Facts When the perception of a stressful situation lessens, the stimulation to the autonomic nervous system decreases and symptoms of stress begin to resolve.

Defining Anxiety

Anxiety is defined as a feeling of apprehension, uneasiness, or uncertainty that occurs in response

BOX 1.2

Common Signs and Symptoms of Stress

- Increased heart rate and blood pressure
- Heart palpitations
- Increased respirations
- Abdominal cramping, nausea, diarrhea
- Headaches
- Insomnia
- Lack of concentration and memory
- Difficulty in making, or inability to make, decisions
- Forgetfulness
- Confusion
- Anxiety
- Nervousness
- Irritability
- Frustration and worry
- Fidgety movements
- Nail-biting
- Smoking or drinking
- Yelling
- Throwing objects

to a real or perceived threat. It is an automatic and unconscious biologic response to a stressor that cannot be controlled by the conscious mind. Anxiety is an unavoidable natural occurrence that is an instinctive response to a threat to the individual's well-being.

Anxiety is a basic emotion and occurs at a deeper level than fear. Fear is a reaction to a specific, defined danger. Normal anxiety is necessary for survival and provides the energy needed to manage daily life and pursue life goals. One may experience acute anxiety when faced with a short-term stressor, such as undergoing surgery or a series of diagnostic testing. When anxiety persists over a long period, such as when an individual experiences a chronic illness, the individual may demonstrate symptoms of chronic fatigue, insomnia, poor concentration, or impairment in work and social functioning. If the feelings of anxiety become too overwhelming, those feelings may then be expressed through behavior.

Anxiety can be thought of as a smoke detector that alerts the senses to the possibility of danger and prepares the individual to respond by either flight or fight. When the "alarm" sounds, it prevents logical thinking about the situation. Therefore, anxiety may be present whether or not an actual danger exists. Anxiety can cause the individual to act impulsively not only when there is actual danger but also when there is the perception of a possible threat, allowing logical and realistic thought processes to be overshadowed. Disorders related to anxiety are discussed in Chapter 9.

> **Just the Facts** Behavior is the result of perceptions and thought processes related to a particular situation.

There are four levels at which anxiety may occur, with each level more severe than the previous one. The levels are mild, moderate, severe, and panic. The severity of the anxiety is determined by an individual's perception of the situation and their reaction to the stressor. This is exhibited in their physical, emotional, and mental behaviors. Regardless of the level of anxiety, the individual experiences an internal need to try to relieve the anxiety as soon as possible.

Mild anxiety is natural and motivating, increasing productivity and improving one's sense of well-being. Anxiety that increases to a moderate level becomes uncomfortable and difficult to tolerate for extended periods. If this level of anxiety is not relieved, it progresses to a severe state that is physically and emotionally exhausting. If steps are not taken to decrease a severe level of anxiety, the state of panic may develop, possibly leading to hysteria, suicide attempts, or violence. The physical and psychological symptoms for each level of anxiety are described in Table 1.4.

Contributing Factors to Stress and Anxiety

An individual can experience both external and internal stressors (Box 1.3). **External stressors** are adverse aspects of the environment, such as an abusive relationship or poverty-level living conditions. **Internal stressors** are from within the individual and can be physical, such as a chronic illness or terminal condition, or psychological, as in continued worry about financial burdens or a disaster that may never happen. Chronic stress is known to have physical consequences on the body. Stress increases the heart rate, blood pressure, and the release of the hormone cortisol. Over time, this can increase the individual's risk for hypertension, myocardial infarction, and cerebral vascular accident (CVA, also called a stroke).

Both positive and negative aspects of life include stress. For example, an individual experiencing their first day on the job after a promotion might experience a pounding heart and tense muscles as they adapt to the new position. By contrast, an environment of everyday stress such as marital discord or a difficult work environment may eventually pose a threat to the individual's health. It is important to recognize that many times external circumstances are viewed as the cause of stress, but in reality, most stress is created from the individual's perception of the circumstances. Irrational thinking tends to overgeneralize and exaggerate the situation, which gives the thoughts an "all or

"Viktor"

YAKOBCHUK VIACHESLAV/ Shutterstock

You are working in the emergency department (ED) when a client, Viktor, is brought in by paramedics after he was involved in a low-speed car accident involving his vehicle and a city bus. You have collected the following data: he did not lose consciousness, denies pain, and there are no apparent injuries. He was restrained and the airbag deployed. His pulse is 102 and bounding, B/P 156/90. He has stated several times that he feels the need to urinate and is mildly diaphoretic. You notice he is quietly lying on the stretcher but is wringing his hands and patting his pockets as if looking for something. As you continue to collect data on Viktor he keeps repeating "I was hit by a bus" and "It was my wife's new car." His speech is slightly increased. You are trying to reinforce the information given to him by the health care provider and he occasionally interrupts with "I was hit by a bus" in a very matter-of-fact manner.

Digging Deeper

1. What signs/symptoms of anxiety does Viktor have?

2. What level of anxiety would he be experiencing?

3. What interventions are important for the nurse to include based on his level of anxiety?

CASE STUDY

TABLE 1.4   Common Signs and Symptoms of Anxiety

Level of Anxiety	Physical Symptoms	Psychological Symptoms
Mild Level	Increased awareness Increased energy Slight discomfort Restlessness Irritability Mild tension-relieving behaviors (fidgeting, nail-biting, foot-tapping, lip-chewing)	Sharp perception of reality Alert and aware of environment Able to identify things producing anxiety Motivated Preoccupied at times Good concentration Reasoning and logical thought processes Attentive
Moderate Level	Voice tremors Muscle tension Rapid speech—change in pitch Difficulty concentrating Shakiness Repetitive questioning Misperception of stimuli Inability to complete tasks Autonomic response Headaches, insomnia Pacing Decreased eye contact	Reduced perceptual ability Decreased attentiveness Needs things repeated to grasp Still functional but problem-solving ability decreased (requires guidance) Decreased motivation and confidence Increased irritability Feeling of being tied in knots Bouts of crying and outbursts of anger Inability to learn or problem-solve
Severe Level	Feelings of impending doom Confusion Purposeless activity Increased somatic complaints Hyperventilation Palpitations Loud and rapid speech Threats and demands Increased pacing Diaphoresis Poor or no eye contact Insomnia Rapid speech Eye twitching Tremors	Distorted perception of reality Attention to details—loses sight of whole picture Focused totally on self and anxiety Defensiveness Oversensitive to comments from others Verbal threats Lacks reasoning or logical thought processes Unable to problem-solve
Panic Level	Hysteria Incoherence Suicide attempts Violent behavior Unintelligible speech Feelings of terror, extreme fear Immobility Dilated pupils Withdrawal Out of touch with reality	Irrational and disorganized thought processes Absent perceptual ability Unaware of reality Unable to perceive environment Depersonalization Delusional thinking Disorientation

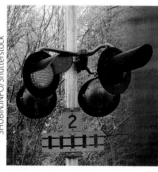
SHUBIN.INFO/Shutterstock

BOX 1.3

Internal and External Stressors

EXTERNAL STRESSORS

- Physical environment (noise, bright lights, weather, crowds)
- Major life events (death of a loved one, divorce, loss of a job, marriage)
- Work-related (rules, deadlines, production pressures, gossip, being short-staffed)
- Social (bossy or aggressive persons, strained friendship, marital affairs)
- Everyday life (schedules, household duties, family conflict)
- Financial (bills, mortgage, bankruptcy)

INTERNAL STRESSORS

- Physical (chronic illness, terminal diagnosis)
- Personality traits (perfectionist, workaholic, worrier, loner)
- Negative self-talk (pessimism, irrational thinking, self-criticism)
- Thinking snags (all-or-none approach, unrealistic and inflexible expectations)

BOX 1.4

Techniques for Managing Anxiety

- Reframing irrational thinking
- Visualization
- Positive self-talk
- Assertiveness training
- Problem-solving skills
- Communication skills
- Conflict resolution
- Relaxation techniques
- Meditation
- Support systems
- Journaling
- Practical attitude
- Sense of humor
- Self-care (diet, exercise, sleep, leisure activities, avoiding caffeine and alcohol)
- Faith in spiritual power and in self

none" frame of thinking (e.g., "Nobody likes me."). This type of thinking also leads to anticipating the worst possible outcome for situations. This is illustrated by an individual who is hit by the car behind them while driving in traffic. Believing that if they ever drive a car again, they will have an accident, the individual no longer drives a vehicle.

Some events create more stress than others. Unpredictability of and lack of control over situations greatly increase the strain the stressor causes the individual. For example, a firefighter faces uncertainty and ongoing threat of danger or injury with each call of duty. Emotional triggers for higher levels of stress are those that are uncontrollable, repetitive, unexpected, and intense in nature. These are seen often in first responders and health care workers in critical care situations. Stress is greater and damage more likely in these situations, and can lead to job-related burnout or mental, physical, and emotional exhaustion.

Just the Facts Job-related burnout is a condition of mental, physical, and emotional exhaustion with a reduced sense of personal accomplishment and apathy toward one's work.

Mind Jogger What types of stress might be more damaging than others?

Managing Stress and Anxiety

Managing stress and anxiety is an ongoing process. To be most effective, techniques often need to be practiced before a stressful or anxiety-causing event occurs. Not every technique is effective for all individuals; therefore, the individual may need to use a "trial and error" approach to see what works best for them. In addition to reframing and visualization, some other effective techniques for managing anxiety are listed in Box 1.4.

Mind Jogger How might failure to achieve one's ambition be seen as a positive experience?

Test Yourself
- ✔ Identify 10 common signs of stress.
- ✔ Name the four levels of anxiety and identify the thinking exhibited in each.
- ✔ What is the difference between internal and external stressors?
- ✔ Give an example of reframing.

Grief and Loss

Grief is defined as the emotional process of coping with a loss. This is often associated with the death of a loved one, such as a spouse, parent, or child, or of any person who is important in the individual's life. In a broader sense, the concept of grief can be applied to the loss of anything that is significant or meaningful to the individual.

With the loss, the attachment bond that is seen as strong and secure is suddenly shattered, making the person vulnerable to the emotional response. Grief is the emotion encountered when an individual is confronted with a loss. It is a feeling of sadness and despondency centered on the loss. These feelings may lead to behaviors such as forgetfulness and crying at unpredictable times. It is helpful for the person to be reassured that this is a common reaction to grief. Tears are accepted as a part of the healing that takes place in the months after the loss. How an individual mourns a loss is also influenced by their personal, familial, and cultural beliefs or customs. The amount of time allotted to the mourning period or how families may view sympathy and support during the time of sadness is often determined by these factors. For example, some prefer to be alone as they mourn a loss, while others may do so openly for a specified time or with specific rituals and family gatherings.

Although a person may experience sadness or sorrow in response to making a mistake or doing something that is hurtful to another, the grief felt as the person adjusts to the absence of the endeared person or object is a deeper and longer-lasting emotion that involves time and emotional energy.

Just the Facts	Grief is the process of working through the emotional response to loss, reorganizing one's life, and accomplishing some degree of resolution or closure.

Loss can be an actual or perceived change in the status of one's relationship to a valued object or person. This concept is easily associated with the death of a valued person or pet. The concept of loss can be applied to a separation or divorce, loss of a body part, threat to one's health, loss of a job or source of income, losses that result from a natural or imposed disaster, and the loss of an ideal (e.g., having a cesarean section when a vaginal delivery was most desired). Losing a home to fire or natural disaster is also a major loss, with a lifetime of memories suddenly gone from view and reality. Another type of loss involves the lack of certainty that a goal or desired outcome will be achieved, such as not receiving a job promotion or experiencing an academic failure.

All of these events or circumstances may leave the person with a sense of emptiness, hopelessness, and detachment from the meaning that previously was found in life. The extent to which emotional energy was previously invested in these objects, persons, and relationships will determine the intensity with which an individual responds to the absence of that object.

Developmental Understanding of Grief and Loss

Children and adolescents respond according to the level at which they understand the concept of death or loss. Table 1.5 shows how the response reflects the age-related cognitive and psychological developments of the child. For example, a toddler may respond to separation from a parent or attachment figure with anxiety but has no concept of loss. Should that attachment figure not return, the child will usually adapt to another attachment figure who is nurturing. The preschool child reacts with magical thinking. In magical thinking, the individual believes their ideas, thoughts, actions or words can cause a real event to happen. An example of this would be a 5-year-old child who says, "Grandpa died because I hit my brother." The concept of death as a finality is not yet understood. An example of this would be the 5-year-old child who says "Grandpa is sleeping. Will he wake up in time to take me to the park"? Associated with the growing moral concept of right and wrong, the school-age child may feel a sense of guilt or responsibility for a loss, such as when a parent is

TABLE 1.5	Age-Related Concepts of Loss
Age Group	**Conceptual Understanding of Loss**
Toddler	Egocentric and concerned with themselves Do not understand concept of loss
Preschool	Use magical thinking and may feel shame or guilt when thinking is associated with loss (i.e., belief that their behavior is reason a parent is gone such as in divorce) Primitive coping mechanisms result in more intense response Do not understand death or its permanence (e.g., believe that the deceased person will come back to play with them)
School-age	Still feel guilt and responsibility in associating negative actions with loss Respond to concrete, simple and logical explanation of death such as in the death of a pet Understand permanence of death and that some losses may be temporary
Adolescent	Able to understand the concept of death, but have difficulty accepting loss Perceive loss as a threat to their identity

absent following a divorce. Although adolescents understand the concept of death as finality, it is difficult for this age group to fit death or loss into their search for an identity.

Adults may view loss as temporary or permanent, and most adults are able to accept their losses and grow from these situations. Acceptance often opens the door of opportunity for new and expanded life experiences. An example of this is seen when one experiences failure in a given situation such as divorce, job promotion, or academic challenges. Failure, if viewed realistically, can allow the individual to try again and achieve more success. Learning what contributed to the loss can open the door to a new challenge. During this time the individual experiences **bereavement**, which is expected reaction of grief and sadness after a loss. It is important to remember that regardless of age or circumstances, bereavement is a natural, healthy, and healing process that emerges in response to any significant loss.

Mind Jogger How might environmental factors during childhood affect a person's ability to cope with loss?

Types of Grief

Anticipatory grief may be seen in individuals and families who are expecting a major loss in the near future. This concept can help nurses understand the reaction of the terminally ill client and the family members who will be left to mourn the death of their loved one. In this case, death is inevitable, and there is a time of preparation and closure that can ease the emotional pain at the actual time of death. This is the premise for hospice care, which provides palliative nursing and supportive interventions to assist the client and family members in coping with the imminent loss. The nurse can also apply this concept to those in the acute care setting who may be anticipating the loss of a body part (e.g., amputation of a limb or a mastectomy) or change in body functioning (e.g., bowel diversion with a stoma creation or a chronic illness such as diabetes) that may inflict a major alteration in lifestyle.

Conventional grief is primarily associated with the grief that is experienced following a loss. The process of bereavement or adapting to loss may take days, weeks, or years, depending on the sense of loss for the person involved. Each person

BOX 1.5

Contributing Factors to Dysfunctional Grief

- Socially unacceptable death such as suicide or homicide
- Missing person related to war, mysterious disappearance, or abduction
- Multiple losses or losses in close succession (loss of several family members in short period with financial loss or disaster loss)
- Ambivalent feelings toward the lost person or object
- Unresolved grieving from a previous loss
- Guilt regarding circumstances at or near the time of death
- Survivor's guilt (the survivor feels that they should have died with, or instead of, the deceased)

responds to loss in a personal and unique way and time. This response is based on the person's level of development, past experiences, and current coping strategies.

Dysfunctional grief is a failure to complete the grieving process and cope successfully with a loss. If the person experiences a prolonged and intensified reaction, they may feel that life has become meaningless and that they are merely existing, longing for what is lost.

Chronic sorrow is seen in a situation where the grief resurfaces at times, but never fully goes away. For example, parents with a child who is developmentally disabled may experience periods of grief when their child does not reach milestones at the same rate, if at all, as others in their age group, such as learning to drive a car or get married.

Unresolved grief describes situations when the grief process is incomplete, and life is burdened with maladaptive symptoms continuing months after the loss has occurred. With unresolved grief, symptoms seen can include consuming feelings of worthlessness with suicidal tendencies; physiologic response to the loss with marked decrease in functioning; or delusional thinking or hallucinations of seeing the image or hearing the voice of the deceased. Factors that may contribute to unresolved grief, which can lead to dysfunctional grief, are listed in Box 1.5.

Grief as a Process

The grieving process includes a series of occurrences in the resolution of the loss. This process provides resolution as an individual works

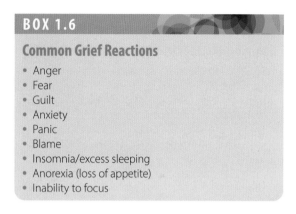

BOX 1.6

Common Grief Reactions

- Anger
- Fear
- Guilt
- Anxiety
- Panic
- Blame
- Insomnia/excess sleeping
- Anorexia (loss of appetite)
- Inability to focus

through the feelings of anger, hopelessness, and futility that accompany loss. It provides time to put things into perspective, to place into memory that which is gone, and to emerge with a new perspective on life. Life is an evolving challenge of events that inevitably requires the individual to cope with disappointment and loss. Learning to deal with these situations in small increments better prepares them to deal effectively with a major loss. The individual can learn to accept loss as part of living or can choose to react negatively. If the anger that is seen naturally in grief is suppressed, the hidden feelings may eventually erupt in negative or maladaptive patterns of behavior such as substance abuse or suicidal ideation. Learning to cope or adapt to loss involves taking advantage of the right to grieve in whatever timeframe is needed to go through the process. The nurse should provide the grieving client with information regarding the feelings that are normal, and appropriate, to grieving (Box 1.6).

Growth occurs as the bereaved person comes to the point of letting go of the past. This does not reduce the importance of the loss but allows the person to continue living with new perspective. In time, the sadness and loneliness felt because of the void left by the cherished object are replaced with an acceptance that the loss is permanent. This acceptance indicates that the grief process is ending.

When the process of grieving becomes prolonged it may be considered atypical or maladaptive with symptoms of a major depressive episode such as extreme sadness, insomnia, anorexia, and weight loss. The person may dismiss emotional symptoms as part of the normal grief process but may seek professional help to treat physical

symptoms like insomnia or appetite loss. In doing so, they can receive treatment for maladaptive emotional symptoms as well.

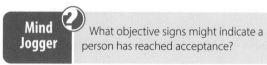

Mind Jogger — What objective signs might indicate a person has reached acceptance?

Stages of Grief

There are several theories that have evolved concerning the grief process, and while not absolute, theories that define distinct stages of grief supply a framework for understanding this process. A person may experience all stages in rapid succession or rally back and forth between stages, remaining in some longer than others. Perhaps the best-known theory of the stages of grief has been described by Dr. Elisabeth Kubler-Ross, a German psychiatrist. Dr. Kubler-Ross identified five stages that humans go through each time they are confronted with a loss or death. The stages are: denial, anger, bargaining, withdrawal/depression, and acceptance (Box 1.7).

The first step is denial that the event is happening, an immediate reaction of "this can't be real." This shock, or disbelief, is driven by an impulse to avoid the reality of the loss. The individual may act as if nothing has occurred or as though the lost object or person is still present. Denial actually allows for an adjustment period in which to gather coping strategies for the grieving work ahead.

Once the individual realizes the loss is real, the denial gives way to feelings of anger. Anger is expressed in many ways, often demonstrated openly in behaviors such as hitting an object or person, blaming someone for the loss (can include self-blame), or expressions of guilt. Some may turn the anger inward, resulting in physical illness or psychological dysfunction.

BOX 1.7

Stages of Grief

- Shock and denial
- Anger and pain
- Negotiation and bargaining
- Withdrawal and depression
- Acceptance and resolution

Anger usually is followed by bargaining as an attempt to postpone acceptance of the loss. As is often seen with terminal illness, this is a time when deals with God or a higher power are attempted as a way to prolong the inevitable. During this period, frequent labile moods are common and are often intermingled with continued anger and unwillingness to accept the loss.

The bargaining period is gradually followed by a deep sense of loss as the reality of what has happened, or is anticipated to happen, settles. At this point the individual may withdraw from social interaction, choosing to spend hours and days alone. Depression, the persistent and prolonged mood of sadness, is a normal response in this process while adjusting to the full impact of the loss and living without the loved object. As opposed to the persistent feelings of sadness and desolation that are seen in depressive disorder, in grief, these feelings may be intertwined with good days of positive emotions. The self-esteem of the survivor is usually intact, and their thoughts are primarily focused on the deceased. For some individuals, this period may be overwhelming, and recovery from the depth of sorrow felt is unlikely without professional support and guidance.

The final stage is acceptance. This is when the person begins to experience peace and serenity. This is the time of letting go and allowing life to provide new experiences and relationships.

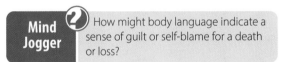

Mind Jogger ② How might body language indicate a sense of guilt or self-blame for a death or loss?

Coping with Grief and Loss

To deal effectively with clients experiencing grief, the nurse must first self-reflect on the reality of their own mortality, the concept of death, and any previous experiences they have had with death and how they perceive those events. The nurse develops their own response pattern toward death and loss that is conditioned by experience and by personal, cultural, and religious beliefs. Most clients experiencing a crisis of major proportion require assistance and support to help navigate the grief process. The nurse needs to respect, and attempt to understand, the unique manner of grieving for every individual.

It is important for the nurse to avoid clichés, such as, "I know how hard it is" or "It was for the best" or "I have been there before." The nurse does not know how the client feels and these statements are unhelpful, can minimize the grief, or may be viewed as hurtful by the grieving person.

Using open-ended statements (e.g., "Tell me what you are feeling now" or "Tell me about what has happened"), can help the nurse determine where the client is in the grieving process. The nurse should also determine what support systems the client identifies as available (e.g., family, friends, religious community) and what coping strategies they may have used in the past that could be used to deal with the present situation.

Using leading statements (e.g., "You seem to regret some things. Tell me about that."), the nurse can determine whether the client has any ambivalent feelings, guilt issues, anger, or feelings of helplessness. Remember that because the process of grieving is individualized, each client will progress in the stages of grieving at a different pace, with some clients taking longer than others.

Interventions that will assist individuals to cope during the grieving process should encourage clients to be open and honest about their feelings with reassurance that they are acceptable and normal as the process follows its course. Having the client journal their feelings or write a letter to the deceased can help to bring closure to the past relationship. Referral to a grief support group can provide additional help. Encourage the client to identify and utilize family, friends, religious, or other groups for meaningful support. Success is measured by the client's progress in establishing new relationships and putting the loss in perspective. A client who expresses hope for the future and reinvestment in personal interests is demonstrating a positive self-image that is separated from the past relationship.

Test Yourself
- ✔ How would a child in each developmental stage view death differently than an adult?
- ✔ Identify four different types of grief and give an example for each.
- ✔ Name the stages of grief.
- ✔ List three interventions that aid coping in the grieving process.

CASE STUDY 1.2

"Art"

fizkes/Shutterstock

The clinic nurse is assessing Art, a 56-year-old farmer, whose wife died 6 months ago from ovarian cancer. He describes himself as "lost, forgetful, and unable to concentrate." He states, "I seem to cry at the most inconvenient moments, so I just stay to myself." The nurse notes his expression is sad and he avoids eye contact. Art says he has no appetite and "doesn't care anymore." When asked about his farming operation, he states he has lost interest in doing anything and has turned the farm over to his son.

Digging Deeper

1. What feelings might be responsible for Art's symptoms?

2. How should the nurse respond to Art?

3. What stage of the grief process is Art likely experiencing?

4. What referrals may be appropriate for Art?

Cultural Considerations

Names of Cultural Healers

Many people seek care from traditional healers for their primary health care. The healer may provide mental, physical, and/or spiritual care. When collecting client data, ask the client who they first go to for care. Do not refer to their healer as a "witch doctor" as this most often has a negative connotation.

Here are a few names for healers from different cultures:

- Curandero/curandera (Hispanic, Latin America)
- Sangoma (Zulu)
- Medicine man (Native American)
- Shaman (North Asian, Native American, Aboriginal Australian)

When a client reports seeing a traditional or complementary healer, ask about the frequency of visits and treatments received including herbal therapies. Document this information, using the client's own words and terms, and report the information to the health care provider or the Registered Nurse (RN).

Sources: van der Watt, A. S. J., van de Water, T., Nortje, G., Oladeji, B. D., Seedat S., Gureje, O., & Partnership for Mental Health Development in Sub-Saharan Africa (PaM-D) Research Team. (2018, April 25). The perceived effectiveness of traditional and faith healing in the treatment of mental illness: a systematic review of qualitative studies. *Social Psychiatry and Psychiatric Epidemiology*, *53*, 555–566. https://doi.org/10.1007/s00127-018-1519-9; World Health Organization. (2013). WHO Traditional medicine strategy: 2014–2023. https://www.who.int/publications/i/item/9789241506096

S U M M A R Y

- Mental health is seen as a state of well-being in which the individual has an awareness of their own abilities and weaknesses, copes with normal stressors of life, works productively, and makes a meaningful contribution to society.
- Mental illness denotes clinically significant behavioral or psychological patterns that occur in an individual causing distress or disability in the person's

life. Disorders manifest as inappropriate behavioral patterns that result from the distortions and discomfort experienced in the mind of the individual. Thinking errors and misconceptions often lead to irrational and unrealistic processing.

- Mental health is achieved as the individual forges a balance between the ups and downs of everyday life. Factors that require them to adapt both physically and emotionally and may affect mental health include stress, anxiety, grief, loss, religion, family, sleep, substance use, trauma, and abuse.

- Stress and anxiety are considered a part of everyday living. Mild stress is motivating and propels individuals to function at optimum levels toward accomplishment and success.
- Acute stress is triggered by an overwhelming sense of danger or threat over which one feels a lack of control. Chronic stress relates to a situation that is experienced on a continuous basis.
- Stress triggers an autonomic nervous system response that results in an unconscious feeling over which the conscious mind has no control. Both internal and external stressors can cause various responses. How an individual perceives a situation directly affects the sense of control felt over the stressor. An individual's response may be either adaptive or maladaptive based on this perception.
- Anxiety in response to stress can range from mild to panic. Coping strategies are learned behaviors. Successful resolution of previous stressful situations will lead to more effective coping methods. Ineffective coping and emotional strategies lead to ineffective and unsuccessful interpersonal relationships.

- If a stressful situation is unresolved, a state of crisis or emotional disorganization can result. The ability to function is impaired and intervention by a support system is required to reestablish homeostasis and control.
- Grief is a response to the anticipation of or the result of a loss. It is the process of mourning for, and coming to terms with, the reality of the loss and putting it into perspective as the individual moves forward. Reaction to loss changes with growth and maturation of individual's cognitive ability.
- Elizabeth Kubler-Ross defined five stages of grief: denial, anger, bargaining, depression, and acceptance. Once the loss is accepted, a new period of growth beyond the object or person can emerge.
- Dysfunctional grief results from a failure to complete the grieving process in which the person experiences a prolonged and intensified sense of loss. Multiple factors may contribute to this unresolved grief.
- Interventions that assist individuals with the grieving process should encourage openness and honesty about their feelings, as well as expressions of hope for the future and reinvestment in life interests.

BIBLIOGRAPHY

Chapman, L. K., & Steger, M. F. (2008). Race and religion: differential prediction of anxiety symptoms by religious coping in African American and European American young adults. *Depression & Anxiety*, 27(3), 316–322. https://doi.org/10.1002/da.20510

Cruz-Ortega, L. G., Gutierrez, D., & Waite, D. (2015). Religious orientation and ethnic identity as predictors of religious coping among bereaved individuals. *Counseling and Values*, 60, 67–83. https://doi.org/10.1002/j.2161-007X.2015.00061.x

Leonhardt, M. (2021). *What you need to know about the cost and accessibility of mental health care in America*. CNBC. https://www.cnbc.com/2021/05/10/cost-and-accessibility-of-mental-health-care-in-america.html

Muriel, A. C. (2021). Preparing children and adolescents for the loss of a loved one. *UpToDate*. Retrieved February 2, 2022, from https://www.uptodate.com/contents/preparing-children-and-adolescents-for-the-loss-of-a-loved-one

National Institute of Mental Health. (2022). *Mental Illness*. Retrieved January 8, 2022, from https://www.nimh.nih.gov/health/statistics/mental-illness#part_2555

Parekh, R. (2018). *Warning Signs of Mental Illness*. American Psychiatric Association. https://www.psychiatry.org/patients-families/warning-signs-of-mental-illness

Pirutinsky, S., Cherniak, A. D., & Rosmarin, D. H. (2020). COVID-19, mental health, and religious coping among American Orthodox Jews. *Journal of Religion and Health*, 59(5), 2288–2301. https://doi.org/10.1007/s10943-020-01070-z

Shear, M. K., Reynolds, C. F., Simon, N. M., & Zisook, S. (2021). Bereavement and grief in adults: Clinical features. *UpToDate*. Retrieved February 2, 2022, from https://www.uptodate.com/contents/bereavement-and-grief-in-adults-clinical-features

Substance Abuse and Mental Health Services Administration. (2019). *Trauma and Violence*. Retrieved January 21, 2022, from https://www.samhsa.gov/trauma-violence

Taylor, R. J., Chatters, L., Woodward, A. T., Boddie, S., & Peterson, G. L. (2021). African Americans' and Black Caribbeans' religious coping for psychiatric disorders. *Social Work in Public Health*, 36(1), 68–83. https://doi.org/10.1080/19371918.2020.1856749

Fill in the Blank

Fill in the blank with the correct answer.

1. Mental health is achieved as individuals forge a _____ between the ups and downs of everyday life.
2. Acute stress is a response to an immediate threat, commonly called the_____ or _____ response in which there is a surge of adrenalin into the blood.
3. When feelings of anxiety become too _____, those feelings may then be expressed through _____.
4. A major factor in whether a stressor becomes a strain on an individual is the _____ of situations over which little or no control is possible.
5. Statements made to the person who is grieving that are seemingly appropriate but tend to be empty and show little support are termed _____.

Matching

Match the following terms to the most appropriate phrase.

1. _____ Anxiety
2. _____ Eustress
3. _____ Adaptation
4. _____ Denial
5. _____ Bargaining
6. _____ Cultural identity
7. _____ Reframing
8. _____ Burnout
9. _____ Distress

a. Positive restructuring of thinking about a stressful event
b. Binding force between members of a cultural group
c. Feeling of apprehension, uneasiness, or uncertainty in response to a perceived threat
d. Adjustment period in which the reality of a loss is avoided
e. Positive and motivating stress
f. Condition of mental and emotional exhaustion
g. Harmful response to a threat or challenge
h. Manner in which individuals manage their anxiety
i. Labile moods and attempts to make deals to postpone a loss

Multiple Choice

Select the best answer from the available choices.

1. Which of the following statements made by a client might indicate a possible problem with the individual's present state of mental health? *(Select all that apply)*
   a. "I am involved in many community activities."
   b. "My children don't care about me anymore."
   c. "I enjoy the solitude of living by myself."
   d. "I try not to let the little things upset me."
   e. "I used to enjoy doing things with my friends."

2. A client diagnosed with a mental illness would demonstrate which of the following?
   a. Rational and realistic thought processing
   b. Ability to function alone or with others
   c. Disrupted interpersonal relationships
   d. Motivation by inner values and strengths

3. An LPN/LVN has worked in the dementia unit of a long-term care facility for the past 8 years. Recently, they have been calling in with various physical complaints and saying "I just don't care about the clients like I used to." It is most likely that the nurse is experiencing:
   a. Distress
   b. Crisis
   c. Burnout
   d. Stress

4. Which of the following statements reframes the irrational thought, "I will always be a failure," into a rational thought process?
   a. "I may fail at some things, but I am not always a failure."
   b. "I don't have to fail at anything."
   c. "I am my own worst enemy."
   d. "I usually fail because most things are just too difficult for me."

5. Your client owns a small business that has recently been experiencing reduced sales and profits. They have obtained a bank loan which will be due for repayment in 6 months. Which of the following describes the client's solution?
   a. Adaptive coping strategy
   b. Palliative coping strategy
   c. Maladaptive coping strategy
   d. Dysfunctional coping strategy

6. A client is scheduled for a radical mastectomy and states to the nurse, "It would be easier if I just didn't wake up from the surgery." Which of the following would be an appropriate response for the nurse to make? *(Select all that apply)*
   a. "You are just afraid now. Everything will look different tomorrow."
   b. "You feel it would be easier to die than to face the loss of your breast?"
   c. "Some people feel the way you do, but this does not mean the end of your life."
   d. "You seem very anxious about your surgery. Tell me more about your feelings."
   e. "Why do you think it would be easier to die than to wake up after surgery?"

7. Your client has been in a comatose state for the past 8 months as a result of an automobile accident. Although doctors have told the family the client does not have brain function, the family insists that the client has purposeful responses. Which stage of grief is the family demonstrating?
   a. Bargaining
   b. Anger
   c. Denial
   d. Depression

8. The nurse is caring for a client who has been told the radiation treatment of their cancer is not working. The client has been placed on hospice care with palliative relief of pain. Which of the following will this client likely soon experience?
   a. Unresolved grief
   b. Conventional grief
   c. Dysfunctional grief
   d. Anticipatory grief

9. The nurse is caring for a client whose wallet was stolen. The client is experiencing palpitations, hyperventilation, diaphoresis, and confusion. Although alert and talking, the client is unable to provide their name and address. How would the nurse document the client's response?
   a. Mild anxiety
   b. Moderate anxiety
   c. Severe anxiety
   d. Panic level

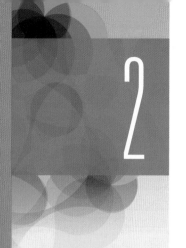

2 The Delivery of Mental Health Care

Historical Advancement of Mental Health Care

Mental health nursing has evolved as a specialized area of nursing practice that applies principles from both scientific theories of human behavior and focused nursing skills and interventions. Mental health care providers have met with numerous challenges in their effort to provide a platform of wellness and treatment for those with mental health issues and to increase public awareness and understanding. Historically, the journey to providing this humane and therapeutic approach has been difficult.

Early Treatment of People with Mental Illnesses

Before the advent of psychotherapeutic medications, now used extensively in the treatment of mental health issues, the available options for controlling symptoms of mental illness were few. Individuals with atypical behavior were considered outcasts of society and harbored in asylums for the remainder of their lives. Many of the more violent patients were referred to as "lunatics" (from the ancient belief that the moon caused insanity) and often became a spectacle for public viewing. The first institution for those with mental illnesses was opened in London as the Bethlehem Royal Hospital in 1247. "The insane," as they were called, received cruel and inhumane treatment and were often forced to wear metal arm and leg irons as they begged for food in the streets.

During the Renaissance, in the early 1400s, there was a growing interest in what led to various atypical behaviors. Early classifications of depression, neurosis, mania, and psychosis were developed by scholars and physicians according to the symptoms they observed. Despite the increased interest in what caused these mental illnesses, the care given to the individuals did not improve.

During the 1600s, care given to people with mental illnesses reached the most inhumane point. Individuals considered to be insane were locked in cells, starved, brutally beaten, and made helpless. In the late 1700s, psychiatry emerged as a separate division of medical science. Those connected with the specialty began to question the way people with mental illnesses were treated. During this time, Europe and the US colonies began to open asylums to house individuals with

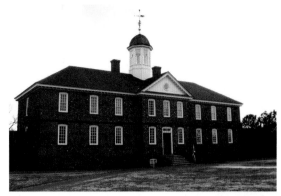

Figure 2.1 The Public Hospital for Persons of Insane and Disordered Minds, originally opened in 1773, was the first mental hospital in North America. The rebuilt structure now stands in Colonial Williamsburg, VA. (Source: Ryan Lintelman/Wikimedia Commons/Public Domain.)

mental illness along with prisoners and orphans (Fig. 2.1). The asylum was considered a place for the rejected members of society. Care was provided by people living in poverty and included such practices as bloodletting, purging, and the use of confinement chairs. Although the study of psychiatry was increasing, the actual treatment of those with behavioral problems remained unjust and cruel.

The Beginning of Change

In the early 1800s, Benjamin Rush (1745–1813) became the first American to advocate change in the conditions for individuals with mental illness. A professor of chemistry and medicine, he theorized that there was a connection between blood circulation and diseases of the mind. For those with these diseases, he advocated for improved conditions, including cleanliness, good air, lighting, and food. In addition, he felt that kindness and improved interaction between the client and care provider would have curative effects.

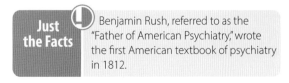

Just the Facts Benjamin Rush, referred to as the "Father of American Psychiatry," wrote the first American textbook of psychiatry in 1812.

In the middle of the 1880s, perspectives changed toward the care provided to those with mental illness. Dorothea Dix, initially a schoolteacher, began to question the treatment of both prisoners and individuals with mental illness. She began a tireless effort to start asylums, expose the poor treatment of people with mental illnesses, and start legislation to help in the construction of mental hospitals. During the Civil War, she was named the Superintendent of Army Nurses for the Union Army. She advocated for training and opportunities for female nurses.

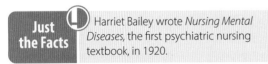

Just the Facts Psychiatric-mental health nursing began in the 1800s.

During the late 1800s and continuing into the 1900s, training programs for nurses were created and provided an option for those interested in caring for the sick. There was also an increasing social awareness of the problems related to mental illness. Although the need for trained nurses was recognized, caring for "the insane" was not seen as a fit occupation for women. Linda Richards (1841–1930) became one of the first trained nurses in America in 1873. Several years later, she traveled to England to receive more training at St. Thomas' Hospital in London, the hospital established by Florence Nightingale in 1860. Here she met and trained under Florence Nightingale. Nightingale encouraged Richards to continue her studies in Europe after which she returned to the United States and began to establish training curricula for schools of nursing. In 1882, Richards opened the Boston City Hospital Training School for Nurses to specialize in training nurses to care for those considered to have mental illnesses. Although this was a beginning, it was not until 1913 that the first psychiatric content was included within the curriculum of a generalized nursing school. As psychiatric content gradually phased into all schools of nursing, the specialized mental health training schools for nursing closed.

Just the Facts Harriet Bailey wrote *Nursing Mental Diseases*, the first psychiatric nursing textbook, in 1920.

Progress During the 1900s

Slowly, a component of psychiatric nursing was included in all nursing curricula. Funds were appropriated by Congress for the National Institute of Mental Health (NIMH), established in 1949, for its support and continued research in the field of mental illness.

These changes began to influence the present and future roles of psychiatric nurses. Although most clients with mental illness were still institutionalized in state mental hospitals, there was a growing trend to provide treatment at inpatient hospitals with units that specialized in the care of mental illness. This meant a growing need for trained nurses to fill both new and expanded roles. By the 1950s, many steps were taken toward improved conditions and treatment methods. In 1953, the National League for Nursing endorsed the inclusion of psychiatric nursing in all nursing programs.

It was during this period that the first psychotherapeutic medications were developed. These medications provided relief of symptoms and put an end to practices of physical restraint in straitjackets and lobotomies (portions of the brain removed to control behaviors). Sedatives were developed and lithium carbonate was found to be effective in controlling mood swings. In 1951, the first antipsychotic medications were introduced to control the atypical behaviors seen in some disorders. Shortly thereafter, antidepressants and anti-anxiety medications were developed.

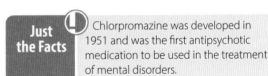

Just the Facts Chlorpromazine was developed in 1951 and was the first antipsychotic medication to be used in the treatment of mental disorders.

Integral to the improvement of the care of, and changing attitudes toward, people with mental illnesses has been the nurse's role in the treatment process. The work of Hildegard Peplau (1909–1999) laid the groundwork for the interpersonal and interactive processes vital to the nurse–client relationship. Peplau believed that when working with the psychiatric client, the nurse acts as a resource person, counselor, role model, and support person for the client.

In 1994, the American Nurses Association adopted standards of clinical practice for psychiatric-mental health nursing. These standards were last revised in 2014. The standards follow the nursing process, implementation of care, and the professional performance of the mental health nurse. Implementation standards include topics such as coordination of care, health teaching and promotion, and therapies. Some of the therapies covered in the standards are pharmaco-logic, milieu, and psychotherapy. Professional performance standards include ethics, evidence-based practice and research, communication, leadership, and collaboration.

The Move Toward Community-Based Care

As this new era of treatment emerged, the movement to deinstitutionalize individuals with mental illness began. Between 1950 and 1980, the number of institutionalized people dropped from more than 500,000 to less than 100,000. With deinstitutionalization, individuals were returned to their homes with follow-up counseling and therapy on an outpatient basis. The focus of care began to be on providing treatment and support systems that provide normalization and allow the client to return to a home setting or structured living situation. The trend toward improved and more compassionate care for those with mental illness was underway. As the need for community-based mental health care gained recognition, federal legislation created funding to establish centers that would offer these services. Table 2.1 identifies significant US legislation that has affected mental health care.

Mind Jogger In what way does the nurse serve as an advocate for those with mental illness?

Test Yourself
- ✔ Compare and contrast early and current treatments and views of mental health clients.
- ✔ What was the first antipsychotic medication?

Barriers to Mental Health Care

The access to mental health care and the way it is delivered has undergone many changes and reforms throughout the centuries. Although mental illness is present in all economic, racial, and ethnic groups, there are disparities in the availability and the utilization of mental health services. There remains a stigma and lack of education regarding mental illness for both the individual and their support system or caregivers. Easily identified barriers to accessing mental health services include lower socioeconomic status, lower educational levels, limited income, differences in language, homelessness, lack of available services,

TABLE 2.1	Legislation Related to Mental Health	
Year	**Legislation**	**Significance**
1946	National Mental Health Act	Provided funds for research, nursing degree programs, and improved community service for individuals with mental illness.
1955	Mental Health Study Act	The Joint Commission on Mental Illness and Health was directed to determine mental health needs and make recommendations for a national program.
1963	Community Mental Health Act	Helped establish community mental health centers to provide care instead of only in hospitals or institutions.
1980	Mental Health Systems Act	Provided grants to community mental health centers and included the Patients' Bill of Rights.
1987	Omnibus Budget Reconciliation Act	Gave residents of nursing homes the right to be free of unnecessary and inappropriate physical and chemical restraints and prevented the inappropriate placement of clients with mental illnesses into nursing homes.
1983	Mental Health Act	Addressed the rights of people admitted to psychiatric hospitals, including their right to refuse being admitted against their will. Also addressed client rights while in treatment, following discharge, and during community follow-up.
1990	Americans with Disabilities Act (ADA)	Prohibited discrimination against persons with mental and physical disabilities.
1996	Health Insurance Portability and Accountability Act (HIPAA)	National standards regarding keeping client information secured, confidential, and private. Clients have the right to know the content of their medical records, what information, and to whom it is being disclosed.
1996 and 2008	The National Mental Health Parity Act and Mental Health Parity and Addiction Equity Act	Created equality in insurance coverage by requiring mental disorder and substance use disorder benefits to be equal to those for other physical disorders and diseases.
2010	Patient Protection and Affordable Care Act (PPACA)	Created mandated benefits for insurance coverage of mental health and substance use disorders.
2016	Mental Health Reform Act	Supported flexibility for states and communities to improve mental health care and promoted increased access including care for at-risk populations.

and the stressors created by the mental health need. Barriers that can prevent an individual from accessing mental health care also include cultural beliefs regarding treatment, travel to appointments, and time off needed from work or extra child-care needs, and the stigma associated with mental illness.

Barriers Related to Culture

Mental illness affects all populations, regardless of race, ethnicity, gender, or economic status. Some marginalized groups are less likely to seek treatment, and those who do often do not receive the same level of care (Abdullah & Brown, 2011; Smedley et al., 2003). Treatment may not be sought because the individual's culture views the symptoms and/or cause of the illness differently than mental health care providers. Cultural beliefs regarding the cause of mental illness can influence whether the individual and/or their support system seeks help. For example, some cultures may believe that the mental illness is a punishment from God, is caused by an evil spirit or curse, is due to a weak character, or means the individual is useless or incompetent. Members of some cultures may be more willing to seek treatment from family, spiritual, or folk remedies than medical providers. Often, treatment from the medical model is sought late in the course of the illness or as a "last resort."

The nurse's personal values, beliefs, and experiences can influence their attitude toward clients. If the client receives care that seems influenced by bias or stereotype, whether perceived or intentional, the client may feel hostile or resentful toward the staff. A client who feels they have received biased care is less likely to follow care instructions. It is vital that the nurse performs ongoing self-assessment and evaluation of their own attitudes and reactions to aid in providing unbiased care.

A lack of trust in the system and fear of the outcome are common feelings of immigrants and both racial and ethnic minorities treated in the US medical system. Immigrants, refugees, and asylum seekers may have endured trauma before coming to the United States and some may have been in refugee camps. These experiences may have also predisposed them to mistrust the system or those seen as authority figures. These individuals are at a high risk for depression, anxiety, and post-traumatic stress disorder (PTSD) (Walker et al., 2021). Age of immigration can influence the risk of developing a mental illness. Rates of mental illness among immigrants who came to the United States during early childhood are comparable to those seen in members of the same ethnicity who were born in the United States. Conversely, those who immigrated during or after adolescence show lower rates than their same-age counterparts who were born in the United States (Alegría et al., 2017).

Cultural misunderstanding of the client's symptoms and their reasons for seeking, or not seeking, mental health care is also a barrier. Problems arise when the mental illness is addressed without considering the individual's cultural and personal beliefs regarding their symptoms and mental health. Progress is being made in understanding cultural bound illnesses or symptoms that may or may not be related to mental health and in understanding the symptoms of mental illness found in other countries that might be viewed as a physical illness in the United States. For example, headaches or seizures might be seen by some cultures as the result of the mind being possessed by a demon.

Multicultural education is necessary for those who care for clients with mental illness. Studies continue to examine the diverse cultural traditions, beliefs, values, and adjustments to acculturation. Cultural awareness and sensitivity in treatment are vital in providing quality care. The nurse must recognize the importance of communicating in the individual's first language, as much as possible, and establishing a therapeutic relationship that includes interventions respectful of cultural traditions.

Barriers Related to Cost of Care

Mental health care is covered by most insurance plans, but the individual must first obtain and pay for the insurance. Visits may be accompanied by copays as well. The visit itself may require time off from work or child-care or transportation costs. For some individuals, these costs are prohibitive to receiving care. For the individual who does not have insurance, the out-of-pocket payments alone can make care unaffordable.

Many inpatient facilities have decreased their bed capacity while others may have waiting lists for treatment. This decreases the number of clients that can be seen by the mental health care providers. Mental health care often receives less funding than other medical specialties. Some facilities or

"Susanna"

Palmer Kane LLC/ Shutterstock

The nurse is caring for a client who is Hispanic. The client and family members are primarily Spanish speaking, although one family member communicates in English. While providing care to the client, the family member, Susanna, tells you she has a brother who has a mental illness, and he often hears voices. Susanna also mentions that he talks a lot to those who have died. She asks you not to say anything about this as the family is very protective of the brother. Susanna admits that she is ashamed of his behavior and feels that he is this way because of things their father has done. You ask if they have taken her brother to get treatment for his mental illness. She replies, "Oh no, my mother would never allow that. She believes the *curandero* is the only one who can help. My grandmother is also a healer. She uses her healing ability to cure him and then he seems to get better for a while."

Digging Deeper

1. What additional information would the nurse need to collect?

2. What cultural issues may be a deterrent for the brother to receive treatment?

3. What steps might the nurse take to encourage the brother to receive treatment by mental health care professionals?

4. Should the nurse encourage the family to have the brother treated by mental health care professionals?

CASE STUDY 2.1

community health centers may not be as well-kept or modern as other specialties, and this can contribute to a negative view of mental health care.

These factors can lead to the reality that those who need these services are unable to secure them. Those living in community settings need ongoing management and support. Without these services, clients often become unstable, and treatment becomes ineffective. This may lead to in-patient hospitalization. Lack of access to treatment has implications for the person with mental illness, their support system, and society.

Those who do receive services but are inconsistent with therapy and medication adherence have difficulties with treatment effectiveness. This may lead to a relapse, further hospitalizations, or longer courses of treatment, which can increase the out-of-pocket or insurance costs or prohibit the individual from further seeking care.

> **Mind Jogger ?** How have the changes in the provision of mental health services affected your community?

Barriers Related to Stigma

Stigma is the negative association and/or perception attached to a disorder or situation. The stigma attached to something can increase and decrease. For example, cancer traditionally had a stigma attached to it which prevented people from discussing cancer treatments, options, or even letting others know someone had cancer. Some went as far as avoiding saying the word and referring to it in code (e.g., "The big C."). Today there is more openness related to discussing, and even having, cancer. However, some individuals or families still have stigmatized views of cancer.

Mental health has a stigma attached to it. This causes an avoidance of discussing the topic, treating individuals with mental health issues differently, avoiding them altogether, or even fear of the person or of "catching" the illness. Stigma can cause families to avoid seeking care for the individual or for themselves. Stigma is also reflected in derogatory statements (e.g., "She's crazy") that hurt the individual and presents their condition in a negative manner. Stigma can cause the individual with a mental health issue to avoid socialization or from seeking help for fear of maltreatment. They may deny their symptoms or delay and/or avoid treatment.

Studies done in many different countries have revealed three similar reactions world-wide toward individuals with mental illness (Abdullah & Brown, 2011). These are physical avoidance, viewing the individual as dangerous and/or aggressive, and self-stigma. **Self-stigma** (also called internal stigma) is when a person believes that, because of their mental illness, they will be rejected personally or when applying for a job; therefore, they begin to avoid others or stop applying for jobs. Self-stigma can lead to feelings of worthlessness, avoidance or poor adherence to mental health treatment, and self-harm.

Additionally, stigma can prevent the topic of mental health from being discussed in open forums or in schools. Schools may say they "don't want to scare the students" to rationalize avoiding the topic. This then causes the teaching of coping skills, explaining behavior, providing resources, and having a known and available support group to be avoided due to stigma. Stigma has prevented some schools from discussing and implementing suicide prevention programs for fear that discussing suicide will cause an increase in suicides (Watson, 2021).

Test Yourself	✔ Identify three barriers to mental health care and give an example of each. ✔ What factors may contribute to the public's attitude, positive and negative, toward those with mental illness?

Legal and Ethical Considerations in Mental Health Care

Laws and standards have been put in place to protect the rights of clients and set guidelines for mental health care providers.

Many decisions of health care professionals involve matters that include both legal and ethical issues. **Ethics** is a set of principles or values that guides behavior, helps determine right or wrong in a situation, and helps determine how the activity should be conducted. Like any other aspect of the health care system, the care of clients with mental health issues involves professional principles and values that provide a guiding philosophy for the ethical and professional care of the client. In some instances, nurses and other mental health care professionals must make decisions that involve conflicting standards and values. These situations sometimes have more than one solution, but the individual client must remain the most important focus in the decision. There are guidelines that assist in resolving these issues, and an ethical review board can help guide the decision-making process.

As members of the health care team, nurses must be familiar with current laws and ethical governance of mental health care delivery. This includes understanding, and protecting, the rights of clients. In addition, the nurse is responsible for maintaining standards within the nursing profession itself. Integrating positivity into client care and adherence to ethics, patient rights, and standards improve the self-esteem of clients, facilitate the therapeutic relationship between the nurse and client, and provide quality nursing care.

Client Rights

All clients entering a mental health treatment facility have rights. Set by the United States government, the rights of the mental health client regarding their treatment are covered in the **Mental Health Patient Bill of Rights** (Box 2.1). Clients are given the opportunity to read, or have read to them, these rights at the time of admission for treatment. The patient bill of rights is also usually displayed in prominent areas of the client care areas to

---

BOX 2.1

The Mental Health Patient Bill of Rights

Included in *U.S. Code Title 42 Chapter 102 Subchapter IV § 9501*, the mental health client has the right to:

- be treated in the least-restrictive setting.
- receive an individualized written treatment plan, receive that treatment, and have the treatment plan reviewed and revised periodically.
- participate, as appropriate, in the planning of mental health services.
- refuse treatment unless there is a court order that dictates otherwise.
- refuse to be a part of experimental therapy or treatment methods.
- be free from restraint or seclusion except in emergency and then only if ordered by a trained medical health professional.
- a humane treatment environment that affords reasonable protection from harm and appropriate privacy to personal needs.
- confidentiality within the limits of the law and to be informed of exceptions.
- access their medical records as appropriate.
- converse with others privately, and have reasonable access to telephone, mail, and visitors.
- be informed of these rights upon admission and periodically thereafter.
- assert grievances and to have grievances considered in a fair, timely, and impartial manner.
- have access to legal representation.

be easily visible to clients and visitors. It is a nurse's responsibility to be knowledgeable of these rights and to ensure that the client's rights are protected.

> **Mind Jogger ❷** In addition to being a responsibility, how does knowledge of client rights protect the nurse?

Informed Consent

Prior to admission to any health care setting, the client receives an explanation of client rights and institutional policies from the agency. In the case of an incompetent or incoherent client, their legal representative is to be given this information. Box 2.2 provides information about legal determination of decision-making ability. These full explanations give the client, or those who may have legal guardianship for the client, the ability to make an informed choice. When the client gives permission to undergo a specific procedure or treatment <u>after</u> being informed about the procedure, risks, and benefits, they are giving **informed consent**. The client must give informed consent before every procedure being performed. At the same time, the client has the right to refuse any aspect of treatment and may elect to withhold consent.

At the time of admission for mental health services, the client, or their representative, receives an explanation of facility policies regarding available services, visitation, phone usage, unit rules,

and provider contact. The facility should provide information regarding payment options. The client should be afforded the opportunity to discuss treatment options with a health care provider. Suggested topics for the client to discuss with their mental health professional are listed in Reinforcing Client and Family Teaching 2.1.

Reinforcing Client and Family Teaching **2.1**

Topics for Clients to Discuss with the Mental Health Professional

- Diagnosis and related information
- Prognosis—both short term and long term
- Details of any testing, medication, or treatment plan
- Alternative options to proposed treatments and their potential outcomes
- Risks and benefits of each option

Confidentiality

Confidentiality refers to the client's right to prevent written or verbal communications from being disclosed to outside parties without authorization. To facilitate a client's trust, nursing students and licensed nurses must assure them that all communication is confidential and will not be communicated to anyone not participating in their care. It is important to let clients know that information they disclose may be shared with other team members if it is relevant to their well-being and treatment progress. The Nurse Practice Act of each state's Board of Nursing requires nurses to protect the client's right to privacy by maintaining confidentiality. Every member of the treatment team has a duty to uphold this ethical standard. In some situations, it may be legally required that client information is disclosed (see Box 2.3).

BOX 2.2

Legal Guide to Decision-Making Capability

- Adults are seen as capable of making informed decisions unless determined "incompetent or incapacitated" by a court of law.
- If it is determined that a person lacks the ability to make informed decisions about health care, another person other than the client will make the decisions.
  - Each state has laws regarding the definition of who this person can be and what types of decisions can be made (e.g., medications, hospitalization, treatment, finances).
  - A family member may or may not be granted the right to make decisions.
  - The term for this position varies. Common terms include Ombudsman, Guardian, Custodian, or Conservator.
- A durable power of attorney for health care allows a person to designate whomever they choose to make health care decisions in the event the person is unable to do so.

BOX 2.3

Legal Situations That May Indicate Disclosure of Client Information

- Intent to commit a crime
- Duty to warn endangered individuals
- Evidence of child abuse
- Initiation of involuntary hospitalization
- Infection by human immunodeficiency virus (HIV)

Note: The nurse is not the professional to notify authorities in these cases. The nurse however has a duty to report any data collected regarding these situations to the proper chain of command as set by their facility policies.

Protecting the client's record from unauthorized personnel is a nursing responsibility. Health care providers who are not consulted by the primary health care provider or who are not providing direct client care do not have the privilege of viewing the client's medical record without permission. Student nurses who are involved in observation or interaction with clients should be cautious not to disclose any clinical information that is used for education purposes. Another way of providing privacy is to conduct the nursing report in a private area where other clients and uninvolved hospital staff cannot hear what is being said. Report sheets should be kept in a discreet place and shredded before leaving the nursing unit. The nurse should never discuss a client's problems or treatment with another client or the nurse's friends or family. Acknowledgment of a client admission should not occur via telephone to outside parties unless a policy and system exists that can be used to ensure confidentiality. Some mental health facilities have code words that are provided to individuals approved by the client.

Mind Jogger ② Would protecting the mental health client's confidentiality be more essential than protecting the confidentiality of a client in another part of the facility?

Appeals and Complaints

Regardless of the setting in which clients receive mental health services, they have the right to receive information about how to submit complaints, either about the care received or the professionals providing their care. This should be explained to the clients at the time services are anticipated, whether in a hospital unit or an outpatient setting. Should the client, or someone on their behalf, wish to file a complaint to a professional board, the person should be advised of the procedure to do so.

Seclusion and Restraint

Because some mental health disorders may cause a person to become extremely agitated or even act violently, seclusion or restraints may sometimes be used if other interventions or therapies are ineffective. The Joint Commission (TJC) and the federal government regulate the use of seclusion and restraints by health care workers. **Seclusion** refers to the involuntary placement of a client alone, in a controlled environment. Many times, this involves placing a client inside a room with a shut door. The room should have a soft floor and walls to prevent the client from injuring themselves and be free from any strangulation hazards such as window blinds or drop-down lights. A window to the room is present for continuous observation of the client. The client being prevented from leaving the room, even if the door is unlocked or if there is no door, also constitutes seclusion.

Physical restraint refers to the use of a method (such as a staff member pinning down a client) or physical device (such as a wrist restraint or straitjacket) to restrict movement by the client. Physical restraints are used only to prevent harm to self or others, never as a punitive means, and require careful monitoring. Physical restraints may be used for the wrist, ankles, chest, waist, or fingers and are made of a soft material or in some cases, leather. **Chemical restraint** refers to the use of medication to restrict a client's behavior.

The use of seclusion or restraint requires a health care provider's order and frequent reevaluation of need. Facility policy guides the steps the nurse takes to obtain and implement the order. Seclusion and restraints are not ordered on a routine basis and cannot be reordered indefinitely. Continuous monitoring of the client in restraints or seclusion is mandatory. Time limits are a part of many state and institutional statutes. These methods are discontinued at any time they are seen as ineffective or at the earliest possible indication that the client has regained control.

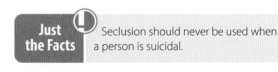
Just the Facts Seclusion should never be used when a person is suicidal.

Just the Facts Restraints are applied only with a health care provider's order and under the supervision of a registered nurse.

These methods are only used when verbal interventions or less-restrictive methods of treatment have been ineffective, and the behavioral issue poses a serious and immediate threat or danger to the individual, staff, or other clients. It is essential that nurses attempt to de-escalate aggressive behaviors before these measures are necessary. Often the environmental situation or other clients have provoked the behavior. In this case, removing the client to another area of the unit allows them the opportunity to regain control without further intervention.

Risks are associated with the use of seclusion and restraints. These risks include increased admission time, readmission, physical and/or emotional harm to the client, harm to staff, and can even cause client death (Substance Abuse and Mental Health Services Administration [SAMHSA], 2019). The use of seclusion and restraint can be traumatic for the client. Safe and alternative approaches to managing agitated or violent clients are encouraged in all areas of mental health treatment. In 2000, the American Psychiatric Nurses Association (2018) released a position statement regarding reducing, and working toward eliminating, the use of seclusion and restraints.

Nurses should be familiar with the legal implications involved in the use of seclusion and restraint. It is important to know the qualifications and training of any person that is delegated the task of assisting with restraint or seclusion. The nurse should know the facility rules and state laws regarding these procedures to avoid any probable cause of wrongful liability. Clients who are confined without justification or who are subject to inappropriate use of seclusion or restraint (either physical or chemical) can take their case to a civil court with a charge of false imprisonment. The restraint of clients with inappropriate use of force can be viewed as assault or battery. It is essential, and ethical, for the nurse to know how, when, and why to use confining methods, as well as knowledge and skills for initial use of least-restrictive interventions. Having a valid health care provider's order; making frequent or continuous observation; noting release, toilet, and meal times; and providing complete documentation of all observations and interventions are vital when caring for the client who is in seclusion or restrained.

Nurse Accountability

Student and licensed nurses are accountable for the care they provide, which means they must take responsibility for what they do. Each level of nursing is responsible for adhering to the standard of care that is acceptable for their level. The Nurse Practice Act of each state identifies the scope and minimum standards of practice for both the LPN/LVN and RN. If the nurse has a question about a statute contained in the practice act, they should contact the board of nursing for the state in which they are practicing.

Nurses have an obligation to maintain current licensure and educational requirements required by their board of nursing. In the area of mental health nursing, the nurse is also responsible for knowing institutional and governmental policies regarding client admission and rights. If uncertainty exists, the nurse is responsible for securing the correct information from other sources such as the facility's nurse leaders or ethics panel, procedure manuals, the state board of nursing, or national nursing organizations.

Nurses may be held accountable, and liable, for an act of incompetence or negligence in the deliverance of care. All actions on the part of the nurse to facilitate appropriate treatment of the client should be documented to provide a written record of events. The nurse also has a legal and ethical responsibility to act as a client advocate to protect the client and their rights.

Test Yourself
- List three ways the nurse can protect the mental health client's confidentiality.
- What are the two types of restraints?
- How would the nurse's role as client advocate pertain to the client who is mentally incompetent?

Practice Settings for Mental Health Care

Mental health care is composed of various approaches and settings that have been developed to meet the needs of individuals with mental health issues and their support systems. Clients with mental disorders are seen in mental health treatment centers. However, they, or other clients with psychological or emotional symptoms, may be seen in other health care settings (e.g., outpatient clinics, hospital units, long-term care facilities, home health care, or correctional institutions) as well. The ability to recognize the symptoms and initiate appropriate nursing interventions is important in any practice setting.

A client has the right to receive treatment in the least-restrictive environment that would promote safety and provide therapeutic care. The type of facility and level of care provided depends on several factors. The client's history has a strong influence on the treatment setting that will be used. The circumstances that led to the current admission also contribute to the setting, treatment plan, and nursing care that will be needed. The health care provider determines whether the client will need to receive inpatient or outpatient treatment and the appropriate setting in which that care can be provided.

> **Just the Facts**
>
> Least-restrictive environments can include locked or unlocked hospital units, community living centers, or outpatient treatment centers, depending on the individual needs of the client.

Although the nurse is not directly responsible for deciding where or what treatment is provided, an integral part of the nurse's responsibility is to ensure that the client receives appropriate care. All clients are entitled to receive care based on a current, updated, and individualized treatment plan that includes a description of the services that are available and those that are offered upon discharge.

Inpatient Mental Health Settings

Depending on the urgency, a referral may be made to a hospital emergency room or inpatient facility for an immediate intervention. A client experiencing acute symptoms of a mental illness may be brought for evaluation by law enforcement officers after an arrest or other altercation with the law. Family members may bring clients out of fear or concern for the welfare of the individual or themselves. In addition, sometimes the client makes an individual decision to seek treatment as an inpatient. Clients may recognize that they are out of control or fear that they will harm themselves or others. In these instances, an admission to inpatient services is usually indicated.

Clients with mental health problems may request admission to a psychiatric center for treatment. A **voluntary commitment** occurs when the client is admitted to the mental health unit based on their own decision for admission. In this situation, the health care provider writes the order for admission, and the client signs and agrees to the terms of treatment. The person is then allowed to sign the appropriate documents and leave when treatment is complete. Policies vary among facilities, but most states have an initial period (e.g., 48 to 72 hours) that allows the provider and other members of the treatment team the opportunity to assess the situation before the client can leave voluntarily. If the client leaves before this time or without a discharge order from the provider, they may be asked to sign an Against Medical Advice (AMA) form that releases the facility from any liability related to the person leaving treatment.

An **involuntary commitment** occurs when a person is admitted to a psychiatric unit against their will. The amount of time a person can be detained is determined by law, which varies from state to state. For an involuntary admission to occur, an evaluation statement that clearly indicates the client's mental state is a danger to self or others is necessary. The order for protective custody is given by a court official. The client can be detained on an emergency status against their will for an interval of 48 to 72 hours. At the end of that period, the client must be discharged, given voluntary admission status, or receive a court hearing to determine if continued involuntary treatment is necessary. Laws may vary from state to state on these options. Involuntary commitment is most commonly used in an inpatient setting but can be ordered on an outpatient basis, such as in substance use disorder programs.

Outpatient Mental Health Settings

In some situations, a client may be referred to a community mental health center, social service agency, or private facility where various outpatient-based treatment options and services are available. This eliminates the need for the client to be admitted while receiving this care. The purpose of outpatient delivery of mental health care is to provide treatment and services to individuals, families, and the community that will promote mental health and support their optimum level of functioning. This allows the individual to remain in a familiar environment and continue their normal daily routine.

An individual may seek help on their own from a private psychiatrist, psychologist, or therapist. These services may include psychotherapy, symptom evaluation, and psychotropic medication evaluation and management. Residential facilities are available for clients who need a therapeutic environment for extended periods of time but are not able to reside in their homes. Individuals who live in a residential environment still attend outpatient treatments or services in the community or from their mental health care provider.

Outpatient Therapies

- Individual therapy
- Marriage or family therapy
- Child/adolescent therapy
- Support groups
  - Divorce therapy
  - Grief and loss
- Group therapy
- Stress reduction and relaxation
- Addiction groups (AA/NA/Al-Anon)
- Biofeedback
- Complementary and alternative medicine (CAM)
  - Acupuncture
  - Biofeedback
  - Imagery
  - Massage
- Art therapy
- Drum circles
- Occupational therapy

A variety of therapies and therapy groups are available to help the individual. Each therapy has a specialized focus to aid mental health. The therapy is led by a trained professional, can be one-on-one or with a group, and has a goal or plan of helping the individual to better understand themselves, their behaviors, or to promote activities that help support mental health. Box 2.4 lists examples of different types of therapies.

Other Health Care Settings

Nurses practice in a variety of settings that are not mental health based; however, emotional and/or psychosocial needs of clients may emerge even in these settings. Settings include health care providers' offices, long-term care facilities, home health care, and hospice care to name a few.

Mental health symptoms may affect a medical condition, which could result in an exacerbation of the illness or a delayed recovery. In some cases, the mental health symptoms may interfere with treatment of the medical condition. An example of this would be the client with altered thought processes who is nonadherent with their diet or medication therapy. Conversely, the physiologic symptoms of a mental health illness may exacerbate a medical issue, as exemplified by a client who is postmyocardial infarction and has severe anxiety that creates a significant elevation in their heart rate and blood pressure.

Regardless of the health care setting, the nurse should recognize behaviors that indicate the client is having anxiety, a situational crisis, or behaviors that are consistent with a mental health issue. The LPN/LVN should notify the registered nurse or the health care provider of their observations. Additionally, they should collect and report data regarding the client's coping ability. Everyone copes with stressful situations differently. What works for one may not work for another. Coping strategies can also include asking questions to obtain information and guidance for treatment, sharing concerns and finding support from others, changing emotional climate with humor, or suppressing fears.

Just the Facts The nurse can strengthen a client's coping strategies with positive reinforcement.

Grief reactions are commonly seen in any health care setting. A physical illness that imposes a severe threat to an individual's health status or a lifetime of chronic disease may elicit a grief response. Additionally, a client in these settings may be faced with a new loss. Examples of a loss could include the client who just received a diagnosis of a long-term illness (e.g., diabetes), a terminal diagnosis, or confirmation of an early pregnancy loss (also known as a miscarriage).

In some situations, the new diagnosis may restrict the client's lifestyle or alter their finances, which may threaten their self-esteem or sense of security. For other clients, future goals and family roles may be altered by the physical needs and/or psychological effects of the diagnosis. Box 2.5

Physical Diseases and Surgeries With Psychological Implications

- Alzheimer/dementia
- HIV/AIDS
- Parkinson
- Multiple sclerosis
- Amyotrophic lateral sclerosis (ALS)
- Hemophilia
- Asthma
- Cancer
- Myocardial infarction
- Hemodialysis
- Quadriplegia/paraplegia
- Radical facial/neck surgery
- Mastectomy
- Prostatectomy
- Colostomy, ileostomy, nephrostomy
- Amputation
- Organ transplant

lists some physical diseases and surgeries that have the potential for psychological effects on the client and the client's family.

Clients admitted to a rehabilitation facility need to be observed for signs of grief, loss, despair, or depression. These are common after a life-altering injury or illness. Residents of long-term care or assisted living facilities can be admitted with an existing mental health diagnosis, or they can develop a mental health issue during their admission. Depression is common in older adults and can be related to end-of-life despair; loss of independence; loneliness; or experiencing the deaths of their spouse, peers, or close family members. It is very important to note that depression is not a normal part of aging.

Among the most common emotional and psychological responses to trauma, physical illness, or loss are depression, fear, anxiety, denial, withdrawal, anger, apathy, regression, and dependency. Levels of these emotions may accelerate as the individual feels a loss of control. This loss of control can occur when pain, disability, hospitalization, or death may be possible outcomes. Threats to independence or self-decision making can also create feelings of a loss of control. The economic impact of health care, in any setting, can also produce anxiety.

Fear of the "unknown" is especially threatening to the client who is experiencing an emotional or psychological crisis. A client may project these fears or their anxiety by exhibiting anger or through self-centered, demanding behaviors such as unreasonable requests of health care providers. Nursing interventions in these situations include therapeutic communication techniques (see Chapter 7), talking softly, acknowledging the client's feelings, offering realistic expectations, and de-escalation techniques if needed. It is important for the nurse to not take the client's behaviors personally, as the client is reacting to their internal feelings and not the nurse.

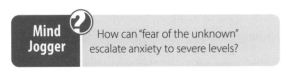

Mind Jogger ② How can "fear of the unknown" escalate anxiety to severe levels?

Acute Care Settings

Clients with a pre-existing mental health diagnosis are admitted to acute care settings for medical or surgical reasons. Additionally, mentally healthy

> ### BOX 2.6
>
> ### Factors Impacting an Individual's Ability to Cope
>
> **Individual factors**
> - Personality
> - Cognitive ability
>   - Age
>   - Developmental level
>   - Presence of developmental disability (e.g., autism spectrum disorder, Down syndrome)
>   - Presence of cognitive disorder (e.g., delirium, traumatic brain injury)
> - Values
> - Cultural beliefs
> - Emotional state
> - Previous experiences
>
> **Environmental factors**
> - Support system(s) available
> - Financial stability
> - Impact on work or home routine
>
> **Illness-related factors**
> - Type of illness
> - Rate of progression
> - Degree of functional impairment
> - Treatments
> - Complications
> - Prognosis

individuals may experience temporary mental health needs due to a situational crisis, such as rape, trauma, abuse, or an environmental disaster. Crisis intervention and supportive nursing strategies can make a major difference in the ability of the client to cope during these difficult situations. Often, the nurse is the one who observes these feelings or behaviors that may demonstrate symptoms of mental health imbalance. Box 2.6 identifies some factors that may impact an individual's coping abilities.

The client with a diagnosed mental illness who is hospitalized can present a nursing challenge due to the nature of the dual diagnoses. Whereas the nurse may prioritize the medical-surgical needs of the client, the secondary mental illness diagnosis must be considered in all aspects of care planning. Critical thinking leads the nurse to ask questions such as: How will the client mentally view this procedure? What environmental stimuli could be misinterpreted? What explanations will be needed to reinforce reality to the client with altered thought processes? How might the client misperceive pain? What approaches could be used if the client exhibits delusional thinking or hallucinations?

Communication techniques and nursing interventions for altered thought processes are critical to the outcome of the client's situation. An altered psychological state complicates adherence to the medical treatment or recovery from surgery. Data collection needs to be done on both the physiologic and psychological needs of the individual client. This includes the client's emotional reaction to the diagnosis or hospitalization, past and current coping abilities, current level of self-care activities, and available support resources. This information provides the nurse with a baseline of the client's status. During this vulnerable time, consistency of caregivers gives the client a sense of security necessary to develop trust in the health care staff and to feel safe in a new environment. Creative approaches to providing nursing care are needed to meet the client's needs, avoid complications, and help them return to their baseline level of functioning. It is most important to reinforce the client's problem-solving skills and provide support for self-care efforts. The increase in self-care responsibilities, as appropriate, helps to preserve self-esteem and provides a sense of control over a situation that may seem overwhelming.

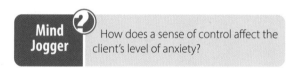

Mind Jogger How does a sense of control affect the client's level of anxiety?

The lack of control over the effects imposed by many of these conditions may be described as a state of helplessness or **powerlessness**. This may be true of both the client and their support systems who are involved. The nurse should assume an empathetic and supportive role as the emotional and psychological defenses of these individuals are lowered by the decision making and coping necessary to deal with the diagnosis, illness, hospitalization, or surgery. The nurse should plan to include time for active listening. This allows and encourages the client to express feelings and concerns. Explanations concerning diagnostic tests, procedures, permits, and consent forms are vital to allow the client to make informed decisions regarding their situation. A sense of empowerment is returned to the client when they are included in planning of their care needs and have the opportunity to make choices. The nurse's sensitivity to the emotions the client is experiencing will also be a major factor in the client's ability to adapt to the situation.

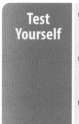

Test Yourself
- ✔ Describe the difference between a voluntary and involuntary commitment.
- ✔ What questions could the nurse ask to collect data on the client's coping strategies?
- ✔ List some of the psychological implications of a major disease or surgery.

Correctional Facilities

Jails or detention centers, where individuals are incarcerated for crimes, provide a large amount of mental health services. When someone arrives at a correctional facility, data is collected on them for both medical and mental health issues. This intake may be done by a paramedic, nurse, or physician depending upon the facility's policy. Mental health data collected in the intake process may include current or previous use of psychotropic medications, family history of mental illness, history of seizures or head trauma, history of suicide attempts, hallucinations, delusional thinking, and any substance use. Further evaluation by a health care provider is done if the person demonstrates symptoms or behaviors of substance use withdrawal, mental health issues, or has a history of previous mental health treatment, suicidal ideation, or attempt.

Continued evaluation and treatment of medical or mental illnesses the client had before incarceration are often the reason the client is seen in the medical unit of the correctional facility. Nursing staff members should be observant for any mental health issues, even when the client is being seen for a nonpsychological complaint, and report observations according to facility policy. The medical unit is a place of respite for the person who is incarcerated, away from confinement of their cell or the general housing areas. Therefore, some clients may begin to view real or perceived ailments as means to seek time away from the areas of confinement. While existing and new medical problems are legitimate health care needs, the client may try to persuade medical personnel to give them special privileges, medications, or movement to a new area. The need for treatment must be separated from nonmedical issues to assure that any legitimate condition receives the appropriate interventions.

Security is always present and the client who is incarcerated must follow the same standards of behavior and rules of the facility while they are in the medical unit. Many people who are incarcerated

CASE STUDY 2.2

"John"

Boonkung/Shutterstock

John is a 38-year-old mechanic who is currently unemployed and has a mental health diagnosis of chronic schizophrenia. He has been living in a group home milieu for the past 6 months. He was admitted to the emergency department, diagnosed with acute appendicitis, and had an open incision appendectomy. Upon admission to the medical-surgical unit, he has a nasogastric tube connected to intermittent suction, a right peripheral IV line, a bulb-suction drainage tube, and a dry abdominal gauze pressure dressing covering the incisional site.

Digging Deeper

1. How do you think John will behave as the effects of anesthesia and sedation wear off?

2. How might he misinterpret the array of "tubes" connected to his body?

3. How do you think John will interpret his pain?

4. What approach might the nurse use to help John understand the cause of the pain?

On the second postoperative day, John begins to question the invasive equipment lines entering his body. The nurse enters his room to find him drinking water with his nasogastric tube lying on the floor beside the bed. He tells the nurse he was thirsty, and "that hose was siphoning all the water out of my body to water the plants neglected by my inability to turn the shower on, and I got some water so I can water the shower."

Digging Deeper

1. What physical assessments related to his surgical care would be important to collect data on and report?

2. What statements could the nurse make to John to help him understand his situation?

are presently dealing with, or have a history of, some type of substance use. Behaviors related to drug use place individuals at risk for Hepatitis B, C, and HIV. Therefore, it is important for the nurse working in a correctional facility to be vigilant in using personal protective equipment (PPE) to protect themselves from blood-borne illnesses.

Nurses who work in a correctional facility must learn to separate what is real from what is a manipulative endeavor by the client who is incarcerated. Manipulation involves behavioral tactics of deceit, devious thinking, or actions used to meet the individual's self-serving needs at the expense of another person. A calm, firm, and matter-of-fact approach is essential to ensure the client adheres to rules and policies of the facility. The empathy and compassion that is integral to nursing may be viewed by the client as an opportunity for manipulation. While it is important to accept them as a person and treat them in an unbiased and ethical manner, the nurse must also be vigilant to avoid being manipulated.

Forensic Psychiatric Nursing

A forensic inpatient unit is for the housing and treatment of individuals who are diagnosed with a mental illness and who have committed a criminal act, usually a felony-level offense such as murder. They are treated in the secured forensic inpatient unit if they have no capacity for liability, meaning their serious mental illness prevents them from distinguishing between good and evil, right and wrong, or from understanding their actions. Their sentence to the unit is court-ordered and involuntary; however, they are not incarcerated. The unit has restrictions on their movement and social interactions that differ from general inpatient mental health units. Mental diagnoses often include schizophrenia, drug-related toxic psychosis, and delusion. Additionally, they may have antisocial behavior, substance use disorders, and poor insight into their crime and treatment. Nurses can find themselves in a role-conflict between that of "care provider" and "guard."

Cultural Considerations

Cultural Values and Stigma

The values a culture views as important have an impact on the expression of stigma toward the individual with a mental illness. Below are some cultural values (shown in bold) and example(s) of how stigma might be expressed.

Collectivism (the need of the group is more important than the individual's need)
- Mental health is seen as a disease of the family or group and therefore other members are tainted by association.
- Physical distance, avoidance, or removal from the group.
- Talking about mentally ill individual (their atypical behaviors or expressing pity for their condition) but not interacting with or talking to them.
- Family or support system do not seek mental health services as they are reluctant, or refuse, to admit the family member has a mental illness.
- Group may deny the existence of mental illness altogether.

Concealing emotions
- Individual is seen as weak when seeking mental health services because they share and make public their emotions.

Family
- Individual seen as not eligible for marriage, unable to have children, or unable to provide for family and therefore viewed as less worthy than others.

Family Honor
- The individual is viewed as betraying or bringing dishonor to the family because of their behavior.
- The individual is a reflection of the family, therefore atypical behavior is seen as the family's shame or as the family's mental illness.
- Emotional detachment from, or actual disownment of the individual from the family.

Family recognition (bringing recognition to family from academics or achievements)
- The individual's inability to bring recognition creates shame on the family/parents who then may disown them.
- Individual is seen to be less worthy or important than others.

Individualism (individual values independence and autonomy)
- If individual requires mental health assistance they are seen as weak or unable to care for themselves.

Respecting and caring for parents
- The individual is unable to financially provide or physically care for parents or elders which brings shame to family.
- The individual is seen as having less social value.

Social harmony (keeping harmony takes precedence over individual's expression of own opinions and values)
- In order to not be a burden on others, the individual intentionally avoids talking about themselves.
- Individual avoids seeking mental health services.

Information adapted from Abdullah, T., & Brown, T. L. (2011). Mental illness stigma and ethnocultural beliefs, values, and norms: An integrative review. *Clinical Psychology Review*, *31*(6), 934–948. https://doi.org/10.1016/j.cpr.2011.05.003

SUMMARY

- Early treatment for people with mental illnesses was inhumane and unjust.
- Dorothea Dix was a 19th-century pioneer in advocating improved standards for mental hospitals and those with mental illness.
- In 1882, Linda Richards opened the Boston City Hospital Training School for training nurses to care for individuals with mental illness.
- The United States has passed legislation to improve the care provided for mental health clients and protect their rights.
- Barriers to mental health care can be related to culture, cost of care, and stigma.
- Clients receiving mental health care should be given an explanation of their rights according to the mental health Patient Bill of Rights and institutional policies.

- Clients must give informed consent, if they are competent, before every procedure is performed. Clients have the right to refuse treatment.
- The Nurse Practice Act of each state and the HIPAA of 1996 hold mental health care professionals to a legal and ethical responsibility of confidentiality.
- Situations that may legally require disclosure of information include intent to commit a crime, duty to warn endangered persons, evidence of child abuse, initiation of involuntary hospitalization, and infection by human immunodeficiency virus (HIV).
- The client receiving mental health care has the right to file a complaint against any professional involved in providing treatment. It is the responsibility of the health care team to provide the contact information to the client.

- Seclusion refers to placement of a client alone in a controlled environment. Continuous monitoring and time limits are required with discontinuance if ineffective or at the earliest indication the client has regained control.
- Restraining a client can include physical restraints such as the use of mechanical devices, or chemical restraints, which refers to the use of medication to restrict a client's behavior.
- Nurses must be familiar with the legal implications, facility rules, and state laws of seclusion and restraint.
- Nurses are accountable for adhering to the standard of care outlined in the Nurse Practice Act for the level at which they are practicing.
- The nurse has a legal and ethical responsibility to act as a client advocate to protect clients and their rights.
- Nurses encounter those who need emotional and psychosocial care in a variety of health care settings other than mental health units.
- Under federal guidelines, the client receiving mental health care must be cared for in the least-restrictive environment possible.
- A voluntary commitment to inpatient mental health care indicates the client's willingness to comply with the treatment program.
- Involuntary commitment occurs when the client is admitted to a psychiatric unit against their will. This requires an order of protective custody issued by a court official.
- The purpose of outpatient mental health care is to provide services to individuals, families, and the community that will promote mental health and quality of life.
- Physical illness can create a psychological response that may impact treatment, result in an exacerbation of the illness, or delay a recovery.
- Psychological responses include grief, depression, fear, anxiety, denial, withdrawal, and anger.
- Clients with a dual diagnosis of a medical condition and a mental illness require that needs related to both situations are assessed and met in systematic care of the client.
- Nurses who work in correctional facilities must learn to separate statements made by clients as attempts to manipulate from those which express a legitimate health care need.

BIBLIOGRAPHY

Abdullah, T., & Brown, T. L. (2011). Mental illness stigma and ethnocultural beliefs, values, and norms: An integrative review. *Clinical Psychology Review, 31*(6), 934–948. https://doi.org/10.1016/j.cpr.2011.05.003

Alegría, M., Álvarez, K., & DiMarzio, K. (2017). Immigration and mental health. *Current Epidemiology Reports, 4*(2), 145–155. https://www.ncbi.nlm.nih.gov/pmc/articles/PMC5966037

American Mental Health Counselors Association. (2020). *AMHCA code of ethics.* (Revised 2020). https://www.amhca.org/HigherLogic/System/Download-DocumentFile.ashx?DocumentFileKey=24a27502-196e-b763-ff57-490a12f7edb1&forceDialog=0

American Psychiatric Association. (2020). *Stigma, prejudice and discrimination against people with mental illness.* https://www.psychiatry.org/patients-families/stigma-and-discrimination

American Psychiatric Nurses Association. (2018). *APNA position statement on the use of seclusion and restraint.* (Revised 2018). https://www.apna.org/resources/apna-seclusion-restraint-position-paper

Betancourt, J. R., Green, A. R., & Carrillo, J. E. (2021). The patient's culture and effective communication. *UpToDate.* Retrieved February 16, 2022, from https://www.uptodate.com/contents/the-patients-culture-and-effective-communication

Bonfine, N., Wilson, A. B., & Munets, M. R. (2019). Meeting the needs of justice-involved people with serious mental illness within community behavioral health systems. *Psychiatric Services, 71*(4), 355–363. https://doi.org/10.1176/appi.ps.201900453

Legal Information Institute of Cornell Law School. (2022). *U.S. Code Title 42 Chapter 102 Subchapter IV § 9501 (Mental Health Patient Bill of Rights).* https://www.law.cornell.edu/uscode/text/42/9501

National Institute of Mental Health. (2019). *Help for mental illnesses.* Retrieved February 24, 2022 from https://www.nimh.nih.gov/health/find-help#part150431

Smedley, B. D., Stith, A. Y., & Nelson, A. R.; Institute of Medicine, Board on Health Sciences Policy, Committee on Understanding and Eliminating Racial and Ethnic Disparities in Health Care. (2003). *Unequal treatment: Confronting racial and ethnic disparities in health care.* The National Academies Press. https://doi.org/10.17226/12875

Substance Abuse and Mental Health Services Administration. (2019). *Trauma and violence: Alternatives to seclusion and restraint.* https://www.samhsa.gov/trauma-violence

Tsunematsu, K., Fukumoto, Y., & Yanai, K. (2021). Ethical issues encountered by forensic psychiatric nurses in Japan. *Journal of Forensic Nursing, 17*(3), 163–172. https://doi.org/10.1097/JFN.0000000000000333

Walker, P. F., Barnett, E. D., & Stauffer, W. (2021). Medical Screening of adult immigrants and refugees. *UpToDate.* Retrieved February 16, 2022, from https://www.uptodate.com/contents/medical-screening-of-adult-immigrants-and-refugees

Watson, T. (2021). *Reluctance to require suicide prevention education could cost lives, but it's complicated.* The Hechinger Report. https://hechingerreport.org/reluctance-to-require-suicide-prevention-education-could-cost-lives-but-its-complicated

Fill in the Blank

Fill in the blank with the correct answer.

1. The development of _____ medications allowed behaviors and symptoms to be controlled without restraints and surgery.
2. _____ or _____ are used to keep the client from hurting themselves or others when de-escalation or distraction techniques are ineffective.
3. _____ refers to a set of principles or values that provide dignity and respect to clients.
4. _____ _____ is a signed statement of understanding that provides protection for both the client and the agency providing the services.
5. _____ refers to the client's right to prevent written or verbal communications from being disclosed to outside parties without authorization.
6. An _____ _____ occurs when a person is admitted to a psychiatric unit against their will.

Matching

Match the following terms to the most appropriate phrase.

1. _____ Chlorpromazine
2. _____ Accountability
3. _____ Nurse Practice Act
4. _____ Seclusion
5. _____ Chemical restraint
6. _____ Manipulation

a. Purposeful self-serving behavior directed at getting needs met
b. Placement in controlled environment
c. First antipsychotic medication developed
d. Taking responsibility for own actions
e. Use of medication to control behavior
f. Defines the scope of nursing practice

Multiple Choice

Select the best answer from the multiple-choice items.

1. Which client statement shows evidence that the client has received stigmatized treatment?
   a. "The nurse asked me what herbal remedies I use at home."
   b. "The nurse asked if I would prefer female caregivers to take care of my mother."
   c. "The nurse asked if I have difficulty paying for my outpatient visits."
   d. "The nurse asked if my family thought I was crazy."

2. In which of the following situations would obtaining an order of protective custody be appropriate?
   a. Client is hallucinating
   b. Client is exhibiting sexually inappropriate behavior
   c. Client's mental state is a danger to self or others
   d. Client is angry and verbally hostile

3. The nurse is caring for a client who has recently been diagnosed with leukemia. Which of the following should the nurse include in the data collection?
   a. Available coping behaviors
   b. Relaxation techniques
   c. Consistency of caregivers
   d. Explanation of diagnostic tests

4. The nurse is collecting data on a client newly admitted to a correctional facility. Which of the following factors would indicate a need for referral and further evaluation? *(Select all that apply)*
   a. Voices current suicidal ideation
   b. Anger toward the justice system
   c. Previous treatment for depression
   d. History of intervention for suicide attempts
   e. Ambivalent feelings about others incarcerated in the facility

5. A client is seen in the emergency room for acute symptoms of anxiety and situational crisis. The health care provider refers the client to a mental health clinic for counseling. Which client right is being upheld?
   a. To accept or refuse treatment
   b. To know qualifications of professionals involved in care
   c. To receive explanations of treatment
   d. To be treated in the least-restrictive setting

6. In which of the following situations would it be considered legally appropriate to disclose client information?
   a. Spouse of client calls and asks for medications they are receiving
   b. Client states they are going to kill their neighbor
   c. Nurse who works part-time on your unit asks about a client's progress
   d. Media inquiries if person involved in accident has been admitted for treatment

7. A client is shouting at others in the hallway. Knowing the shouting client has a history of aggressive behavior, what would be the nurse's initial action?
   a. Check the provider's orders for sedative medication directive
   b. Warn the client seclusion will be necessary if action continues
   c. Attempt to de-escalate the situation and redirect other clients
   d. Allow the clients to work through the conflict on their own

8. After repeated attempts to secure cooperative behavior from a client who is aggressively acting out, the nurse notifies the health care provider and receives restraint orders. Which order would be the least-restrictive?
   a. Sedating medication
   b. Seclusion until behavior is controlled
   c. Sedation followed by seclusion
   d. Five-point physical restraints

9. For which behavior would the nurse recognize seclusion as an inappropriate intervention for behavior management?
   a. Continued verbal aggression toward staff and other clients
   b. Physical aggression toward nurse and other personnel
   c. Threatening suicidal intent
   d. Throwing chairs during sessions of group therapy

10. The nurse is admitting a client to the unit and observes a lack of orientation with delusional thought processes present. What would be important to do when explaining client rights and unit policies?
    a. Go over the information more than once to reinforce content
    b. Wait until a later time when the client is more rational
    c. Include a family member or guardian in the explanation
    d. Ask a coworker to witness the conveyance of information

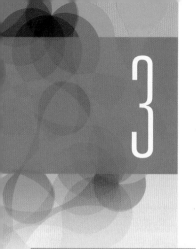

3 Theories of Development

LEARNING OBJECTIVES

After learning the content in this chapter, the student will be able to:

1. Describe the factors that shape an individual's personality.
2. Identify the levels of Maslow's hierarchy of needs.
3. Define temperament and name three types of temperament.
4. Describe the difference between transference and countertransference.
5. Define defense mechanism and list examples.
6. Identify the eight stages of Erikson's theory and give an example for each stage.
7. Explain the relationship between cognitive and moral development.
8. Describe Peplau's nursing model of interpersonal development.
9. Discuss the Family System theory and how it applies to mental health.

KEY TERMS

anal stage
concrete mental operations
conscious
countertransference
defense mechanism
ego
formal operations
genital stage
hierarchy
holistic
id
latency stage
oral stage
perseverance
phallic stage
preconscious
preoperational
psychosocial
sensorimotor
superego
temperament
transference
unconscious

Personality

An individual's personality is made up of experiences, behaviors, thinking patterns, perceptions, relationships with others, and thoughts about themselves and the world in which they exist. Personality is exhibited in patterns of perceiving, relating to others and society, and thinking about oneself. Individuals have personality traits which are established characteristics and consistent behavioral responses. Not everyone has the same personality make-up or personality traits. This explains why not all people act the same in similar situations.

From the moment of conception, human development is influenced by forces that ultimately shape the way in which an individual responds to the world around them. The individual's innate tendencies result from a combined transmission of personality traits from both parents and a unique blend of inherited multigenerational family personality patterns. However, personality and development are not solely based on familial traits and genetics. There are also many societal and environmental influences. Patterns of behavior are formed as one responds to the awareness and perception of the self as autonomous and capable of individual control. Relationships with others, thought processes, and moral beliefs contribute to development. Much research has been done regarding personality development, which has resulted in different theories. These theories help to provide understanding regarding how an individual's personality develops.

There are many theories about what shapes a person's personality. One of these is the holistic approach where all aspects of the individual are viewed as the sum of the individual. This holistic view not only applies to understanding personality and its development but also is the foundation of the nursing model of comprehensive care. The **holistic** concept of nursing care incorporates the entire scope of human needs, addressing the physical, emotional, psychosocial, cultural, and spiritual issues of the client.

Individual Needs and Behavior

Abraham Maslow, a humanistic psychologist, theorized that one acts in response to certain needs that are unchanging and innate in origin. He defined these needs as a **hierarchy** in which some needs are more basic or more powerful than others. As the more basic needs are satisfied, the

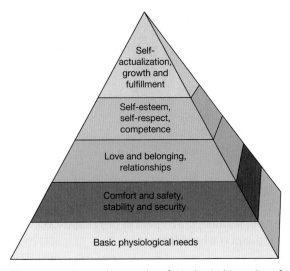

Figure 3.1 Pyramid example of Maslow's hierarchy of needs.

individual can move upward to meet other higher needs. Physiologic needs form the first level, or those considered essential for basic functioning (Fig. 3.1). These basic needs include oxygen, food, sleep, elimination, and sex. Comfort, safety, stability, and security are sought once the physiologic needs are met. The need for a sense of being loved and belonging is achieved through relationships with others. Feeling loved and accepted promotes a feeling of self-respect and esteem that leads to confidence in oneself. Self-actualization, growth, and fulfillment occur at the top level of the hierarchy. It was Maslow's opinion that movement to a higher-level need cannot occur unless the previous level of needs is satisfied. He believed that a personal identity is formed as conscious choices are made to seek certain things that provide value or meaning to life. These experiences and choices may cause the individual to vacillate between levels and disrupt personal growth toward self-fulfillment.

William Glasser, the founder of Reality Therapy and Control Theory, described four basic psychological needs that determine a behavioral response in any given situation (Box 3.1).

BOX 3.1

Glasser's Four Basic Psychological Needs

- Love and belonging
- Power and control
- Freedom and choice
- Fun and relaxation

He theorized that individuals seek to satisfy a void in their lives on a continual basis driven by the need for love and belonging, power and control, freedom and choice, and fun. The need to love and belong is internal, a hunger or void that may be filled by other people, pets, or even inanimate objects. The drive for power often conflicts with the need for love as the individual seeks to exert control over their world. Glasser asserts that when the individual's desire to exercise control over their existence is hindered, they will respond or behave to regain the power that provides a psychological homeostasis. He also theorizes that a measure of fun and playtime evens out the personality. In an effort to meet these needs, Glasser advocates that people have a choice regarding how to behave. From the moment of birth, mental pictures accumulate from experiences. This photo album provides the individual with a basis for future behavioral choices in response to a given situation. Behavior is a constant attempt to decrease the incongruence between what the person wants (pictures in their head) and what they have (their perception of the situation). Glasser found that mental health is improved when individuals learn to meet their needs with responsible choices.

As children develop, their environment grows increasingly more complex, expanding beyond the basic family unit to include the influence of society and culture and this can impact temperament.

> **Test Yourself**
> ✔ What are the components of a holistic view of the individual?
> ✔ According to Maslow, which is more important, love or sex?
> ✔ What adult behaviors might reflect a slow-to-warm-up or a difficult temperament?

> **Just the Facts**
> Hippocrates, in one of the earliest documented medical theories, identified four temperaments related to bodily secretions. Some traditional medicines continue to follow this theory or a variation of it. The four temperaments (first called "humors") are sanguine, choleric, melancholic, and phlegmatic. Choleric individuals are said to be irritable and quick to anger, melancholic individuals are sad and anxious, sanguine are positive and outgoing, and phlegmatic individuals being slow to rise in emotion and action.

Temperament

Some individuals respond to a situation with anger but defuse it quickly, while others may show milder emotional reactions, and others may show no reaction at all. **Temperament** is the inherent way an individual behaves or reacts to stimuli, self-regulates (the ability to manage disruptive stimuli), and the intensity of their emotions and reactions. It is partially genetic, meaning it is present at birth, but is also influenced by experiences, social factors, culture, and maturity. Temperament, sometimes referred to as disposition, is an innate aspect of the developing personality and influences interpersonal relationships.

Stella Chess and Alexander Thomas (1977) studied temperament in babies starting in the early 1960s and described the three types of temperament in babies that are still commonly used. *Easy* babies, who comprise the largest group, are seen as playful and adaptable. By contrast, a smaller number of babies are seen as *difficult* or irritable and unable to adapt well. A third group, *slow-to-warm-up* babies, show lower activity levels and slower adaptation to any new situation.

Perseverance and Determination

Along with temperament, there are other personality traits that can influence how an individual reacts to a situation including perseverance and determination. **Perseverance** is when an individual continues to do, or follows through with, something that is difficult, even when they are faced with obstacles or a delayed outcome. An individual who exhibits perseverance in a situation may be described as steadfast. This can be a positive trait when it aids the individual. A person who attends therapy appointments for several years to improve parenting skills is exemplifying perseverance as a positive trait. However, perseverance can also be a negative trait. An example of when it would be negative is the individual who has unrealistic expectations of their spouse and continually tries to change the spouse's behavior.

Perseverance occurs over a longer time than determination. Determination is when an individual has a goal and works toward achieving that goal. An example of determination as a positive trait would be an athlete who is training for a specific competition and trying to improve their performance. However, determination can "run out" and the individual may give up on their goal or when they achieve their goal, they no longer pursue it. This differs from perseverance where the goal may not ever fully be achieved.

> **Just the Facts**
> Temperament, perseverance, and determination are personality traits that can be helpful for the individual when responding to a new or unfamiliar life situation.

Developmental Theories

Why do humans think and behave in the way they do? This question is a main concept in the study of psychology. Many have studied and developed theories about the human mind, development, and human behavioral responses. The following theories are some of the ones that provide the foundation of nursing's understanding of the individual and also provide the basis for therapeutic approaches to mental health and its treatments. It is important to remember that development is an ongoing process throughout the lifespan.

Freud's Psychoanalytic Theory

Sigmund Freud is considered the founder of psychoanalytic theory. Although some of the theories he developed in the late 19th and early 20th centuries have been criticized by other theorists and health professionals, his work laid an important foundation for the development of other theories.

The Role of the Unconscious

Freud proposed that the psyche is made up of three components: the **conscious** or present awareness, the **preconscious** (also referred to as subconscious) or that which is below current awareness but easily retrieved, and the **unconscious**, which he cites as the largest part of the psyche. The unconscious includes past experiences and the related emotions that have been completely removed from the conscious level. This level is largely responsible for contributing to the emotional discomfort and disturbances that threaten the individual, even though they are unaware of unconscious thoughts and feelings.

Freud also identified the concept of **transference** or the unconscious transfer of feelings and attitudes from a person or situation in one's past to a person or situation in the present. It may be a current expression of a previous experience or need (e.g., client may transfer romantic feelings to the therapist or nurse that was once felt for a person who was previously in their life). Freud noted that clients tended to unconsciously transfer distressing thoughts and personal feelings to the therapist as the content was being analyzed. **Countertransference** is the response that is elicited in the person receiving the transferred feelings or communications. It is important for the recipient (including nurses) to be aware of the exchange in order to maintain insight into the client's problem.

Personality Components

Freudian theory divides personality into three parts. The **id**, which operates on the pleasure principle and demands instant gratification of drives, is present at birth and contains the instincts, impulses, and urges for survival. These drives include hunger, aggression, sex, protection, and warmth. The **ego** begins to develop during the first 6 to 8 months and is fairly well developed by 2 years of age. The ego is the conscious self, which develops in response to the wishes and demands of the id that require appropriate exchanges with the environment. It is here that sensations, feelings, adjustments, solutions, and defenses are formed. The **superego**, often referred to as the conscience, starts developing at about 3 to 4 years of age and is fairly well developed by the age of 10 to 11 years. It controls, inhibits, and regulates those impulses and instinctive urges whose unrestricted expression would be socially unacceptable. The values and moral standards of parents are incorporated into this control along with the norms and moral codes of the society in which one lives and grows. The superego operates at both the conscious and unconscious levels, decides right from wrong, and offers both critical self-evaluation and self-praise.

When environmental stressors create conflicts between the id and the superego, the ego is the peacemaker and balance between the instinctual drives and the societal demands influencing the superego (Fig. 3.2). For example:

Id—I want a piece of chocolate cake.
Superego—There are too many calories in that cake.
Ego—Be satisfied with a small piece.

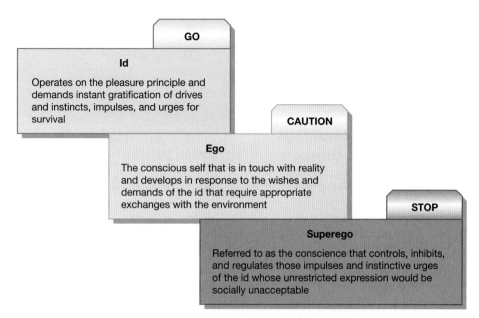

Figure 3.2 Freud's three divisions of the personality.

Ego Defense Mechanisms

The constant need for the ego to reconcile the conflicts between the id and superego leads to increased anxiety. This anxiety creates a dilemma in which stability is needed to preserve the individual's sense of self. Freud theorized that for the ego to remain in control, automatic psychological processes called **defense mechanisms** are mobilized to protect the person from anxiety and the awareness of internal or external stressors (Table 3.1). Most of these mechanisms are utilized at the unconscious level. High levels of anxiety can disturb perception and performance, which compromises the individual's ability to problem solve and learn. These unconscious defense mechanisms provide the protection from unacceptable thoughts and impulses while continuing to meet personal and social needs in acceptable ways.

According to Freud, defenses are a major means of managing conflict and emotional response to environmental situations. These mechanisms differ from one another and may be adaptive as well as maladaptive. Used short-term, defense mechanisms can be utilized in an adaptive way that allows the individual to work toward a realistic outcome or solution. Maladaptive defense mechanisms, on the other hand, may lead to distortion of reality and actual self-deception that can interfere with personal growth and interaction with society. For example, a person may continue their maladaptive use of alcohol, using the mechanism of projection to blame their spouse and children for the behavior, while using denial to avoid self-blame and damage to their own ego. This maladaptive use of mechanisms interferes with an honest self-appraisal of reality and the detrimental effects of substance use. By contrast, a person may temporarily deny their spouse's extramarital affair by telling themselves and others the spouse is just busy, yet projects their feelings onto their children by punishing them for things they did not do. Unlike the person in the first example, when this person realizes that they are projecting, they apologize to the children and change their own behavior. The determinant for whether defense mechanisms are effective and healthy is based on the frequency, intensity, and length of time they are used.

Human beings sometimes behave in ways that provide a means of escape from the realities and responsibilities of life. These patterns of adjustment are common to everyone and are used to resolve conflicts and provide relief from the anxiety and stress of everyday existence. Most of the time, individuals are not aware that a defense mechanism is being used to adapt to a situation. However, when this escape becomes habitual, it becomes a dangerous inability to deal with reality and constitutes a problem.

 Just the Facts Ego-defense mechanisms help justify behavior in a seemingly logical way that allows self-respect to remain intact. However, habitual use can cloud the view of reality.

TABLE 3.1	Ego Defense Mechanisms—Freud	
Mechanism	**Description**	**Example**
Sublimation	A socially acceptable behavior replaces one that is not acceptable or attainable. Primitive impulses are not acceptable to the ego and are rechanneled into a constructive outlet.	*Aggressive desire to attack another person is rechanneled into a sport activity such as football.*
Intellectualization	Person using reasoning and facts or logic to block unconscious conflict that creates stress and uncomfortable emotions.	*Person explains the signs of abuse to another person while ignoring their own abusive situation.*
Suppression	Voluntary exclusion from conscious awareness anxiety-producing feelings, thoughts, or situations.	*Nurse who argues with a family member during breakfast sets the incident aside while caring for clients at the hospital.*
Humor	Temporary reprieve of laughter to ease an anxiety-producing situation or stressor.	*Individual who is fired from their job laughs and says, "I've always wanted to go on a cruise and now I can!"*
Denial	Conscious act of rejecting reality or refusal to recognize facts of a situation. Ego refuses to see the truth because it causes severe mental pain.	*Person continues to set the table for two as if deceased spouse will be present for dinner.*
Displacement	Transfer of hostility or other strong feelings from the original cause of the feelings to another person or object.	*Person who has a confrontation at place of employment goes home and argues with their family.*
Fantasy	Conscious distortion of unconscious wishes or needs by using imagination to solve problems.	*Young child who sees parent physically abused may imagine they are attacking a wild animal and saves parent from harm.*
Repression	Involuntary distancing of events or thoughts that are too painful or unacceptable to one's ego into the unconscious level.	*Person who was sexually abused as a child is unable to achieve a meaningful intimate relationship as an adult.*
Regression	Returning to an earlier more comfortable and less stressful stage of behavior.	*Child who is weaned returns to drinking from a bottle during hospitalization.*
Projection	Unacceptable traits, feelings, or attitudes are blamed on something or someone else. The person refuses to admit own weakness or accept responsibility for own actions.	*Person who drinks alcohol blames spouse for doing something to make them get drunk.*
Compensation	Emphasizing capabilities or strengths to make up for a lack or loss in personal characteristics.	*Person who is not talented in athletics excels in scholastic achievement.*
Introjection	Unconsciously integrating ideas, values, and attitudes of another into own mannerisms and actions.	*Without awareness, a child begins to talk and act like their parent.*
Reaction formation	A conscious attempt to make up for feelings or attitudes that are unacceptable to the ego by replacing them with the opposite feelings or beliefs.	*Parent who secretly dislikes their child becomes overprotective and outwardly affectionate toward the child.*
Conversion	Transfer of emotional conflicts into physical symptoms.	*Person who dislikes boss at work develops migraine headaches to avoid going to work.*
Undoing	A positive action is initiated to conceal a negative action or to neutralize a previously unacceptable action or wish.	*Employer offers to take their assistant to lunch after verbally attacking them earlier in the day.*
Rationalization	Substituting false reasoning or justification for behavior that is unacceptable or threatening to the ego.	*Employee who is not given a promotion tells coworkers they did not want the position.*

Freud's Psychosexual Development Theory

Freud believed that as the personality develops, there is an increasing self-identification and changing self-perception of sexuality and sexual identification. In his psychosexual theory, he proposed five major stages of development. The **oral stage** occurs during the first 2 years as the child seeks pleasure from sucking and oral gratification of hunger. The **anal stage** takes place from 2 to 4 years of age, during which pleasure is achieved as the child develops an awareness and control of urination and defecation. In the **phallic stage**, around the age of 4 years, the child discovers pleasure in genital stimulation and also struggles to accept a sexual identity. Freud believed these feelings are put into the **latency stage** during middle childhood when the sexual desires remain subdued. The **genital stage** occurs as the child enters puberty and adolescence. It is at this stage that Freud believed sexual feelings reemerge and become directed toward establishing a relationship.

According to Freud, at any point during psychosexual development, the child can become fixated and frustrated, resulting in exaggerated adult character traits that reflect the arrested growth. Although Freudian theory has been the subject of much controversy regarding its sexual orientation it provided the groundwork for future developmental theories. Table 3.2 outlines the stages of

TABLE 3.2	**Stages According to Major Developmental Theories**	
	Signs of Successful Resolution	**Indicators of Unsuccessful Resolution**
Freud (Psychosexual)		
1. Oral stage	Satisfaction—gratification	Dependent on and easily influenced by others, manipulative cocky attitude, gullible
2. Anal stage	Giving, openness, self-control	Stinginess and orderliness Stubborn and rigid meticulousness
3. Phallic stage	Sexual identity accepted	Vanity and brashness, flirtatious
4. Latency	Sexual urges suppressed—expansion of social contacts beyond family	Unsuccessful attempts at expanding social relationships
5. Genital	Sexual energy channeled toward peers	Unconscious sexual conflict and undesired inability to form intimate sexual relationship
Erikson (Psychosocial)		
1. Trust versus mistrust	Hope	Suspicion and fear of people and relationships Extreme self-doubt and fear of independence
2. Autonomy versus shame and doubt	Will	Sense of inadequacy and defeat
3. Initiative versus guilt	Purpose	Inadequate problem-solving skills
4. Industry versus inferiority	Competence	Manipulating others, no regard for the rights of others (such as in the workplace) Feeling unworthy, fear of failure
5. Identity versus role confusion	Fidelity	Uncertainty and loss of one who is in relationships with others
6. Intimacy versus isolation	Love and commitment	Emotional withdrawal into oneself
7. Generativity versus stagnation	Caring and giving	Inability to grow as an individual
8. Integrity versus despair	Wisdom	Disillusioned with life and inability to view death as reality
Piaget (Cognitive)		
1. Sensorimotor	Growth of abilities related to senses and motor skills Goal-directed behaviors Egocentric thinking	Focus only on what one wants without regard for possible consequences of those actions
2. Preoperational	Exploration motivated by magical and imaginative thinking	Decisions based on intuition, fantasy, or superstition with inability to make choices rooted in reality
3. Concrete	Base cognitive connections on actual events or objects Begin to think logically Think in terms of intentional moral response	Resistant to change with meager attempts at risk-taking strategies in which the outcome is unknown
4. Formal operations	Abstract thinking Problem-solving ability Symbolic reasoning with conceptual theoretical thinking	Unable to visualize possibility or solution to a problem Unwilling to formulate or accept reality-based decisions
Sullivan (Interpersonal)		
1. Infant	Satisfaction of needs	Anxiety develops as a result of unmet physiologic needs Lack of bonding between infant and caregiver
2. Childhood	Self-control in gratification of needs	Increasing anxiety experienced with delay in gratification of own needs
3. Juvenile	Successful relationships with peer group	Difficulty in relating to others and developing interpersonal group relationships/workplace interaction
4. Preadolescent	Beginning appropriate interactions with persons of other genders	Inability to relate in a meaningful way to persons of other genders
5. Early adolescent	Sense of personal identity in intimate relationships	Fear and withdrawal of intimate relationships
6. Late adolescence	Satisfying intimate relationship with another	Inability to form a long-term intimate relationship with another person

some of the major developmental theories that will be discussed and signs of successful or unsuccessful resolution for each stage.

Erikson's Psychosocial Development Theory

Erik Erikson viewed personality as **psychosocial**, meaning it relates to both psychological and social factors. His theory proposes that individuals develop in a pattern of eight psychosocial stages throughout their lifespan (Box 3.2). Each stage consists of two developmental markers. One indicates a successful completion of the stage and the other indicates the stage is not resolved (these are sometimes referred to as developmental crises). Resolution of this critical period will enhance a healthy continuation of the process. If unresolved, the progression to subsequent stages of development could be adversely affected. Erikson's view emphasizes, however, that an unresolved stage can be corrected by successes at a later stage.

Erikson maintained that if each developmental crisis was not resolved in sequence, the personality would continue to manifest this conflict into the adult years (refer back to Table 3.2). Although critics of the stage theory say that psychological development may be influenced and altered by experiences throughout life, many have found Erikson's theory useful for continued study of personality development.

Stage I: Trust versus Mistrust (Birth to 1 Year)

A sense of trust results in a feeling of comfort and reassurance that the world is a safe and pleasant place in which the child can live with minimal fear and apprehension. Consistency and responsiveness by the caregiver in providing for the infant's needs of nourishment, comfort, and nurturing are essential to the development of trust. Babies who do not have a trusting relationship with their

caregivers are less responsive to them and show less effort in exploring the environment and world in which they exist.

Mind Jogger How might failure to develop a sense of trust have implications in the establishment of adult relationships and one's interaction with society?

Stage II: Autonomy versus Shame and Doubt (Ages 1 to 2 Years)

This stage is characterized by a period of increased self-confidence and independent striving to do more on their own. The most important developmental task during this stage is toilet training. Children also try to do new things such as feeding or dressing themselves. It is essential that caregivers positively reinforce these efforts while avoiding the urge to be overprotective and critical. Erikson believed that if caregivers do not show a consistent and reassuring attitude during this phase, children will experience too much self-doubt and shame about their abilities, resulting in a lack of confidence that will persist throughout life.

Stage III: Initiative versus Guilt (2 to 6 Years)

During these years, children are challenged with increasing responsibilities including care of their physical needs, managing their behavior, beginning friendships, and caring for belongings such as toys and pets. This requires children to be assertive and creative in assuming the new tasks. The child is eager to do things, and it is essential that caregivers praise and recognize the child's efforts no matter how small they may be. On the other hand, children must also learn to accept that in their quest for independence, there are some things that are not allowed or safe for them to do. It is important they be reassured, however, that being imaginative and pretending to take on adult roles are okay. If they are not given the chance to do things safely on their own and to be responsible, a sense of guilt may result. The child will learn to believe that what they want to do is not good enough or is always wrong.

Stage IV: Industry versus Inferiority (6 to 12 Years)

In this stage of development, children are learning to be productive and to accomplish things on their own, both physically and mentally. This is a period when they master their ability to succeed in peer relationships, school, and activities. It is essential for children to receive encouragement and support in their drive for success from parents and others. Children learn by repeated efforts driven by self-confidence in their own abilities. If children have difficulty relating to others outside of the home or in achievement of skills, a sense of inferiority and self-doubt may result.

Stage V: Identity versus Role Confusion (12 to 18 Years)

During the years of adolescence the individual searches for identity and purpose in their life. Erikson postulated that a basic sense of trust and self-confidence was necessary to provide the foundation for the adolescent to make conscious choices about a vocation, relationships, and life in general. Failure to resolve previous conflicts successfully would result in an inability to make these decisions and choices. As a result, adolescents might experience role confusion as to who they are and where they belong as they move into adulthood.

Stage VI: Intimacy versus Isolation (Ages 19 to 40 Years)

In the years of young adulthood, the most important developmental goal, according to Erikson, is to form a committed relationship with another. A true intimate relationship requires sincerity and open sharing of feelings. Having a sexual relationship does not imply intimacy. A person can be sexually intimate without feeling for and commitment to the other person. Conversely, an individual can have strong relationships that do not involve sex. Love relationships are strengthened by the ability of partners to relate on a deep personal level. The young adult who is unable to be open and committed to another may retreat into isolation and fear a giving and sharing relationship.

Stage VII: Generativity versus Stagnation (Ages 40 to 65 Years)

As individuals enter middle adulthood, the task is related to parenting and supportive involvement in providing for the next generation. This role includes being an active participant in issues that will make this world a safer and better place for the future. The inability to nurture and make an attempt to ensure this progressive stability may lead to stagnation and decreased meaning for one's life.

Stage VIII: Integrity versus Despair (Over 65 Years)

The important event during these years is seen as a reflection on and acceptance of one's life. According to Erikson, a positive outcome is demonstrated by a sense of fulfillment about a life lived and acceptance of death as an inevitable reality. This involves accepting responsibility for and being satisfied with choices that have been made over a lifetime. The older adult who has successfully reached this stage is able to put the past in perspective and achieve a sense of self-satisfaction with the present. Those who are unable to reach this sense of fulfillment and wholeness will despair about life accomplishments and fear death.

Test Yourself	✔ Identify and describe four defense mechanisms. ✔ Name a developmental task for each of Erikson's stages.

Just the Facts	The aim of progress in emotional development is not to get rid of the negative personality quality but to move toward the positive personality quality as a dominant trait.

Piaget's Cognitive Development Theory

Jean Piaget theorized that personality is the result of increasing intellectual ability to organize and integrate experiences into behavior patterns. His observations led him to conclude that this organization tended to occur at certain age groups. Physical and psychological growth or maturation occurs in the child during a specific stage as the child thinks and experiences interaction with the environment. As the child begins to distinguish the self as a separate being, social experiences become a part of this learning. Piaget proposed that cognitive development occurs in four stages (Box 3.3) and once the child has entered a new stage, the process is irreversible, with each stage building on the previous level of development.

BOX 3.3

Piaget Stages of Cognitive Development

- Sensorimotor: Birth to 2 years
- Preoperational: 2 to 7 years
- Concrete: 7 to 11 years
- Formal operations: 11 years and older

CASE STUDY 3.1

"Anthony"

Rawpixel.com/
Shutterstock

Anthony is a 32-year-old client who is being seen in an outpatient clinic for symptoms of depression and anorexia. He states he has had no success in finding a job and his girlfriend "ditched" him several months ago. Anthony states he has been living out of his car and on the street since his girlfriend left him. When asked about his family, he states, "I basically don't have one." He then adds, "I can't seem to get along with anyone—they all act like they are out to get me one way or another."

Digging Deeper

1. *Based on Erikson's theory of psychosocial development, at what point might Anthony's personality development have been disrupted?*

2. *How is this preventing him from advancing according to Erikson's theory?*

3. *What other questions might you ask?*

4. *According to the Hierarchy of Needs, what would be a priority for this client?*

In the first 2 years of life, the **sensorimotor** stage involves the growth of abilities related to the five senses and motor functions. Early responses are primarily reflexive in nature, with a gradual increase in skill as children adapt to their environment. These responses tend to reflect only a perception of that which is visible to the child. The perception that what is gone from view still exists (object permanence) begins to develop at about 9 months of age and is well developed by 1 year.

The **preoperational** stage of development occurs from 2 to 7 years. The child communicates their thoughts; however, these thoughts are largely egocentric without regard for another point of view. Language and actions reflect a focus on thinking that the world exists solely to meet the demands of the child's ego. As children grow, they explore and try out many new activities motivated by increasing magical and imaginative thinking.

Just the Facts Most children in the preoperational stage are impulsive and cannot distinguish between actions and feelings. Unable to understand that others may see their actions differently than they do, they react to conflict with egocentric hitting, shoving, whining, and hiding behaviors.

From 7 to 12 years of age, Piaget saw children as able to perform **concrete mental operations** based on their accumulated thoughts and memories. The phrase "seeing is believing" is descriptive of the child's need to base these cognitive connections on actual events or objects. Facts and routines with one way of doing things are a characteristic of this age group. The child begins to think logically, classify objects, and recognize that objects and people can have more than one label (e.g., Daddy can also be a husband, a brother, and an uncle all at the same time). Although they are capable of thinking more logically, children of this age still depend on concrete cues to develop these thoughts.

According to Piaget, the person moves into the stage of **formal operations** during the years of 11 to 12 and older. This period of growth involves abstract thought processes, problem solving, and systematic purposeful mental relationships. Adolescents are capable of symbolic thinking and comprehension of theoretical concepts. They are able to visualize beyond what is known and formulate hypothetical reasoning.

Kohlberg's Moral Development Theory

In his research on cognitive development, Piaget concluded that changes in the child's level of thinking also affect the moral decisions the child makes. Motivated by Piaget's studies, Lawrence Kohlberg

BOX 3.4

Kohlberg's Levels of Moral Development

- Preconventional Level: Influenced by environmental pressure
- Stage 1: Acts or behaves to avoid punishment
- Stage 2: Is motivated by personal reward (what is in it for me?)
- Conventional Level: Influenced by societal pressure
- Stage 3: Values the opinion of the peer group and acts to meet the expectations of others (peer group)
- Stage 4: Is motivated by the laws of society/legal system
- Postconventional Level: Influenced by standards and shared principles
- Stage 5: Acts for the good of society or the most people
- Stage 6: Bases actions on moral principles and ethical values (the right thing to do)

developed his own theory based on six stages of moral reasoning included in three levels. Box 3.4 outlines these levels and stages. Basic to Kohlberg's theory is the belief that the choices one makes do not determine the stage of moral logic, but rather the reasons one gives to justify the behavior establish the level of ethical development. Like Piaget, Kohlberg believed that the intellect and the child's emotional development occur in a parallel pattern of stages during which the child changes their concept of self in relation to interaction with others. The level of cognitive development determines how the child perceives a situation and what is learned from that experience. Each of the three levels builds on the one prior with increasing complexity in the individual view of a moral issue.

Sullivan's Interpersonal Development Theory

Nurses in the mental health setting develop therapeutic relationships with clients in an attempt to help them develop the skills to interact successfully with others. Harry S. Sullivan believed that behavior and personality developments are the direct result of these interpersonal relationships. Unlike Freud, who believed that all behavior is the result of unconscious drives and unfinished agendas, Sullivan believed that human behavior could be seen in the social interaction between people. The major concepts of his theory include the following:

- Anxiety is a major force that develops because of unmet needs and interpersonal dissatisfaction.

- Fulfillment of needs occurs when all physiologic, comfort, and security needs are met.
- The concept of self incorporates those experiences and behaviors developed to protect the child against anxiety and provide security for the self. As a result, three images of self develop:
  - *Good-me* develops in response to positive feedback
  - *Bad-me* develops in response to criticism from caregivers
  - *Not-me* develops in response to intense anxiety and dread with resulting denial and repression of the situation to avoid the anxiety (this avoidance of emotions can result in mental disorders in the adult)

Sullivan divided development into six stages. During *infancy* (birth to 18 months), the child is concerned with oral satisfaction of needs. In *childhood* (18 months to 6 years), children learn to delay personal gratification with a minimum of anxiety. The *juvenile* (6 to 9 years) is learning to develop satisfaction in relationships with the peer group, while the *preadolescent* (9 to 12 years) is striving to develop successful interactions with persons of the same gender. During *early adolescence* (12 to 14 years), a sense of personal identity is formed as relationships with persons of other genders are sought. In *late adolescence* (14 to 21 years), the person is working to develop satisfying and meaningful long-term relationships with others.

Sullivan believed that the attainment of successful interpersonal relationships was dependent on the formation of interaction skills at each level of development (refer again to Table 3.2).

Peplau's Psychodynamic Nursing Theory

Hildegard Peplau applied the interpersonal theory to nursing and the nurse–client relationship. She saw the stages of developmental growth as the basis for therapeutic interaction with clients, including many whose behaviors reflect a failure to understand their own feelings and actions, and the results of those actions.

Peplau's theory identified four stages of development. In *infancy*, the child is learning to count on others, while the *toddler* is learning to delay self-gratification. At the same time, the toddler derives much pleasure in a positive response to their actions from others. *Early childhood* is a time of developing the skill of behaving in a way that is acceptable to others, preceding *late childhood* in

"Denise"

fizkes/Shutterstock

You are interacting with Denise, a young female client who repeatedly apologizes for saying "the wrong thing." In response to your question about her family, she answers, "I really don't have a family. I'm sorry, that was a bad thing to say." She goes on to say that she has never done anything good enough for her parents. She feels that regardless of how hard she tries, she is always telling them she is sorry for disappointing them. Denise states that she is so afraid of failure that she is unable to follow through with a job application and cancels them before the scheduled appointment.

Digging Deeper

1. What other information about Denise's interpersonal relationships might be important?

2. How are past relationships with her parents affecting her present interpersonal relationships?

3. How is Sullivan's theory of interpersonal development reflected in this situation?

4. How would you follow up to continue the conversation?

which the child learns to compromise, compete, and cooperate in participation and interactions with others. Learning to practice self-control and compromise in relationships with others is a precedent to living successfully and interacting as a member of society.

> **Test Yourself**
> ✔ What do the stage theories have in common and how do they differ?
> ✔ What are the implications of interpersonal relationship development in the nurse's interactions with clients?

Other Theories Important to Mental Health Treatment

In addition to the developmental theories discussed in this chapter, other approaches are integral to the overall understanding of human development and behavior related to mental health. These theories look at the individual's family relationships, how their development influences their behavior, or how their behavior can be influenced. Common to these theories is the view that an individual's actions are deeply rooted in their development. Each theory has its specific focus, and these theories are also important to the current treatment approach to mental health treatment.

Bowen's Family Systems Theory

The Family Systems theory asserts that one can change behaviors based on an awareness of the impact that present and past family patterns of behavior have on the choices one makes. This awareness can lead to an intentional desire to make changes and a refusal to function in the way that has been perpetuated by members of the family.

Family is defined as the nuclear family of origin and extending to past relationships and family histories. Murray Bowen saw this family as a single emotional unit composed of relationships that intermingle over several generations. He felt the dynamics of these family relationships held the key for understanding current behaviors. Integral in Bowen's theory are the biologic, genetic, psychological, and sociologic factors in the determination of behavior. Actions are seen as preceded by feelings that to some degree can be controlled by the ability to think. People are able to predict their own patterns of response based on an awareness of the dynamics that are evident in the family system.

The person whose behavior is based on internal convictions and principles is defined as a *solid self*, as opposed to the *pseudoself* whose behavior reflects an external locus of control. Individuals described as a solid self are more adaptable, more flexible, and more effective in coping with stressful situations, while those defined as a pseudoself are less adaptable, less flexible, and less able to rely on internal sources of strength to cope with anxiety.

Family systems are classified as either open or closed. An open family system is made up of people who are predominantly solid selves. This promotes flexibility and exchange of ideas within an accepting environment. They are comfortable with being visible and are free to clearly define themselves and their belief system. By contrast, individuals who are willing to compromise their values when pressured by external sources make up the closed family system. The result of these relationships is one of dysfunction, tension, and rigid standards in which one person gains control and the other loses self. An increase in tension increases the anxiety within the system. As anxiety escalates, the emotional ties of family members become frayed and one or more people feel overwhelmed. The family members who feel out of control tend to be the ones who give in to reduce tension in others. This absorption of the family anxiety issue leaves the individual most vulnerable to psychological problems and dysfunction. Some people deal with the anxiety through emotional distancing and cutting ties with parental conflict, which eventually results in continuation of the conflict. Those who attempt to reduce tension in their current family relationships by distancing from the nuclear family issues will eventually see the patterns they are trying to escape emerging in their present relationships. Triangles are created that draw a third party into the conflict, further dismantling the homeostasis of the family unit. The interactive patterns in a triangle tend to shift with two members being close and "inside" and one being excluded and "outside." Involving others tends to make the situation more complicated and resolves nothing. Those within the triangle tend to become emotionally involved and take sides in the conflict.

The differentiation of people within the family system is projected onto other members of that family, creating a spiral effect as children marry and create another generation with similar characteristics and value systems. Marital conflict may result as a second generation of dysfunction is shaped. A union that pairs one spouse who repeatedly yields to a controlling or abusive partner in order to prevent family discord will result in the dysfunction of that individual. In addition, one or more children of the family will absorb the tensions and anxiety that perpetuate the dysfunction and demonstrates the continuation of the cycle.

This theory provides a way for us to understand how families function and how people are affected by the dynamics in this multigenerational process. Once clients are aware of how they are influenced by dysfunctional patterns of behavior, they can be supported in an effort to effect change and break the cycle.

Just the Facts Within a family, a change in one person's functioning is typically followed by give-and-take changes in the behavior of others.

Mind Jogger In what way do children become involved in a triangle formed by marital conflict between parents?

Skinner's Behavioristic Theory

B. F. Skinner theorized that behavior, both adaptive and maladaptive, is the result of conditioning which is shaped by a system of reward, punishment, and reinforcement. Conditioning strengthens and weakens behaviors automatically without regard to the individual's conscious thought processes. Skinner also showed that people will exhibit consistent patterns of behavior that will continue if the action is rewarded by a response. If no reinforcement is given, the behavior will decline.

Bandura's Social Learning Theory

Albert Bandura theorized that individuals can act to change their surroundings as a result of both internal and external forces that influence each other. He felt social learning is based on the observation and imitation of others. Both children and adults tend to imitate people they like or respect (called models) more than those who are less appealing. Models whose behavior leads to a desirable outcome (in the individual's mind) are more likely to be copied. Self-confidence develops as the expected outcome of the imitated behavior becomes reality in the individual's actions.

Beck's Cognitive-Behavioral Theory

Aaron Beck's theory places the focus on the individual's abilities to think, analyze, and decide on certain behavior rather than acting on feelings.

The individual's actions that are the result of distorted perceptions and thoughts can be changed. This is unlike Freud's theory that viewed mental disturbances as being the result of childhood experiences. In Beck's theory, self-defeating behaviors are maintained because of irrational thoughts and erroneous beliefs. Self-concept and evaluation of social image are affected by how the individual thinks others see them. Self-talk is used to praise or criticize and interpret situations. This is reflected in both typical behaviors and mental disorders. Negative self-talk can be changed into more positive thoughts, leading to a more positive self-image and more productive outcomes.

Cultural Considerations

Temperament Across Cultures

It is important to understand the role the client's culture has on temperament. Some cultural expressions of temperament include:

- Some cultures value quiet, even temperaments while others value being boisterous and even argumentative. Clients from cultures that value the latter type of temperament might ask repeated questions in a raised voice when given discharge instructions.
- Some cultures feel it is not necessary to speak if there is nothing of importance to say, and instead value being quiet yet present. For example, when the nurse talks about the weather outside and what is being served for the meal, a client from such a culture may consider this as unimportant talk and may remain silent and not respond.

- Being very quiet around medical staff and agreeing with what is presented, even if the client does not understand or agree with the information or diagnosis, may also be influenced by cultural norms where quiet behavior is seen as demonstration of respect. An example of this would be a client who nods and remains silent when the health care provider gives the client information about their condition and changes to the plan of care.
- Some social groups (such as the military) also have a tendency toward specific temperament patterns. Clients who have spent many years adhering to norms regarding schedules and were expected to arrive 15 minutes or more prior to a scheduled appointment may become very upset with the nurse who shows up 15 minutes after the nurse stated they would arrive.

SUMMARY

- An individual's personality is made up of experiences, behaviors, thinking patterns, perceptions, relationships with others, and thoughts about themselves and the world in which they exist. Patterns are the result of genetics and the influence of social and environmental forces throughout the lifespan.
- The holistic concept of nursing care incorporates the entire scope of human needs, addressing the physical, emotional, psychosocial, cultural, and spiritual issues of the client.
- Maslow theorized actions are in response to a perceived internal or external force determined by a hierarchy of needs that are innate and unchanging.
- In the hierarchy, basic needs must be met before the individual can achieve higher level needs. Basic needs include oxygen, food, sleep, elimination, and sex. Higher needs include love and belonging, self-esteem, and self-actualization.
- Glasser identified the basic needs of love and belonging, power and control, freedom and choice, and fun and relaxation as the driving forces that drive us to interact with the environment.
- Temperament is the inherent way an individual behaves or reacts to stimuli, self-regulates (the ability

to manage disruptive stimuli), and the intensity of their emotions and reactions. These are identified as the easy or adaptable disposition, the slow-to-warm-up disposition, and the difficult (irritable) or unadaptable disposition. Temperament is inherent at birth through genetics but is also shaped by social factors and experiences.

- Personality development is most often described by stage theories that divide the lifespan into age-related periods that correlate with physical growth and development.
- Freud proposed the psyche is made up of three parts: the conscious (current awareness), the preconscious (just below the awareness and easily retrievable), and the unconscious (buried and removed from conscious awareness and responsible for much of the individual's emotional discomfort).
- Freudian theory divides the personality into three parts: The id, present at birth, operates on the pleasure principle, demanding instant gratification of drives, impulses, and urges for survival. The ego is the conscious self that develops in response to the wishes and demands of the id that require boundaries for appropriate exchange with the environment. The

superego, or the conscience, controls, inhibits, and regulates the impulses and urges of the id, which, if unchecked, may be socially unacceptable.

- For the ego to remain in control, automatic psychological processes called defense mechanisms are mobilized to protect from anxiety and awareness of internal or external stressors.
- Freud proposed five stages of psychosexual development: oral, anal, phallic, latency, and genital.
- Erikson identified eight psychosocial stages of development. Each stage consists of a developmental crisis, indicating a period of vulnerability. Erikson proposed that if each development crisis is not resolved in sequence, the individual will continue to show this conflict into the adult years.
- Erikson's eight stages are: trust versus mistrust, autonomy versus shame and doubt, initiative versus guilt, industry versus inferiority, identity versus role confusion, intimacy versus isolation, generativity versus stagnation, and lastly, integrity versus despair.
- Piaget theorized that cognitive growth occurs as the child thinks and experiences interaction with the environment. The four stages of cognitive development that align with chronologic age periods are sensorimotor, preoperational, concrete mental operations, and formal operations.
- Kohlberg focused his theory on the moral development, dividing growth into three levels (preoperational, conventional, and postconventional) that center on the reasons one gives to justify choices and behaviors.
- In the preoperational level, values indicate environmental pressures to avoid punishment and receive personal reward. The conventional level demonstrates influence by societal pressures to meet the expectations of others or the legal system. The postconventional level reflects influence by ethical values and shared moral principles that show actions for the good of society or most people.

- Sullivan's theory states that behavior and personality develop as a direct result of interpersonal relationships. Anxiety is the major force that results from unmet needs and dissatisfaction.
- Sullivan's concept of self incorporates experiences and behaviors developed to protect against the anxiety and provide security. Positive response builds the "good-me," while negative criticism creates a sense of "bad-me" that over time can lead to repression and avoidance of emotions.
- Peplau applied the interpersonal theory to nursing and the nurse–client relationship with a focus on client behaviors that reflect understanding of their own feelings, actions, and the results of those actions.
- In Family Systems theory, Bowen asserts that a person is able to change behaviors based on an awareness of the impact that present and past family patterns of behavior have on the choices they make. Behavior based on internal convictions and principles defines the solid self, while a pseudoself reflects an external locus of control.
- Behaviorist, social learning, and cognitive-behavioral theories contribute significantly to the overall current views underlying the current approach to treatment of mental health.

BIBLIOGRAPHY

Brennan, D. (2021). *What to know about Erikson's 8 stages of development*. WebMD. https://www.webmd.com/children/what-to-know-eriksons-8-stages-development

Center for Early Childhood Mental Health Consultation. (2022). *Infant toddler temperament tool (IT3): Supporting a "Goodness of fit."* Georgetown University. https://www.ecmhc.org/documents/CECMHC_IT3_Booklet_Infant.pdf

Chess, S., & Thomas, A. (1977). Temperamental individuality from childhood to adolescence. *Journal of the American Academy of Child Psychiatry, 16*(2), 218–226. https://doi.org/10.1016/S0002-7138(09)60038-8

Lewis, R. (2020). *Erikson's 8 stages of psychosocial development, explained for parents*. Healthline. https://www.healthline.com/health/parenting/erikson-stages

McLeod, S. A. (2018). *Sigmund Freud's theories*. Simply Psychology. https://www.simplypsychology.org/Sigmund-Freud.html

McLeod, S. A. (2020). *Maslow's hierarchy of needs*. Simply Psychology. https://www.simplypsychology.org/maslow.html

Petiprin, A. (2020). *Hildegard Peplau—Nursing theorist*. Nursing-Theory.org. https://nursing-theory.org/nursing-theorists/Hildegard-Peplau.php

Fill in the Blank

Fill in the blank with the correct answer.

1. Patterns of perceiving, relating to, and thinking about ourselves and the world around us define the concept of _____.
2. Oxygen, food, and sleep are considered _____ _____ by Maslow.
3. _____ is the inherent way an individual behaves or reacts to stimuli, self-regulates, and the intensity of their emotions and reactions.
4. Automatic psychological processes that are mobilized to protect the person from anxiety and the awareness of internal or external stressors are called _____ _____.
5. The individual who is learning to master their peer relationships, to be productive, and accomplish things on their own is said to be in the stage of _____ versus _____.
6. Peplau's psychodynamic nursing theory looked at the _____ – _____ relationship.
7. The person whose behavior is based on internal convictions and principles is defined as a(n) _____ _____.

Matching

Match the defense mechanism with the appropriate behavior.

1. _____ Rationalization
2. _____ Denial
3. _____ Repression
4. _____ Regression
5. _____ Projection
6. _____ Displacement
7. _____ Reaction formation
8. _____ Sublimation

a. Unhappy with her boss for his criticism, Clara turns around and takes her anger out on her husband.
b. David is unable to remember a boating accident in which his friend was killed.
c. After going to the movie the night before an exam, Molly states that she failed the exam because she did not study the right chapter.
d. An adolescent wants his mother to stay with him during a hospital stay.
e. After an injury that will require him to use a wheelchair for the rest of his life, Jack becomes a computer specialist.
f. A young man who secretly desires to harm his wife appears on a television show against spousal abuse.
g. When Martha is confronted about her alcohol problem, she states she can quit anytime she chooses.
h. After taking funds out of their savings account to buy golf clubs, Hank tells his wife that the bank must have made a mistake.

Multiple Choice

Select the best answer from the multiple-choice items.

1. A 70-year-old client states to the nurse, "My life is a pile of shambles with nothing to show for it." The client is demonstrating what Erikson would term:
   a. Doubt
   b. Inferiority
   c. Despair
   d. Stagnation

2. A client experiencing homelessness is brought into the emergency department with hypothermia. What would their primary need be?
   a. Oxygen
   b. Shelter
   c. Food
   d. Security

3. A child states, "I'll believe my dad is home from military deployment when I see him." What stage is the child in according to Piaget?
   a. Sensorimotor
   b. Preoperational
   c. Concrete operations
   d. Formal operations

4. A person refrains from telling the truth to a friend whose partner is having an affair with a coworker to avoid hurting their friend. According to Kohlberg, this demonstrates which level of moral development?
   a. Preconventional
   b. Conventional
   c. Postconventional
   d. Preconscious

5. A client has been arrested for physical assault of another individual. They have a history of an abusive childhood and previous aggressive offenses. Behavioral theory would explain this behavior as:
   a. Feelings of repressed hostility
   b. A diminished sense of self-esteem
   c. An innate impulsive drive for survival
   d. Reinforcement of early learning experiences

6. Surveys show that cigarette smoking and alcohol consumption are common among the adolescent population. These results reflect peer behavior and provide support for which of the following theories?
   a. Social learning theory
   b. Conditioning theory
   c. Psychosexual theory
   d. Behavioristic theory

7. A client tells the nurse they realize most of the things that happen to them are the result of their own choices. They indicate a desire to make changes that will lead to better outcomes. According to Bowen, this client seems to have:
   a. A strong superego
   b. An internal locus of control
   c. A strong pseudoself
   d. Strong unconscious drives

8. A young adolescent client is seen in the emergency room after they were raped by their brother. Calm and laughing, the client says, "I don't know why the big deal. Nothing happened." The nurse would identify the use of which defense mechanism?
   a. Projection
   b. Conversion
   c. Denial
   d. Rationalization

9. A client is being seen who is unable to maintain employment. They state that there is always an ulterior motive in company policies that affect them. Which of the following psychosocial stages is likely unresolved?
   a. Trust versus mistrust
   b. Autonomy versus doubt
   c. Initiative versus guilt
   d. Industry versus inferiority

10. A client is sitting upright in bed while listening to the health care provider. They nod and do not ask any questions. On the third hospital day the client is smiling, asking a few questions, and calls the nurse by name. How would this client's temperament be described?
    a. Easy
    b. Difficult
    c. Slow-to-warm-up
    d. Adaptable

Unit II | Mental Health Care

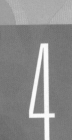

4 Treatment of Mental Illness

LEARNING OBJECTIVES

After learning the content in this chapter, the student will be able to:

1. Define what is meant by a therapeutic milieu.
2. Differentiate between roles and responsibilities of the mental health team members.
3. Discuss the roles of the nurse in the psychotherapeutic process.
4. Identify the basic principles of common psychotherapy treatment methods.
5. Identify different adjunctive therapies used in the treatment of mental health issues.
6. Identify the function of psychopharmacology in the psychotherapeutic treatment regimen.
7. Name five classes of psychotropic medications.
8. Describe the path neurotransmitters take.
9. Discuss effects of psychotropic medications in older clients.

KEY TERMS

behavioral therapy
biofeedback
clinical psychologist
cognitive behavioral therapy
contracting
electroconvulsive therapy (ECT)
group therapy
humanistic therapy
neurotransmitter
postsynaptic receptors
presynaptic compartment
psychiatrist
psychodynamic therapy
psychopharmacology
psychotherapy
psychotropic agents
reuptake
synaptic cleft
telehealth
therapeutic milieu

Introduction

The treatment of mental health issues aims to reduce the symptoms and to allow the individual to live and function in society with improved personal and interpersonal skills. Trained professionals help clients to identify and change current behavior or thought patterns that adversely affect their lives. This treatment gives the client the opportunity to set realistic goals for living. Specific treatment goals are set collaboratively by the health care team and the client.

Various approaches to treatment have evolved to meet the individual needs of clients and their families. Treatment methods may include medications, counseling, various types of psychotherapy, or other therapies. This chapter will discuss these components of mental health treatment. Integral to the development of a treatment plan in mental health care are the therapeutic milieu, the professionals who serve as members of the treatment team, and the more common modalities or types of therapy that are used.

Establishing a Therapeutic Milieu

In mental health care, a **therapeutic milieu** is a safe and structured environment that facilitates the therapeutic interaction between clients and members of the professional team. This combination of a social and encouraging environment provides a supportive network in which there is a sense of common goals. All components of the environment contribute to the milieu including physical objects, colors, lighting, people, stimuli present, and treatments. In one situation, this setting might be the client's individual room, or in another, it could be a day room designed to encourage interaction between clients and the support team. Dayrooms often include furniture; tables and chairs for games, puzzles, reading; and arcade games such as air hockey or pool tables. These types of activities help clients meet goals and participate in acceptable social behaviors and communication skills. Group activities are scheduled that maximize the functional ability of each client, and clients are encouraged to be as independent as possible during treatment. The nurse is often in a position to maintain the milieu as a place where dignity and acceptance allow the client to practice skills without reprimand.

Because of time spent with the client, the nurse is also a role model for social behaviors and

---

BOX 4.1

Topics to Cover With Clients

- Hours of visitation and client approval for visitors
- Times for therapy sessions
- Personal free time
- Times for meals, snacks, and lights out/bedtime
- Caffeine and smoking restrictions
- Available food, or snack items
- Shaving or cosmetic items allowed
- Sharp items, cords, and belts not allowed
- No tolerance for violent or threatening behaviors
- Medication schedule
- Activities
- Telephone privileges
- Restricted areas

---

communication skills, which reinforces the trusting relationship needed for successful treatment. The nurse is seen as someone who will listen and assist the client with difficult situations that arise in their day-to-day efforts toward improved mental functioning. The support provides an encouraging climate for growth and change.

To establish a safe and structured therapeutic milieu, rules are often needed. Initially explaining unit rules or policies to the client and support persons help to establish a mutual understanding of routines and accepted behaviors and helps develop in the client a sense of trust. These rules may vary from facility to facility. See Box 4.1 for typical topics to discuss with the client that help establish a safe and therapeutic milieu.

Close supervision is necessary to maintain compliance with all unit rules. It is important for each member of the mental health team to maintain consistency in enforcing these rules to establish limits and boundaries for behavior. Clients are encouraged to comply with all the rules and to attend all activity and therapy sessions.

In outpatient settings such as therapeutic community groups, the security of a safe environment to express these feelings is essential as clients often voice complaints, concerns, or feedback regarding the staff, other clients, or the environment in general. The group leader establishes and maintains guidelines for behavior in a consistent manner. This structured milieu helps the client toward normalization, improved social skills, and functioning as a member of society. The client learns how to express concerns in a rational and acceptable manner as well as tolerance and acceptance of the views of others.

Client behaviors such as aggression and physical violence, lewd sexual gestures, foul language, or inappropriate confrontation are not tolerated in a therapeutic milieu. Clients are encouraged to express thoughts and feelings they experience during times when these actions occur. Interventions are used to help the client identify the unacceptable behavior and develop constructive approaches to deal with similar situations in the future. This provides the client with a way to effectively manage self-control toward behavior modification.

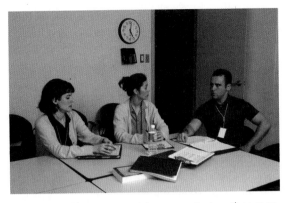

Figure 4.1 The treatment team meets together regularly to coordinate client care. (Source: Mohr, W. K. [2013]. *Psychiatric-mental health nursing: Evidence-based concepts, skills, and practices.* Wolters Kluwer Health/Lippincott Williams & Wilkins.)

Just the Facts ① Nurses collect data on both adaptive and maladaptive behaviors and collaborate with clients to identify behaviors that need to change.

Mind Jogger ② What benefit could there be to moving a client who has been discharged from an inpatient setting to a group home milieu instead of returning to the general social climate?

Treatment Team

Within the various mental health care settings, medical and other professionals work together to provide a diversified treatment plan of care with a common goal. Each team member has a specific role in the treatment process. Because each of the members may have contact with the client in a different circumstance, it is important to have collaborative meetings in which each member can provide insight and any new information about the client (Fig. 4.1). Such meetings enhance the holistic approach to optimize the treatment pathway. The frequency of the meetings will depend on the individual needs or problems the client is experiencing, but they are often daily or weekly meetings. Not all members will attend every meeting, for example, the dietitian may only be consulted if there are specific nutritional needs or if medications interact with certain foods. The exchange of ideas focuses on what will be the best approach to facilitate a positive outcome for each person. Discharge planning is also a topic during the meeting. From time of admission, all strategies are aimed toward discharge as an outcome.

Interdisciplinary Team Members

While the health care provider, usually a psychiatrist, is often considered the primary leader of the multidisciplinary team, there can be other primary leaders and there are many other professionals who contribute to working toward the best possible outcome for any particular client. Box 4.2 lists members of the treatment team.

Psychiatrist

A **psychiatrist** is a licensed physician who specializes in psychiatric or mental disorders. A psychiatrist can evaluate, diagnose, and treat all types of mental illness. As medical doctors, psychiatrists are licensed to prescribe medications in addition to providing individual psychotherapy. Some psychiatrists subspecialize in the pediatric, adolescent, or geriatric populations. Others may specialize in the area of substance use and addiction disorders. The

BOX 4.2

The Mental Health Treatment Team

- Psychiatrist
- Clinical psychologist
- Registered nurse (RN)
- Licensed practical/vocational nurse (LPN/LVN)
- Mental health technician
- Social worker
- Licensed professional counselor
- Case managers and outreach workers
- Therapeutic recreation specialist
- Occupational therapist
- Religious advisor

settings in which they offer services may include hospitals, outpatient clinics, geriatric–psychiatric units, private practice offices, schools, correctional facilities, or other organizations as consultants.

Clinical Psychologist

Clinical psychologists administer and interpret psychological testing that can be used in the diagnostic process. Most licensed clinical psychologists have received a master's or doctoral level degree specializing in psychology with advanced training and field requirements. A clinical psychologist also provides individual, family, marital, and group therapies to assist in the resolution of mental health issues. Licensed psychologists can work independently or as members of the mental health team. They work in private practice settings, hospitals, outpatient clinics, schools, research institutions, and other settings that provide mental health services. Some, but not all, clinical psychologists have prescribing authority for certain medications.

Psychiatric Nurse

Psychiatric nursing is a specialized area of nursing practice that focuses on the prevention and treatment of mental health–related problems. Most psychiatric nurses are registered nurses (RNs), with advanced-practice nurses (APRNs) working in specialized areas such as geriatric psychology, mental health centers, correctional institutions, or consultation.

The RN may have an associate degree, diploma, or bachelor's degree in nursing. In the mental health care setting, the RN is accountable for both the physical and mental health care of the client. The RN is responsible for developing the individualized care plan and ensuring that it is implemented within a safe and therapeutic environment. APRNs have at least a master's or doctoral degree in nursing. APRNs may diagnose and treat mental illnesses in some settings and work under the supervision of a physician, in this case, a psychiatrist.

The licensed practical/vocational nurse (LPN/LVN) assists in all aspects of the nursing care of the mental health client. Responsibilities of the LPN/LVN include basic nursing care such as observing behaviors and collecting data, administering medications, monitoring for vital signs and symptoms after medications are administered, reporting these observations to the RN or health care provider in charge, participating in therapeutic communication with clients, and documenting in the client record.

The nurse, RN or LPN/LVN, is often able to establish and maintain a therapeutic relationship with the client while performing basic nursing interventions such as vital signs, dressing changes, or assisting with hygiene needs. The nurse works closely with other members of the mental health care team to develop a client-centered plan of care. (See the section titled Role of the Nurse later in the chapter for a more detailed discussion of specific nursing responsibilities.)

Mental Health Technician

A mental health technician assists clients with physical and hygiene needs as needed, observes and documents unit activities, and assists with group or recreational activities. Technicians usually receive on-the-job training. Technicians do not administer medications or perform treatments but do assist with safety interventions as needed. Their observations are also important to the mental health treatment team.

Social Worker

Licensed clinical social workers (LCSWs) are trained as client advocates and usually have a master's or doctoral level degree in their discipline. They are responsible for providing referrals, acting as a client liaison with government and civil agencies, and helping individuals with daily living problems and readjustments to living in society. The LCSW often works with placement agencies, such as community group homes and nursing homes, to secure a continued support and care system for the client who is unable to live in an independent or home setting. Some LCSWs specialize in specific areas such as domestic violence, rape and abuse, or substance use disorders.

Licensed Professional Counselor

Licensed professional counselors have a master's level degree in psychology with specialized training and licensure in professional counseling. Counseling incorporates approaches that best meet the needs of the client to resolve problem areas toward a more satisfying and rewarding lifestyle. Counselors may specialize in areas such as marital and family counseling or substance use, and they may work in various community settings and schools or in private practice.

Case Manager and Outreach Worker

Agencies such as mental health centers, psychosocial rehabilitation programs, and government agencies employ case management and outreach workers to monitor and ensure that a client's needs are met. Most individuals with severe mental illness need medical care, social services, housing, and financial assistance. Case managers and outreach workers provide assistance in securing these services. They also provide follow-up support to ensure the client's ability to live in the community setting. RNs function as case managers in some facilities.

Religious Counselor

Pastoral or religious counselors provide spiritual support and counseling for clients and their families. They participate in treatment team meetings, therapy sessions, and discharge planning.

Therapeutic Recreation Specialist

Therapeutic recreation specialists use various approaches such as art, music, leisure education, and recreation participation to help clients make the most of their lives physically, mentally, and socially. These specialists have either a bachelor's or a master's degree, receive national certification, and are licensed or certified by the state in which they work. Recreation therapy provides ways for people to help themselves and to feel good about their improvements in the areas of concentration, decision-making, and completion of task-oriented projects. These accomplishments help to enhance the client's self-confidence and improve their ability to work in a team environment with improved social and communication skills. Participating in tasks that require concentration, such as making a collage or coloring, can help minimize some mental illness symptoms such as hearing voices, or can provide a calming environment.

Occupational Therapist

Occupational therapists have a bachelor's or master's level degree in occupational therapy and work with clients to improve their level of functioning for everyday living. Occupational therapists use activities such as cooking, money management, grocery shopping, and transportation to improve the client's self-esteem and promote a realistic level of independent living. Occupational therapists work with other members of the treatment team toward rehabilitation and discharge planning.

Dietitian

Dietitians usually have a master's level degree in nutrition and serve as resource persons by providing nutrition information and counseling to clients with specific nutritional problems and needs. Some psychotropic medications have side effects related to appetite, either increased or decreased, which can impact nutritional status. Also, some medications have food interactions that need to be avoided such as grapefruit juice or alcohol.

SeventyFour/Shutterstock

"Marsha"

Marsha has been admitted to your mental health unit for evaluation of a possible eating disorder. Marsha uses a wheelchair to move about but can take several steps and transfer with assistance. The unit has recently been remodeled. There are large maroon overstuffed chairs in the common room and small tables between the chairs. A large TV is secured to the wall of the common area. The unit has vinyl flooring and soft overhead lighting. Large windows that face a garden-like courtyard provide viewing of the unit's outdoor basketball court and covered patio with picnic tables. There are two wings to the unit, one for female clients and one for male clients. Each client room has a single floor-mounted bed, open shelves for personal belongings, and a bathroom with a toilet and shower but no door. Central to the two wings is an L-shaped nurses' desk. The community phone for client use is located at the nurses' desk. The multidisciplinary treatment team conference room is also located between the two dormitory wings.

Digging Deeper

1. Identify the components of the milieu of the mental health unit Marsha has been admitted to.

2. Which members of the multidisciplinary treatment team would you expect to attend daily meetings regarding the client's treatment plan of care?

3. Are there any members of the team you would expect to attend on less frequent basis than those who meet daily?

4. Would the client be involved in the meetings with the treatment team? Explain why or why not.

CASE STUDY 4.1

Role of the Nurse

At the hub of the mental health team, the nurse functions in a variety of different roles (Box 4.3). The LPN/LVN collects data, interacts with clients, and serves as a liaison between the client and the RN and health care provider. The nurse–client relationship provides multiple opportunities for the nurse to obtain information that is often a vital resource to other team members. The nurse is a vital component of maintaining a therapeutic milieu that supports and encourages clients in appropriate behavioral responses. In addition, the nurse models and assists the client with communication skills and social interactions with others in the milieu (Fig. 4.2).

The nurse is an important source of unbiased and nonjudgmental support for the client. How the nurse perceives the client and the client's behavior can be influenced by the nurse's psychological state at the time of the interaction. The nurse can maintain an objective view of the client's situation by recognizing and understanding their feelings and emotional responses toward the client. This is known as self-assessment. Ongoing self-assessment allows the nurse to separate reaction from therapeutic action and remain focused on ways to promote a positive outcome for the client and their family.

Just the Facts The nurse's psychological state can influence the nurse's perception of the client and the intended behavioral message.

The Nurse as Caregiver

The nursing process provides the foundation for the implementation of all nursing interventions. Basic to data collection is the observation of appropriate and inappropriate behaviors, noting both precipitating factors and situational reinforcers. The nurse documents this information in the client record and provides feedback for other members of the mental health care team for evaluating effectiveness and progress of the treatment plan. The nurse often observes a response to therapy while performing other nursing interventions such as medication administration, data collection, or personal care assistance. It is important for the nurse to positively reinforce appropriate behavior and encourage clients to participate in all aspects of the psychotherapeutic process.

The Nurse as Counselor

Nurses are often the members of the mental health team who are most available and willing to provide an attitude of genuine concern for the client through active listening and therapeutic communication. The nurse should encourage the client to openly express feelings and thoughts without fear of judgment. Not all behavior is acceptable and the nurse must call out inappropriate behavior expressed by the client. Unconditional acceptance of the client as a person is imperative to a therapeutic outcome.

The Nurse as Educator

Nurses are often the link between clients and information about their illnesses and treatment. Adherence to treatment is more probable when clients are informed about the problem and how the treatment works. The nurse needs to provide information at the client's level of understanding through verbal explanation, demonstration, and printed materials about the illness and treatment regime. It is important for the nurse to determine

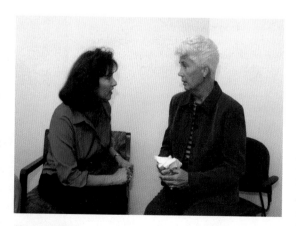

Figure 4.2 The nurse communicating with the client. Note how the nurse is eye level with the client and facing the client at an angle, not directly face to face. (Source: Shives, L. R. [2011]. *Basic concepts of psychiatric-mental health nursing*. Wolters Kluwer Health/Lippincott Williams & Wilkins.)

the client's understanding of the instructions by verbal response or return demonstration.

The Nurse as Advocate

As a client advocate, the nurse functions to protect the rights of the client through acceptance and support for decisions that are made. Adherence to treatment usually improves as the nurse demonstrates an empathetic positive regard for client needs. Empathy involves the nurse's willingness to understand the situation from the client's perspective. By being willing to listen, the nurse can view a problem through the client's eyes and assist in providing the resources necessary for the client to make a decision.

> **Test Yourself**
> ✔ What makes up a therapeutic milieu?
> ✔ Who makes up the interdisciplinary team and what are their roles?
> ✔ How would the nurse support a client's decision if that choice is contradictory to the suggested treatment? What role of the nurse would this be?

Types of Therapy

Specific types of therapies are selected based on the treatment plan and goals determined by the mental health treatment team and the client. Common types of treatment for psychiatric disorders include pharmacologic treatment, psychotherapy, electroconvulsive therapy (ECT), and others. The most common treatment approach in the United States for individuals with mental illness is the use of psychotherapeutic medications in conjunction with psychotherapy.

Psychotherapy

Psychotherapy is a dialogue between a mental health practitioner and the client with the goal of reducing the symptoms of the emotional disturbance or disorder and improving that individual's personal and social well-being. The aim of this dialogue is not to give advice, but to allow clients to learn about themselves, their lives, and their feelings, and to make choices toward change. The intent is for clients to rediscover their identities, priorities, and inner courage to act on these priorities. Credible psychotherapy fosters insight into feelings, behavior, and interpersonal skills with

success resting in the quality, not the type, of therapy method used. Most clinical licensed mental health practitioners embrace an eclectic approach, meaning they believe in using components of many types of therapies in their practice. People are complex beings with diverse and unique individual problems that are more successfully addressed by a flexible multimethod, rather than a single-method approach. There are five main approaches to individual therapy: psychodynamic, humanistic, behavioral, cognitive, and contracting.

> **Just the Facts**
> Therapeutic intervention begins with the assumption that everyone can experience functional growth in interpersonal relationships and the demands of daily living.

Psychodynamic Therapy

Psychodynamic therapy is primarily based on psychoanalytic theory, or the assumption that when a client has insight into early relationships and experiences as the source of their problems, the problems can be resolved. It is further assumed that these experiences can be analyzed to resolve current emotional problems. This Freudian-based therapy characteristically lasts several years with biweekly sessions.

Humanistic Therapy

Humanistic therapy centers on the client's view of the world and their problems. The goal is to help clients realize their full potential through the therapist's genuineness, unconditional positive regard, and empathetic understanding of the client's point of view, which foster the client's sense of self-worth. This therapy is nondirective but focuses on helping the client to explore and clarify their own feelings and choices, while emphasizing potential and individual strengths.

Behavioral Therapy

Behavioral therapy does not foster awareness but emphasizes the principles of learning with positive or negative reinforcement and observational modeling. The goal is to bring about behavioral change within a relatively short time. In this therapy, the behavior or symptom is the problem. The underlying belief is that the original causes of maladaptive behavior may have little to do with present factors invoking the behavior. It is primarily used to treat mood and anxiety disorders, but can also be used successfully in other disorders such as attention deficit hyperactive disorder (ADHD) and some addictive conditions.

The therapist formulates and executes a plan of treatment, often with a variety of exercises for the client to perform between sessions. Gradual exposure or systematic desensitization to an anxiety-producing situation (such as in phobias) may be used along with relaxation exercises (e.g., breathing, visualization, or meditation). The therapist teaches and models skills for real-life situations with emphasis on what works best in specific symptom situations. Other techniques that may be used include contracting and role-playing scenarios. **Contracting** is a behavioral technique in which the client and therapist draw up a contract to which both parties are obligated. The contract requires the client to demonstrate specific behaviors that are included in the therapy and also defines what the therapist is responsible for doing. The criteria for success are clearly outlined in the contract. It is important that reinforcement schedules, limits, contracts, and consequences be consistently followed.

Cognitive Behavioral Therapy (CBT)

Cognitive behavioral therapy (CBT), is based on the cognitive (cognitive = thinking) model that focuses on identifying and correcting distorted thinking patterns that can lead to emotional distress and problem behaviors. Cognitive therapists believe that clients respond to stressful situations based on their subjective perception of an event. Once the misperception is identified, clients can change their behaviors by changing their maladaptive thinking about themselves and their experiences.

Albert Ellis was the first to consider the client's irrational thoughts as the cause of existing psychological problems. He developed the pioneering form of cognitive behavioral therapy (CBT) called rational emotive behavior therapy (REBT). REBT is based on the idea that it is primarily the individual's thinking about the world around them that leads to emotional and behavioral distress. These irrational thoughts tend to be in the form of "musts," "oughts," or "shoulds" that create anger, depression, low self-esteem, and other psychological problems. Individuals often choose to respond to these unreasonable thoughts with behaviors in which they actually create their own consequences and disappointments. REBT therapists attempt to help clients to identify and change these unrealistic

thoughts and beliefs and replace them with positive rational thinking that can lead to a more reasonable and satisfying way of living. REBT continues to be used and has been shown to be effective in the treatment of obsessive-compulsive disorder (OCD), social anxiety, and depression.

Aaron Beck also based his cognitive therapy on the premise that how an individual thinks influences their feelings and actions. Cognitive behavioral therapy (CBT) is a combination of using this approach to help the client modify their dysfunctional thinking which will subsequently change the client's feelings and behavior. Cognitive behavioral therapy (CBT) therapists teach clients problem-solving skills and stress-reducing methods. Techniques may include self-monitoring logs and homework that work toward mutually set goals. Clients learn that their psychological difficulties or problems can be solved through cognitive processing.

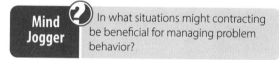

Mind Jogger In what situations might contracting be beneficial for managing problem behavior?

Telehealth

Current trends have increased the use of telehealth. **Telehealth** is the use of electronic and telecommunication technology to interact with clients. In mental health, there is growing research that suggests this type of therapy may be more successful, especially with children and adolescents, than traditional face-to-face intervention.

When telehealth is determined to be a desired approach, an initial in-person visit should occur that consists of identification of the individual, a face-to-face intake history, and a head-to-toe assessment. This initial interaction is usually done by a psychologist or other health care provider. Once the client is established, video meetings via a phone or computer camera, where both the client and mental health care provider can view each other, can be used to monitor progress toward goals and review medication effectiveness. The client, family, and/or other significant individuals can participate as identified in the initial meeting. This allows the provider to view behavior and/or symptoms that relate to that client's situation. In the case of children, there may be specific toys or tables that allow the clinician to observe development and other behaviors. For those who are reluctant to seek traditional psychotherapy, tele-health may offer a more cost-effective alternative by which the client can answer questions more honestly on a camera or computer than face-to-face. On the other hand, some clinicians are concerned that camera-based intervention lacks the ability to establish an effective rapport with the client that in turn promotes a successful clinical relationship and compliance with treatment.

Regardless of the method used, psychotherapy is successful when issues in the person's life are uncovered and client work is done to allow constructive change. An important variable in this success is the relationship between the client and therapist, as well as how the client views this relationship. Various types of approaches have proven to be comparably effective, although each may have its advantages and disadvantages in different client situations.

Group Therapy

In **group therapy**, a trained therapist leads a small group of people with similar problems who discuss individual and common issues. Remedial groups are concerned with individuals who are not coping effectively with the stresses and strains of living. These groups can assist individuals in learning age-appropriate ways to manage behavior or regain self-control, skills for conflict resolution, problem solving, and interpersonal socialization and communication. Groups often must work through negative content before positive results can surface. The success of the group interaction depends on the degree of trust, openness, and interpersonal risk taking among the members. Interaction between members allows each to hear from others about their perceptions and behavior, either confirming or contradicting these self-views. Arguments and debates often indicate the attempt of each member to validate their own sense of reality.

Couples therapy is a highly effective group model used in helping couples resolve interpersonal conflict and initiate enhanced communication skills. In cases of marital conflict, the therapy tends to be most effective if the differences are of short-term duration. The therapist facilitates by listening to points of view and reality expressed by both partners.

Family therapy involves discussions and sessions designed to assist members with problem-solving skills within the family system. The problem may lie with all family members (e.g.,

troubled communication among family members) or center on the behavior of one particular person. The underlying belief is that individual problems originate from the family system. To treat the basic issue, the whole family must undergo therapy. The goal is to facilitate and encourage the family to work together, listen to, and respect each other as they gain an understanding of how their behaviors affect the entire family.

Electroconvulsive Therapy

Electroconvulsive therapy (ECT) is a treatment using low-voltage electric shock waves passed through the brain to induce short periods of seizure activity. The seizures appear to aid in restoring a chemical balance within the brain, which helps to relieve the serious symptoms of mental illness. Some conditions where this type of therapy may be used include severe major or treatment-resistant depression, psychosis, bipolar disorder, catatonia, severe agitation and aggression in dementia, and severe suicidal ideation. Electroconvulsive therapy (ECT) is generally reserved for clients with severe mental illnesses that are unresponsive to medications and other forms of therapeutic intervention. Treatment is voluntary, and the client must give informed consent. Some clients are reluctant to try electroconvulsive therapy (ECT) due to its historical stigma and its slang name "shock therapy."

During electroconvulsive therapy (ECT), the electric shock is given for several seconds to cause the seizure activity. It is administered along with general anesthesia and muscle relaxants to minimize the risk and negative impact on the client. The combined use of the two different types of medications helps to prevent the seizure from impacting the entire body and to prevent severe muscle contractions that can inadvertently result in fractures or dislocated bones. An electroencephalogram (EEG) records electrical activity in the brain during the procedure. Electroconvulsive therapy (ECT) is usually given two to three times a week, typically lasting no longer than 6 to 12 treatments. A newer technique called unilateral ultrabrief pulse electroconvulsive therapy may be done daily on weekdays. Use of therapy may vary in the electrode placement and the type and exposure time of the electrical stimulus. Adverse effects include temporary memory loss, headache, hypotension, tachycardia, and confusion. Most confusion clears within hours after the treatment, while memory loss may be more persistent. Studies continue regarding the long-term effects of electroconvulsive therapy (ECT). Nursing care of the client undergoing electroconvulsive therapy (ECT) includes supportive caring interventions in addition to data collection and monitoring of vital signs.

Adjunctive Therapies

There have been many other types of adjunctive therapies that have been shown to be helpful and therapeutic in the treatment of mental health issues. Each therapy should be individually considered for the client's condition or symptoms and the client's willingness to participate in the therapy. Adjunctive therapies can include biofeedback, agitation therapy, play therapy, pet therapy, and complementary and alternative medicine (CAM).

Biofeedback is a training program used for specific types of anxiety that is designed to develop the client's ability to control heart rate, muscle tension, and other autonomic or involuntary functions of the nervous system by using monitoring devices during situations that trigger this reaction. This is followed by an attempt or feedback that allows the person to reproduce the desired change and control these body functions under the anxiety-producing emotional circumstances. Biofeedback works best if used consistently. Neurobiofeedback is currently being used in the treatment of attention deficit hyperactivity disorder (ADHD).

Agitation therapy may be used in people who display problematic and aggressive behavior and do not respond positively to other therapies. In this form of therapy, the person is exposed to external agitation from other clients in a controlled atmosphere. This is designed to increase that person's self-awareness of maladaptive behavior and limitations. The goals of this therapy are to teach sublimation of aggression and anger impulses with insight and a willingness to change. The desired outcome is for the client to achieve control over their behavior and assume responsibility for emotional and social growth. It is often used in combination with other types of therapy.

Play therapy is often used with children and allows the therapist to treat the child during the dynamic process of play. The therapist assesses the child's internal affective state and psychological response during the various stages of the treatment process. With the activity techniques used, the child can more easily express emotions and feelings if they are unable to do in words.

The attachment that is formed between humans and animals has led to the use of pet therapy. Old and young alike are drawn to the unconditional response and affection of animals. An animal can stimulate a client to interact with another person by creating a subject for conversation. Petting the animal also brings the comfort of touch and the acceptance the client feels from the animal. Pet therapy may be used in treating children and adolescents and has widespread use in nursing homes and geriatric psychiatric facilities. Additionally, studies have been done on the relaxing benefits, lowering of blood pressure, and reduction of feelings of stress that occur with pet therapy.

Complementary and alternative medicine (CAM) therapies include acupuncture, herbal remedies, yoga, spirituality and religious activities, and meditation. Other adjunctive therapies may include occupational, recreational, and creative art therapies. These provide a relaxed atmosphere in which the client is often able to express emotions and feelings that may be subdued during other forms of therapy. Recreational therapy provides an outlet for sublimating frustration and internal drives of emotion, along with encouraging social interactive skills. In the clinical setting, participation in all forms of therapy sessions is encouraged to provide the client with every opportunity for maximum benefit of treatment.

Drum circles/therapy groups have been shown to positively help clients with post-traumatic stress disorder (PTSD), anxiety, grief, depression, and behavioral issues. Drumming techniques require focus and help with impulse control and decision-making skills. Clients can utilize the drum circle as a safe area for expression of feelings including grief, anger, and impulsiveness.

Test Yourself
- ✔ How can telehealth help the client with a mental health issue?
- ✔ Describe the difference between behavioral therapy and cognitive behavioral therapy (CBT).
- ✔ Name three adjunctive therapies.

Pharmacologic Medications and Mental Illness

Throughout history, there have been efforts that aim to treat psychiatric disorders using both medications and various approaches in psychotherapy. Early pharmacotherapy used plants (e.g., the purple foxglove, *Digitalis purpurea;* the opium poppy; and the antimalarial compound quinine from the bark of the cinchona tree), mineral salts, and herbs. Over time, a more scientific approach evolved in understanding the molecular components of medications taken from natural sources. These advances in chemistry and human physiology led to the modern branch of pharmacology and the laboratory origin of most medications.

Today, the major approach to the treatment of psychiatric disorders is the use of psychotherapeutic medications used in conjunction with psychotherapy. Developing medications to treat the cause of a particular psychiatric disorder is difficult because the actual causes of most disorders have not been identified; in most cases, a pattern of both genetic and environmental factors predisposes a person to the development of a particular illness. Regardless of the etiology, the psychiatric disorders are considered to be medical illnesses with typical signs and symptoms. Therefore, pharmaceutical companies have focused on treating the symptoms of these disorders, rather than the causes.

Categories of Mental Health Disorders

A group of medical symptoms seen in combination together are referred to as a syndrome. Much as a group of symptoms characterize the illnesses such as diabetes or gastroesophageal reflux, the symptoms of the psychiatric disorders are recognizable and linked to a particular diagnosis that the health care provider makes. See Box 4.4 for the common mental illness categories.

Since the 1950s, the development of medications for psychiatric disorders has provided symptomatic relief for many people. **Psychotropic agents** are medications that have their impact on target sites or receptors of the nervous system to induce changes that affect psychiatric function, behavior, or experience. **Psychopharmacology** refers to the study of the changes that occur as

the medications interact with the chemicals in the brain. These medications have provided a sense of normalcy for many clients with altered feelings, perceptions, and thinking. The use of psychotropic agents has also expanded our understanding of how the brain and mind are affected by mental health disorders. These medications do not cure or resolve the underlying problem. Rather, they are used in combination with counseling and other therapeutic modalities to reduce the atypical symptoms and promote restoration of a manageable and functional level of existence. Most clients with mental health disorders require a combination of two medications to maintain stability.

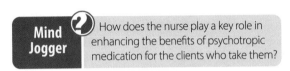

Mind Jogger ② How does the nurse play a key role in enhancing the benefits of psychotropic medication for the clients who take them?

Classification of Psychotropic Medications

Medications used to treat mental disorders fall into five major categories

- Antianxiety medications
- Antidepressants
- Mood stabilizers
- Antipsychotic medications
- Antiparkinson (anticholinergic) medications

Although each medication has an individual chemical composition, each group of psychotropic agents includes medications that are similar in their desired effect, side effects, adverse effects, and related properties. The categories and their characteristics, along with normal dosage ranges and related nursing responsibilities or interventions, will be discussed in Chapters 9 to 11.

Action of Psychotropic Medications on Neurotransmitters

Psychotropic medications have their primary effect on neurotransmitter systems of the body. **Neurotransmitters** are the chemical messenger proteins stored in the **presynaptic compartment** located before the nerve synapse. There are many types of neurotransmitters that combine with individual receptors of the body. The neurotransmitter is released into the **synaptic cleft** (the space between two neurons) where it crosses the cleft and attaches to a **postsynaptic receptor** (a cell component located in the neuron distal to

BOX 4.4

Categories of Mental Illness

- Mood alterations
- Irritability and anxiety
- Altered thought processes
- Misperceptions of the environment
- Impaired and illogical communication or interaction patterns
- Disorientation and confusion

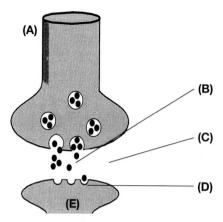

Figure 4.3 A presysnaptic neuron (**A**) releasing neurotransmitters (**B**) into the synaptic cleft (**C**) that will be bound to receptors (**D**) on the postsynaptic neuron (**E**) (see related Figure 10.1). (Source: *Foye's Principles of Medicinal Chemistry*. [2013]. Lippincott Williams & Wilkins.)

TABLE 4.1	Basic Relationship of Neurotransmitters to Mental Disorders
Neurotransmitter	**Relationship to Mental Disorder**
Acetylcholine	Decreased in Alzheimer disease
Dopamine	Decreased in Parkinson disease
	Increased in schizophrenia
Gamma-aminobutyric acid (GABA)	Decreased in anxiety disorders
Norepinephrine	Decreased in depression
	Increased in mania
Serotonin	Decreased in depression
	Increased in mania

the synapse) where it will continue to activate a response until the neurotransmitter is inactivated (Fig. 4.3). Neurotransmitters can be inactivated either by enzymatic action or by reuptake. In the case of **reuptake**, the neurotransmitters are absorbed back into the presynaptic compartment of the previous neuron.

Psychotropic medications are effective because they either enhance or decrease the brain's ability to use a specific neurotransmitter. Some medications, such as the antiparkinson medications, cause the release of the neurotransmitter acetylcholine, which is thought to contribute to the transmission of nerve impulses at the synapse and myoneural junctions. Others, such as the antipsychotic medication clozapine, interfere with the binding of chemical messengers to the intended receptors in the brain. Lithium carbonate, a medication used in the treatment of bipolar disorders, accelerates the destruction of monoamine neurotransmitters (dopamine, norepinephrine, and serotonin), inhibits their release, and decreases the sensitivity of postsynaptic receptors. Table 4.1 identifies the link between the specific neurotransmitters and the deficiency or excess seen in common mental disorders.

Just the Facts Monoamine neurotransmitters stored in presynaptic compartments of neurons in the central nervous system (CNS) include the chemical messengers norepinephrine, dopamine, and serotonin.

Not all medications penetrate the brain cells equally. The chemical property known as *lipid solubility* is a major determinant of a medication's molecular infusion into the brain tissue. The selectivity of the barrier between the blood and the brain further protects the brain by regulating the extent to which the medication penetration can occur. Substances such as alcohol, heroin, and diazepam have high lipid solubility and are readily absorbed into the cerebral cells through the blood–brain barrier, increasing their potential for addiction and misuse. By the same token, the rate at which a medication is absorbed affects its efficacy. Scientists continue to study the specific effects of individual psychotropic medications on psychological processes and the use of these medications in treating psychiatric disorders.

Psychotropic Medications and the Older Client

For older clients who have dementia-related aggression, distressing repetitive behaviors, catastrophic reactions, delusions, hallucinations, or agitation, the use of antipsychotic medications has become a common approach to reducing and managing the incidence of these symptoms. The Omnibus Budget Reconciliation Act (OBRA) of 1987 limited the use of psychotropic medications for residents in long-term care facilities. These guidelines have been modified but with specific diagnostic and monitoring specifications. Antipsychotic medications can cause serious side effects such as extrapyramidal symptoms and tardive dyskinesia. The newer generation of psychotropic medications is associated with fewer side effects, and they have now become medications of choice for older clients. Guidelines set by OBRA specify that these medications can

"Lynn"

Lynn is 48 years old and is being evaluated for symptoms of mood alteration. Her symptoms have been present for over 2 months.

Digging Deeper

1. Which category of the psychotropic medications would you expect Lynn to be prescribed by the healthcare provider?

2. What types of therapies would you expect the treatment team to plan for Lynn?

3. Which neurotransmitter(s) is/are most likely related to Lynn's mood alteration?

4. What would you need to collect data on why Lynn was receiving a psychotropic medication?

5. How would you expect Lynn's psychotropic medication treatment to be different if she was 70 years old instead?

CASE STUDY 4.2

---

only be used for specific diagnoses and when behavioral and environmental measures are unsuccessful in managing symptoms. Research data on the safety and response of the older client to psychotropic medications is limited further suggesting a cautious approach to the use of these medications.

> **Senior Focus**
> In the older adult, the half-life of a medication tends to increase by as much as five to six times, increasing the risk of toxicity. The effects accumulate slowly and may not be apparent for days or weeks following the initiation of the medication.

The impact of age-related physiologic changes on antipsychotic medication therapy accounts for many of the serious side effects that occur in older adults. Many antipsychotic medications, either by themselves or in interaction with other medications, can cause the very symptoms they are prescribed to treat, such as agitation or delusions. Many older clients commonly take medications for several illnesses, and all medications they are taking need to be reviewed by a pharmacist for interactions. In addition, the adverse effects of one medication can be mistaken as symptoms of another condition and needlessly treated. Older adults have a higher body fat-to-lean ratio, less serum albumin, less total-body water, fewer brain cells, and slower liver metabolism and renal clearance than young adults, so they need far less of these medications to produce a therapeutic effect. The higher fat composition of tissue increases retention of the medication resulting in effects and side effects that persist longer, sometimes even after the medication is discontinued. Because older clients have less protein to bind with the medication, more of the medication is free to circulate. A slowed metabolic rate and renal excretion time allow the medication to remain in the body longer. Table 4.2 shows these physiologic changes and their imposed risk when administering a psychotropic agent.

All of these factors highlight the importance of monitoring the response to and recognizing the adverse effects of psychotropic medications in the older client. It is extremely important that all alternative approaches be considered before the use of medications, and that, if used, treatment is discontinued if the person is adversely affected by the medication.

> **Senior Focus**
> In the older client, always consider that a new symptom or behavior may be related to medication therapy.

> **Test Yourself**
> ✔ Name the five categories of psychotropic medications.
> ✔ Describe how the action in the presynaptic neuron differs from the postsynaptic neuron.

TABLE 4.2   Age-Related Physiologic Changes and Psychotropic Medications in Older Clients

Physiologic Change	Risk
Higher body–fat-to-lean ratio	Increased risk of cumulative effects
Less serum albumin and protein-bound medication	More free (unbound) medication circulating in bloodstream. This can lead to higher blood levels and the therapeutic effect(s) of the medication may be decreased
Less total body water	Dehydration increases concentration of medication in body
Decreased liver metabolism	Clearance of medication is delayed or slowed (alprazolam, chlordiazepoxide, desipramine, diazepam, imipramine, nortriptyline, trazodone, triazolam)
Decreased renal elimination	Slowed elimination of medication from system (risperidone)

Cultural Considerations

Cultural Attitudes and Knowledge Regarding Electroconvulsive Therapy (ECT)

There have been many studies that look at a specific culture's beliefs and knowledge regarding electroconvulsive therapy (ECT). There have also been studies that compare two or three cultures to determine if there were differences between them regarding the treatment. Results from the studies show common themes. Low to lack of knowledge about the procedure was seen in most studies. In most cultures, the primary information source about electroconvulsive therapy (ECT) was identified as the media and movies. Common attitudes experienced by families regarding the procedure included a less positive attitude, a lower willingness to consent to the procedure, and low knowledge. Some college students felt the procedure was painful, ineffective, or even illegal (Kramarczyk et al., 2020). Another common theme was that some family members and patients who consented to the procedure felt they were coerced to consent and have the treatment.

SUMMARY

- Mental health care includes a variety of therapeutic treatment methods directed toward relieving the symptoms of mental illness and empowering the individuals to live and function within society.
- A therapeutic milieu describes an environment that is conducive to providing therapeutic interaction between clients and members of the professional team. Within this atmosphere, there is a supportive network to help the client establish common goals within safe and secure surroundings.
- The treatment team consists of professionals who work together to provide a diversified approach toward a common outcome of improved access and outcome to mental health care.
- The health care provider, often a psychiatrist, is usually considered the primary leader of the multidisciplinary team. There are many other professionals who contribute to the client's care, with each team member having a specific role. The multidisciplinary team provides a holistic approach to treatment.
- Collaborative team meetings, where each member can provide insight from their perspective, are held daily or weekly to discuss new and continuing needs or problems of individual clients. The exchange focuses on the best approach to facilitate a positive outcome for each person.

- The nurse often serves as a liaison between the client and health care provider.
- The psychological state of the nurse can influence how the client or client behavior is perceived. Understanding these feelings and emotional responses will assist the nurse in maintaining an objective view of the client situation.
- Nursing roles in the treatment milieu include caregiver, counselor, educator, and client advocate.
- Various types of psychotherapy are used to allow clients to interact with practitioners toward a goal of reducing the symptoms of the emotional disturbance or disorder and improving the individual's personal and social well-being.
- Therapeutic intervention begins with the assumption that everyone can experience functional growth in interpersonal relationship and the demands of societal living.
- Regardless of the method, psychotherapy is successful when issues in the person's life are uncovered and the client experiences constructive change.
- Electroconvulsive therapy (ECT) may be used to treat clients with severe mental illness unresponsive to other methods of treatment.
- Other types of therapy may include biofeedback, agitation, play, pet, occupational, recreational, or

creative art therapy, all of which are designed to support varied opportunities for the client to improve their functioning.

- Psychotropic medications affect psychiatric function, behavior, or experience. They are not curative, but are used in combination with counseling and other therapeutic modalities to reduce the atypical symptoms to a manageable and functional level, allowing them to function in an adaptive role within society.

- Psychotropic medications have a primary effect on neurotransmitter systems, either enhancing or decreasing the brain's ability to use a specific neurotransmitter.

- All psychotropic medications are used with caution in the older client because of age-related physiologic changes. The medication effects persist longer and remain in the body longer. Careful monitoring is mandated to avoid the adverse consequences of their use.

BIBLIOGRAPHY

Bystritsky, A. (2022). Complementary and alternative treatments for anxiety symptoms and disorders: Herbs and medications. *UpToDate*. Retrieved on Feb 25, 2023, from https://www.uptodate.com/contents/complementary-and-alternative-treatments-for-anxiety-symptoms-and-disorders-herbs-and-medications

Bystritsky, A. (2021). Complementary and alternative treatments for anxiety symptoms and disorders: Physical, cognitive, and spiritual interventions. *UpToDate*. Retrieved on March 28, 2022, from https://www.uptodate.com/contents/complementary-and-alternative-treatments-for-anxiety-symptoms-and-disorders-physical-cognitive-and-spiritual-interventions

Dickerson, D. L., D'Amico, E. J., Klein, D. J., Johnson, C. L., Hale, B., Ye, F., & Dominguez, B. X. (2021). Drum-assisted recovery therapy for Native Americans (DARTNA): Results from a feasibility randomized controlled trial. *Journal of Substance Abuse Treatment, 126,* 108439. https://doi.org/10.1016/j.jsat.2021.108439

Kellner, C. (2021). Overview of electroconvulsive therapy (ECT) for adults. *UpToDate*. Retrieved on March 28, 2022, from https://www.uptodate.com/contents/overview-of-electroconvulsive-therapy-ect-for-adults

Kramarczyk, K., Ćwiek, A., Kurczab, B., Czok, M., Bratek, A., & Kucia, K. (2020). Does pop-culture affect perception of medical procedures? Report on knowledge and attitude towards electroconvulsive therapy among Polish students. *Psychiatria Polska, 54*(3), 603–612. https://doi.org/10.12740/PP/109157

Mulvaney-Roth, P., Jackson, C., Bert, L., Ericksen, S., & Ryan, M. (2022). Using pet therapy to decrease patients' anxiety on two diverse inpatient units. *Journal of the American Psychiatric Nurses Association.* https://journals.sagepub.com/doi/abs/10.1177/1078390321999719

Ragg, D. M., Soulliere, J., & Turner, M. (2017). Drumming and mindfulness integrations into an evidence-based group intervention, *Social Work with Groups, 42*(1), 29–42. https://www.tandfonline.com/doi/abs/10.1080/01609513.2017.1402401

Ruscin, J. M., & Linnebur, S. A. (2021). *Overview of drug therapy in older adults*. Merck Manual for the Professional. https://www.merckmanuals.com/professional/geriatrics/drug-therapy-in-older-adults/overview-of-drug-therapy-in-older-adults

Fill in the Blank

Fill in the blank with the correct answer.

1. A therapeutic milieu combines a _____ and _____ environment.
2. The mental health _____ _____ is a multidisciplinary group made up of the health care provider, nurse and other professionals.
3. The nurse is an important source of _____ and _____ support for the client.
4. _____ is described as a dialogue between a mental health practitioner and the client with a goal of reducing the emotional symptoms and improving the client's personal and social well-being.
5. _____ agents are medications that affect psychic function, behavior, or experience.
6. The chemical property known as _____ _____ is a major determinant of a medication's molecular infusion into the brain tissue.
7. Older clients have less _____ to bind with the medication therefore _____ of the medication is free to circulate.

Matching

Match the following terms to the most appropriate phrase.

1. _____ Neurotransmitter
2. _____ Synaptic cleft
3. _____ Therapeutic milieu
4. _____ Contracting
5. _____ Cognitive therapy
6. _____ Electroconvulsive therapy (ECT)
7. _____ Behavioral therapy

a. Focuses on identifying and correcting distorted thinking patterns
b. Psychopharmacological and electroconvulsive methods of treating mental disorders
c. Behavioral method with a mutually obligated agreement between therapist and client
d. Supportive network providing a sense of common goals within safe and secure surroundings
e. Space between two neurons where neurotransmitter activity occurs
f. Chemical messenger proteins stored in presynaptic compartments
g. Fosters reinforcement and observational modeling to resolve problems

Multiple Choice

Select the best answer from the multiple-choice items.

1. The role of the nurse working with the client who has a mental disorder includes:
   a. Conducting psychological testing
   b. Daily individual psychotherapy sessions
   c. Monitoring behavioral responses to therapy
   d. Acting as a liaison with government and civil agencies

2. When caring for the client with outbursts of uncontrolled anger, which nursing action would most reinforce the desired outcome?
   a. Model an appropriate response to the situation
   b. Provide insight into the cause of the observed response
   c. Reprimand the client for the inappropriate actions
   d. Observe and document a detailed description of the incident

3. The nurse is working with a client who is to be discharged in the next few days. Which mental health team member will be most involved in securing placement for the client?
   a. Mental health technician
   b. Licensed professional counselor
   c. Licensed practical/vocational nurse
   d. Clinical social worker

4. The nurse demonstrates an empathetic positive regard for the client's needs. This is an example of which role of the nurse?
   a. Educator
   b. Advocate
   c. Counselor
   d. Caregiver

5. The nurse observes a client having thrusting tongue movements that were not present on admission and reports this to the charge nurse and the health care provider. This is an example of which role of the nurse?
   a. Caregiver
   b. Counselor
   c. Educator
   d. Advocate

6. A client has contracted with a therapist to demonstrate decreased inappropriate language outbursts on the nursing unit. Which of the following nursing actions would best support the client toward a positive outcome?
    a. Ignoring negative behaviors and reporting to the therapist
    b. Separating the client from other clients if outbursts occur
    c. Modeling appropriate ways to communicate feelings
    d. Reprimanding the client for language outbursts

7. A newly diagnosed client with bipolar disorder is prescribed several psychotropic medications. Which of the following would best guide the nurse to reinforce teaching to the client about the actions of the medications?
    a. Psychotropic medications will resolve the underlying problems of the disorder
    b. They will reduce symptoms and assist to restore functional levels of living
    c. These medications will restore the client to a symptom-free level of existence
    d. The medications can help to cure this illness if they are taken correctly

8. The nurse is caring for an older adult client who is taking a psychotropic medication. Which of the following is a contributing factor to the increased risk of adverse effects in this client?
    a. Slowed metabolic rate and renal excretion time
    b. Decrease in the fat composition of body tissue
    c. Increase in protein-bound medication in the bloodstream
    d. Increase in total serum albumin available for binding

9. A nurse working in an outpatient clinic is preparing an older adult client to be seen by the provider. Which of the following statements by the client would alert the nurse to a need for further questioning? *(Select all that apply)*
    a. "I take all my medicine in the morning so I don't have to later."
    b. "I just don't understand why I have to take all this medication."
    c. "I take so much medication every day but I just seem to feel worse later."
    d. "I just had my medication refilled so I hope the doctor doesn't change anything."
    e. "It takes me a long time to take all this medication since I take one or two at a time."

10. A nurse working in a long-term care facility is preparing to administer an antidepressant medication to an older adult client. Which of the following would alert the nurse to an increased potential for accumulated effects of this medication?
    a. Client requires a walker for ambulation to the bathroom
    b. Client takes more naps than usual during the day
    c. Client shows lack of interest in participating in group activities
    d. Client has dry skin with decreased intake of fluids

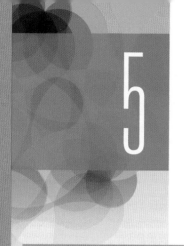

5

Establishing and Maintaining a Therapeutic Relationship

The Therapeutic Relationship

The holistic concept of nursing looks at all areas of the client including physical, psychosocial, cultural, and spiritual. Each person is influenced by a different combination of genetic and environmental issues. They also view the environment subjectively as it relates to their past experiences and relationships. A person learns to adapt to life and the environment by observing the world in which they exist. The complex nature of each individual is a factor in the development of a therapeutic relationship. Because of the psychosocial differences between clients and nurses, there is no one effective model for establishing the therapeutic relationship. Clients with the same medical diagnosis may even have a different pattern of symptoms based on their past experiences, current situation, and individual needs. The external demands of the environment and the internal forces of each person will require an individual approach to the nurse–client interaction.

The **therapeutic relationship** is a helping bond in which one person assists in the personal growth and improved well-being of the other. In this relationship, a series of interactions between the nurse and the client provides information about the client's needs and problems. The nurse works in collaboration with other members of the mental health team toward a common goal of assisting the client toward adaptive and improved functioning within their personal life and society.

Important Characteristics for Establishing a Nurse–Client Relationship

The establishment of a therapeutic nurse–client relationship is dependent on certain consistent characteristics of the nurse. Box 5.1 lists components that are essential to this professional relationship. One of the most important is that of **empathy**, which is the ability to hear what another person is saying, to have temporary access to that person's feelings, and to perceive the situation from that person's perspective. Empathy is vital to the establishment of trust. At the same time, it is important for the nurse to maintain enough distance from the situation to be objective and remain in touch with their own feelings. To become sympathetic and overidentify with the client's problem and feelings is nontherapeutic. In order to reach an understanding of the client's view, the nurse must engage in active listening that attentively

uses both the mind and the body. A seated distance of approximately 3 feet allows personal space but is close enough that interest is communicated and barriers can be avoided. Eye contact with a relaxed open posture facing the client shows a willingness to listen to what the other person is saying. Sitting at an angle to the client instead of facing them directly is viewed as less threatening by the client. These positioning techniques allow the nurse to maintain a mental focus on meaningful interaction with the client.

Trust is vital in the nurse–client relationship because of the vulnerable position in which the client is placed. Because it can be easily broken, the establishment of trust comes slowly and without guarantee until it is proven. The client may perceive the nurse as an authority figure and associate them with power. Since many clients with mental health issues do not trust those in authority, the nurse must earn their confidence by being consistent in following through with strategies that reinforce that the client can trust the nurse. **Genuineness**, or realness, is an attribute that comes from feeling concern about the client, which fosters an honest and caring foundation for trust.

The nurse's acceptance of the client as a person with worth and dignity, who is not judged or labeled by the nurse's standards, is also necessary for the establishment of a trusting relationship. The nurse's willingness to recognize the client with a mental health issue as one who deserves respect and needs approval helps the client to accept the environment. The foundation of the relationship is based on dependable interactions that demonstrate honesty, integrity, and consistency. Involved in this honesty is the establishment of boundaries

---

BOX 5.1

Essential Components of a Therapeutic Relationship

- Empathy
- Caring
- Acceptance (unconditional positive regard)
- Mutual trust
- Honesty
- Integrity
- Consistency
- Genuineness
- Self-awareness
- Limit-setting
- Reassurance
- Explanations

BOX 5.2

A Tool for Self-Assessment/Awareness

- What topics or ethical issues do I have strong feelings about?
- Are there topics I avoid or am uncomfortable discussing?
- Are there clients or diagnoses that I have strong reactions to?
- What is it about that client or diagnosis that makes me react strongly?
- How do I respond when I disagree with others?
- How do others react when I disagree with them?
- Who can I discuss work issues with?
- Do I have close relationships? With whom?
- What type of stressor is most recurrent in my life?
- How do I respond to stress?
- What coping mechanisms do I use to adapt? Do I use them frequently or occasionally?
- Do I usually think of myself first, or do I consider others?
- What type of personal space is my comfort zone?
- If I am threatened or scared, how do I respond?
- How do I respond to others who are withdrawn, anxious, or aggressive?
- Do I blame others for my problems and anxiety?
- What changes can I make to improve my interactions with others?

It is this same self-assessment clients do to help them view themselves and their behavior more realistically.

Mind Jogger How can self-awareness assist the nurse to help clients view themselves and their behavior more realistically?

Just the Facts Caring involves compassion, confidence in one's own abilities, a desire to do the right thing, and the courage to intervene as indicated. The nurse needs to also care for themselves. This includes enjoying their work, being knowledgeable in their role, taking pride in their work and accomplishments, recognizing the limitations of the amount of care they can provide at one time, and finding a colleague or mentor to share their experiences with.

and limit setting with predetermined consequences. This assists the client in self-control and management of behavior. The client needs constant reassurance to develop a sense of emotional security within their surroundings.

Self-awareness is a consciousness of one's own individuality and personality. The nurse cannot understand others unless they learn about themselves, how they respond to different issues, and potential pitfalls when working with clients. Box 5.2 provides a tool with questions for the nurse to ask themselves when doing a self-assessment. The awareness of oneself comes with an attitude of openness and wanting to come to an honest evaluation of behavior with a willingness to make changes. The nurse would also take note of their self-talk, acknowledge it, and be willing to change the recurrent negative scripts they themselves are subject to (e.g., "If I was smarter I would have gone to nursing school sooner in life."). When an individual moves beyond themselves and sees the world from the perspective of others, they open the door for growth. Insight into the connection between *thinking* and *behavior* provides the opportunity for the individual to change their behavior.

Phases of a Therapeutic Relationship

The therapeutic relationship is dependent on the situation and needs of the individual client. Interpersonal interaction in this relationship requires the nurse working with the client with a mental health issue to use observation and communication skills based on a knowledgeable understanding of human behavior. This is not a social interaction, but one that focuses on identifying the client's problems, developing goals for the client to improve on, and promoting their highest achievable level of functioning.

The phases of the nurse–client relationship must center on the client's ability to participate in the process. The relationship may vary in intensity, length, and focus depending on the particular client's needs. There are three phases of the therapeutic relationship: orientation, working, and termination.

Orientation Phase

The **orientation phase** involves meeting and getting to know the client. It involves an explanation of the purpose for the nurse–client interaction as a means of building trust, establishing roles, and identifying the client's problems and expectations. The nurse and client contract a time and place for a meeting and outline the roles of each person. The focus of the meeting is the client's self-identified problem. The nurse's role is to be a facilitator. Confidentiality is explained in terms of information that is shared only with members of the treatment team as it applies to the client's well-being. Rules and boundaries are explained to provide structure with guidelines for behavior. This gives the client an organized environment that resembles what is seen in society. It is important to document any negative feelings or comments the client expresses when behavior limits are discussed. The nurse can also use this time to observe other client behaviors, immediate concerns and needs, and the client's perceived reason for treatment. The initial data provides a baseline for the next phase of the relationship. It is essential for the nurse to convey a caring and honest concern for the client and to send a congruent message through both verbal and nonverbal communication. By showing a genuine interest and supportive attitude, the nurse helps the client to feel worthwhile, respected, and deserving of treatment.

> **Just the Facts**   Establishing rules and setting limits for behavior are consistent with behavior patterns in society.

Working Phase

The **working phase** is a period in which goals are set and interventions are planned for behavior change and to improve the client's well-being. This involves work by both the nurse and the client to develop an awareness of the problem and possible solutions to it. Through the use of problem-solving skills, the nurse assists the client to express feelings and thoughts about the present situation. It may be useful for the client to keep a journal of feelings and progress made between sessions. During this phase, the nurse becomes a role model and reinforces teaching about appropriate coping skills. The client is encouraged to practice adaptive responses and evaluate the effectiveness of changes. Every effort should be made to reinforce and support each small step of the client's progress toward change. Helping the client to set priorities provides a way of accomplishing short-term gains toward a bigger step or challenge. Helping the client recognize their accomplishments and achievement of goals helps foster self-confidence and self-esteem in the client.

Termination Phase

The third phase or **termination phase** of the relationship is necessary to allow the client to depend

on their own strengths while continuing to use their adaptive skills. The nurse should encourage the client to have increased social interaction and participate in all activities. This promotes independence in getting along with others in preparation for discharge and a return to the demands of society. It is important to discuss the termination with the client and respond to any feelings or concerns the client may express. It is not uncommon for nurses to feel like they are abandoning the client's trust as therapeutic closure occurs. However, when taken to extremes, traits found in nurses such as commitment, selflessness, and responsibility can hinder progress toward client independence. The nurse should stress that the relationship has been valued and purposeful in helping the client toward relying on their own ability to deal with problems. Some clients may be so fearful of becoming more independent or leaving the safety of the therapeutic relationship that they may self-sabotage their progress in order to remain in the comfort of the known environment.

> **Test Yourself**
> ✔ _____ is vital to the establishment of trust.
> ✔ What are the main tasks in each phase of the nurse–client relationship?
> ✔ What behaviors might indicate the client's dependence on the nurse–client relationship?

Professional Boundaries

Nursing is a helping profession, one in which compassion and concern are integral to the care provided. However, for the mental health nurse, the emotional and psychological problems of the client are especially challenging. The desire to help the clients or ease their burden can easily draw the nurse into personal involvement that crosses the line of professionalism.

Within the therapeutic nurse–client relationship, it is the nurse's responsibility to initiate and maintain limits or **professional boundaries**. The guidelines for professional behavior are centered on a condition of helpfulness. Too much concern or not enough can both cross this standard. According to the National Council of State Boards of Nursing, professional boundaries are the "spaces between the power of the nurse and the vulnerability of the client" (NCSBN, 2018). It is important for the nurse to set boundary standards that provide for safe interactions with the client.

It is vital for the nurse to remember that the needs of the nurse are distinctly different from those of the client. Some interventions are helpful and promote independence of the client, but others actually cause the client to develop a dependence on the relationship. Clients need an explanation to help them understand where the line of distinction lies in the nurse's response to the client's needs and requests. Clarification of the nurse's role may be necessary in situations in which the boundary may be violated. Situations such as involvement in personal relationships of the client, financial affairs unrelated to the treatment process, or a third-party liaison that is not treatment related are issues that must be clearly understood. The nurse must identify and reinforce explanations to the client where the boundaries are. For example, if a client asks the nurse to relay a personal message to their girlfriend who happens to live next-door to the nurse, the nurse must decline and explain to the client that the request is outside their professional role. Events surrounding any situation that deviates from the baseline of helpfulness and involves professional boundaries should be clearly documented in the client's clinical record.

> **Just the Facts** When taken to extremes, qualities such as commitment, selflessness, and responsibility that are found in nurses can hinder the client's progress toward independence.

As clients improve, they are expected to function independently to the highest level of which they are capable. When nurses allow a strong sense of commitment and personal need to help the client overshadow a focus on the client's needs, professional boundaries have been crossed. The nurse cannot let the relationship fulfill a personal need and remain objective about the client's needs at the same time. Anytime the nurse shows more concern for one client over another, they are at risk for becoming too involved. When focus on the client is maintained, it is less likely that the nurse will be manipulated into violating professional ethics. The nurse–client relationship must not extend beyond the therapeutic termination phase. Any further contact by phone, mail, e-mail, or socialization is in violation of the professional code of ethics. If former clients are seen outside of the mental health setting, it is important to avoid recognition or speaking to them unless the client recognizes the nurse and speaks to them first. Detailed conversation or other interactions should be avoided.

> **Just the Facts** Client-specific interactions and actions in which boundaries are clarified should be documented in the client medical record.

> **Mind Jogger** ❷ How might a nurse's strong sense of commitment lead to a violation of professional boundaries?

Violations of professional boundaries can occur when gray areas exist in the delivery of mental health care. The deviation from the standard is often an unintentional act that was intended to be helpful but crosses that line. Acts that may fall into this category of boundary violations include unnecessary personal disclosure by the nurse, secrecy, sexual misconduct, over-helping, controlling, and role reversal in the nurse–client relationship. Personal experiences and feelings associated with an issue can be transferred to the client situation and influence how the nurse responds. The nurse should never share personal feelings or experiences to the client even in an attempt to show they understand how the client feels. The nurse must maintain constant vigilance and mentally review their own feelings in order to separate themselves from the client. The nurse must also avoid flirtation in any manner or giving specialized individual attention to any one client. A nurse becoming overinvolved in the client's problem, to the point where other team members are excluded, clearly departs from the integrity of the professional role. Box 5.3 provides some guidelines for professional behavior from the NCSBN.

> **BOX 5.3**
>
> **Nursing Guides for Professional Behavior**
> - Be aware
> - Be cognizant of feelings and behavior
> - Be observant of the behavior of other professionals
> - Always act in the best interest of the client
>
> Source: National Council of State Boards of Nursing (NCSBN). *Professional boundaries: A nurse's guide to professional boundaries.* https://www.ncsbn.org/public-files/ProfessionalBoundaries_Complete.pdf

"Sammy"

You have been assigned to an older adult client, Samson. When you introduce yourself to him, he asks you to call him "Sammy." You establish a time each day to meet to discuss what he wants to accomplish for the day and what activities he can participate in to meet those goals. After several shifts you look forward to working with Sammy. His daily jokes remind you of your favorite uncle who is the same age as Sammy. On your day off you wonder if the staff will help him with his daily goals like you always do.

Digging Deeper

1. What questions would it be important to ask yourself?

2. What action should you take on your day off?

3. Have you done anything improper?

4. What would be an appropriate action to take when returning to work?

CASE STUDY 5.1

Response to Difficult Client Behaviors

The nurse–client relationship may involve situations in which the nurse is challenged with brief periods of inappropriate or difficult client behaviors, especially when working with clients who have mental health issues. It is important for the nurse to observe and anticipate behaviors that may require an immediate or directed response. Most client displays of excessive behavior response are the result of personality problems or in response to other issues such as their mental illness or heightened anxiety levels. The basic dynamic at the root of these difficult situations is the client's individual response to anxiety created by environmental or internal stressors. The reaction may reflect personality characteristics, or it may be totally out of character for the person. Under high levels of stress, a person may respond in a manner atypical of the normal expected behavior for that individual. Some of the more common difficult client situations include manipulation, violence or aggression, altered thought process (e.g., hallucinations, illusions, delusions), and sexually inappropriate behaviors or aggression.

Manipulation

Clients who exhibit manipulative behaviors usually tend to be impulsive and are unable to tolerate frustration or inattention to their requests. They may demand instant gratification of their needs and lack of self-control. The nursing approach is to recognize what the client is attempting to do and reinforce limits. It is important that limits are maintained by all the nursing staff in a consistent manner. A client who displays manipulation can recognize when the boundaries are not firmly enforced. This leaves open the opportunity for the client to plot strategies that undermine the care plan.

Limits should be fair and explained thoroughly to the client. In response to manipulation, nurses should avoid reinforcing the negative behavior and focus on the feelings the client is experiencing at the present time. For example, a response to the client who is constantly asking the nurse to come to their room might be, "You seem to be uncomfortable being by yourself." Further interaction can then be aimed toward the client's thoughts and response.

Mind Jogger ② How could limit setting be used to effectively establish behavior parameters in a way that is nonpunitive?

Violence or Aggression

Clients may become hostile or violent without warning. Typical triggers for violence or aggression include poor self-regulation, feelings of having lost control, having had limits recently imposed upon them (e.g., told they cannot use the phone until a certain time or cannot smoke inside the building), being under the influence of a substance, or reactions to internal stimuli (e.g., hearing voices or having a hallucination). There are also certain time frames on the unit when a client may act on their aggression. Predictable times for violence or aggression include when the staff are distracted such as during shift change, during the admission of a new client, or when another client is being aggressive or violent. It is not unusual for nurses to be concerned for their personal safety, or the safety of others, when a client is being hostile or violent. Important safety measures to protect the nurse are listed in Box 5.4.

It is most important to keep in mind the safety of the client and other persons in the immediate area. Clients usually exhibit an increasing state of

---

BOX 5.4

Safety Measures

PRECAUTIONARY MEASURES TO ALWAYS PERFORM

- Maintain at least two-arm's–length distance between you and the client.
- Do not turn your back to the client.
- Do not wear lanyards around your neck whenever possible—if worn they must be the break-away type. Avoid necklaces.
- Position yourself closest to the exit or stand in the doorway.
- The client should not be allowed to sit between you and the exit (do not allow yourself to be "trapped").
- Do not attempt to touch the client without their approval.
- Be vigilant:
  - to client behavior and cues (clenching fists, kicking chair, etc.).
  - during shift change.
  - when setting limits.

INTERVENTIONS TO TAKE WHEN A CLIENT IS ACTIVELY AGGRESSIVE OR VIOLENT

- Call for assistance—many units have a code for this situation.
- Do not provoke the behavior or threaten the client with action.
- Do not enter a room alone when a client is out of control.
- Move other clients away from the area.

TECHNIQUES THAT MAY HELP DECREASE CLIENT AGITATION OR HOSTILITY

- Lower your voice.
- Acknowledge their feelings ("You seem angry.").
- Offer the client time to regain control and stop the behavior.
- Eliminate excess stimuli if possible (have someone turn off the TV or radio, dim lights).

---

anxiety prior to any aggressive behavior. The nurse who recognizes these signs in the early stages can often de-escalate the behavior using communication and a calm approach that provides the time and space the client needs to regain control. In some situations, it may be best to ensure the safety of other clients and move them away from the immediate location, which allows space and time for the agitated client to defuse.

Altered Thought Process (Hallucinations, Illusions, Delusions)

Clients with altered thought processes are often suspicious and guarded in their behavior. Because the basic feelings of the client are fear and mistrust, the nurse should be especially careful to provide explanations in a language and context the client can understand. During a therapeutic encounter, it is important to impart a feeling of genuine concern for the discomfort that the client may be experiencing. All movement by the nurse should be purposeful and carefully executed to avoid actions that can be misinterpreted. Touch should be avoided and personal space maintained so that the client does not feel threatened or trapped.

Initially, if the client is seeing or hearing something that is not apparent to the nurse, the nurse should acknowledge and clarify the content. For example, if a client is seeing someone in the room who is not obviously present, the nurse can respond with, "I don't see anyone in the room except you and me. Tell me what the person is doing." If the client is hearing voices, a response such as, "I don't hear anyone talking. Tell me what they are saying to you" is appropriate. Once the nurse has insight into the content, the focus should be diverted from the hallucination or delusional thought. It is nontherapeutic to allow the client to continue the description. It is ineffective to argue or tell the client that what they are experiencing is not real. Remember that these are symptoms of the illness and are real to the person who is experiencing them. The nurse should reestablish the client's contact with reality and focus on the feelings the client is presently experiencing. For example, a client tells the nurse, "They are laughing at me and saying ugly things about me." Once the nurse has clarified the content, an appropriate reply might be, "I understand that is hard to hear. Tell me about what you are feeling now." If the content of the altered thought process is threatening to the client or another individual

"Connie"

Connie is 35-year-old woman with a diagnosis of bipolar disorder. She is brought to the psychiatric unit after being detained in the county jail for disruptive behavior. In her present manic state, Connie is aggressive both verbally and physically. She has just removed all of her clothing in the hallway while loudly inviting male attention. She has not sat down in the 6 hours she has been on the unit, nor has she eaten any food. She claims she is "Queen of the Nile in the body of a shark." Several of the other clients appear anxious and fearful as they observe her behavior.

Digging Deeper

1. *What would be the best approach to this situation?*

2. *What is your responsibility to Connie? What is your responsibility to the other clients?*

3. *What can the nurse do to begin a therapeutic relationship with Connie?*

4. *How could limit setting be used to manage Connie's behavior?*

CASE STUDY 5.2

(e.g., "They are telling me to stab myself."), every effort should be made to protect the client and others from injury.

Sexually Inappropriate Behaviors or Aggression

Most clients will refrain from making suggestive or sexually oriented comments or advances once they are asked to stop. The nurse should be direct in letting the client know that the actions are unacceptable. Once the limits have been established, the client has a choice to use self-control. The nurse can then proceed to discuss the underlying issue with the client. If the behavior continues, the nurse can terminate the session, citing the behavior as the reason (e.g., "I will not tolerate this behavior. I am going now. I will come back at a later time."). This will allow the client time to reflect on the actions and leave open the option of discussing the behavior at a later point. If the situation becomes unmanageable, the nurse should consult with a supervisor or colleague.

> **Test Yourself**
> ✔ Give two examples of behaviors seen in manipulative clients.
> ✔ Name four precautionary safety measures you would perform.
> ✔ How would you respond if a client asks if you want to go on a date?

Cultural Considerations

Cultural Differences in Communication

A therapeutic relationship requires the nurse to effectively communicate with the client. This includes determining the language the client is most comfortable speaking. The use of an interpreter may be needed if the nurse does not speak the client's preferred language. Nonverbal communication also impacts the therapeutic relationship. Some nonverbal communication may be culturally appropriate to either the nurse or client but offensive to the other. Other examples of cultural differences in communication include:

- Pointing a finger can be seen as giving a direction or as an insult.

- When confronted by an unacceptable topic, the individual may completely stop talking and avoid looking at the other person.
- A woman making eye contact with a man may be viewed as flirtatious.
- Personal space, either sitting or standing close to, or further away from, each other may be perceived as rude or intrusive.
- Showing emotions can be seen as inappropriate as it burdens the other person.
- Sticking out one's tongue can be a greeting.

SUMMARY

- The therapeutic relationship is a helping, interactive exchange between a client and a mental health professional. This compact is formed with the goal of improved functioning and well-being for the client.
- The nurse–client relationship is based on trust with honest communication that focuses on the client's feelings and problems. An empathetic and accepting approach is necessary to see the client as a unique person with individual needs and issues. Empathy allows the nurse to grasp and view the present situation from the client's perspective. Active listening engages the nurse attentively in both mind and body to capture what the client is conveying in both verbal and nonverbal messages.
- Self-awareness is a process of self-evaluation and an attempt to see oneself through the eyes of others. This provides insight into how the nurse responds to their environment and how others react to the nurse's behavior.
- The willingness to see oneself realistically can open the door for positive change and improved interpersonal relationships. This same awareness is encouraged in the client with mental health issues.
- Although it may be difficult for clients to identify problems related to their behavior, doing so can allow them to take ownership of the problem and commit to a plan for change.
- The therapeutic nurse–client relationship consists of the phases: orientation, working, and termination.
- The initial contact with the client identifies the purpose and guidelines for the interaction. In addition, it ensures a safe and trusting milieu designed to facilitate and encourage the client to express needs and problems without criticism or reprisal.
- A series of interactive sessions is conducted with therapeutic communication techniques designed to explore and identify client problems and possible options for resolution. These sessions maintain a client focus to help set priorities for short-term goals that lead to improved functioning.
- The relationship is terminated at a point when the client is seen as having adequate skills and emotional resources to function independently. This is an important step to helping the client move back into society in an adaptive manner.
- Professional boundaries are the gaps that exist between the indirect power of the nurse and the vulnerable state of the client. Because the nurse has the knowledge and control inherent in a professional role, it becomes vital that a perspective of helpfulness be maintained.
- Client needs must be foremost and the focus of all therapeutic nursing interventions. The nurse must be cautious not to reverse these roles in the process of maintaining the relationship.
- To avoid an unintentional violation of the ethical standards of behavior, the nurse should maintain a constant vigilance and awareness of actions that might be perceived as overly involved in the client's situation.
- Some client situations may pose a threat or challenge to the nurse. It is important for the nurse to remain focused and anticipate behaviors that may demand an immediate or directed response. Manipulation, violence and aggression, altered thought processes, and sexually inappropriate behaviors can all require acute nursing observation and interventions.
- The nurse can take precautionary measures to help provide for their safety. The nurse can also institute interventions when a client is actively aggressive or violent. There are also techniques the nurse can implement that may help decrease client agitation or hostility.

BIBLIOGRAPHY

Moore, G. P., & Pfaff, J. A. (2022). Assessment and emergency management of the acutely agitated or violent adult. *UpToDate*. Retrieved April 3, 2022, from https://www.uptodate.com/contents/assessment-and-emergency-management-of-the-acutely-agitated-or-violent-adult

National Council of State Boards of Nursing. (2018). *Professional boundaries: A nurse's guide to professional boundaries.* https://www.ncsbn.org/public-files/ProfessionalBoundaries_Complete.pdf

National Institute for Occupational Safety and Health. (2022). *Violence occupational hazards in hospitals.* Centers for Disease Control and Prevention. https://www.cdc.gov/niosh/docs/2002-101/default.html

Occupational Safety and Health Administration. (2015). *Guidelines for preventing workplace violence for healthcare and social service workers.* U.S. Department of Labor. OSHA 3148-06R 2016. https://www.osha.gov/sites/default/files/publications/osha3148.pdf

Skodol, A., & Bender, D. (2018). Establishing and maintaining a therapeutic relationship in psychiatric practice. *UpToDate*. Retrieved March 31, 2022, from https://www.uptodate.com/contents/establishing-and-maintaining-a-therapeutic-relationship-in-psychiatric-practice

Fill in the Blank

Fill in the blank with the correct answer.

1. The ability to hear what another person says and to borrow those feelings to perceive a situation from that person's viewpoint is referred to as _____.
2. _____ is a consciousness of our own personality and behavior in response to the world around us.
3. Therapeutic relationships are dependent on the _____ and _____ of the individual client.
4. The termination phase of the therapeutic relationship promotes _____ for the client in getting along with others as preparation for discharge.
5. When nurses allow a need to "help" to overshadow a focus on the needs of the client, professional _____ have been crossed.
6. Clients usually demonstrate an increasing state of _____ prior to aggressive behavior.

Matching

Match the following terms to the most appropriate phrase.

1. _____ Self-awareness
2. _____ Holistic
3. _____ Orientation phase
4. _____ Working phase
5. _____ Active listening
6. _____ Professional boundaries

a. Listening attentively using both mind and body
b. Period of planning outcomes and interventions toward behavior change with improved client well-being
c. Consciousness of own individuality and personality
d. Totality of biologic, psychosocial, cultural, and spiritual functioning of an individual
e. Gaps between the control of the nurse and the vulnerable state of the client
f. Time of building trust, establishing roles, and identifying problems and expectations

Multiple Choice

Select the best answer from the multiple-choice items.

1. When establishing a therapeutic environment, which of the following factors would be most important in forming the foundation for a trusting nurse–client relationship? *(Select all that apply)*
   a. Nonjudgmental approach to client
   b. Sympathetic attitude of the nurse
   c. Educational background of the client
   d. Amount of time spent with the client
   e. Honesty and consistent integrity of the nurse

2. The nurse is working with a client who says, "You are the only one who really cares about me. I feel like everyone else is giving me the shove just because I am getting out of here this week." What does the client's statement demonstrate?
   a. Avoidance
   b. Withdrawal
   c. Ambivalence
   d. Manipulation

3. The client suddenly starts shouting and tightening their fists. What would be an appropriate action for the nurse?
   a. Acknowledge the client's change in behavior
   b. Tell the client they will be secluded if the behavior continues
   c. Touch the client's arm and ask them to calm down
   d. Walk away from the client without responding

4. What can the nurse do to promote a safe environment? *(Select all that apply)*
   a. Perform a self-assessment
   b. Sit at the back of the common room to observe all client behaviors
   c. Lead the clients to the cafeteria so they don't get lost
   d. Observe a client after they were told that meals do not come with soft drinks
   e. Have only two of six oncoming staff receive hand-off shift report at a time

5. The nurse is explaining the content of a contract with behavior guidelines to a client. Which phase of the therapeutic relationship is the nurse facilitating?
   a. Orientation
   b. Working
   c. Termination
   d. Evaluation

6. Which statement best describes the role of the nurse in terminating the therapeutic relationship with the client?
   a. To reduce the amount of time spent with the client
   b. Encouraging independence and self-reliance of the client
   c. Reinforcing continued support following discharge
   d. Discussing possible solutions to the present problem

7. Which situation shows the nurse violating professional boundaries in the nurse–client relationship? The nurse:
   a. Encourages the client to discuss feelings of remorse over rejection by another client
   b. Agrees to relay personal information about the client to the therapist
   c. Calls a client who was discharged 2 weeks earlier to see if they are attending therapy
   d. Assists a client who is disabled with physical hygiene and bathing

8. A client tells the nurse, "I feel so secure when I am with you. Don't tell the others, but you are the best nurse here." What is the nurse's most appropriate response?
   a. "I am glad you feel secure with me. I will try to spend more time with you."
   b. "You don't mean that. There are many good nurses here."
   c. "Why do you feel more secure with me than the others?"
   d. "It seems as though you are feeling anxious. Tell me about that."

9. Which of the following behaviors by the nurse would be considered a violation of professional boundaries in the nurse–client relationship?
   a. Accepting a gift from a client
   b. Showing genuine concern for the client
   c. Listening while client talks about a problem with intimacy
   d. Talking with client in privacy of client's room

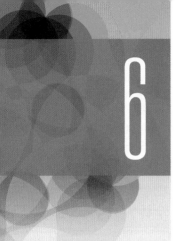

6 Dynamics of Anger, Violence, and Crises

Anger and Aggression

Negative human emotions tend to disrupt feelings of internal comfort. They can range from a mild feeling of discontent to a volatile degree of hostile and potentially harmful outrage. Anger is a universal emotion. Sometimes this emotion can have a short-term positive effect. However, not everyone is able to harness their feelings before they get out of control. The spiraling effects of this escalation in emotion are often at the root of abuse and violence. Although aggressive behavior may be seen as one way of expressing anger, it is not an acceptable outlet for negative emotions. Acting out in a violent manner is never a positive way to handle the feelings associated with anger or its associated emotions.

Defining Anger

Anger is an emotion triggered in response to threats, insulting situations, or anything that seriously hampers the intended actions of an individual. In one sense, anger is a natural adaptive response needed for survival in the face of a threat or danger. In most instances, however, the reaction may be directed at a specific person or, in a generalized sense, toward a group and even society itself. The anger builds into bitterness and becomes an unconscious hurt that breeds a desire to get even. These negative feelings are often expressed through hurtful words or actions toward another individual. The feelings can also be self-directed, resulting in varying degrees of guilt, anxiety, and depression. A mild form of anger may be described as annoyance that, if provoked, can escalate to a more volatile state. Anger can also be expressed aggressively, either verbally or nonverbally in the form of hostility, or can spiral to intense anger or rage that may result in violence toward the subject.

Trait Anger

Trait anger is often referred to as a general biologic leaning toward a volatile personality that may be described by the person themselves as a "quick-temper," a feeling of becoming "hot," feeling their heart rate accelerate, or behavior that reflects a quick response of irritation and fury. The individual with this type of personality typically has a habitual response to frustrating circumstances that trigger a negative social outcome. They may have difficulty interacting and encountering new relationships or social situations without preformed opinions or biases. This makes it more difficult to avoid conflict and tense atmospheres, while those with low trait anger may be able to compromise and develop longer solid relationships.

Just the Facts An individual who is easily frustrated and angered usually has a history of being irritable, touchy, and quick-tempered from an early age.

Expressing Anger and Resentment

Both anger and resentment originate in the mental perception of a situation. This perception usually includes feelings of being wronged, ignored, cheated, or abused in some way. When an individual feels insulted, their reaction generates the need to fight back. This unconscious frustration becomes their private battle within the mind where emotions follow the thoughts. Anger can be used in a manipulative way to cause an emotional reaction in another in order to get them to act in accordance with the thinking of the angry individual. Often, perceptions of anger are formed during the vulnerable years of childhood and the perceptions carry over throughout one's lifetime. Other situations such as cases of intimate partner violence (IPV), rape, and abuse can instill the desire for retribution. Suppressed over time, the hurt turns into resentment and often is expressed in a destructive means of resolution. Effects of anger include a clouded assessment of the situation, a change in focus, energy depletion, creation of painful emotions, and a destruction of teamwork. Concealed hurt is often turned inward resulting in depression. It can also be a reason someone becomes involved in an unhealthy relationship. Suppressed or concealed anger can lead to both physical and psychological disorders.

In many instances, the outward reaction fueled by the emotions may be directed at a specific object or person, or in a generalized sense, toward a group and even society itself. The indirect expression of resentment or chronic anger is often seen in the projection of the negative feelings toward another object or person. The anger builds into bitterness and becomes an unconscious hurt that breeds a desire to get even. These feelings can also be self-directed resulting in varying degrees of guilt, anxiety, and depression.

Unrestrained Anger and Violence

Anger and its associated emotions are expressed in different ways. The individual with high trait anger is more likely to respond with aggressive behavior or violence. Anger-based aggressive behavior is termed **hostility,** or an intense feeling of animosity toward someone or something. Hostility can be a precursor to a confrontation, which can result in physical aggression and violent behavior. **Aggression** can include behavior that may result in both physical and psychological harm to oneself or another that can occur both verbally and nonverbally. **Violence** is an expression of anger or resentment in an attempt to maintain power in a situation or relationship. This may be related to a misconstrued belief of entitlement, manipulation, rationalization, or indifference toward the feelings of another.

Rooted in a feeling of being wronged is the desire to retaliate or "get even." Given fuel, this bitterness and anger will send the individual into an aggressive overdrive. In this emotional state, the individual is capable of inflicting harm on another person or themselves. In other words, the anger is in control. Although inappropriate, violence and abusive behaviors are often learned responses in an environment where this is the norm. Growing up, the child learns to deal with frustration and disappointment by observing patterns modeled by the family members. Since the conditioned response may be reactive and automatic, neutralizing efforts to dissolve the intensity of the emotion, or to resolve the situation through problem solving, may be ineffective, especially during an intense expression of the feelings.

Along with family influence, the effect of peer relationships and the community are major in the learned anger response. The individual who is constantly subjected to violent verbal or physical responses learns this behavior to be the normal or accepted reaction. The individual may also be the object of the anger and receive both verbal and physical results of adult fury. With continued exposure to this negative world, they are given few chances to develop trusting, positive relationships to counteract the cycle. When they are faced with their own feelings of anger, their immediate impulse is to utilize the defense that was modeled to them.

> **Just the Facts** Explaining anger in a logical way to oneself defeats the fury of the emotion. Anger, even if justified, is an irrational means to an end.

Violence has become a central theme to many shows on television, movies, and video games. Because these are seen as fictional and action-packed, they are accepted as entertainment. Much research has been done to see if there is a link between an individual who plays violent video games and commits violent crimes. Many individuals who play violent video games never commit violence. This would suggest other factors than violent video games lead an individual to be violent.

Large-scale acts of violence, such as mass shootings, are committed by an individual or individuals who use the violence as a response to their own provocations and/or feelings of being wronged by someone or society in general. When the life experiences of the individual are reviewed after the large-scale act of violence, it is often revealed they had one or more of the following: a troubled childhood, experienced repeated bullying during their school-age years, difficulty getting along with others, truancy at a young age, history of harming animals, or a significant loss they felt someone needed to be punished for. It is important to recognize that none of those factors alone automatically predispose an individual to violence. One or more of these factors combined with poor coping skills or a personality that is easily angered increases the risk that an individual for externally reacting to a stimulus.

> **Test Yourself**
> ✔ Describe the difference between anger and trait anger.
> ✔ Give an example of aggression.
> ✔ What can happen to a child who has continued exposure to aggression or violence?

Constructive Methods of Managing Anger

An instinctive reaction to anger is aggression; however, the individual also has the ability to be in control of their behavior. They can choose a negative response or can elect to develop steps toward managing or redirecting the anger in a constructive way. Some people learn to manage their anger earlier in life than others. Other people may need guidance in learning this skill. For clients who receive treatment related to their anger, the nurse may ask them questions such as "What is it that sets you off or makes you angry?" or "How do you react when you get really angry?" This can help the client in starting to recognize the origin or triggers of their anger and how these relate to their behavior. Stating these thoughts out loud can help the client understand why they respond as they do. This awareness gives them the opportunity to assume control of their anger.

Restructured Thinking

Putting the situation in perspective with restructured thinking can help prevent the individual from overdramatizing the facts. Sensible reasoning can diffuse anger. Anger that is left unchecked will accelerate and can lead to negative and harmful consequences. The feelings created do not resolve the situation underlying the emotion, but rethinking the worst possible scenario can make it more palatable. For instance, if one feels like other people in the workplace are "always saying things behind my back," one might restructure it by replacing it with "maybe I can turn this around by saying nice things to them." This approach requires self-control to restrain one's volatile feelings before they lead to actions one regrets later (see Fig. 6.1).

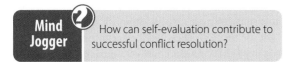

Mind Jogger How can self-evaluation contribute to successful conflict resolution?

Physical Activity

One way to manage the anger is to engage in some form of physical activity such as walking, jogging, or playing tennis or a game of volleyball.

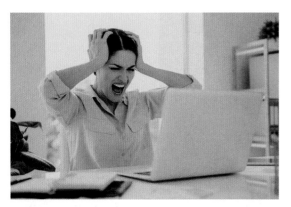

Figure 6.1 Recognizing the sources of anger can help a person regain control. When the emotion of anger is elicited in a person, the result is both an emotional and an internal physiologic combination that stimulates and accelerates the nervous system. In order to control the emotion, the individual must also take steps to decrease the body's response.

The activity utilizes energy for a constructive purpose rather than an emotional outburst. People who know their temperament is easily irritated may want to plan a "time-out" period each day for exercise and meditation. Separating oneself from the situation allows the mind time to reflect and think about the cause of the feelings. Sometimes changing the timing surrounding the conflict (e.g., parental confrontation after school or at meal-time, arguing with a spouse when both are tired) and allowing a cool-down period before discussing issues can allow time to think about the emotions before the interaction and separate reaction from an impulsive action in words or deeds.

Assertion

Anger can also be managed through assertion. **Assertion** is standing up for one's rights, beliefs, or values in such a way that it does not hurt others in the process. This demonstrates a form of respect for oneself and for those with whom one interacts. Thinking about the situation usually precedes assertive behavior. This gives the individual an opportunity to restructure and replace negative thoughts with more rational ones. For example, a young couple is arguing over their vacation plans. One says, "You never want to do what I want. I'm going to my parents' and you can go by yourself!" Restructured into a more rational approach, they might say, "I really want to see my parents on this trip. Could we work that into your plan?" Recognizing that anger will not solve a problem can help address the issue and find a solution.

"I" Statements

Using "I" statements allows for feelings and thoughts to be expressed in a way that avoids attacking the other person. Volatile emotions can often be diffused when there is a mutual willingness to view a situation from more than one perspective. This approach of conflict resolution and improved communication can rechannel the negative feelings into a situation where all participants benefit.

Expressing Feelings

Talking with someone who will listen is also a positive means of reducing the intensity of emotions. Sometimes in talking with someone else, humor can add a dimension that lightens the impact of the feelings. An objective view from another person can sometimes help the individual to see the situation from another angle. If another person is not available, the individual can use a tape recorder to provide the listening ear. Writing or typing a letter but never sending it can allow the individual to express their thoughts and feelings without hurting the other person. Feelings are brought outward and mellowed by acknowledging them in print. This prevents the buildup of resentment or animosity over time that results in hostile feelings.

Counseling in anger management allows time to reflect and discover reasons behind the anger and learn new ways of coping with the feelings. Anger management groups also allow the individual to not only to learn how to cope and control their anger but also to see that other people also struggle with similar feelings and problems and how they handle them. Anger management classes may help perpetrators in intimate partner violence (IPV) situations to address issues of power and control which are central to the abuse.

Forgiveness

Perhaps the most effective means of dealing with the negative feelings of anger is forgiveness, both of someone else or oneself. Holding on to anger or bitterness is like a chronic disease that is harmful both physically and psychologically. True joy and happiness become diminished by the negativity and animosity that come from holding grudges. Forgiveness allows the individual to let go of the hurt and to heal the bruises of emotional pain and bitterness. True forgiveness is cleansing and brings peace within. Forgiving oneself often involves apologizing or confessing to another person for something one may or may not have done. Learning to forgive is difficult, but once done will lift the burdens one has been carrying.

Test Yourself
- ✔ Give two examples of an "I" statement.
- ✔ Name five different constructive methods an individual can use to manage their anger.

Bullying

Violence and aggression can also manifest as **bullying,** which is psychological harassment or physical confrontation used repeatedly to intentionally bring harm or humiliation to one seen as weak or different. This form of abuse gains strength because of the power imbalance, whether real or perceived, between the perpetrator (bully) and the person being bullied. Bullying increases school absenteeism and poor scholastic performance, anxiety, sleep difficulties, violence at schools, and adolescent suicide. Box 6.1 lists some information related to bullying. It is a frightening experience for the recipient that may be done

---

"Kendall"

From an early age, Kendall has had what most people called a "short fuse." Because he would always argue and start fights, it became difficult for him to make friends during his school years. In addition, nothing seemed to curb the angry response Kendall displayed when his parents tried to discipline him. Aside from his inability to control his temper, Kendall was intelligent and athletic. He made good grades and engaged in competitive sports. Social relationships remained an issue as he was controlling and impulsive.

After graduating from college, Kendall works in a pharmaceutical laboratory. Coworkers describe him as "touchy" and "easily ticked off," but brilliant and efficient at what he does. One day, Kendall is unable to contain his anger over an incident in which a lab technician makes an error in a chemical formula. Kendall becomes so irate and angry that he throws the flask across the room, narrowly missing the young technician's head. The technician runs out of the lab screaming that "He's lost it this time!" Kendall is put on leave from the company and is required to enter treatment for anger management.

Digging Deeper

1. How are anger and aggression evident in Kendall's situation?

2. In what ways might Kendall's behavior be a conditioned response?

3. What methods might be used to help him defuse some of his anger before it controls him?

CASE STUDY 6.1

BOX 6.1

Bullying Incidence

- 1 out of 5 students report being the victim of bullying
- Male students report being victims of physical bullying more than female students, and female students report being bullied more by social means.
- Cyberbullying has negative impacts on self-esteem, friendships, physical health, and schoolwork.
- Middle-school students report being victims of cyberbullying more than high school students.
- The types of cyberbullying most often reported are hurtful comments and rumors spread online.
- Males report that they were threatened online more than females.
- Students with disabilities are more worried about being bullied than students who do not have disabilities.
- LGBTQ students report being bullied because of their sexual orientation or gender expression and report feeling unsafe at school.
- Observing bullying has also been linked to mental health issues.
- Peer supportive actions to bullying (spending time with person being bullied, talking to them, or giving advice) were perceived as more helpful than teacher actions.

Adapted from PACER's National Bullying Prevention Center. (2022). *Bullying statistics by the numbers.* Retrieved April 15, 2022, from https://www.pacer.org/bullying/info/stats.asp

in different ways. Bullying can occur in the following forms: physical (hitting, pushing, kicking, tripping), verbal (name-calling, teasing), social (excluding from group, spreading rumors, texting), or destroying property belonging to the targeted individual. Cyberbullying is another form of bullying, in which damaging entries may be posted on the internet or social network that can cause serious and often irreparable harm.

The perpetrator usually surrounds themselves with allies who enhance the bully's feeling of power. The bully continues to pick on the target daily while seeming to enjoy the obvious fright and fear of the victim. Timing of the harassment is usually during a time when an authority figure is not present. This pattern of repeated intent to diminish the victim and harm them distinguishes bullying from other types of conflict. The bullying can cause the victim to drop out of school and can even lead to mental health issues as a result of the psychological abuse. The problems experienced by these individuals may extend into adulthood with difficulties in

the individual's ability to function both in relationships and society in general.

Mind Jogger With the increase in cyberbullying, what can be done by parents or the victims themselves to reduce the harmful effects?

Those who experience bullying develop a feeling of low self-esteem and helplessness as a result of the repeated threats and taunting hurtful abuse. This sense of decreased self-worth can be devastating and lead to serious depression and emotional problems. There is a strong association between bullying and self-harm, suicidal ideation, and suicide. When suicide occurs as a result of bullying there are often other additional factors such as depression or substance use. Some instances of suicide occur after the victim has been encouraged to end their life or told that that the world would be better without them.

Intimate Partner Violence and Abuse

Intimate partner violence (IPV) is seen in all social, economic, and educational levels and can affect anyone regardless of gender, ethnicity, race, religion, income, sexual orientation, or age. The effects leave the victim with a sense of fear and hopelessness that is often shrouded in secrecy caused by intimidation from the abuser. Children who grow up in families where abuse and violence are common experiences tend to continue the modeled behaviors in adult relationships either as an abuser or as a person experiencing abuse.

Intimate Partner Violence Defined

Intimate partner violence (IPV) is a pattern of behavior displayed by a current or former intimate partner using physical or sexual violence, psychological intimidation, aggression, or stalking. Intimate partner violence (IPV) was previously called domestic abuse or domestic violence. The **abuser** (formerly called the batterer) inflicts harmful or offensive conflict, the abuse, on their partner. The abuser gains power and control over their partner through violence that causes the partner to be fearful and intimidated. The violence can take the form of threats or emotional, physical, economic, or sexual abuse. It is estimated that 1 in 4 women and 1 in 10 men have experienced some form of intimate partner violence (IPV) (CDC, 2021b).

Physical abuse is an intentional injury to another person and can include slapping, pinching, choking, scratching, stabbing, shooting, and homicide. **Emotional abuse** inflicts psychological trauma as words and nonverbal language are used to criticize, demean, or humiliate another person. Each incident further deteriorates the self-esteem of the victim. The batterer often blames the victim for the abuse which leads to feelings of guilt in the victim. **Sexual abuse** and/or rape often accompanies other forms of abuse and refers to any behavior using forced or unwanted sexual acts that are inflicted on an unwilling participant. Any of these situations can also be accompanied by **stalking** which involves harassing or threatening phone calls, e-mails, texts, voice mails, mail, or unwanted appearances at the victim's place of employment, home, or other location. Stalking can also involve vandalism or forced entry of the victim's place of residence or vehicle. Abuse of a partner or parent also puts children in the home at risk for abuse and emotional and/or physical problems. Some research indicates that because of the trauma, the child may be at greater risk for emotional problems or substance use disorder.

Just the Facts | Intimate partner violence (IPV) and abuse are patterns of behavior used by one person to control or have power over another through fear and intimidation using threats or acts of violence.

Risk Factors

Individuals who abuse others tend to have experiences from their past that have provided the basis for their behavior. Certain personality traits can also lead to abusive behavior. These experiences and personality traits put an individual at risk for harming others. Conversely, there are protective factors that can help prevent an individual from becoming an abuser. Box 6.2 lists these risk and protective factors. Abusers tend to exhibit similar behaviors as a result of their experiences and personality traits (Box 6.3). Recognizing these characteristics and their potential to trigger destructive behavior can help avert the continued escalating incidence of violence-related events.

BOX 6.2

Factors of Abusers

Risk factors that might lead to an individual becoming an abuser:
- Family history of violence
- History of physical or emotional abuse as a child
- Excessive drug or alcohol use
- Low self-esteem
- Poor impulse or behavioral control
- Antisocial beliefs and attitudes
- Association with delinquent peers or gangs
- Social rejection
- Economic stress

Protective factors than can help prevent an individual becoming an abuser:
- Intolerant attitude toward deviance
- Positive self-esteem
- Highly developed social skills or competencies
- Realistic expectations of themselves and others
- Connectedness to family or friends outside the family
- Constructive coping strategies
- Religious beliefs

Adapted from Centers for Disease Control and Prevention. (2021). *Risk and protective factors for perpetration.* https://www.cdc.gov/violenceprevention/intimatepartnerviolence/riskprotectivefactors.html

Cycle of Violence and Abuse

Abusers do not start the relationship with violence. Often the beginning of the relationship is seen as ideal and the partner is seen as attentive and loving. As the relationship progresses, subtle behavior changes of the perpetrator begin occurring. Box 6.4 lists warning signs that the partner might be abusive.

Violence toward an individual starts with verbal or physical threats and assaults that quickly victimize the person into going along with the

BOX 6.3

Traits Exhibited by Abusers

- Moody and overly sensitive to criticism
- Power-seeking or overly competitive
- Blame others for their problems or feelings
- Rationalize the use of violent behavior as necessary to resolve a situation
- Expect others to meet their needs or wait on them
- Frequent arguing, cursing, or physical fighting
- Verbal threats against others
- History of degrading or putting down women

Warning Signs of an Abusive Partner

- Excessive jealousy (even imagining infidelity or flirtation, jealous of attention given to children)
- Being possessive of their partner's attention, time, and belongings
- Temper that is "set off" by minor inconveniences
- Verbal abuse, yelling, or calling their partner names
- Controlling behavior (checking phone call history, text messages, monitoring car mileage, regulating money, preventing partner from talking to or visiting friends or family, determining what the victim can or cannot wear)
- Controlling all household finances
- Blaming victim for anything that happens
- Demeaning the victim in private or publicly
- Cruelty to animals

Adapted from National Coalition Against Domestic Violence (NCADV). *Signs of abuse.* https://ncadv.org/signs-of-abuse

abuse. There may be blaming, insults, name-calling, or accusations of infidelity. Often the abuser will be extreme in controlling the family money, stopping the partner from getting a job or furthering their education, and isolating the family from relatives and friends. Stalking, threats of divorce, taking the children, and killing or harming the victim are ways the abusive partner seeks power. During these violent episodes, the abuser may punch walls or doors, throw objects, break mirrors or windows, tear clothing or furniture, block driveways or take keys, and take money or means for independence of the victim. The abused individual may attempt to protect themselves as the intensity of the attacks increases.

The emotional or verbal abuse often appears before the physical harm occurs. The contact level may include pushing, shoving, twisting limbs, slapping, punching, choking, hair pulling, forced sex, or threats with a weapon. Once major physical and emotional harm has been done to the victim, the abusive partner usually tries to offer some type of gift or loving gestures of remorse and promises it will not happen again. Ironically, this demonstration of sorrow sets the victim up for the next step of abuse in which the perpetrator justifies the behavior by blaming the victim. The victim feels guilt and accepts the blame. Each incident of this violence cycle further depletes the victim's self-esteem and sense of worth as they feel trapped and powerless to end the cycle. Figure 6.2 shows the cycle of violence.

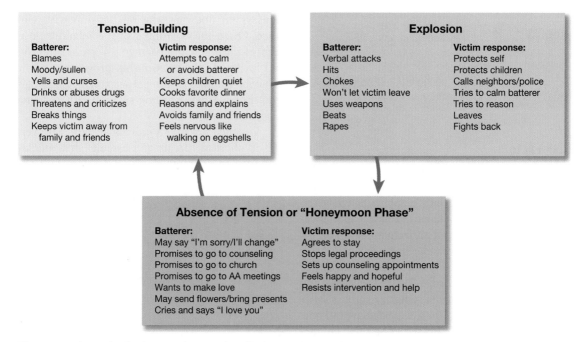

Figure 6.2 The cycle of violence with examples of behaviors that may be exhibited by the abuser or the victim. (Adapted with permission from Wolters Kluwer Health, Inc.: Kincheloe, C. A., & Hatfield, N. T. [2018]. *Introductory maternity & pediatric nursing* [4th ed.]. Wolters Kluwer.)

Just the Facts

Many women report that their intimate partner violence (IPV) started or intensified when they became pregnant. Pregnant women who experience intimate partner violence (IPV) during pregnancy are at a greater risk for postpartum depression, preterm birth, and low–birth-weight infants. All pregnant clients should be screened repeatedly during their pregnancy for intimate partner violence (IPV).

Source: Goodman, S. (2021). *Intimate partner violence endangers pregnant people and their infants*. National Partnership for Women & Families. https://www.nationalpartnership.org/our-work/health/moms-and-babies/intimate-partner-violence.html#

BOX 6.5

Help for Intimate Partner Violence and Abuse

- National Domestic Violence Hotline
  https://www.thehotline.org
  1-800-799-SAFE (7233)
  Text "START" to 88788
- Safe Horizon Domestic Violence Hotline
  https://www.safehorizon.org/hotlines
  1-800-621-HOPE (4673)
- Americans Overseas Domestic Violence Crisis Center
  Toll-free: 1-866-USWOMEN (879-6636) (International Crisis Line)
- National Resource Center on Domestic Violence
  https://www.nrcdv.org
- Rape, Abuse & Incest National Network (RAINN) Hotline
  https://www.rainn.org
  1-800-656-HOPE (4673)

There are many misconceptions about those who perpetrate and those who experience intimate partner violence (IPV). As stated earlier, violence is a character trait and not the result of the relationship. The person who is abused is not responsible for triggering the abuse. Ownership of the subsequent violent response solely belongs to the abuser. It is important to point out that mental health issues of depression, low self-esteem, anxiety, and fear are the result of abuse and not the cause. The abuser will continue to abuse until they get help. It is necessary for the abuser to recognize and take responsibility for their own actions.

The partner who has been abused often separates from an abusive partner only to return to the situation. This may be the result of fear of the abuser, feelings of guilt that it is their fault, lack of support or resources, or because they are encouraged to "try again" to make the relationship work. Sometimes the victim feels a dependency on the abuser for an income or because it would be detrimental to the children to break up the home. Abusers often search their partner's belongings for business cards or handouts with information on leaving the abuser and will destroy the information. Computer internet search histories are often monitored for any suggestion that the victim might be looking for a way to leave the abusive situation.

It is also important that intervention in this situation involves providing a safe environment and counseling to help build a sense of power, self-worth, and support for the person who has experienced abuse. The victim is usually in greatest danger right after the separation occurs as the abuser is flooded with a surge of anger and blame. There is a very real possibility of a tragic ending to this scenario. It is estimated that 1 in 5 homicides are committed by an intimate partner (CDC, 2021b). Some available links and hotlines are listed in Box 6.5.

Teen Dating Violence

Teenagers can also experience intimate partner violence (IPV). It is often referred to as teen dating violence. Teenage abusers have the same risk factors and traits as adults who are abusers. However, teens are less likely to report the dating violence for fear of telling friends or family. Teens who experience dating violence are more likely to experience symptoms of depression and anxiety, use drugs and alcohol as a coping mechanism, and think about suicide. It is important to recognize that teens who experience dating violence establish relationship patterns that can continue into adulthood. Reinforcing Client and Family Teaching 6.1 lists red flags that are seen in an abusive relationship that should be shared with teens who are in a relationship.

Test Yourself

✔ List four different forms intimate partner violence (IPV) can take.
✔ Identify four risk factors that an abuser might have.
✔ Describe the cycle of violence and abuse.
✔ How can nurses help to prevent, or advocate for a survivor of, intimate partner violence (IPV)?

Crisis and Intervention

A **psychological crisis** differs from stress and anxiety in that a state of disorganization and disarray occurs in the individual as usual coping strategies fail or are not available. The total inability to control the situation and to function in daily activities leads the person to seek a way out. The level of anxiety increases to a severe or panic level during which the individual feels helpless and lost. Attempts to cope may meet with little success. The state of dysfunction is usually receptive to the right intervention that can help the person stabilize and regain a sense of power and control over their own being.

Types of Crises

A model for crisis intervention developed in the early 1960s by Linder Mann and Gerald Caplan identifies two primary types of crisis situations. A **developmental crisis** may occur at a predictable time period in an individual's life related to maturational stages (e.g., teenage, mid-life, or old-age crises) and changes. The other type, a **situational**

crisis, is unpredictable and sudden without warning such as a fatal illness diagnosis, plane crash, natural disaster, or sudden death. Thoughts are dismantled and behavior changes in response to these crisis situations. People become confused, feel helpless and lost, and are easily angered and agitated.

It is important to note that intervention is not intended to correct the actual event or situation but to help the individual deal with their response to that situation. Intervention is an attempt to offer help to the client in the way of support, resources, and short-term stabilization.

Just the Facts Disorganization may result from an unrealistic perception of a threatening event, lack of a support system, or inadequate coping ability.

Crisis Intervention

A state of psychological crisis is intolerable if help is not received. Resolution will usually allow the person to either emerge at a higher and more productive level of functioning, at the same level, or at a lower level of coping ability. The outcome depends on the actions taken by the individual to cope with the crisis and those taken by others to intervene. During a crisis, an individual is often more receptive to support from others and can learn adaptive coping strategies to assist in the resolution. Reassuring the person that they are mentally healthy and encouraging them to remember how they have coped with difficulties in the past often helps them to reinvest in their ability to face the current crisis.

Intervention deals with the present situation and resolution of the immediate issue. It is important to assess the events that led up to the crisis. Listening to what the client says both verbally and nonverbally gives insight into the event or problem from the client's perspective. It is important that the intervention offers hope to the individual and a plan for resolution of the crisis with specific steps. Focusing on the present situation and keeping a reality-based approach helps the person to concentrate on a specific task. At this point, the person may be able to make a temporary form of resolution that allows them to function and move on with daily activities.

Early intervention in assisting the individual to manage the current situation promotes the best chance for a positive outcome. Once the anxiety level is reduced to a tolerable level, the individual can be assisted in defining the problem, determining available support, and setting realistic goals for resolution of the issue. The nurse is integral in providing support and returning control to the client. This allows the nurse to help the client identify alternative ways of reducing the anxiety and feelings of powerlessness. It is important for the nurse to remain nonjudgmental and to resist letting personal feelings interfere with an objective view of the client's problem. Establishing a sense of trust and respect will help the client focus on their feelings. The nurse should allow the client time to sort through their thoughts as questioning begins. Using open-ended statements (e.g., "Tell me what happened right before you started feeling this way.") will also help the client work through the details that led up to the current crisis. Listen for meaning behind statements that help to define the situational trauma the client is experiencing. If the person is suicidal, protective measures must be initiated to provide a feeling of safety and security. This feeling will allow the individual a temporary sanctuary in which the inner resources can be stabilized. Outcomes are aimed at promoting optimum psychological and physiologic functioning. Therapeutic strategies are designed to assist in mobilizing the client's currently available coping mechanisms and developing new strategies to assist in preventing future emotional states of dysfunction.

 Mind Jogger How would the need for intervention increase for someone experiencing several potential crisis situations at one time?

Suicide

Each year, there are many people who contemplate or complete suicide, or self-inflicted death. Although some people are at a greater risk, people of all ages, races, and socioeconomic status die by suicide. In 2020 suicide was the 12th leading cause of death in the adult population of the United States, claiming the lives of more than 45,000 people (averaging about 125 suicides per day). Approximately 11 attempted suicides occur for every suicide that ends in death. Statistics show that about four times as many males die by suicide as females. Males and older adults are more likely to have attempts that end in death than females and youth. Firearms, suffocation, and poisoning tend to be the most common methods used (American Foundation for Suicide Prevention, 2022). A familial history of mental disorders is shown to increase the risk for suicidal behaviors. Research also demonstrates that the risk increases when depression, other mental disorders, or substance-related disorders are involved. It is estimated that most of those who

"Nathan"

 Nathan feels that his world is coming to an end. Seventeen years ago, his fiancé was badly beaten by an intruder and left with multiple scars and a loss of vision in one eye. Last week, Nathan learned that the intruder was due to be released from prison and would be returning to the community. Nathan is so worried about further danger to his now-wife that he cannot sleep, eat, or function. Nathan feels that he will not be able to control his impulse to kill the man if he sees him.

Digging Deeper

1. How does Nathan's problem demonstrate a crisis situation?

2. What is the first step of the intervention to help Nathan?

3. Why is it so important to listen to what Nathan says both verbally and nonverbally?

CASE STUDY 6.2

succeed in ending their life by suicide have one of these problems.

Risk Factors

Some identifiable factors can put a person in a mindset leading to the actual decision to end their life. These factors can be intrinsic (a mental illness or depression) or extrinsic (loss of job). For example, a person may distance themselves from others with a feeling of hopelessness and worthlessness. This despondency may be related to loss of a love object, loss of health, or pressures related to the demands on them. Other factors may include substance use or loss of control over situations that seem hopeless. Risk factors for adolescents and youth include depression, alcohol and drugs, bullying, physical or sexual abuse, and behavior disorders. Box 6.6 lists some risk factors that are associated with suicide. There are also factors that are protective to help reduce the risk of suicide (Box 6.7).

Suicidal erosion, or the long-term accumulation of negative experiences throughout an individual's lifetime, can lead to suicidal thoughts. This occurs not as a result of a single factor that leads to suicidal thoughts but instead because of a combination of situations over time. Any kind of loss has the potential to precipitate depressive symptoms. In a person who is depressed, the symptoms may go undetected by family members or friends. Most suicide attempts are an expression of severe internal and mental distress. Box 6.8 provides a list of warning signs that may indicate the person may be considering suicide.

There are four levels of risk that apply to the person who may be contemplating suicide. A verbalized thought or idea that indicates the person's desire to do self-harm or destruction is **suicidal ideation**. This person may have recurrent thought processes that center on death as a means of ending mental and physical anguish. A further step is taken if the person has devised a plan for ending their life. A statement of intent is considered a **suicidal threat** and is usually accompanied by behavior changes that indicate the person has defined their plan. Action that indicates the person may be

---

BOX 6.6

Risk Factors Associated With Suicide

- Previous suicide attempt
- Mental illness especially depression
- Substance use disorder
- Family history of suicide
- Chronic pain
- Military service
- Serious illness
- Hopelessness
- Financial, criminal, or legal problems
- Bullying

Adapted from American Foundation for Suicide Prevention. (2022). *Risk factors, protective factors, and warning signs.* https://afsp.org/risk-factors-protective-factors-and-warning-signs#protective-factors; National Institute of Mental Health. (2022). *Suicide prevention.* https://www.nimh.nih.gov/health/topics/suicide-prevention; Centers for Disease Control and Prevention. (2021). *Suicide prevention risk and protective factors.* https://www.cdc.gov/suicide/factors/index.html

---

BOX 6.7

Protective Factors Against Suicide

- Access to mental health care and being proactive about mental health
- Feeling connected to family, friends, and community
- Positive problem solving and coping skills
- Limited access to lethal means
- Cultural and religious beliefs that discourage suicidal behavior
- A strong sense of purpose or self-esteem

Adapted from American Foundation for Suicide Prevention. (2022). *Risk factors, protective factors, and warning signs.* https://afsp.org/risk-factors-protective-factors-and-warning-signs#protective-factors; National Institute of Mental Health. (2022). *Suicide prevention.* https://www.nimh.nih.gov/health/topics/suicide-prevention; Centers for Disease Control and Prevention. (2021). *Suicide prevention risk and protective factors.* https://www.cdc.gov/suicide/factors/index.html

---

BOX 6.8

Suicide Warning Signs

- Talking about suicide
- Expressing feelings that life is not worth living or of being a burden
- Difficulty eating and sleeping
- Increased substance use
- Social withdrawal
- Loss of interest in school, work, or pleasure activities
- Giving away prized possessions
- Previous suicide attempt
- Unnecessary risk-taking
- Recent major loss
- Preoccupation with death and dying
- Lack of attention to personal hygiene

BOX 6.9

If You Think Someone Might be Suicidal

- Do not leave the person alone—stay with them.
- Ask directly if they are thinking about suicide.
- Take them seriously.
- Tell them you care about them.
- Avoid debating the value of life, minimizing their problems, or giving advice.
- Try to get the person immediate medical help.
- Call 911.
- Eliminate access to firearms or other potential suicide tools.
- Remove any unsupervised access to prescription or over-the-counter (OTC) medications.

Adapted from American Foundation for Suicide Prevention. (2022). *What to do when someone is at risk.* https://afsp.org/what-to-do-when-someone-is-at-risk; Centers for Disease Control and Prevention. (2022). *Suicide prevention.* https://www.nimh.nih.gov/health/topics/suicide-prevention

Other signs to consider are reports from family or friends that the individual may have recently expressed a desire to die or wanting to kill themselves, or about being a burden to family. The person may feel trapped in a presumably inescapable situation, such as an individual who is caught stealing money from the company they work for and faces litigation and an uncertain future. The person may also have exhibited reckless behavior or an increased use of alcohol or drugs. Withdrawal from friends and family events or giving away items that previously had significant meaning to the individual can also indicate a loss of the will to live.

 Just the Facts To the person who is unable to see any other way of improving their present situation, suicide may seem to be a logical and rational solution.

about ready to carry out the plan is considered a **suicidal gesture**. If the person actually carries out a **suicide attempt**, it is possible they will succeed. This is often the last desperate cry for help by a person who sees no other alternative. To the person who is unable to see any other way of improving the present situation, suicide seems to be a logical and rational solution. It is important that any person who appears to be suicidal is not left alone and is assisted in securing immediate mental health treatment (Box 6.9).

Suicide Risk Assessment and Intervention

A risk assessment should be done on the first contact with the individual. It is important that this assessment determines the lethality and immediacy of the crisis. Is the person thinking about suicide now or have they thought about it in the past few months? If the answer is yes, was it a passing thought or a continuing thought (suicidal ideation)? Does the person have a plan (suicidal threat) and do they have the means available to carry out their plan (suicidal gesture)? Has the individual actually attempted to carry out the plan (suicide attempt)? The assessment should address the suicidal desire, suicidal capability, suicidal intent, available support system, and the individual's sense of purpose. Once a crisis intervention assessment has been made, the risk designation can be assigned and a plan for treatment can be initiated.

Prevention of Suicide

Individuals who indicate that they are thinking about suicide or wanting to die by suicide need help. It is imperative to listen and find support for the person. Box 6.9 provides steps that an individual can take if they feel that another person is suicidal. Suicide crisis centers have hot lines that can provide assistance from medical and mental health professionals. Talking to someone who is trained to lend a listening ear is often a lifesaving intervention. Reinforcing Client and Family Teaching 6.2 provides information for the National Suicide Prevention Lifeline and Veteran's Crisis Line.

It is important that interventions focus on the immediate danger to and safety of the individual. The person in an acute crisis situation should

Reinforcing Client and Family Teaching 6.2

988 Suicide & Crisis Lifeline

If you are in a crisis and need immediate help, dial 988. Help is available 7 days a week, 24 hours a day. You may call or anyone else may call for you. All calls are confidential and answered immediately.
https://988lifeline.org

Veteran's Crisis Line
988 then Press 1
OR
Text to 838255
https://www.veteranscrisisline.net

never be left alone. A rapport should be established that conveys a calm and caring attitude or genuine concern for the person's life and story. If the individual has called the crisis line, the person is asking for help—the help-seeking should be validated as the first step in a solution to their problems and treatment can be initiated.

Test yourself

✔ Describe the difference between a developmental and a situational crisis.
✔ Identify five different factors that place an individual at risk for suicide.
✔ Describe suicidal ideation.
✔ Name five steps to take if you feel someone is suicidal.

Cultural Considerations

Anger Across the World

Anger is a universal emotion; however, its cultural expression varies. Cultural scripts are unwritten expectations of how emotions should be expressed. Expressing anger varies on the spectrum from being inappropriate to being an acceptable show of emotion. Ultimately the individual and their unique experiences dictate their emotional expression, not solely their culture. Below are some examples of cultural reactions regarding anger.

- In some cultures, it is expected to control and suppress anger (East Asian and Indian). This is often seen in cultures where social harmony and well-being of the group (interdependence) are valued. However, in some instances it may be permitted if the individual has a high social status; for example, a Japanese executive who yells at a janitor may be seen as having anger privilege and therefore the yelling is permitted.
- In North American and Western European cultures where independence and the uniqueness of the individual are valued, outward expressions of anger may be seen as culturally permitted or socially justified.
- Americans who face more societal pressures tend to express more anger. As frustration levels increase, the individual expresses more anger.
- In honor cultures (where defending one's honor or that of one's group is valued), the expression of anger is acceptable in certain circumstances. These cultures may also have strong politeness norms, even in frustrating or confrontational settings.
- Public displays of anger or yelling at another person may be viewed as an insult (Egyptian).
- Some cultures have a norm for how males and females can express their anger (machismo and marianismo seen in some Latin American cultures).
- Silence is used by some to maintain autonomy (Native American) and not engage in anger-provoking situations. Silence can also be used to show respect to other individual (Native American). In other cultures becoming very silent is an indication of anger (Greek).
- In some cultures, raising one's voice at someone in public is seen as disrespectful or reserved only to warn of danger (Afghan) while in other cultures it is a norm during conversation (Greek, Afrikaners, and Black South African). Continuing a conversation by shouting across the room or even from another room (Black South African) may be acceptable.
- Some cultures avoid conflict in order to save face (Cambodian and Filipino) while others dislike conflict and will attempt to avoid it (Portuguese).
- Swearing may be considered offensive and a sign of anger but it also may be socially acceptable (Australian).

SUMMARY

- Anger describes the emotion elicited in response to a threat, insult, or circumstance that prevents individuals from following through with intended actions or desires. Anger drives the response of aggression and bitterness that can lead to hostility and outward attacks toward another person or object.
- Trait anger is often referred to as a general biologic leaning toward a volatile personality. A person with trait anger may describe themselves as quick-tempered.

- Anger is outwardly expressed as hostility, aggression, or violence.
- Bullying is a form of psychological harassment or physical confrontation used to intentionally bring harm or humiliation to one who is seen as weak or different. It can take the form of physical, verbal, or social harassment, or destruction of property belonging to the victim.
- Both the victim and family members may be affected in some way by bullying. Victims report low

self-esteem, increased school absenteeism, and physical symptoms. Bullying can even lead to depression, mental health issues, and suicide.

- Constructive methods of managing anger include restructured thinking, physical activity, assertion, use of "I" statements, expressing feelings, and forgiveness.
- Intimate partner violence (IPV) is a pattern of behavior that is used by the abuser to gain power and control over another person through fear and intimidation that often includes threats or use of physical violence. This form of violence can take the form of emotional, physical, economic, or sexual abuse, and/or stalking.
- Risk factors for abusers include family history of violence, history of physical or emotional abuse as a child, drug or alcohol use, low self-esteem, poor impulse or behavioral control, antisocial beliefs and attitudes, association with delinquent peers or gangs, social rejection, or economic stress.
- Traits of abusers include being moody and over sensitive to criticism, being power-seeking or overly competitive, blaming others for their problems or feelings, rationalizing the use of violent behavior as needed to resolve a situation, expecting others to meet their needs or wait on them, frequent arguing, cursing, or physical fighting, and making verbal threats against others.
- Warning signs that might indicate the partner is abusive include excessive jealousy, possessiveness, short temper, verbal abuse, name calling, controlling acts, blaming victim for anything that happens, demeaning the victim in private or publicly, or being cruel to animals.
- The cycle of abuse is seen in intimate partner violence (IPV). It begins as put-downs and verbal accusations. As control escalates, physical attacks that can endanger the victim and cause serious bodily harm occur. The abuser seems remorseful and gives gifts followed by a pause in the violence, which is soon resumed with blaming and further abuse that repeats the cycle. Fear of the abuser and the unknown holds the victim captive in the repetitious sequence.
- A psychological crisis can take the form of a developmental crisis or situational crisis. A developmental crisis can occur at a predictable period of a person's life such as being a teenager or a new parent, whereas a situational crisis is unpredictable and happens suddenly such as a natural disaster or a car crash.
- The goal of crisis intervention is to reduce the anxiety to a level that will allow the client to look at the situation more realistically toward a resolution.
- Risk factors for suicide include a previous suicide attempt; mental illness, especially depression; substance use disorder; family history of suicide; chronic pain; military service; serious illness; feelings of hopelessness; financial, criminal, or legal problems; and bullying.
- A suicide risk assessment includes determining the lethality and immediacy of the crisis. The assessment should address the suicidal desire, suicidal capability, suicidal intent, available support system, and the individual's sense of purpose. Once a crisis intervention assessment has been made, the risk designation can be assigned and a plan for treatment can be initiated.
- Prevention of suicide includes staying with the individual, directly asking if they are thinking about suicide, taking them seriously and telling them you care about them, getting immediate help, and eliminating access to lethal weapons.

BIBLIOGRAPHY

American Foundation for Suicide Prevention. (2022). *Suicide statistics*. Retrieved April 15, 2022, from https://afsp.org/suicide-statistics/

Cancio, R. (2020). Experiences with machismo and pain: Latino veterans. *American Journal of Men's Health*, *14*(6). https://doi.org/10.1177/1557988320976304

Centers for Disease Control and Prevention. (2020). *Web-based Injury Statistics Query and Reporting System (WISQARS) Fatal Injury Reports*. Retrieved April 16, 2022, from https://wisqars.cdc.gov/data/lcd/home

Centers for Disease Control and Prevention. (2021a). *Preventing bullying*. https://www.cdc.gov/violenceprevention/youthviolence/bullyingresearch/fastfact.html

Centers for Disease Control and Prevention. (2021b). *Fast facts: Preventing intimate partner violence*. https://www.cdc.gov/violenceprevention/intimatepartnerviolence/fastfact.html

Centers for Disease Control and Prevention. (2021c). *Intimate partner violence*. https://www.cdc.gov/violenceprevention/intimatepartnerviolence/index.html

Centers for Disease Control and Prevention. (2021d). *Risk and protective factors for perpetration*. https://www.cdc.gov/violenceprevention/intimatepartnerviolence/riskprotectivefactors.html

Centers for Disease Control and Prevention. (2021e). *Suicide prevention risk and protective factors*. https://www.cdc.gov/suicide/factors/index.html

Centers for Disease Control and Prevention. (2022). *Violence prevention*. https://www.cdc.gov/violenceprevention/

Hedegaard, H., Curtin, S. C., & Warner, M. (2021). *Suicide mortality in the United States, 1999–2019 (NCHS Data Brief No. 398).* Centers for Disease Control and Prevention. https://www.cdc.gov/nchs/data/databriefs/db398-H.pdf

Hendy, H. M., Hakan Can, S., & Heep, H. (2021). Machismo and Caballerismo linked with perceived social discrimination and powerlessness in U.S. Latino men. *Journal of Cross-Cultural Psychology, 53*(1), 109–121. https://doi.org/10.1177/00220221211054206

Malti, T. (2020). Children and violence: Nurturing social-emotional development to promote mental health. *Society for Research in Child Development, 33*(2), 1–27. https://doi.org/10.1002/sop2.8

National Coalition Against Domestic Violence (NCADV). (2022). *Signs of abuse.* https://ncadv.org/signs-of-abuse

National Domestic Violence Hotline. (2022). *Power and control: Break free from abuse.* https://www.thehotline.org/identify-abuse/power-and-control/

National Institute of Mental Health. (2022). *Suicide.* Retrieved April 12, 2022, from https://www.nimh.nih.gov/health/statistics/suicide

National Institute of Mental Health. (2022). *Suicide prevention.* https://www.nimh.nih.gov/health/topics/suicide-prevention

PACER's National Bullying Prevention Center. (2022). *Bullying statistics by the numbers.* Retrieved April 15, 2022, from https://www.pacer.org/bullying/info/stats.asp

Shao, R., & Wang, Y. (2019). The relation of violent video games to adolescent aggression: An examination of moderated mediation effect. *Frontiers in Psychology.* https://doi.org/10.3389/fpsyg.2019.00384

U.S. Department of Veterans Affairs, Office of Mental Health and Suicide Prevention. (2020). *2020 National veteran suicide prevention annual report.* https://www.mentalhealth.va.gov/docs/data-sheets/2020/2020-National-Veteran-Suicide-Prevention-Annual-Report-11-2020-508.pdf

Wamser-Nanney, R., Walker, H. E., & Nanney, J. T. (2019). Trauma exposure, posttraumatic stress disorder, and aggression among civilian females. *Journal of Interpersonal Violence, 36,* 17–18. https://doi.org/10.1177/0886260519860894

STUDENT WORKSHEET

Fill in the Blank

Fill in the blank with the correct answer.

1. _____ _____ is often referred to as a general biologic leaning toward a volatile personality.
2. _____ involves harassing or threatening phone calls, e-mails, texts, or voice mails.
3. _____ is used repeatedly to intentionally bring harm or humiliation to another person who is seen as weak or different.
4. _____ _____ _____ can take the form of physical, emotional, economic, and/or sexual abuse.
5. Substance use disorder is a _____ factor for suicide while a strong sense of purpose or self-esteem is a _____ factor.
6. _____ is standing up for one's rights, beliefs, or values in such a way that it does not hurt others in the process.

Matching

Match the following terms to the most appropriate phrase.

1. _____ Crisis
2. _____ Hostility
3. _____ Stalking
4. _____ Suicidal erosion
5. _____ Trait anger
6. _____ Aggression
7. _____ Suicidal gesture

a. Action that indicates that self-harm may be imminent
b. Verbal or nonverbal behavior that can result in harm to oneself or another
c. General biologic leaning toward a volatile personality
d. State of emotional disorganization and loss of control
e. Abuse that involves harassment or threatening behaviors
f. Intense feeling of animosity toward someone or something
g. Long-term accumulation of negative experiences throughout a person's lifetime

Multiple Choice

Select the best answer from the multiple-choice items.

1. A client is brought to the emergency room in a state of crisis following a motor vehicle accident in which their parent was killed. Which of the following statements by the nurse would be most appropriate to determine the client's coping ability for this crisis?
   a. "What family members are available to be here with you?"
   b. "Tell me what brought you to the hospital today."
   c. "How have you handled difficult experiences before?"
   d. "What was your relationship like with your parent?"

2. A call is received by the crisis hotline with the person stating, "I have a gun and I am going to shoot myself." What is being demonstrated by this individual?
   a. Suicidal erosion
   b. Suicidal ideation
   c. Suicidal gesture
   d. Suicidal attempt

3. The client is having severe symptoms of headaches, crying episodes, and anorexia. They state they separated from their partner, lost their job because of excess absences, and now have been evicted from their apartment. What is the client experiencing?
   a. Situational crisis
   b. Maturational crisis
   c. Developmental crisis
   d. Identity crisis

4. Which statement would be correct in describing the perpetrator in a situation of intimate partner abuse? *(Select all that apply)*
   a. History of degrading or putting down women
   b. Family history of alcohol use disorder and violence
   c. Enjoyment of watching action-packed movies on television
   d. Frequent involvement in fights and vandalism
   e. Having had numerous intimate relationships

5. A 16-year-old tells their parent that they are being bullied by other kids at school. They are distraught and don't want to go to school. Which statement by the adolescent would indicate bullying?
   a. "They were teasing me all day yesterday about my hair cut!"
   b. "I can't do what the gym teacher wants and they make fun of me."
   c. "They wait for me in the hall every day and make fun of me in front of everyone."
   d. "Someone posted a picture of me on Facebook—I look so fat in that picture!"

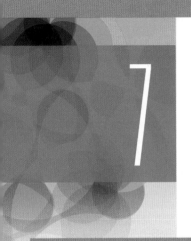

Unit III | Fundamental Nursing Roles in Mental Health Nursing

7

Communication in Mental Health Nursing

LEARNING OBJECTIVES

After learning the content in this chapter, the student will be able to:

1. Discuss how communication is used as a therapeutic tool to interact with clients.
2. Identify effective verbal communication techniques that facilitate communication between the client and the nurse and give an example for each one.
3. Describe examples of nonverbal communication and how they impact communication.
4. Identify nontherapeutic or blocked communication techniques and describe how each technique blocks communication.
5. List common speech patterns common to clients with mental illness and give an example for each one.

KEY TERMS

active listening
blocking
circumstantiality
clang association (rhyming)
echolalia
flight of ideas
focusing
loose association

neologism
objectivity
reflection
restating
silence
validation
word salad

Communication in Mental Health Nursing

Communication is a process of exchanging information involving the person sending a message, the person receiving the message, and the message itself (Fig. 7.1). Thinking is the way a thought is developed, but thinking in itself does not communicate that thought. The thought content must be communicated by one of various methods, which may be verbal or nonverbal. Verbal communication is the exchange of information using words, such as through speaking, listening, writing, or reading. Nonverbal communication is the exchange of information without using words, for example, through body language, space, or touch. These processes of communication occur in response to an instinctive drive for connection to other human beings.

In nursing, communication is purposeful and is centered on the needs and problems of the client. Through communication, the nurse builds the therapeutic relationship and establishes trust. To do this effectively, the nurse must develop effective therapeutic communication skills, which are described in this chapter.

Therapeutic Communication

Therapeutic communication is an interaction between the nurse, or other team personnel, and the client that is conducted with the specific goal of learning about the client and their problem. This type of skilled communication is learned and requires practice. Although the focus is on the client, the exchange is planned and guided by the nurse. The goal is to use both verbal and nonverbal techniques to facilitate active involvement by the client and to encourage the client to express feelings and thoughts that are contributing to their problem.

To do this, it is important to view the relationship between the nurse and the client as part of a complex environment influenced by individual experiences, culture, values, and beliefs. Many cultural and ethnic factors relating to both the client and the nurse impact the quality of this exchange. In addition, educational background, gender, and personal emotions all impact the dynamics of this interaction. Each message within the communication exchange is filtered through the mental processes of both the sender and the receiver. Differences in communication style or expression of one's feelings can easily cause the message to be misinterpreted. **Objectivity**, or the ability to view facts and events without distortion by personal feelings, prejudices, or judgments, allows the nurse to remain unbiased and open to what clients say about their problems and about themselves. Therapeutic communication is integral to establishing trust within the nurse–client relationship.

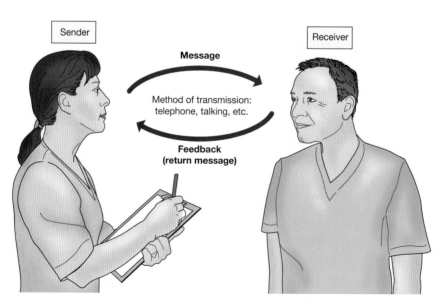

Figure 7.1 Communication is a process of exchanging information involving the person sending a message, the person receiving the message, and the message itself. This interaction occurs both verbally and nonverbally in response to an instinctive drive for connection to other human beings.

The nurse must be vigilant, demonstrating awareness and sensitivity to the needs of the client. The perceived power of the nurse may at times relay a condescending attitude to the client. It is essential for the nurse to be constantly aware that manner of speech and actions are being observed and interpreted by the client. Many clients are mistrustful and are especially suspicious of those in authority. Nurses are seen as authority figures. Keeping this in mind, the nurse must continuously monitor their own actions as well as the client's response to maintain a therapeutic climate within the relationship. It is important to be flexible and make the client physically and emotionally comfortable during the therapeutic interaction. Learning to anticipate the client's needs and meet them as completely and consistently as possible within therapeutic guidelines is important.

Verbal Communication

Verbal communication is enhanced by speaking clearly, using vocabulary the listener can understand, and avoiding ambiguous statements. Both the sound of the voice and the tone of the conveyed message have an impact on the way in which the message is received. Because of the differences between participants, the meaning intended by the sender is never exactly the same as the meaning understood by the receiver. Meanings are interpreted based on individual experiences and knowledge. Verbal communication can be either enhanced or undermined by the nonverbal dynamics that accompany the verbalization.

When engaged in verbal communication with a client, **silence**, in which the nurse remains quiet with an attentive manner, conveys a willingness to continue listening. It allows both the nurse and the client time to collect thoughts. A client may also find that emotions override the ability to convey feelings verbally. Silence shows respect for the emotions and offers the client time to regain control and continue the conversation.

Table 7.1 describes some effective verbal communication techniques. These techniques are used with the specific intent of facilitating interaction

TABLE 7.1	Effective Verbal Communication Techniques	
Effective Technique	**Example**	**Therapeutic Effect**
Clarification	**Nurse:** "Did I understand you correctly..." "Let me see if I have this correct..." "I seem to have missed something. Could you repeat that?"	Clears up any possible misunderstanding and ensures message intended is message received
Validation	**Nurse:** "You seem anxious." "I get the feeling that something is bothering you." "You look down this morning. Would you like to talk about it?"	Attempts to verify the nurse's perception of feeling conveyed by either verbal or nonverbal message of the client
Reflection (also called parroting)	**Client:** "I don't think my daughter will need me after she gets married." **Nurse:** "You are afraid you won't be needed after your daughter's marriage?" **Client:** "I am sick of all this mess." **Nurse:** "Sick of this mess?"	Shows nurse's perception of the client's message in both content and feeling areas—paraphrases the message that the client has conveyed to nurse
Restating	**Nurse:** "You have told me something about the problems between you and your wife."	Repeats to the client the content of interaction and serves as lead to encourage further discussion
Focusing	**Nurse:** "Let's get back to the problem with your son."	Helps the client concentrate on a specific issue
Using a general lead	**Nurse:** "Go on..." "And then..." "Continue..."	Shows the nurse is listening and interested—encourages the client to continue talking
Giving information	**Nurse:** "The doctor has ordered a new medication for you. Let me go over this information with you."	Increases client involvement in plan of care—helps to demonstrate team effort to improve the client's well-being
Using silence	Nurse remains silent with attentive manner.	Conveys willingness to continue listening—allows both the nurse and client time to collect thoughts
Explore alternatives	**Nurse:** "How else could you spend some time alone with your wife?"	Guides the client to possible options for problem solving
Offering of oneself	**Nurse:** "I will be here awhile if you wish to talk."	Reassurance of interest and presence in the client's problem
Reinforcing reality	**Nurse:** "I know you hear the voices, but I do not hear them. You and I are the only ones in this room."	Provides reassurance that voices are symptoms of illness—helps the client to trust the nurse as real

with the client. The method used will depend on the situation and the client's ability to communicate verbally. For example, if the purpose is to encourage the client to discuss feelings about a current problem, the nurse would use methods of **reflection** (communication technique that paraphrases message client has conveyed to nurse) or **validation** (verifying the nurse's perception of the verbal or nonverbal message conveyed by the client). On the other hand, if the nurse is unsure of the message being conveyed by the client, the nurse might choose clarification, **restating** (repeating back to client the content of interaction for the purpose of leading and encouraging further discussion), or **focusing** (communication technique that helps client concentrate on a specific issue). Whatever the situation, it is important to consider what technique will best encourage a therapeutic outcome for the client.

Test Yourself	✔ How is therapeutic communication different than social communication? ✔ Name three effective verbal communication techniques. ✔ Give an example of each of the three identified techniques.

Nonverbal Communication Techniques

Nonverbal communication is an exchange of information without the use of words. It can confirm, strengthen, or emphasize what is being said verbally. It can add emotional color to spoken words, but it can also contradict the message that is being sent. The behavior that accompanies a verbal message is often more important and more powerful than what is said aloud. The nonverbal message will go beyond verbal content and convey unconscious emotions or thoughts than can negate the verbal message.

Nonverbal aspects of a therapeutic exchange must convey a sense of genuine caring and interest in what the client has to say. Body movements such as hand gestures, facial expressions, and other mannerisms can invite the trust of the client or block further interaction. Effective use of nonverbal techniques must be a conscious choice for the nurse to maintain a therapeutic relationship with the client. Nonverbal techniques the nurse can employ to improve communication in a therapeutic exchange with the client are listed in Table 7.2.

Use of therapeutic touch can help to communicate caring and understanding. However, when working with the client who has a mental illness, the nurse must use caution and forethought about how the client might interpret actions. A client who is suspicious, for example, might react with aggressive actions toward a simple pat on the shoulder. A client who is sexually preoccupied might misinterpret any form of touch as having seductive connotations. Some cultures (e.g., certain Islamic and Japanese cultures) may

TABLE 7.2	Nonverbal Communication Techniques
Nonverbal Aspect	**Message Conveyed**
Appearance	• The nurse models socially appropriate behaviors.
Eye Contact	• Intermittent eye contact helps provide reassurance that the nurse is interested and concentrating on what the client is saying.
Facial Expression	• A facial expression that is congruent with other verbal or nonverbal messages assures the client of the nurse's interest and attention. • Inconsistency between verbal and nonverbal messages leads to misinterpretation of the intended meaning. ◦ Example: the nurse is smiling when they say, "That sounds like an awful experience."
Gestures	• Hand gestures can convey inconsistency between messages. • Drumming of fingers conveys a message that the listener is bored or uninterested in the conversation. • Pointing has different meanings in different cultures.
Personal Space	• In most people, personal space is an arm's length, which is about 2 to 4 feet. • Respecting the physical or personal space between the client and the nurse helps the client feel safe. • The anxiety level, suspiciousness, distorted thinking, and personal comfort zone of the client will all influence the proximity of this distance. • Aggressive or violent client behavior requires the nurse to be further away from the client than 4 feet.

Stance	• Vertical conversations (the nurse is standing while the client is sitting or lying down) can be intimidating and block further communication.
	  ◦ Lateral conversations with both the nurse and client at eye level are more conducive to therapeutic communication.
	  ◦ Arms or legs that are not crossed convey a sense of openness to the client.
	  ◦ Crossed arms and/or legs send the message that the nurse is not interested or open to the client's point of view.
	  ◦ A seated position with legs together and both feet on the floor with arms uncrossed reflects an attitude of acceptance and genuineness.
	  ◦ A standing position with legs spread apart conveys an authoritarian attitude.

also view personal touch as inappropriate except in certain circumstances.

Mind Jogger ② What body posture would reflect an attitude of acceptance and genuineness?

Test Yourself
✔ Name three nonverbal communication techniques.
✔ Describe how each identified technique impacts communication.

Active Listening

Active listening is a learned skill that includes observing nonverbal behaviors, giving critical attention to verbal comments, listening for inconsistencies that may need clarification, and attempting to understand the client's perception of the situation. Active listening by the nurse demonstrates care and a desire to help the client. It allows the client to express feelings and thoughts without fear of being judged or criticized. The nurse must constantly listen and cognitively review the comments and behaviors of the client before responding. Because clients tend to view the nurse as someone with power who cares and is available, the opportunities for interaction are more likely. Some responses by the nurse may not be effective or correct. The intended message can be misread by either the client or the nurse. It is important that both participants remain open to the possibility of error. Sometimes this actually allows the nurse to apologize and model appropriate behavior. Willingness to try another approach can also reinforce the genuineness of the nurse's efforts to help the client.

Just the Facts ① Accept that as a nurse, you may have feelings of irritation and impatience toward a client. Doing a self-assessment of your feelings and response to the client situation can help you to grow and be more effective.

Nontherapeutic Communication

It is important to recognize that there are also ways that communication can be sidetracked so that it does not accomplish the intended goal of helping the client. In contrast to effective therapeutic communication, nontherapeutic communication involves messages and behaviors that actually hinder the therapeutic process. For example, closed body language with arms folded and appearing busy or uncomfortable with the conversation would send a message to the client that the relationship is superficial. If the nurse interjects opinions or personal

"Olivia"

BigPixel Photo/Shutterstock

Olivia is a 26-year-old married mother of three children who is brought to the emergency room of a local hospital following a suicide attempt using an excessive ingestion of a prescribed antidepressant. After Olivia has been stabilized the nurse monitoring her notes that Olivia is avoiding eye contact. She turns her head to the side, but the nurse sees that tears are consistently running down her cheeks. She tells the nurse in a quiet voice, "I never seem to do anything right. My family would be so much better off without me. Why don't you just let me die?"

Digging Deeper

1. *What would be an appropriate reflection response by the nurse to Olivia at this time?*

2. *How can the nurse validate Olivia's feelings at this time?*

3. *What techniques would encourage Olivia to tell the nurse more about her feelings and thoughts leading up to her suicide attempt?*

CASE STUDY 7.1

TABLE 7.3 Blocks to Therapeutic Communication

Ineffective Technique	Example	Blocking Effect	Therapeutic Response
Arguing or disapproving	**Client:** "I want to try to get my girlfriend back." **Nurse:** "Why would you want to do that after what she did to you?"	Expresses opinions or interjects the nurse's values of right and wrong on the client's actions—may prevent the client from working through options in solving the problem	**Nurse:** "Tell me more about that…"
Giving advice	**Nurse:** "You should not be so hard on your kids." "If I were you, I would do what the doctor says."	Implies the nurse's values are correct and devalues the client's actions	**Nurse:** "It seems your kids are a problem for you…" "Tell me about what the doctor has told you."
False reassurance	**Nurse:** "You are going to be out of here before you know it."	Minimizes the client's feelings and concerns—conveys superficial attitude	**Nurse:** "We are here to help you get stronger and feel better."
Use the word "why"	**Nurse:** "Why did you act that way?" "Why are you getting so upset?"	Puts the client on the defensive— demands an answer Invasive and direct probing of issue	**Nurse:** "Tell me more about what you are feeling right now." "You seem to be upset about something. Tell me about it."
Closed-ended questions	**Nurse:** "Do you want to talk about it?" "Are you feeling better this morning?" "I don't think that's a good idea, do you?"	Allows a "yes" or "no" response without encouraging further information from the client (If the client replies with a "yes" or "no," nurse can use a more effective response to elicit more conversation)	**Nurse:** "Tell me about that…" "Tell me how you are feeling this morning…" "Let's talk about that…"
Changing the subject	**Client:** "I really don't think I can handle going back home." **Nurse:** "Let's talk about the incident that occurred yesterday during art therapy."	Minimizes importance of client concerns—discourages further exploration of feelings and thoughts May show the nurse's insecurity in talking about the issue	**Nurse:** "Tell me what bothers you about going home…"
Agreeing or approving	**Nurse:** "You are absolutely correct." "I think that is a great idea." "You should do that."	Can set the client up for failure if the idea doesn't work Can be seen as judgmental	**Nurse:** "Tell me more about your idea…" "Let's look at that again…"
Minimizing or belittling	**Nurse:** "That is how everyone feels when they are admitted." "We all resent being told what to do."	Conveys an attitude that the client's feelings are common and devalues the uniqueness of the person	**Nurse:** "I'm sure it is difficult for you to be told what to do…tell me what you are feeling."
Focusing on the nurse	**Client:** "I just broke up with my boyfriend a few weeks ago." **Nurse:** "That has happened to me several times…"	Pulls focus from client problem and delays further exploration or information regarding the client's feelings	**Nurse:** "That must have been difficult…tell me about that time…"
Stereotype statements	**Nurse:** "Tomorrow will be a better day." "Hang in there."	Empty clichés close the client to further response	**Nurse:** "You seem rather low today; would you like to talk about it?"

values, or minimizes the client's feelings, a condescending attitude is presented that puts the client on the defensive. This type of approach denies the client the chance to trust the nurse as a resource of help and hope. Table 7.3 demonstrates how ineffective responses can block therapeutic communication along with suggested therapeutic alternatives.

Just the Facts If a communicative response is intimidating, judgmental, or demeaning, it is NOT therapeutic.

In addition, there are several factors that can prevent an intended message from being understood. Variances in age, language, or ethnic and cultural differences can produce barriers to the correct interpretation of a message. Differences in ability to see and hear can also interfere with the transfer of information. Background noise or confusion can be distracting and hinder attentive listening. Communication is only therapeutic when the client is actively involved in the process. The nurse must be alert to any indication that communication is being misunderstood and make provisions or adjustments to improve the outcome.

A supportive approach is needed to aid the client with mental health issues in working toward resolution of their own problems. The nurse should refrain from offering advice or responding to the client with criticism. While the ability to be empathetic is necessary, giving appropriate feedback is just as important. Clients need to feel valued, respected, and accepted by the nurse. The nurse should recognize that they may not always get the response or cooperation anticipated. Used consistently however, these techniques can help accomplish the goal of initiating and maintaining a therapeutic nurse–client relationship.

Mind Jogger How could the use of silence by the nurse be nontherapeutic?

Test Yourself
- ✔ What is the overall effect of a nontherapeutic technique on communication?
- ✔ Name three nontherapeutic techniques.
- ✔ How do the three identified techniques impact communication?

Speech Patterns Common to Clients with Mental Illness

It is important to understand speech patterns that are common to the clients who have mental illness. These speech patterns often reflect distorted thoughts and processing flaws that occur as the person is attempting to process or transmit a message. Not all of these speech patterns are exhibited by each client. As you learn about individual disorders, you will become familiar with those patterns that are more common to each. Common abnormal speech patterns include the following:

- **Blocking**—The client unconsciously blocks out information, which results in loss of thought process and causes the client to stop speaking (e.g., "Then my father. . . What was I saying?").
- **Circumstantiality**—The client cannot be selective and describes in lengthy, great detail (e.g., when asked, "Do you have any physical illness?" client replies, "My head hurts, but my nose has been leaking, my hair just won't stay in place, I have this cramping in my joints.").
- **Clang association (rhyming)**—Words that rhyme are used but do not have meaning ("Shake to bake to fake a bake cake.").

"Gerome"

Media/ Shutterstock

Gerome is a 21-year-old man who has been admitted to the inpatient mental health unit after he was found crawling in a park wearing only tennis shoes and underwear. When the nurse makes the morning check, Gerome is sitting in a corner of the room covering his head and making head motions as if he is avoiding being hit in the head. Periodically he stops and turns his head to the side, cups his ear, and nods. When the nurse introduces themselves Gerome states, "Bing bang the sing sang. Windy is Cindy. Whoo whoo a boo boo."

Digging Deeper

1. *How would the nurse document Gerome's speech pattern?*

2. *How can the nurse respond to Gerome's statements?*

3. *What other documentation should the nurse include?*

4. *What other data should the nurse collect during this interaction?*

CASE STUDY 7.2

- **Echolalia**—The client imitates words or phrases made by others (e.g., "Please wait here" is responded to with, "wait here, wait here").
- **Flight of ideas**—The client rapidly shifts between topics that are unrelated to each other (e.g., "My cat is gray. The day is gray. The food here is good. My hair needs a perm. Do you think my pants are too tight? What color should I dye my hair?").
- **Loose association**—The client exhibits continuous speech, shifting between loosely related topics (e.g., "Martha married Jim. You know Jim is a good cook. I can cook. Chickens are something we can cook. The cook comes here before daylight. I get up in the daylight. Do you know Jim?").
- **Neologism**—The client creates new words and definitions (e.g., "Hiptomites are real powerful people" in reference to a large statured mental health technician on the unit.).
- **Word salad**—incoherent mixture of words and phrases that have no connection (e.g. "Spring flowers…purple…I am farmer….train whistle….good fun.").

Cultural Considerations

Eye Contact

One part of nonverbal communication is eye contact. However, people from different cultures and communities have different norms for eye contact. As with any cultural description, care must be taken not to stereotype an individual's behavior based upon their cultural identification as other factors can impact the expression of the behavior. Below are some ways people from different backgrounds might view eye contact.

- People from the United States
  - Strong eye contact can be seen as bold or a sign of self-confidence.
  - Little or no eye contact can be seen as a sign of low self-esteem.
  - Prolonged eye contact can be viewed as intimidating or even aggressive.
  - A lack of eye contact can sometimes be interpreted as the person is not being truthful.
- People from Hispanic, Asian, Middle Eastern, and Native American cultures
  - A lack of eye contact does not mean the person is not paying attention. Instead, it may mean that the person sees prolonged eye contact as a sign of disrespect.
- People from Middle Eastern and Muslim cultures
  - Anything beyond brief eye contact between people of different genders can be viewed as flirtatious or inappropriate.
- People from Asian, African, or Latin American cultures
  - Occasional or brief eye contact may be seen as polite and respectful especially when there is a difference between the status (e.g., the nurse and the client).
- People with cognitive disabilities such as dementia
  - The individual may no longer be aware of eye contact and cultural norms surrounding it. They may stare directly at an individual without looking away or may make direct eye contact with a member of another gender in cultures where such contact is discouraged.
- People with autism spectrum disorder
  - May find eye contact uncomfortable and will look down or somewhere other than the other person's eyes.

Source: Raeburn, A. (2021). *10 places where eye-contact is not recommended (10 places where the locals are friendly)*. The Travel. https:// www.thetravel.com/10-places-where-eye-contact-is-not-recommended-10-places-where-the-locals-are-friendly/

SUMMARY

- Therapeutic communication includes both verbal and nonverbal techniques in the exchange of information between the nurse and the client.
- Communication techniques are as diverse as the situations themselves. No one approach will work in every circumstance or with all clients.
- Successful attempts rely on the willingness of the client to reveal personal information and the nature of their problem. The goal is then to use techniques that guide the client to express emotions and thoughts that surround the situation.
- It is important to recognize that the client's communication is formed from many factors including age and gender, culture, beliefs and values, educational background, and experiences. These factors form the basis for communication.

- The tone of voice and manner of speaking can convey either a message of caring and concern or one that is intimidating and condescending.
- Silence allows the client to regain composure or collect thoughts and is a way of showing respect and concern for what the client has to say.
- Active listening and open posture are vital to projecting a genuineness and willingness to help the client. Eye contact should be intermittent and attentive without staring or fixating to the point of intimidation.
- The nurse should maintain an awareness of mannerisms that could imply power that is nontherapeutic. Many clients are mistrustful, especially of those in authority.
- Communication can occur in ways that do not evoke a therapeutic interaction with the client.

Closed-ended questions, putting the client on the defensive, or disapproving of the client's statements can impede the communication exchange. Statements that devalue the client and interject the opinions or judgments of the nurse are nontherapeutic. Clichés that offer a stereotyped response usually close the client to further response.
- Communication used effectively will open the door for the therapeutic relationship to grow and produce an outcome that will aid clients in accomplishing their goals for improvement.
- Clients with mental illness tend to demonstrate atypical speech patterns that reflect the distortion in their thoughts and processing of thought content into verbal transmission.

BIBLIOGRAPHY

Amoah, V. M. K., Anokye, R., Boakye, D. S., Acheampong, E., Budu-Ainooson, A., Okyere, E., Kumi-Boateng, G., Yeboah, C., & Afriyie, J. O. (2019). A qualitative assessment of perceived barriers to effective therapeutic communication among nurses and patients. *BMC Nursing, 18*, 4. https://doi.org/10.1186/s12912-019-0328-0

Betancourt, J. R., Green, A. R., & Carrillo, J. E. (2021). The patient's culture and effective communication. *UpToDate*. Retrieved February 16, 2022, from https://www.uptodate.com/contents/the-patients-culture-and-effective-communication

Burke, A. (2021). *Therapeutic communication: NCLEX-RN*. Registered Nursing. https://www.registerednursing.org/nclex/therapeutic-communication/

Cherry, K. (2021). *Types of nonverbal communication*. Verywell Mind. https://www.verywellmind.com/types-of-nonverbal-communication-2795397

Current Nursing (2020). *Therapeutic communication in psychiatric nursing*. https://currentnursing.com/pn/therapeutic_communication.html

Roscoe, L. (2022). *Therapeutic communication in correctional nursing*. National Commission on Correctional Health Care. https://www.ncchc.org/correctional-nursing-practice-what-you-need-to-know/therapeutic-communication-in-correctional-nursing/

Sharma, N., & Gupta, V. (2022). Therapeutic communication. In: *StatPearls [Internet]*. StatPearls Publishing. https://www.ncbi.nlm.nih.gov/books/NBK567775/

Fill in the Blank

Fill in the blank with the correct answer.

1. It is important for the nurse to convey a _____ message through both verbal and nonverbal communication.
2. _____ eye contact will provide reassurance that the nurse is interested and concentrating on what the client is saying.
3. _____ is when the client unconsciously blocks out information, which results in loss of thought process and causes the client to stop speaking
4. The coining of new words and definitions of words is referred to as _____.
5. _____ _____ describes continuous speech with shifting between loosely related topics.
6. _____ _____ such as hand gestures, facial expressions, arm placement, movement and other mannerisms can invite or block interaction with the client.
7. In most people, personal space is _____ _____ which is about 2 to 4 feet.

Matching

Match the following terms to the most appropriate phrase.

1. _____ Blocking
2. _____ Neologism
3. _____ Loose association
4. _____ Flight of ideas
5. _____ Echolalia

a. "Your hair is red—I have a red dress—I like red apples—apples, oranges, pears—you are shaped like a pear…"
b. "And I need help—help—help—help—help…"
c. "Whymothig" is used to describe a puzzle.
d. "I like to go camping—that book is old—my necklace is broke—the sky is cloudy—fish are lucky…"
e. "I have not seen my mother in 5 years…I need to go to the bathroom…"

Multiple Choice

Select the best answer from the multiple-choice items.

1. A client tells the nurse, "The voices say that I am evil and I am going to be punished." What is the nurse's most therapeutic response?
   a. "The voices are not real so why are you worrying about it?"
   b. "I don't hear the voices, but the words must be frightening for you."
   c. "You are imagining the worst when nothing is going to happen."
   d. "How can you hear voices when you and I are the only ones in this room?"

2. The nurse is caring for a client who says, "I feel like I will never be able to leave this place." The nurse's most therapeutic reply would be:
   a. "You don't need to worry about that. We can only keep you for a certain length of time."
   b. "You keep working on your problem and you will be out of here before you know it."
   c. "Everyone feels like it is hopeless, but we will discharge you when you are better."
   d. "You feel as though you will not get better and leave the unit?"

3. During conversation a client tells the nurse, "My husband left me 6 months ago." The nurse notes that the client is repeatedly twisting strands of their hair. The most appropriate technique for the nurse to utilize at this time would be:
   a. Silence
   b. Verification
   c. Restating
   d. Focusing

4. When initiating interaction with a client, which of the following would be most appropriate to open the communication?
   a. "How would you describe what you are feeling today?"
   b. "Tell me about your family."
   c. "Do you always look at things in such a negative way?"
   d. "You are sad today because no one is talking to you?"

5. A client who will be having several diagnostic tests the following day reports being unable to sleep and says, "I am so afraid something is really wrong with me." What is the nurse's most therapeutic response?
   a. "You seem worried about the results of your tests. Would you like to talk about it?"
   b. "It is important that you get some sleep. I will see what the doctor ordered to help you rest."
   c. "You really need to believe that everything will turn out okay."
   d. "Your doctor performs these tests every day. Everything will be fine."

6. A client jokingly says, "You nurses are bossy just like my wife. In fact, everyone I know tries to put me in a dog chain." Which of the following would best clarify the nurse's perception of the client's statement?
   a. "Why do you think other people try to push you around?"
   b. "I can't believe someone can do that to someone like you!"
   c. "You don't have to put up with that kind of treatment."
   d. "You feel a lack of control in your life. Is that correct?"

7. A client with a history of excessive alcohol use tells the nurse, "I haven't always drunk this much, but lately my life is so bad." The nurse notes the client is rubbing their hands together and squirming in the seat. Which of the following responses would be appropriate at this time?
   a. "Go on…"
   b. "Why do you think your life is so bad?"
   c. "Are you blaming someone else for your drinking?"
   d. "What could be so bad that you need to drink more?"

8. A client is talking about their family and suddenly changes the subject to what television show is their favorite. Which of the following strategies by the nurse would best elicit more information about the client's family situation? *(Select all that apply)*
   a. "Is there some connection between the TV show and your family?"
   b. "Tell me more about your family…"
   c. "Why did you change the subject?"
   d. "Are you uncomfortable talking about your family?"
   e. "Let's get back to your family…"

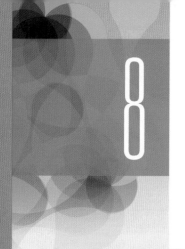

8

The Nursing Process in Mental Health Nursing

Understanding the Nursing Process for Mental Health Nursing

The **nursing process** is a scientific and systematic method for providing effective individualized nursing care and serves as an aid in resolving client problems. The nursing process consists of five components: assessment (data collection), nursing care focus (sometimes called nursing diagnosis), planning, intervention, and evaluation (Fig. 8.1). This problem-solving approach allows the nurse to help the mental health client achieve a maximal level of functioning and well-being. It is accepted by the nursing profession as a standard for providing ongoing nursing care that is adapted to individual client needs. Integral to this approach is an organized method called the nursing care plan. Use of the nursing care plan also allows nurses to share information that is important to the continuity of client care and treatment. The nurse can revisit each component of the nursing process to adjust, revise, or terminate the plan of care based on new or added information. It is important to remember that each client's response to therapy and treatment may be different. Adjustments can and must be made as the level of illness and dysfunction affects their independence and well-being.

During the nursing process, the nurse collects the data and, based upon that information, identifies the client's problems and determines the nursing care focuses (nursing diagnoses) in collaboration with the client when possible. Based upon the nursing care focus that is selected, the nurse identifies outcomes and plans and implements nursing interventions to help reach the outcome. The nurse then compares the client's actual outcome with the goal that was set. The nursing process, however, does not end at this point. The nurse revisits the data collection component and adjusts the nursing care focuses and goals as needed.

Vital to the nursing process is the therapeutic climate of interaction between the client and members of the mental health team. The nurse is often the first member of the team that is in contact with the client. It is at this point that a therapeutic milieu is established. The environment is modified to create a setting in which the client feels safe, secure, and free to express feelings and thoughts without fear of rejection, retaliation, or punishment. The nurse can best build a relationship and establish a sense of trust by approaching the client in an accepting and nonjudgmental manner. A trusting link is vital to the successful outcome of the client's improved functioning and well-being.

As in other areas of nursing, the nursing process in mental health nursing is the foundation of providing care to the client through a systematic, organized approach. Since the mental health nurse is in frequent contact with the client, they

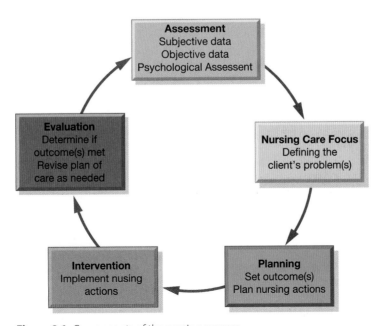

Figure 8.1 Components of the nursing process.

are in an optimum position to provide new data, implement the care plan, and observe the response to treatment.

Assessment (Data Collection)

Assessment involves the collection of psychosocial, subjective, and objective data about the client. **Subjective data** is data spoken by the client or family and **objective data** is data the nurse observes. Data collected forms the basis of all nursing care for the client. Collection of data is a skill that takes study and practice. Although the assessment is usually the responsibility of the registered nurse (RN), assisting with the collection of data and observation of the client's response to treatment is integral in the role of the licensed practical/vocational nurse (LPN/LVN). Often, the client's past medical and psychiatric histories help to identify potential problems related to the present situation.

Assessment begins when the client is admitted to a health care facility or contact is made for the first time, and it continues as the cycle of the nursing process progresses and new information is gained. Because the nurse is often the first person to do an admission physical assessment of the client, they have an opportunity to begin gathering information informally by observing nonverbal behaviors and using direct questioning. To be effective at data collection, the nurse needs to understand the concepts of communication, growth and development, the influence of culture, and the effects medications can have on the client.

Test Yourself	✔ What are the components of the nursing process? ✔ What are the three types of data that are collected during the assessment component? ✔ What is the difference between subjective and objective data?

Psychosocial Assessment

A psychosocial assessment is usually conducted within the psychiatric setting. However, symptoms of psychosocial needs can be seen in any health care setting and therefore are part of any nursing assessment. A psychosocial assessment is an important part of any nursing assessment,

but for the mental health nurse, its purpose is to assist in specifically identifying any problems in the individual's life that could have a psychological impact on their immediate well-being or indicate mental health dysfunction. Social issues may include relationships, personal or family history of mental illness, religious and cultural beliefs, and specific health practices.

The nurse uses a standard assessment tool to gather cognitive, emotional, and behavioral data, which helps to categorize the information obtained during collection. A basic psychosocial assessment usually includes the client's history and mental or emotional status. Table 8.1 provides a summary of the different components covered in a psychosocial assessment.

TABLE 8.1	Components of Psychosocial Assessment
Assessment Component	**Examples of Observations**
Appearance	Grooming, dress, hygiene, eye contact, skin markings, posture, facial expression
Motor activity	Pacing, slow, rigid, relaxed, restless, combative, gait, hyperactive, aggressive
Attitude	Cooperative, uncooperative, friendly, hostile, apathetic, suspicious
Speech pattern	Speed, volume, articulation, congruence, confabulation, slurring, dysphasia
Mood	Intensity, depth, duration, anxious, sad, euphoric, labile, fearful, irritable, depressed
Affect	Flat or absence of emotional expression, blunted, congruent with mood, appropriate, inappropriate
Level of awareness	Level of consciousness, attention span, comprehension, processing
Orientation	Time, place, person
Memory	Recent or short term and remote or long term
Understanding of illness	Insight or ability to perceive and understand their illness and symptoms as related to the illness
Description of stressors	Ability to describe any internal or psychological/physical stress factors they are experiencing or an actual loss or crisis occurring in their life
Thought processes	Speed, content, organization, logical, illogical, delusions, abstract, concrete
Perception	Hallucinations, illusions, depersonalization, distortions
Judgment	Problem-solving and decision-making ability
Adaptation	Available coping mechanisms, adaptive or maladaptive coping
Relationships	Attainment and maintenance of interpersonal and social relationships

Subjective Data

Subjective data are provided by the client and typically include the client's history and perception of the present situation or problem, in addition to feelings, thoughts, symptoms, or emotions that they may be experiencing (Box 8.1). Sometimes the client's information is called into question or contradicted by information received from other sources and may need to be validated by family, friends, law enforcement officers, or others who are involved with the client.

Just the Facts Input from the client's family can provide information about family dynamics, any present turmoil or disruption within the family, and how the client's problem may be affecting other members of the family.

When collecting subjective data, it is important for the nurse to be as accurate and descriptive as possible. Citing direct quotes from the client is a way of reporting what the client is saying without attempting to interpret the intended meaning. Using the client's own words to describe feelings or thoughts often provides insight into perceptual distortions or illogical thought processes.

The subjective information gathered during the initial assessment will allow the nurse to establish a baseline used to formulate the nursing care plan. By asking direct, focused, and leading questions, the nurse gets a clear picture of certain problems or issues concerning the client. Providing a climate that ensures privacy and confidentiality affords the client the freedom to communicate personal feelings openly. The nurse's willingness and ability to listen actively to the client are vital to the outcome of this step. Leading questions can be used to obtain data from the client during the assessment interview (Box 8.2).

Objective Data

Objective data are observed and gathered by the nurse or provided by others who are familiar with the client including additional members of the health care team (Box 8.3). A standardized facility-based assessment tool is often used to compile this information. It is very important to note both verbal communication and nonverbal mannerisms, expressions, and emotions. The nurse should look for congruence between what the client is saying and what is displayed in the accompanying behavior.

It is also important to recognize if the client poses any immediate threat or danger to self or others, in which case safety becomes a priority and must be secured. Ensuring safety includes the following actions by the nurse: not positioning themselves toward the back of a room where the exit is then blocked; refraining from being alone in a room with the door shut when a client is known to act violently or pose a safety risk; wearing identification badge or lanyards around their neck, avoiding leaving sharp objects including pens, pencils, silverware (even plastic ones), syringes with needles or even long strangulation hazards such as shoelaces unattended around the client.

Data collected also includes the factors that put the client at risk emotionally and psychologically (i.e., recent changes or stressors, history of mental disorder, drug use or misuse) and those positive factors that suggest the likelihood that the client can improve from the current situation, such as positive coping strategies, a strong support system, and willingness to receive treatment. Objective data resulting from a review of the client's previous medical records includes the client's medical history, past illnesses or surgeries, medication history, allergies, diet, and physical assessment.

| **Mind Jogger** | Describe how a past medical and psychiatric history would help to identify potential problems. |

Nursing Care Focus (Nursing Diagnosis)

Establishing a nursing care focus from collected data is the second step in the nursing process.

The **nursing care focus** is an identification of a client problem based on an actual or a potential problem that falls within the range of the nursing scope of practice. The nursing care focus *is not* a medical diagnosis. The LPN/LVN helps to develop a nursing care focus with the RN based upon the data collected. The nursing care focuses change as the client's condition changes; they are in a continuous cycle of being reevaluated and updated or resolved based upon the evaluation and assessment (data collection) stages. Determining the client's problem, which becomes the nursing care focus, provides the groundwork for planning nursing interventions to meet the client needs for which the nurse is responsible.

Nursing care focuses can be classified as actual or risk. An actual nursing care focus identifies an existing client problem. A risk nursing care focus identifies a problem that the client is vulnerable to experiencing. An actual nursing care focus statement usually consists of three parts:

1. The actual or potential problem related to the client's condition
2. The causative or contributing factors
   a. A medical diagnosis is *never* used as the etiology (cause) of a nursing problem
3. Data collected that supports the problem

CASE STUDY 8.1

"Ray"

mirelasantiagophoto/Shutterstock

Ray is admitted to your unit after he was brought in by the police for involvement in a physical altercation. As you collect data during the admission you note that he has a 5 cm circular and red contusion on his right cheek, a 3 cm cut on his forehead that is not actively bleeding but covered with dried blood, and his right knuckles are swollen and red. His heart rate is 104, respiratory rate is 24, and blood pressure 156/88. He states his normal blood pressure is 140/82. He denies loss of consciousness, headache, and visual changes. The police state they removed a knife from his waistband. The x-ray of his right hand and wrist is negative for a fracture per the health care provider's report. Ray provides a urine sample that is clear and is sent from a toxicology screen. As you ask questions, he periodically checks the door as if looking for someone. You notice that his pupils are not dilated or pinpoint and they both react to the lights in the room. When you ask him what occurred prior to the altercation he states "I'm just mad. Is that OK with you?" You ask Ray about the motorcycle tattoos on his arms and what they mean and he replies, "It's who I am."

Digging Deeper

1. What subjective data did you collect?

2. What leading questions were asked?

3. What objective data did you collect?

4. What further information would you want to gather or questions to ask?

An example of a correctly written actual nursing care focus statement is: *Overweight related to medications as evidenced by a 20-pound weight gain since starting antipsychotic medication 3 months ago.* In this example the actual problem is being overweight, the causative factor is the antipsychotic medication, and the supportive data is the 20-pound weight gain over a 3-month period.

An example of a correctly written risk nursing care focus statement is: *Suicide Attempt Risk related to suicidal ideation.* In this example the potential problem is the suicide attempt risk and the supportive data is the suicidal ideation. There is no causative factor listed in a risk nursing care focus as it is a potential problem; only supportive data is listed to show why it is a potential problem.

Once applicable nursing care focuses have been determined, they are prioritized. **Prioritization** is the act of deciding the order in which to address the issue, or individual, based upon the intensity and immediate urgency of the problem. Any health condition that endangers life will receive a high priority. Situations that are recurrent or chronic might be given a lower priority to be addressed at a later time. A client with suicidal ideation or intent, for example, would have an immediate risk for self-harm. This problem would require the nurse's attention first.

Based on Maslow's hierarchy of needs, basic physiologic needs such as oxygen, food, water, warmth, elimination, and sleep must be met before other higher-level needs can be addressed. This model can be seen as a staircase in which a client may vacillate between steps. Given that the client can move up and then back down, the nurse should understand that the priority given to a problem can change at any time during the treatment process. To illustrate this concept, a client who has begun to identify strengths and display positive self-talk (self-esteem level need) is told by another client that they are "stupid and ugly." Since then, the client has refused to eat for 2 days. At this point the nutritional needs of the client become the priority.

It is important to include the client in determining and prioritizing their nursing care focuses. It is not unusual for the client's prioritization of their needs to be different than the nurse's. Whenever possible, and safe to do so, the client's prioritization should be followed. It is also important to give priority to the problem that the client is currently experiencing (actual) over a problem that may happen (risk). An actual problem has priority over one that could possible occur during the course of the illness. Acute withdrawal symptoms in the client with substance use disorder would have priority over the potential for social isolation in that individual.

Just the Facts Nursing care focuses and implementations should be planned to include religious and cultural practices of the client.

"Matthew"

Matthew is a 26-year-old carpenter who, up until 5 days ago, was employed by a building contractor. At the time of his termination, Matthew was told by his supervisor that his work had not been consistently satisfactory and to avoid legal problems, he was being fired. Matthew has been living with his girlfriend and her two children for the past 3 years. Two days after he lost his job, his girlfriend told him she was seeing someone else and wanted him to move out. Matthew is brought to the emergency room by the police who state he was wandering around a parking lot at 2:00 AM. He is disoriented and unable to tell the nurse who he is or what he was doing in the parking lot. He states he is lost and doesn't know where he should go.

CASE STUDY 8.2

Digging Deeper

1. *What subjective data has been gathered?*

2. *What objective data has been gathered?*

3. *Using the nursing process, how would you develop the following nursing care focuses?*

Acute Anxiety, related to _____, *evidenced by* _____

Coping Impairment, related to _____, *evidenced by* _____

Memory Impairment, related to _____, *evidenced by* _____

Outcome Identification and Planning

The next phase of the nursing process involves identifying outcomes in cooperation with the client and planning appropriate nursing interventions that will help to achieve the outcomes. **Outcomes** are specific, measurable, and realistic goals. In addition, the outcome should include a time frame for accomplishing it. The outcomes help to measure the resolution of the problem identified in the nursing care focus. They should be determined in collaboration with the client, to increase cooperation and adherence to therapeutic interventions. Clients who do not have input in their plan of care are less likely to cooperate or follow through with the interventions.

Listed below are examples of outcomes for a common mental health nursing care focus: *Depression*

- Client reports an increase in energy levels
- Client identifies two personal strengths
- Client consumes at least 75% of each meal
- Client attends unit activities
- Client sleeps no more than 8 hours at night
- Client performs activities of daily living (ADLs) independently
- Client does not report feeling or thought of self-harm

Timelines are not given in the sample outcomes as they will vary based upon individual client situations. It is important to note that not all outcomes listed for each nursing care focus will be realistic or appropriate for every client. Select the most appropriate one (or ones) or develop individualized outcomes. Then choose appropriate interventions that will help meet the outcome that was set.

Implementation

In the implementation component of the nursing process, the nursing plan of care is put into action. The nursing interventions that were planned in the previous step are carried out. **Nursing interventions** are actions taken by the nurse to assist the client in achieving the anticipated outcome. It is important to plan actions that are appropriate for the individual client and take into consideration the level of functioning that is realistic for them. What may be realistic for one client may be unattainable for another. The written plan of care is a collaborative effort between all members of the health care team and is communicated to each health care worker. This helps to ensure the continuity of care and consistency in the implementation of interventions by all personnel. Consistency is a vital component of the therapeutic milieu.

Some nursing interventions are independently performed based on the nurse's judgment (such as observing a client during a group activity) while other nursing interventions are dependent upon a health care provider's order (such as administering a medication). Other nursing interventions are interdependent between the nurse and another member of the health care team (such as working with the occupational therapy department). The nurse must understand their scope of nursing practice as set by their state board of nursing.

There are many clinical units that use standardized or computer-generated care plans or clinical pathways. These are designed to reflect current standards of care, be cost-effective, and improve the efficiency with which treatment is carried out. Regardless of the method used, the nursing plan of care identifies those interventions for which the nurse has responsibility. It is imperative that the unique needs and problems of each client are retained as central to their plan of care.

Mental health nursing interventions do not involve intensive physical care nursing skills. Rather, the nurse focuses on observing behaviors and symptoms, improving communication strategies, and assisting the client in problem solving with improved overall functioning. Nursing interventions are implemented according to the nurse's level of practice. Achievement of the anticipated outcomes is difficult for clients with mental illnesses and many require extensive reinforcement and reassurance to change behaviors and understand the underlying emotional issues. Box 8.4 provides a list of strategies for working with mental health clients.

Just the Facts Nursing interventions are intended to encourage, maintain, and reestablish a level of mental and physical functioning that promotes the well-being of the client.

Mind Jogger How can the nurse increase the client's motivation to participate in the plan of care?

BOX 8.4

Nursing Strategies for Mental Health Nurses

- Respect and accept each client as they are.
- Allow the client opportunity to set own pace in working with problems.
- Nursing interventions should center on the client as an individual, not on the medical diagnosis. Safety interventions should be included and usually take priority.
- Remember, *all behavior has meaning*. Behavior is an attempt to prevent the occurrence or decrease the intensity of anxiety.
- Recognize your own feelings toward clients. Address your feelings in a professional manner with another nurse.
- Go to the client who needs help most—prioritize which client needs to be seen first.
- Do not allow a situation to develop or continue in which a client becomes the focus of attention in a negative manner.
- If client behavior is atypical, base your decision to intervene on whether the client is endangering self or others.
- Ask for help—don't be the only staff member present when dealing with a client who is out of control.
- Avoid highly competitive activities between clients or clients and staff.
- Make frequent contact with clients—let them know they are worth your time and effort.
- Remember to assess the physical needs of your client.
- Be patient. Move at client's pace and ability.
- Suggesting, requesting, or asking work better than commands.
- Therapeutic thinking is not to think about or think for the client, but *with* the client.
- Be honest and truthful so the client can trust you.
- Make reality interesting enough so the client prefers it to their fantasy.
- Compliment, reassure, and model appropriate behaviors.

The implementation step of the nursing process should focus on helping clients redirect their energies in a constructive manner. The nursing interventions should be based on scientific principles for resolving the identified problem and should be safe for the client and others involved. Other chapters in this text will include appropriate nursing actions for clients with the various types of mental health issues and illnesses. As nursing actions are implemented and documented, a picture of client progress evolves. Data collection is continuous during this phase. Client response to interventions provides valuable information that assists the nurse in determining whether the client is making progress toward the defined outcome criteria. Additional data also aids in the planning of ongoing nursing care.

Test Yourself
- ✔ How is prioritization determined?
- ✔ List the four criteria that should be part of an outcome.
- ✔ What is the importance of including the client in the plan of care?

Evaluation

Measuring whether the nursing plan of care was achieved occurs in the **evaluation** component of the nursing process. Here the nurse determines if the outcome was met, partially met, or not met at all. The evaluation of the outcome can be stated as one of the following: "the goal has been achieved," "some progress has been made toward the intended outcome," or "no steps forward have been observed or documented." If a goal has been partially met, there may be supporting data to indicate continuance of the current plan of care. This approach recognizes that the client may need more time to make changes and adjust to them. A distinction must be made between a lack of client motivation and the need to continue the current plan to help the client achieve the outcomes. Some interventions may have been ineffective and new strategies may be needed to help meet the client's needs. It is also important to determine if the expected outcome was not actually achievable for the client.

The evaluation phase is a form of validation for the entire nursing process in the delivery of care to the client. Continued data collection may indicate new problems or alterations in the original nursing care focuses. Outcomes are clarified to reflect realistic and measurable terms for the client. Nursing interventions are reevaluated for effectiveness. The nursing process helps in maintaining a therapeutic approach and continuity of nursing care for the mental health client.

Just the Facts   The nurse is the only member of the mental health team who can evaluate client response to the nursing care plan.

Documentation

While not part of the nursing process, documentation of information about the client in the permanent record is a vital component to the nursing care. The client's medical record is a legal document and must be factual, accurate, and complete. Documentation must occur as soon after the instance as possible to ensure the actions are communicated to all members of the treatment team. It helps to provide a history of the client's problems and their response to nursing interventions. It also gives an accurate history of the client's admission dates, medications, dosages, and response to the medication and other therapies. Documentation must be free from the nurse's opinion and feelings. Nursing care and the client's response to it and the medical interventions must be documented. All documentation requires a date and time. Handwritten notes must be legible, in ink (not pencil), and there should be no instances of scratched out entries or words. Handwritten errors should have a single line drawn through them with the nurse's initial, date, and time written above the line.

The form of documentation depends on the facility's policy. Some facilities use a computerized format and others use written notes. Documentation includes the data collected regarding the daily observations, client's behavior and responses during activities, physical data (e.g., vital signs, weight, hours of sleep), and any unexpected interventions and client observations (e.g., when a client becomes aggressive and the staff response and safety measures instituted as a result of the aggressive behavior). Other types of documentation include reinforcing teaching that was done by the RN and the client's response, discharge checklists, and medication administration records.

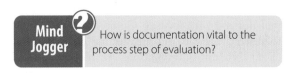

Mind Jogger How is documentation vital to the process step of evaluation?

Example of Application of the Nursing Process

Chapters 9 to 19 each have a section that applies the nursing process to the specific mental health disorders discussed in the chapter. An example of a client situation is shown below to help facilitate understanding of the nursing process as it relates to the mental health client.

Client Situation

Freda is a 47-year-old public school teacher who received word several days ago that her only child, 23-year-old Benjamin, was arrested for armed robbery. Benjamin is married and the father of two small children. Two months ago, Freda discovered that her husband of 26 years is having an affair. Freda blames herself for the affair, stating that she is "overweight and unattractive." She says that he would be better off without her anyway. She states, "I'm a failure as both a mother and a wife." She is unable to concentrate in the classroom and has considered a leave of absence from her job. Last night Freda's husband told her he was leaving her and wants a divorce. Freda was brought to the emergency room this morning after being found unresponsive by her daughter-in-law. First responders found beside her an empty bottle of alprazolam that was filled 2 days ago. The daughter-in-law tells the nurse that Freda has been drinking a lot of wine in the past few months. After initial treatment and several days of stabilization on a medical–surgical unit, Freda is admitted to the mental health unit for follow-up.

Data Collection

The mental health nurse obtained the additional data:

- Is overweight and has unkempt appearance
- Has two small grandchildren she loves
- "I don't blame him for finding someone else. I am so fat and ugly."
- "He would be better off without me anyway. I'm such a mess."
- "I must have done something wrong for my son to be in so much trouble. I can't do anything right."
- "I can't even think clearly enough to teach my class. I might as well quit."
- "The only good thing in my life is my little grandkids. They deserve better than me."

Table 8.2 demonstrates the application of the nursing process to Freda's situation for three applicable nursing care focuses.

TABLE 8.2	Sample Nursing Plan of Care		
Nursing Care Focus	**Goal** **The Client:**	**Nursing Interventions**	**Evaluation of Goal/** **Desired Outcome**
Self-Harm Risk, evidenced by suicide overdose with use of alcohol and statements of low self-worth	Does not engage in self-harm behavior while hospitalized	Assess for social withdrawal or isolation Assess for self-destructive thoughts Remove potentially dangerous items from room Monitor mood, affect, and behavior Provide suicide watch if client states active thoughts of self-harm	Has not harmed self during hospitalization Expresses feelings about suicide attempt
Coping Impairment, related to life events, as evidenced by increased drinking, self-blame, and inability to meet role expectations	Communicates feelings about current situation within 2 days of admission Identifies and uses one adaptive coping strategy within 4 days of admission	Encourage expression of feelings Help to identify internal factors of self-blame Teach and model adaptive coping strategies Encourage to use adaptive coping skills Praise efforts and successes in coping observed on unit	Openly discusses feelings and emotional response to life situations Demonstrates use of adaptive coping strategies
Situational Low Self-Esteem, related to husband's infidelity and son's arrest evidenced by feelings of self-blame and inadequacy	Refrains from self-blame and negative self-talk by discharge Identifies positive life accomplishments and personal strengths within 3 days of admission	Establish trusting relationship Encourage to discuss life events Assist to distinguish between life situations over which she does and does not have control Help to recognize negative self-talk and self-defeating statements Encourage to keep journal of negative and defeating thoughts Assist to identify personal strengths and accomplishments Provide positive reinforcement for expression of positive feelings and thoughts	Reframes self-blame and negative self-talk with more realistic perspective Uses positive statements to describe self Identifies strengths and acknowledges accomplishments Identifies self-talk that is destructive

Cultural Considerations

Culture and the Psychosocial Assessment

It is important for the nurse to consider the client's culture when doing a psychosocial assessment to make accurate observations. Below are some parts of the psychosocial assessment, a response that might be seen among members of some cultures or groups that would be viewed as appropriate within those groups, and what it should *not* be documented as. If the nurse is unsure if the expression is a cultural norm or not, they should verify from the client's support people how the client usually responds or consult with the registered nurse (RN).

Assessment Component	Cultural Value/Norm	Don't Document as:
Affect	Concealing or not showing emotion	Flat affect
Speech Pattern	Rapid pace	Pressured speech
	Pausing before or during speaking	Slowed speech
	Avoiding unnecessary conversation	Refusal to participate in care
Orientation	Not focused on what day of the week it is or not using a clock for describing time	Disorientation
Perception	Speaking to deceased individuals (saints or ancestors)	Hearing voices or hallucinations

Sources: Lim, L. (2016). Cultural differences in emotion: differences in emotional arousal level between the East and the West. *Integrative Medicine Research, 5*(2), 105–109. https://doi.org/10.1016/j.imr.2016.03.004; Shearer, C. (2020). The cultural implications of silence around the world. *Culturewizard.* https://www.rw-3.com/blog/cultural-implications-of-silence

SUMMARY

- The nursing process is a scientific, organized, problem-solving method that has five components.
- The five components of the nursing process are: assessment (data collection), nursing care focus (sometimes called nursing diagnosis), planning, intervention, and evaluation.
- Assessment involves the collection of psychosocial, subjective, and objective data about the client. Subjective data is data spoken by the client or family and objective data is data the nurse observes.
- A psychosocial assessment is an important part of any nursing assessment, but for the mental health nurse, the purpose is to assist in specifically identifying any problems in the individual's life that could have a psychological impact on their immediate well-being or indicate mental health dysfunction.
- A basic psychosocial nursing assessment usually includes the client's history and mental or emotional status including both subjective and objective data.
- The nursing care focus is an identification of a client problem based on an actual or a potential problem that falls within the range of the nursing scope of practice.
- Nursing care focuses are formulated by relating them to the cause or contributing reason for the symptoms.
- The three parts of a nursing care focus statement are: the problem, the causative factor, and the supportive data.
- Prioritization is the act of deciding the order in which to address the issue, or individual, based upon the intensity and immediate urgency of the problem.

- Prioritization in nursing care would be seeing and addressing the needs of the client with the most urgent or life-threatening problem. Any condition that endangers life will receive the highest priority.
- Prioritization of nursing care focuses gives highest priority to the ones that threaten health or that the client identifies as a priority. Situations that are risk, recurrent, or chronic might be given a lower priority.
- An outcome needs to be specific, measurable, realistic, and have a timeline for completion.
- Planning measurable and realistic outcomes that anticipate the improvement or stabilization of the identified problem provides a strategy for nursing interventions to be developed.
- Nursing interventions are intended to encourage, maintain, and reestablish a level of mental and physical functioning that promotes the client's well-being.
- The evaluation phase is a form of validation for the entire nursing process in the delivery of care to the client. Continued data collection and revisiting the plan of care allows the nurse a system of addressing client problems in the most effective manner toward resolution.
- The nursing process is an ongoing continuum from admission to discharge and outpatient status.
- Documentation ensures the nurse's actions are communicated to all members of the treatment team. It helps to provide a history of the client's problems and their response to nursing interventions. It also gives an accurate history of the client's admission dates, medications, dosages, and response to the medication and other therapies.

BIBLIOGRAPHY

Hatfield, N. T., & Kincheloe, C. A. (2022). *Introductory maternity and pediatric nursing* (5th ed.). Wolters Kluwer.

RegisteredNursing.org Staff Writers. (2022). *Integrated processes: NCLEX-RN*. RegisteredNursing.org. https://www.registerednursing.org/nclex/integrated-processes/#nursing-process

Toney-Butler, T. J., & Thayer, J. M. Nursing process. [Updated 2022 Apr 14]. In: *StatPearls [Internet]*. StatPearls Publishing. https://www.ncbi.nlm.nih.gov/books/NBK499937/

Tyerman, J., Patovirta, A-L., & Celestini, A. (2021). How stigma and discrimination influences nursing care of persons diagnosed with mental illness: A systematic review. *Issues in Mental Health Nursing*, 42(2), 153–163. https://doi.org/10.1080/01612840.2020.1789788

Fill in the Blank

Fill in the blank with the correct answer.

1. The scientific and systematic method for providing effective individualized nursing care is the _____ _____.
2. Information that is provided by the client is _____ data.
3. Information that is observed by the nurse client is _____ data.
4. A nursing care focus statement consists of a _____ its contributing factor, and supportive _____.
5. _____ should be specific, measurable, realistic, and have a time-frame.

Matching

Match the following terms to the most appropriate phrase.

1. _____ Assessment
2. _____ Prioritization
3. _____ Nursing care focus
4. _____ Nursing interventions
5. _____ Evaluation
6. _____ Outcome

a. Actual or potential client problem
b. Measurable and realistic goal that will help to resolve the client problem
c. Collection of subjective and objective data
d. Defining immediacy or intensity of problems to determine the order in which they will be addressed
e. Actions taken to assist client to achieve desired goal
f. Determines effectiveness of strategies used in meeting anticipated criteria

Multiple Choice

Select the best answer from the multiple-choice items.

1. The nurse is assessing a client with chronic schizophrenia who has stopped taking medication and is being admitted with acute psychotic symptoms. The client's perception of the present problem would best be documented by the nurse using:
   a. The client's exact words and statements
   b. Information obtained from the family
   c. Client behavior that was observed for several hours
   d. Interpretations about the client's thoughts

2. Which of the following is most important in establishing a trusting environment for the organized delivery of nursing care to a client?
   a. Cooperation of the client
   b. A therapeutic milieu
   c. The client's perception of the current situation
   d. An accepting and nonjudgmental attitude by the nurse

3. Which of the following is a component of the client's mental status nursing assessment?
   a. Past medical history
   b. Mood and affect
   c. Medical diagnosis
   d. Nursing care focus

4. Which of the following terms would be descriptive of a client's attitude? *(Select all that apply)*
   a. Cooperative
   b. Friendly
   c. Uncooperative
   d. Depressed
   e. Apathetic

5. What is true regarding a nursing care focus? *(Select all that apply)*
   a. It reflects only actual problems.
   b. It is based upon the medical diagnosis.
   c. It remains unchanged throughout the client's admission.
   d. It contains a problem, the causative factor, and supportive data.
   e. It determines the therapies the client attends.

6. The nurse and client have set an outcome as, "Verbalizes thoughts that precipitate anxiety by discharge." Which part of the outcome statement is missing?
   a. Measurable
   b. Specific
   c. Timeline
   d. Realistic

7. After reinforcing teaching to a client about a newly prescribed medication, the nurse asks the client to explain how they will take the medication and what side effects to watch for. The nurse is executing which step of the nursing process?
   a. Assessment
   b. Planning
   c. Intervention
   d. Evaluation

8. Validation of the nursing process in the delivery of care is most evident in which phase of the care plan?
   a. Assessment
   b. Nursing care focus
   c. Interventions
   d. Evaluation

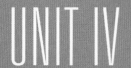

UNIT IV | Specific Psychiatric Disorders

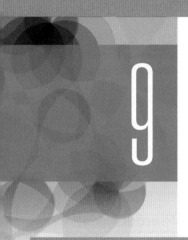

Anxiety Disorders

LEARNING OBJECTIVES

After learning the content in this chapter, the student will be able to:

1. Distinguish between common anxiety and generalized anxiety disorder.
2. Describe the relationship between panic disorder and agoraphobia.
3. Differentiate between specific phobia and social phobia in terms of causative factors and signs and symptoms.
4. Identify the four categories of symptoms seen in post-traumatic stress disorder (PTSD) and examples for each category.
5. Describe the relationship between obsessions and compulsions that are seen in obsessive-compulsive disorder (OCD).
6. Identify different classifications of medications used to treat anxiety.
7. Identify nursing interventions for the client receiving antianxiety medications.

KEY TERMS

agoraphobia

antianxiety agents (anxiolytics)

anticipatory anxiety

automatic relief behaviors

compulsion

cued

emotional numbness

free-floating anxiety

obsession

panic attack

social phobia

specific phobia

uncued

Anxiety

As the stimulus of an actual or perceived threatening situation is processed by the brain, the result is fear. Anxiety is felt as the fear is realized. Anxiety is a vague, uneasy emotional feeling experienced by a person in response to the threat or danger. When anxiety increases to the point of discomfort or distress, then the person senses something is wrong. Sometimes the person can identify the stimulus that is causing the uncomfortable feeling, but in other cases, a cause cannot be identified. **Free-floating anxiety** occurs when the individual is unable to connect the anxiety to a stimulus. This inability to identify a cause of the anxiety can sometimes create additional anxiety for the individual.

The manifestations of anxiety can take many forms. Experiences range from vague discomfort to extreme panic. Increased levels of anxiety can be experienced continuously or periodically. Thoughts, feelings, and behavior are all affected as anxiety increases. Anxiety can be expressed through repetitious behaviors such as counting continuously or repeated handwashing. It can also cause a brief change in behavior such as acting "out of character." This is illustrated by a person who is late for an appointment and delayed in traffic. When a police officer approaches, stating that there is an accident scene that will be cleared in about 30 minutes, the individual starts shouting at the officer.

In other situations, subtle manifestations of anxiety such as clenching the jaw, tapping fingers on a table, or fidgeting may be evident. These **automatic relief behaviors** are unconscious behaviors aimed at relieving the anxiety. Although the individual may be unaware of their actions, others may also be affected. For example, a person sitting at a conference is constantly clicking their ballpoint pen. This continues for nearly 30 minutes, until the person next to them asks them to please stop as they cannot hear the speaker. Unaware that they were doing this behavior, they stop clicking the pen and state, "I'm very nervous with all these people around me." Both individuals in this example are experiencing anxiety, but the anxiety being experienced by the person who is uncomfortable in a crowded room will most likely continue to be felt unless they leave the room. Unless measures are taken to remove the cause, the anxiety will continue to be experienced and can even escalate.

 Mind Jogger What physiologic symptoms usually accompany an increase in anxiety?

Beyond the everyday experiences of anxiety, anxiety disorders are characterized by uncontrolled anxiety that leads to an impairment in social, interpersonal, or work functioning. Although signs and symptoms may vary from disorder to disorder, the common thread or feature of these conditions is overwhelming anxiety that is uncontrolled. Unlike anxiety felt briefly during a traffic stop, the level of anxiety that leads to a disorder is disabling and progressive unless treatment is obtained.

Types of Anxiety Disorders

Generalized Anxiety Disorder

In generalized anxiety disorder, the individual experiences an increased level of anxiety and worry about various situations on most days over a period of at least 6 months. The individual has difficulty controlling the anxiety and experiences considerable discomfort, lack of concentration, and impaired ability to function that cannot be attributed to the physiologic effects of a substance or another medical condition.

Signs and Symptoms

In addition to the excessive worry and anxiety over several different activities or events, the person also experiences at least three other symptoms. See Box 9.1 for signs and symptoms of generalized anxiety disorder. The existence of continued tension and feeling on edge can lead to a reduced quality of life and overall dissatisfaction with self and others. The anxiety impacts the individual's daily functioning and is typically chronic, but in some individuals, it may occur in a cyclical pattern.

 Just the Facts Typical fears of the individual with generalized anxiety disorder include physical injury, major illness or death, mental illness, loss of control, and rejection.

Incidence and Etiology

Generalized anxiety disorder is the most common anxiety disorder seen in the United States, affects approximately 3% of the country's adult population

BOX 9.1

Signs and Symptoms of Generalized Anxiety Disorder

PSYCHOSOCIAL

- Chronic excessive worry and anxiety with no particular stimulus
- Negative self-talk
- Difficulty falling or staying asleep
- Increased startle reflex
- Feeling on edge, inability to relax
- Restlessness
- Irritability
- Inability to control the anxiety
- Anticipating the "worst"
- Inability to concentrate

SOMATIC (PHYSICAL)

- Tremors
- Chest pain
- Hyperventilation
- Muscle tension
- Headaches
- Fatigue
- Breathing difficulties
- Gastrointestinal disturbances and urinary frequency
- Teeth grinding (bruxism)

(approximately 6.8 million persons), and is more common in women than men (Anxiety and Depression Association of America [ADAA], 2022a). However, less than half of individuals with generalized anxiety disorder receive treatment. Most people who are diagnosed with generalized anxiety disorder have felt excessive worry and anxiety all their life, although most do not request treatment until their mid-30s. Onset is usually in childhood or early adolescence. A family history of generalized anxiety disorder, as well as stressful life experiences, can increase the individual's risk for developing the disorder. A coexisting diagnosis of depression is commonly seen with generalized anxiety disorder.

 Mind Jogger What psychosocial factors might contribute to the familial tendency of generalized anxiety disorder?

Panic Disorder

A **panic attack** is described as an intense feeling of fear or terror that occurs suddenly and intermittently without warning. The individual experiencing the panic attack is unable to determine when these attacks will occur or reoccur. When they are unable to connect any particular stimulus with the panic attack, this is known as an **uncued** attack. An attack is said to be **cued** when an identified trigger can be associated with the attack. Some people may only experience a single attack, while others go on to develop a panic disorder.

A panic disorder is characterized by recurrent, unexpected panic attacks. The frequency and severity of these attacks may vary. Some people

---

"Josephine"

shisu_ka/ Shutterstock

Josephine is a 46-year-old female admitted with depression after the loss of her job has left her despondent. She states, "I don't blame my boss—I could not concentrate or get anything done. I did not want to make any decisions because I was afraid any decision I made would hurt someone's feelings." Josephine is tearful, jumpy, and on edge during the assessment interview. She states, "I don't know what I'm going to do. I have to pay the bills because my husband can't work. The kids need clothes for school. I must be the most terrible mother and wife on earth. I can't sleep. Everything I try to do is a disaster. I'm such a failure. My family would be better off without me." You notice her speech is rapid and she has dark circles under her eyes. She is constantly fidgeting with a tissue in her hand.

Digging Deeper

1. What data was collected that supports that Josephine has anxiety?

2. How can the nurse help to lower Josephine's anxiety level?

3. What statements would be therapeutic for the nurse to make?

CASE STUDY 9.1

may be able to endure brief exposure to the situation that causes panic. Others may not be able to expose themselves to the situation at all. When this occurs, the consequences of the disorder are much greater, and the functional capacity of the individual decreases significantly.

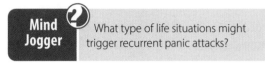

Mind Jogger ❷ What type of life situations might trigger recurrent panic attacks?

Signs and Symptoms

A state of panic results in sympathetic nervous system symptoms of heart pounding, palpitations, shortness of breath, dizziness, sweating, weakness, and numbness. The individual may also feel shaky and chilled with accompanying nausea, chest pain, tingling or numbness of the hands, feelings of suffocation, and being out of control. Many individuals feel they are having a heart attack or even dying when they first experience a panic attack. Attacks may occur daily, weekly, or monthly. Attacks may also occur during the night. Many last only a few minutes, but they may last longer. People experiencing panic attacks often have a fear of "going crazy" or "losing it." Self-esteem may also be affected in varying degrees. Many clients seek medical attention because of their fear of having a life-threatening illness. Fear of having the "next attack" can cause significant impairment in the individual's overall functioning. The signs and symptoms for panic disorder are found in Box 9.2.

Just the Facts Individuals who become aware of their anxiety learn to identify specific fears that overwhelm them during a panic attack.

BOX 9.2

Signs and Symptoms of Panic Disorder

- Rapid and pounding heart rate
- Increased perspiration
- Chilling or flushing
- Tingling or numbness of hands, shaking
- Nausea
- Chest pain, shortness of breath
- Feeling of being suffocated
- Fear of being out of control
- Fear of dying or having a heart attack
- Agoraphobia
- Depression

Individuals with panic disorder often develop **agoraphobia**, or an avoidance of certain places or situations where escape is impossible. Because they fear a reoccurrence of the panic state, they often restrict their activities to avoid the possibility of this happening. Everyday activities such as shopping for groceries and attending church or family events may be avoided because of fear that escape from these situations might be difficult or embarrassing. They may have fears of being in a crowd or on a bridge, or traveling in a bus, airplane, or automobile. Should they be entrapped in this situation, the anxiety experienced would lead to a feeling of helplessness and panic. By limiting the possibilities that this would happen, the person often becomes homebound, or restricted to home surroundings.

Unemployment and school drop-out are common. Decreased work functioning is evidenced by the inability to complete tasks, repeated absences, and difficulty interacting with others. Up to two thirds of those with this disorder also experience depression or engage in excessive substance use to cope with the anxiety.

Incidence and Etiology

Although panic disorders can occur at any age, the typical onset is between late adolescence and the mid-40s. Individuals with an immediate biologic relative who has a panic disorder are more likely to also develop the disorder. Panic disorder affects approximately 2.7% of the United States population (about 6 million adults) and is twice as common in females as males (ADAA, 2022b). Most of those diagnosed with agoraphobia have an accompanying diagnosis of panic disorder. Common coexisting diagnoses include depression and obsessive-compulsive disorder (OCD).

Test Yourself
- ✔ How does free-floating anxiety differ from the anxiety felt after being in a car accident?
- ✔ What is the difference between generalized anxiety disorder and panic disorder?
- ✔ How would agoraphobia impact an individual's lifestyle and day-to-day functioning?

Specific Phobia

A **specific phobia** is characterized by an excessive and persistent irrational fear of specific objects or situations that pose little threat or danger. The

"Jack"

Jack loves baseball. He has a fear of crowded places from which there is no accessible exit. When he attends baseball games, Jack usually gets a seat close to the exit ramp. Today, however, he discovers that his ticket is not for an aisle seat. He suddenly becomes very aware that the stadium is crowded, and he will have to move between many people to get to his seat. He begins to feel his heart throb and has a general flushed feeling. Sweat begins to form on his scalp and down his back. Instead of going to his seat, he quickly goes to exit the stadium. Attempting to leave, he has to weave around and in between people the entire trip. Jack begins to panic and feels a sense of terror. He cannot find the exit and feels nearly paralyzed. A staff member notices his distress and the stadium health team is notified. When asked if he is willing to be transported to the hospital Jack manages to nod "yes" but is unable to verbalize which hospital.

Digging Deeper

1. How does Jack's behavior support the presence of a panic disorder?

2. In what way is Jack's behavior different from free-floating anxiety?

3. How is this problem impairing his ability to function in a social setting?

CASE STUDY 9.2

---

common categories of phobias include animals, height, water, storms, blood or needles, flying, or spaces. Box 9.3 lists examples of specific phobias.

Just the Facts Specific phobias usually cause little concern because the person can usually plan ahead to avoid the feared stimulus.

Signs and Symptoms

When an individual encounters the object or situation that causes the fear, they usually experience an immediate anxiety reaction. The reaction can be mild, severe, or even result in a panic attack. The distance between the person and the feared object will affect the level of response. A person who fears dogs will experience the most anxiety while near the animal but may have a less severe response when viewing a picture of a dog. Whether or not there is a way to escape from the feared stimulus also plays a role in the intensity of the anxiety the person feels. A person who has a fear of going over bridges, for example, will have the most anxiety if there is no way to avoid crossing the bridge. Although children may not be aware of the stimulus causing the anxiety, adolescents and adults are usually aware that their response is extreme and unrealistic. Those with intense fears may experience anxiety symptoms when just thinking about or seeing a picture of the precipitating factor.

Some people avoid the activities of everyday life because they experience discomfort or increased anxiety when faced with the feared stimulus. During times when there is no exposure to the feared object or situation, however, their anxiety level is no higher than it would normally be. It is when this avoidance significantly impairs the person's ability to continue functioning in social and work settings that the diagnosis of specific phobia is made. The signs and symptoms for specific phobia disorder are listed in Box 9.4.

Incidence and Etiology

Specific phobias affect 8.7% of the United States population (over 19 million adults) and are twice

---

BOX 9.3

Examples of Specific Phobias

- Fear of germs—mysophobia
- Fear of spiders—arachnophobia
- Fear of snakes—ophidiophobia
- Fear of heights—acrophobia
- Fear of thunder and lightning—astraphobia
- Fear of confined spaces—claustrophobia
- Fear of flying—aerophobia
- Fear of dogs—cynophobia
- Fear of blood—hematophobia
- Fear of injections—trypanophobia
- Fear of the number 13—triskaidekaphobia

BOX 9.4

Signs and Symptoms of Specific Phobia Disorder

- Irrational and persistent fear of an object or situation
- Immediate anxiety, including physical symptoms, when encountering the feared object or situation
- Loss of control, fainting, or panic response
- Avoidance of activities involving feared stimulus
- Worry with anticipatory anxiety
- Possible impaired social or work functioning

Just the Facts Individuals with social anxiety disorder may try to decrease the overwhelming anxiety felt in the feared situation by using drugs and/or alcohol.

as common in females as males (ADAA, 2022b). Although phobias are common, they are rarely severe enough to be diagnosed. Symptoms usually have an onset during childhood or adolescence and persist throughout adult life. The fear of a particular stimulus is usually present for some time before it is severe enough to be considered a disorder. Phobias following a traumatic event, such as the fear of water after a near-drowning situation, can develop at any age.

Mind Jogger How would fear of germs or injections affect the nursing care of a hospitalized client?

Social Anxiety Disorder (Social Phobia)

Social anxiety disorder, also known as **social phobia**, is characterized by an excessive fear of any social situation in which embarrassment is possible. The person with this disorder experiences intense discomfort when being watched or at risk of being judged or ridiculed by others. This experience typically occurs during social activities where the person will be speaking, dining, or writing in public (such as a student working out a math problem in front of the classroom). Although the person may recognize that the fear is extreme and unrealistic, they are unable to stop it. Social anxiety may be related to a specific situation, such as indoor activities or loud music, or it may be related to social occasions in general. Symptoms may be severe enough to interfere with the individual's work or school functioning. Social isolation may result in which the person has limited friends or contacts.

Just the Facts In some cultures, a person's anxiety stems from the fear of embarrassing others rather than embarrassing themselves. For example, in taijin kyofusho, common in Japan and Korea, the fear is related to offending other people.

Signs and Symptoms

Physical symptoms of anxiety are usually experienced by the person with social anxiety disorder (Box 9.5). The person may be embarrassed by the symptoms, which adds to their discomfort. Most people will avoid the difficult situation altogether, while others will tolerate the activity but with intense anxiety.

Anticipatory anxiety is anxiety that occurs in advance of a feared situation (such as a public speech or social event). This leads to thoughts of dread leading up to the event. The added anxiety results in actual or perceived failure in the situation, leading to embarrassment and further anxiety. This pattern sets up a vicious cycle of persistent discomfort that can be incapacitating. Many people who have social phobia may also have test anxiety, poor job performance, or poor communication skills related to the effects of their anxiety on interactions in the feared situation. The signs and symptoms for social anxiety disorder are listed in Box 9.5.

Incidence and Etiology

Social anxiety disorder affects approximately 6.8% of the United States population (about 15 million adults) and tends to be equally distributed between men and women (ADAA, 2022b). The

BOX 9.5

Signs and Symptoms of Social Anxiety Disorder (Social Phobia)

- Hyperventilation
- Sweating
- Cold and clammy hands
- Blushing
- Palpitations
- Confusion
- Gastrointestinal symptoms
- Trembling hands and voice
- Inability to speak correctly
- Urinary urgency
- Muscle tension
- Diarrhea
- Anticipatory anxiety
- Fear of embarrassment or ridicule

"Kim"

BublikHaus/
Shutterstock

Kim is a 22-year-old college student who comes to the student health center. She states she has difficulty participating in class group activities. She feels that everyone will laugh at her and criticize her for the way she looks and talks. She states she has not been eating well and her friends have to encourage her to leave her room to go to class, but she would prefer to stay in her dorm room. Her professors have told Kim that her grades are poor due to a lack of participation. During the initial interaction with Kim, the nurse notes that the client's hands are trembling and that her respiratory rate is increased.

Digging Deeper

1. *What approach would you use to establish a therapeutic relationship with Kim?*

2. *What objective symptoms support the diagnosis of social phobia disorder?*

3. *What can the nurse do to help decrease her level of anxiety?*

4. *How can the nurse support Kim in her attempts to interact with others?*

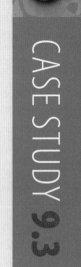

CASE STUDY 9.3

---

disorder usually has an onset in early adolescence. Onset may be abrupt, following an embarrassing event, or may be insidious or slow in onset. There is a tendency for this condition to run in families.

Post-Traumatic Stress Disorder (PTSD)

Post-traumatic stress disorder (PTSD) is a disorder that develops in some individuals after a traumatic event. The traumatic event may be directly experienced by the person or from witnessing a traumatic event. Symptoms are seen as early as several months after the event but in some individuals, it can take years for the symptoms to be exhibited. Box 9.6 lists examples of traumatic

> ### BOX 9.6
>
> ### Traumatic Events That Can Cause Post-Traumatic Stress Disorder (PTSD)
>
> - Military combat experience
> - Physical assault
> - Being the victim of a robbery or mugging
> - Sexual assault
> - Childhood sexual abuse
> - Being kidnapped or taken hostage
> - Being the victim of a terrorist attack
> - Being caught in a natural disaster
> - Observing or being involved in a fatal or severe accident

events. It is typical for any individual to have short-term reactions to these events. The person with post-traumatic stress disorder (PTSD) experiences an intense feeling of fear and dread with each recurring mental rerun of the event.

Signs and Symptoms

The person with post-traumatic stress disorder (PTSD) is plagued with increased anxiety that was not present before the precipitating event. Some may feel extreme guilt for surviving when others did not survive. People, activities, or places that may be connected to the situation are avoided because of the **emotional numbness** (not feeling or expressing emotions) that accompanies the exposure. This numbness is shown by an expression of little or no emotion soon after the event as an attempt to prevent future mental pain. The person may continue to show a lack of affect for the remainder of their life. It is common for the person to re-experience the event mentally or to re-encounter the trauma in dreams. This may lead to insomnia, inability to concentrate, and impaired social or work functioning. The duration of symptoms must be seen in all four categories for longer than 1 month and impair relationships and/or work to be given the diagnosis of post-traumatic stress disorder (PTSD). See Box 9.7 for the four categories and the signs and symptoms in each category.

BOX 9.7

Signs and Symptoms of Post-Traumatic Stress Disorder (PTSD)

Re-experiencing symptoms (at least one from this category must be present)
- Flashbacks
- Bad dreams
- Frightening thoughts

Avoidance symptoms (at least one from this category must be present)
- Avoidance of people, places, or things associated with the event
- Avoiding thinking or talking about the event

Arousal or reactive symptoms (at least two from this category must be present)
- Startles easily
- Insomnia
- Feeling tense or "edgy"
- Angry outbursts

Cognition or mood symptoms (at least two from this category must be present)
- Difficulty remembering details of the event
- Negative thoughts about self
- Exaggerated guilt or blame
- Loss of interest in previously enjoyed activities

Information modified from National Institute of Mental Health (2022). *Post-traumatic stress disorder.* https://www.nimh.nih.gov/health/topics/post-traumatic-stress-disorder-ptsd

It is not uncommon for people experiencing the symptoms of post-traumatic stress disorder (PTSD) to dissociate or depersonalize as a result of the mental anguish they experience (see Chapter 14 for information on dissociation). Persons with post-traumatic stress disorder (PTSD) may experience a general lack of trust that impairs their ability to interact with others. Panic attacks, perceptual alterations or hallucinations, and depression may also result. Some people may resort to violence, drugs, or suicide to deal with the recurring disturbing mental pictures. Exposure to similar events can also impose flashbacks or mental images that increase the chances of these complications. This return to the trauma may increase the likelihood the person will resort to extreme means of dealing with the continued emotional pain.

 Just the Facts During a flashback, the person feels as though they are reliving the traumatic experience. The flashbacks can be very terrifying for the individual or may even incapacitate them from thinking, speaking, or moving.

 Mind Jogger Why might an individual with post-traumatic stress disorder (PTSD) tend to engage in aggressive verbal or physical behavior toward others, or reckless, self-destructive behavior?

 Just the Facts Post-traumatic stress disorder (PTSD) can disrupt a person's job performance, relationships, physical and mental health, and everyday life.

Incidence and Etiology

Post-traumatic stress disorder (PTSD) affects approximately 3.5% of the United States population (about 7.7 million adults) (ADAA, 2022b). Not everyone who is exposed to a traumatic experience develops post-traumatic stress disorder (PTSD). Factors that contribute to the likelihood include the sudden occurrence of the event (e.g., a plane crash or fatal accident) and the severity of the situation (e.g., a mass shooting or natural disaster). Post-traumatic stress disorder (PTSD) can be seen in any age group and is most common after a sexual assault. When seen in children, the child may be unaware of the thoughts but demonstrates the trauma through repetitive play. There is evidence that post-traumatic stress disorder (PTSD) is more common if there is a family history of the disorder.

Test Yourself
- ✔ How are specific phobias alike and how are they different?
- ✔ How might social phobia prevent or interfere with a person's goals in life?
- ✔ What are the four categories of symptoms seen in post-traumatic stress disorder (PTSD)?

Obsessive-Compulsive Disorder

Obsessive-compulsive disorder (OCD) is characterized by a combination of obsessions and compulsions. **Obsessions** are the reoccurrence of persistent unwanted thoughts or images that cause the person intense anxiety. Table 9.1 provides common types of obsessive thought themes. **Compulsions** are the repetitive behaviors or rituals the person engages in to reduce their anxiety. In obsessive-compulsive disorder (OCD), the obsessions and compulsions severely impact the individual's level of functioning. The compulsive actions consume at least 1 hour of the individual's day.

TABLE 9.1	Common Types of Obsessive Thought Content
Contamination	Thoughts of being polluted with germs (e.g., by touching doorknobs or shaking hands with others)
Repeated doubts	Questioning thoughts as to whether one did or did not do something (e.g., turning off the stove or locking the door)
Orderliness	Thinking that one must have everything in a particular order (e.g., placing things symmetrically on the desk or dresser, placing shoes in alphabetical order by color in a closet)
Impulses that are aggressive or horrific in nature	Recurring thoughts about doing actions that could bring great distress to others (e.g., hurting someone who is completely defenseless such as a baby or a person who is physically impaired)
Sexual imagery	Thoughts about sexually revealing images or pornography (e.g., a person obsessively imagines people wearing see-through clothing or a monogamous married person thinks about sexual activity with multiple partners)

Information modified from Mayo Foundation for Medical Education and Research (MFMER). (2022). *Obsessive-compulsive disorder (OCD). Mayo Clinic.* https://www.mayoclinic.org/diseases-conditions/obsessive-compulsive-disorder/symptoms-causes/syc-20354432#

Other types of obsessive-compulsive disorders (OCD) include hoarding disorder, body dysmorphic disorder, trichotillomania, and excoriation disorder. In hoarding disorder, the individual excessively gathers and keeps possessions, regardless of their actual value, and becomes very anxious whenever they are forced to get rid of them or even think about giving them up. Possessions can include inconsequential items such as newspapers or in some cases, even trash. In body dysmorphic disorder, the individual has a preoccupation with an imagined defect in appearance or an overconcern with an existing slight physical defect and experiences distress over the imagined or existing defect. An example of this is an individual who has a mole on their chin and is so concerned that they will be considered ugly because of the mole that they wear a scarf whenever they are around other people so no one will see it.

Trichotillomania is also referred to as hair-pulling disorder and involves recurrent and uncontrollable urges to pull hair out from the scalp. In some cases, the individual may have significant bald spot and may wear a wig, scarf, or hat to disguise the hair loss. The bald patches may also lead to anxiety which can increase the hair pulling. The individual may also pull out their eyebrows or eyelashes. Trichotillomania can also be seen in individuals with attention deficit hyperactivity disorder (ADHD) or as a side effect from some attention deficit hyperactivity disorder (ADHD) medications (see Chapter 18). Excoriation disorder, sometimes called skin-picking disorder, is seen when the individual has uncontrollable urges to pick at their skin, often causing sores and bleeding. In trichotillomania and excoriation disorder, the individual experiences anxiety before the pulling or picking occurs or if they try to prevent themselves from doing so. Afterward, the person feels a sense of pleasure or relief with a decrease in anxiety. The behavior is often done in private. In some cases, the pulling or picking is unconscious; the person is not aware that they are doing it.

Just the Facts Hoarding may impose complications such as unsanitary living conditions, risk for falls or injury, fire hazards, and social isolation.

Signs and Symptoms

It is common to have some recurring uncomfortable thoughts or concern such as whether a car is locked, or if the garage door closed. However, in obsessive-compulsive disorder (OCD), the thoughts tend to be focused on one theme. The thoughts are pervasive and dominate the person's thinking at times. The person may recognize the thoughts as atypical and self-generated but has no ability to control them. This lack of control leads to the extreme anxiety.

In an attempt to deal with the anxiety, the person performs repetitive acts that serve no purpose other than to relieve the anxiety. The person who feels contaminated with sexual thoughts may wash their hair repeatedly until the scalp is bleeding. The person with violent thoughts of harming their family may check door locks and gas knobs every few minutes. In the person with obsessive-compulsive disorder (OCD), the symptoms severely interfere with social and occupational functioning. The ability to finish a task is impaired by lack of concentration, invasion of the obsessive thoughts, and need to perform the actions. Symptoms may be intermittent or get worse over time. Signs and symptoms for obsessive-compulsive disorder (OCD) are found in Box 9.8.

BOX 9.8

Signs and Symptoms of Obsessive-Compulsive Disorder (OCD)

- Recurrent unwanted thoughts referencing a theme such as contamination, sexuality, aggression, need for perfection, or excessive doubt
- Attempts to reduce the effect of the thoughts with other thoughts
- Repetitive acts, impulses, or rituals such as showering, washing hair or hands, checking, hoarding, rearranging things for perfect alignment, or repeating words or phrases
- Recognition that the thoughts are produced in their own mind
- Lack of concentration and task completion
- Impaired social or work functioning

Incidence and Etiology

Obsessive-compulsive disorder (OCD) affects approximately 1% of the United States population (about 2.2 million adults) (ADAA, 2022b) and is evenly distributed between males and females. Onset is usually in childhood or adolescence. Most adults with the disorder have experienced the symptoms since childhood. There tends to be an occurrence of the behavior pattern in families.

Treatment of Anxiety Disorders

Treatment of anxiety disorders focuses on reducing the client's anxiety level. The two main approaches to the treatment of the anxiety disorders include medications and psychotherapy, either alone or in combination. Antianxiety medications (anxiolytics), including benzodiazepines, may be prescribed. The largest percentage of success is experienced when antianxiety medications are used in combination with psychotherapy sessions.

Psychotherapy

Research demonstrates that cognitive-behavioral therapy is the most effective therapy in helping the individual to replace negative thoughts and behaviors with more positive and productive ones. The basis for the outcome is that individuals can control and change their thinking and consequently their actions. Anxiety support groups can also provide sharing of experiences and offer suggestions for coping.

Antianxiety Agents

Antianxiety agents (anxiolytics) are medications used to counteract or diminish anxiety. Current

CASE STUDY 9.4

"Yumi"

GaudiLab/Shutterstock

Yumi is a 25-year-old college student. She has an older brother, Kenji, who is a practicing lawyer. Yumi's parents have always told her that she "can't measure up to Kenji." No matter what she does, or how well she does in her college courses, she never does as well as her brother did. Recently, Yumi has begun having recurring thoughts that if her brother was not around, maybe she could be "important" to her parents. She finds herself constantly wishing her brother would be killed in an accident or struck by lightning. She realizes the extreme and unreasonable nature of these thoughts but cannot control their continuous intrusion in her mind or the anxiety they create. She has begun calling Kenji 20 to 30 times throughout the day to make sure he is okay. He cannot convince her there is nothing wrong with him. Yumi is having difficulty maintaining her concentration and has been skipping classes to make the phone calls. Kenji does not understand what is wrong with Yumi but is annoyed by the many phone calls. He has his mobile and home phone numbers changed and asks his secretary to screen calls at his office. This action increases Yumi's anxiety. She has decided to drop out of her college classes and wants to move to a location adjacent to Kenji's home.

Digging Deeper

1. How is Yumi's behavior characteristic of obsessive-compulsive disorder (OCD)?

2. What impact is this behavior having on her functioning?

3. What effect did Kenji changing his phone numbers have on Yumi?

4. How do her earlier feelings of inadequacy continue to influence her current behavior?

5. What types of positive reinforcement could the nurse use to help Yumi decrease her anxiety?

TABLE 9.2	Benzodiazepine Medications	
Medication	**Length of Action**	**Duration of Action**
Alprazolam	Short	7–15 hours
Lorazepam	Short	8–15 hours
Oxazepam	Short	5–15 hours
Clonazepam	Long	20–40 hours
Clorazepate	Long	30–40 hours
Diazepam	Long	20–50 hours
Chlordiazepoxide	Long	5–30 hours
Prazepam	Long	30–100 hours

antianxiety medications were preceded by studies involving the calming effects of alcohol on the level of discomfort caused by anxiety. The effects of alcohol were limited by its rapid metabolism by the body, the tendency for tolerance to develop, and the tendency for rebound anxiety to occur. Researchers attempted to find chemical agents that would produce the calming effects without the toxic and addictive qualities of alcohol. In the 1950s medications chemically related to the barbiturates were developed and remain in existence. Their use, however, has been replaced by more effective medications that are less addicting than the barbiturates and produce lesser side effects. The earliest of these medications were the benzodiazepines, chlordiazepoxide, and diazepam. Table 9.2 lists common long- and short-acting benzodiazepines and their length of action.

Senior Focus Sensitivity to benzodiazepines is increased in older adults. Smaller doses may be effective as well as safer. The long-acting benzodiazepines have a long half-life (sometimes days) in the older adult, causing prolonged sedation and increased risk of falls and injury. Ambulation should be supervised for at least 8 hours after the administration of an injectable form to avoid injury. If needed, short- or intermediate-acting agents (Table 9.2) and decreased dosages are preferred.

Medications in the benzodiazepine group are more useful in stopping acute, severe anxiety symptoms, like those seen in panic disorders. Because of their potential for tolerance and addictive tendencies, they are most suitable for short-term treatment. Used continuously, and without adjunctive psychotherapy, their anxiety-reducing effects tend to diminish, and tolerance develops. Their usefulness lies in the rapid onset of symptom relief because they enhance the binding of gamma-aminobutyric acid (GABA) receptors, which causes an inhibitory or calming effect on the excited response in the brain. Higher doses can create a more profound effect, inducing sleep or perhaps even coma, indicating their depressive action on the subcortical levels of the central nervous system (CNS).

Antidepressants, including some selective serotonin reuptake inhibitors (SSRIs) and serotonin–norepinephrine reuptake inhibitors (SNRI) are often the first choice in treating generalized anxiety symptoms for long-term treatment. These medications help the absorption and use of serotonin and other neurotransmitters in the brain to improve mood, anxiety, and often the accompanying depression.

Other agents that may be used to treat anxiety disorders include gabapentin (an anticonvulsant medication) and propranolol (a beta-blocker commonly used to treat heart conditions and hypertension). Propranolol is used to control the heightened anxiety encountered with social phobia, such as when a client has stage fright prior to a public appearance or speech. Commonly used antianxiety agents and their more common side effects are listed in Table 9.3.

Indications for Use

Antianxiety medications are used in the treatment of anxiety disorders, anxiety symptoms, acute alcohol withdrawal, skeletal muscle spasms, convulsive and seizure disorders, status epilepticus, neuropathic pain, and preoperative sedation. Because these medications have a potential for misuse with the development of tolerance, dependence, and withdrawal, they are usually prescribed for short periods of time. Although some clients may require long-term treatment, most antianxiety medications are recommended for only several days or weeks. Discontinuance of long-term usage should be done with health care provider supervision and should occur gradually with tapered doses rather than abruptly ending treatment.

Contraindications

Antianxiety agents are contraindicated in clients with hypersensitivity, narrow-angle glaucoma, pre-existing central nervous system (CNS) depression, or psychosis, and in clients who are pregnant and lactating, or younger than 12 years. They should not be taken in combination with other

TABLE 9.3	Antianxiety (Anxiolytic) and Antidepressant Medications	
Chemical Group	**Medication**	**Adverse Reactions and Side Effects**
Antihistamines	Hydroxyzine	Dry mouth, drowsiness, pain at site of intramuscular injection
Benzodiazepines	Alprazolam Chlordiazepoxide Clonazepam Clorazepate Diazepam Lorazepam Oxazepam Prazepam	Drowsiness, dizziness, ataxia, lethargy, hypotension, blurred vision, nausea, vomiting, anorexia, sleep disturbance, tolerance, physical/psychological dependence
Sedative	Meprobamate	Drowsiness, dizziness, ataxia, reduced seizure threshold, tolerance, and dependence Not recommended in older adult clients
Antidepressants	Fluoxetine Paroxetine Citalopram Escitalopram Sertraline Mirtazapine	Anxiety, agitation, dizziness, migraine, depression, fatigue, dry mouth, nausea, diarrhea, increased or decreased weight
Miscellaneous	Buspirone	Drowsiness, dizziness, excitement, fatigue, headache, insomnia, nervousness, weakness, blurred vision, nasal congestion, palpitations, tachycardia, nausea, rashes, myalgia, incoordination

central nervous system (CNS) depressants. They should be used with caution in older adults, those with hepatic or renal dysfunction, a history of drug dependence or substance use disorder, and depression. Physical dependence is indicated by withdrawal symptoms if discontinued abruptly. Severe withdrawal symptoms are most likely in clients who have taken higher doses for a period of more than 4 months. The symptoms are caused by the acute separation of the drug molecules at the receptor site and the acute decrease in gamma-aminobutyric acid (GABA) neurotransmitters. These symptoms most commonly include increased anxiety, psychomotor agitation, insomnia, irritability, headache, tremors, and palpitations. In severe cases, psychotic manifestations and seizures may occur.

 Mind Jogger How do the effects of withdrawal from antianxiety agents resemble those experienced from alcohol withdrawal?

Nursing Interventions for Antianxiety Medications

The nurse needs to monitor the client taking antianxiety medications for the effectiveness of the medication. This includes collecting data on the client's mood and level of anxiety. The nurse should observe the client's reactions to anxiety-provoking situations such as being in a group, their response to news items on the television or social media, or fixation on a body part. The nurse should also observe for an increase or decrease in compulsions, sleeping, or participation in group activities. These observations can help gauge if the client's level of anxiety is decreasing or increasing. The nurse also reinforces teaching related to antianxiety medications (see Reinforcing Client and Family Teaching 9.1).

The nurse must also monitor the client for side effects of antianxiety medications. Monitor the client's blood pressure for orthostatic hypotension, observe for signs of dry mouth and offer ice chips, hard candy, frequent sips of water, or sugarless gum as appropriate. Administer medication

Reinforcing Client and Family Teaching 9.1

Important Information About Antianxiety Medications

- The most common side effects are drowsiness, fatigue, confusion, and loss of coordination.
- Do not combine with alcohol or other medications such as muscle relaxants, antidepressants, or prescribed pain medications.
- Smoking decreases the effects of benzodiazepine medications.
- Avoid driving or operating dangerous machinery while taking the medication.
- Do not discontinue taking the medication abruptly. Abrupt withdrawal can be life-threatening. (Symptoms may include depression, anxiety, abdominal and muscle cramps, tremors, insomnia, vomiting, diaphoresis, convulsions, and delirium.)
- Rise slowly from a reclining position.
- Clients taking buspirone may experience a delay of 10 days to 2 weeks between onset of therapy and reduction of anxiety symptoms. Continue taking the medication during this time.
- Do not take over-the-counter (OTC) medications without the permission of your health care provider.
- Report any symptoms of fever, sore throat, feeling "run-down," easy bruising, bleeding, or increased motor restlessness to your health care provider.

with food or milk to prevent nausea and vomiting. Observe for symptoms that could indicate a blood dyscrasia such as sore throat, fever, malaise, easy bruising, or unusual bleeding.

> **Just the Facts** Reduced dosages are recommended for older adults with antihistamines and benzodiazepines

> **Test Yourself**
> ✔ What types of behaviors are seen in obsessive-compulsive disorder (OCD)?
> ✔ Name four disorders that are related to obsessive-compulsive disorder (OCD).
> ✔ Name five classifications of medications that are used to treat anxiety.

Nursing Process and Care Plan *for the Client With an Anxiety Disorder*

When establishing a nurse–client relationship with the person experiencing anxiety, it is important to initially take steps to help the client lower their anxiety level. The person cannot identify the problem, or causative factor of the anxiety, until this is accomplished. The nurse can best encourage trust by a calm and reassuring approach.

> **BOX 9.9**
>
> ### Leading Statements That Encourage Client Participation in Providing Information
>
> - Tell me what happened.
> - Tell me what was going through your mind when that happened.
> - Describe how you felt at that time.
> - Give me a specific example of what that was like for you.
> - Tell me more about that.
> - Go on…And…
> - Tell me how you feel right now.
> - What is helping you to decrease that feeling?
> - What can you do to decrease that feeling when this situation happens again?

Assessment (Data Collection)

When collecting data, observe basic characteristics that help identify the client's level of anxiety (Table 9.4). Use leading statements to elicit subjective information about how the client is currently feeling and what happened before the onset of symptoms. Box 9.9 provides examples of leading statements to use to gain an understanding of the situation from the client's perspective. Ask the client about other somatic symptoms such as muscle aches, eating patterns, bowel habits, sleeping

TABLE 9.4	**Components of Data Collection That Reflect Level of Anxiety**	
Component	**Examples Seen in Low or Moderate Levels of Anxiety**	**Examples Seen in Elevated to High Levels of Anxiety**
Thought process	• Able to complete one thought before continuing to next thought • Thoughts are logical and orderly • Able to focus on current situation • Follows directions • Able to problem solve	• Thoughts jump from one topic to another often rapidly • Incomplete thoughts expressed before going on to next topic • Distracted • Unable to follow multiple or complex directions • Unable to problem solve or make simple decisions
Affect	• Appropriate to situation	• Wide-eyed/scared look • Blank, unfocused look • Frightened
Communication	• Coherent speech • Able to answer questions • Able to follow conversation	• Incoherent speech, may "babble", uses incomplete sentences • Unable to answer questions, even simple ones • Needs frequent reorientation to conversation
Physiologic response	• Vital signs normal for client • Absent to slight perspiration • Steady hands and voice • Able to be led to a different location • Subtle to no fidgeting/nervous behaviors	• Increased heart and respiratory rates • Perspiration present including palms of hands • Tremors noted in hands • Voice shaky • Inability to move from current spot ("frozen in place") • Excessive fidgeting, wringing hands, bouncing legs • Rapid back and forth eye movements
Task completion	• Able to complete one task before progressing to next task	• Unable to complete a task—jumps from one to the next

patterns, and fatigue that might further indicate a psychological origin for the complaints.

Observe the client during activities of daily living and interaction with others to determine when symptoms are most obvious. Assessing the client during usual activities can also provide clues about the client's thought processes. Even though something may not mean much to others, it may be very meaningful to the client. For example, while sitting in the dayroom watching a movie with other clients, one client leaves the room quietly and does not return. When gathering information on what happened, the nurse finds out that part of the movie took place in a circus, similar to the circus where the client had been raped as a child. Although seeing a circus in a movie was insignificant to the other clients, it was very significant to that client. Withdrawing from the stimulus was an attempt to lower anxiety.

When questioning a client, consider that your questioning may increase the client's anxiety and interfere with their ability to answer. When faced with a frightening situation, a person's anxiety levels increase and their thoughts can become more disorganized or extremely focused. The client may report not being able to collect their thoughts or not being able to control the thoughts. Either way, the client is unable to think, speak, or perform tasks as effectively as compared to when they are not in the frightening situation. While taking a test, for example, a student previously was able to state the answer to a question but now cannot recall it; the student can remember what page the answer is on and which paragraph it is in but still cannot recall it. This is an example of increased anxiety affecting thought processes of memory. Thought blocking or inability to recall information is a common response when suddenly faced with increased anxiety. After relaxing at home later that evening, the student may be able to recall the answer without difficulty. Similarly, when questioning clients, remember that thought blocking may occur and further increase the client's anxiety. The clients may approach the staff later stating the information asked of them earlier.

It is important to note the client's affect. Facial expressions are not easily disguised and may provide more meaningful insight into the client's feelings. A client may report that they are fine but have a facial grimace. The facial expression usually reflects true feelings before behavior does. The nurse may note a flat affect several times during the day when the client is unaware that they are being observed. Observe for congruence of nonverbal and verbal messages during each observation or contact with the client.

Determine how well the client is able to communicate. When assessing for interactive skills, take into consideration the client's level of education. For example, a client who has been in the hospital for 4 days consistently complains about the food and asks the staff to order something different for them. While observing the client selecting food for the next day from the menu, a nurse notices that the client is very anxious and unable to make decisions or direct thought processes long enough to mark the menu. Using a sensitive approach, the nurse determines that the client is illiterate and is unable to understand what food choices are available. Determining how well the client is able to communicate thoughts is also relevant. If the client's speech is choppy and pressured, the client may be experiencing anxiety and subsequent distress from impaired communication skills. During interaction with the client, the nurse should be aware of their own verbal and nonverbal message. Anxiety is contagious and can contribute to the client's difficulty in communicating.

Also observe the client's ability to perform and complete tasks. Psychomotor responses can reach a hyperactive level and be counterproductive when anxiety is high. On the other hand, when anxiety is extremely high, psychomotor responses can become slowed and decrease functional ability. Collecting observations helps to determine if the client's inability to perform tasks is the result of impaired thought processes or impaired motor responses. For example, when observing a depressed client attempting to get dressed, a nurse notes several articles of clothing lying on the bed. The client is across the room crying and wringing her fingers. At this point, the nurse concludes the client may be experiencing increased anxiety about deciding between choices of what to wear; this would be an impaired thought process.

Observation of the client with particular attention to specific anxiety-reducing behaviors should be part of the initial and ongoing assessment for each client. Sometimes symptoms are expressed in subtle ways, such as leaving group therapy to go to the bathroom or avoiding an activity where several clients are participating. It is important to note if behaviors are improving with the administration of antianxiety medications or if the client is experiencing any side effects from the medication.

Nursing Care Focus

Once the assessment is made and data are collected, the information is reviewed and sorted into meaningful clusters. From this data, problems are identified to determine applicable nursing care focuses. Nursing care focuses for the client with an anxiety disorder are directed at reducing the client's anxiety and providing for their safety.

Outcome Identification and Planning

Once the nursing care focus is made, appropriate outcomes for clients can be determined. Careful consideration should be given to a realistic time-frame in which the outcomes can be achieved. Outcomes are always client-centered and time-limited. Goals may need to be short term initially. A goal of "Client will not experience any anxiety during hospitalization" would be inappropriate for a client with generalized anxiety disorder. A short-term goal of "Client will participate in 50% of unit activities" would be more appropriate.

Nursing Care Focus

- Chronic Anxiety related to a feeling of actual or perceived threat

Goal

- The client reports that anxiety has been reduced to a manageable level.

Implementations for Chronic Anxiety

When dealing with anxiety in clients, the nurse should take into consideration their own anxiety level and how it may affect nursing care. Subtle behaviors such as a change in the tone of voice, rushed movements, or spending less time with the client can communicate anxiety to the client. This in turn can generate increased anxiety in the client resulting in a decreased ability to function. Establishing a sense of trust includes maintaining a calm and supportive environment in which the client feels a sense of safety and security. It is important to use caution when touching or approaching the person having a panic attack. Doing so may pose an additional threat to the client or an invasion of their own personal space.

Interventions should include only what the client is able to do at that time. It may be difficult for the client to take more than small steps toward reaching expected outcomes. Overwhelming the client with unrealistic expectations may indicate anxiety on the nurse's part and lead to counterproductive results in the client. Observing the client's tolerance for change is essential for planning appropriate client-centered nursing interventions. Efforts should be made to assist the client in identifying the issues that precipitate the feelings of anxiety. Linking the behavior exhibited by the client to a particular situation can help the client to develop an awareness of feelings that precede the anxiety attacks. The nurse should model positive coping strategies and help the client to identify and try new, more adaptive coping strategies.

Specific nursing interventions for the client with anxiety include:

- Encourage participation in social interaction and exercise activities.
- Give positive reinforcement for the client's efforts to participate.
- Reinforce stress-management techniques (progressive relaxation, music therapy, deep breathing).
- Assist the client experiencing compulsive behaviors to find ways to set limits on the rituals.
- Acknowledge the behaviors but do not focus on them—it is important to express an empathetic response rather than criticize the behavior. For example, in response to a client who has shampooed their hair four times in 2 hours, the nurse might say, "I am sure your scalp is getting sore from washing your hair so much," rather than, "You only need to wash your hair once a day."
- Observe for automatic relief behaviors.
- Encourage open discussion of feelings and thoughts.
- Monitor for indications of escalating anxiety.
- Avoid giving advice to client.
- Reinforce client teaching regarding anxiety and precipitating factors.
- Provide sources of information about anxiety disorders such as those found in Reinforcing Client and Family Teaching 9.2.

Effectiveness of planned interventions will be demonstrated in the client's ability to recognize and deal with the anxiety-producing factors. Once the client identifies the relationship between unreasonable thoughts and subsequent behaviors, it is more realistic to anticipate the client to use more effective coping strategies to reduce their anxiety. It is important for the client to openly express feelings and thoughts related to the situation. This can also be demonstrated as the client shows relaxed behaviors, participation in activities, and reports longer periods of restful sleep. It is anticipated that through learning what precipitating factors can be changed and steps that can be taken to lower anxiety for those that cannot be changed, the client will demonstrate less focus on the anxiety itself.

Evaluation of Goal/Desired Outcome

The client will:

- identify initial signs and symptoms of anxiety.
- identify effective coping methods to use when anxiety begins to occur.
- look at pictures of a phobic stimulus without excessive anxiety.
- describe measures to reduce their anxiety when faced with phobic stimulus.
- demonstrate effective strategies to lower anxiety.

Nursing Care Focus

- Injury Risk

Goal

- The client will be free from harm while taking antianxiety medications.

Implementations for Safety

The client taking antianxiety medications is at risk for injury due to side effects of the medication. Because it is not possible to identify which client will experience side effects, it is important to reinforce client teaching regarding the medications. Provide the client with explanations about their medications, expected effects, and potential side effects.

Observe the client's blood pressure every 4 hours at a minimum when initially administering a benzodiazepine or buspirone due to potential hypotension. Encourage the client to rise slowly from a sitting or reclining position as many antianxiety medications can cause dizziness. Also, due to the potential for dizziness or incoordination, the client should not drive or operate dangerous machinery until they have established their personal response to the medication. Avoid administering sedatives, prescription pain medications, or multiple antidepressants concurrently with antianxiety medications to prevent over-sedation. Administer antianxiety medications on a regular schedule to maintain therapeutic levels. Older adult clients taking antihistamines or benzodiazepines should receive a reduced dosage rather than the recommended adult dosage.

Evaluation of Goal/Desired Outcome

The client will:

- not suffer an injury from a fall or loss of balance.
- not experience increased sedative effects.
- tolerate usual activity without excessive sedation.
- notify their health care provider if symptoms of an infection are noticed.

Cultural Considerations

Words for Anxiety

There are differences in the way that anxiety is named based upon the individual's culture. Cultures that commonly utilize psychological terms will use the term "anxiety" with very similar understandings of how that word is expressed in an individual's behavior and emotions. Some other cultural terms used that refer to anxiety or an anxiety disorder include:

- nervios/ataque de nervios (Hispanic, Latin America, and Caribbean Latino cultures)
- taijin kyofusho (Japan)
- khyâl cap (Cambodia)
- May not have a specific term but is expressed in physical symptoms (headache or upset stomach)
- May be expressed in spiritual terms

SUMMARY

- Anxiety is an unconscious uneasy feeling that everyone experiences at some time. When aware of the cause, the individual manages to cope and manage the anxiety-provoking situation.
- The level of anxiety that results in a disorder is intense and disabling to some degree.
- Generalized anxiety disorder involves an increased level of anxiety and worry about various situations on most days over a period of at least 6 months.
- Panic disorder results in a sense of terror and fear that is exhausting and emotionally draining. Some individuals with panic attacks develop agoraphobia and will avoid events or places that trigger the fear.
- Specific phobias are demonstrated in those who experience intense anxiety when exposed to the object or situation. Specific phobias usually do not require treatment as the individual does not experience the anxiety when the feared stimulus is not present.
- Social phobia (social anxiety disorder) occurs in situations when embarrassment may result from the exposure and the individual is unable to control the symptoms.
- Experiencing or witnessing a traumatic event can result in post-traumatic stress disorder (PTSD) that leaves a reaction of emotional numbing. Reminders or triggers of the traumatic event can cause flashbacks in which the individual relives the experience and its associated emotions in their mind.
- Obsessive-compulsive disorder (OCD) is characterized by obsessions (recurring, persistent, unwanted thoughts or images that cause intense anxiety), coupled with compulsions (repetitive behaviors or rituals the person engages in to reduce the high level of anxiety).
- Actions in obsessive-compulsive disorder (OCD) are repetitive and ritualistic in nature and have a negative effect on work, social, and interpersonal relationships. Although aware that the thoughts are psychological, the person is unable to control them.
- Treatment of anxiety focuses on reducing the anxiety level to a point at which the person can identify the precipitating factors and their connection to the resulting behaviors.
- Antianxiety medications used in combination with psychotherapy have proven to be the most beneficial treatment approach.
- Antianxiety agents (anxiolytics) are used in the treatment of anxiety disorders, anxiety symptoms, acute alcohol withdrawal, and convulsive or seizure disorders.
- Different classifications of antianxiety medications include antihistamines, benzodiazepines, antidepressants, anticonvulsants, and beta blockers.

BIBLIOGRAPHY

Anxiety and Depression Association of America. (2022a). *Generalized anxiety disorder (GAD)*. https://adaa.org/understanding-anxiety/generalized-anxiety-disorder-gad

Anxiety and Depression Association of America (ADAA). (2022b). *Anxiety Disorder: Facts and Statistics*. https://adaa.org/understanding-anxiety/facts-statistics

Back, S. E. (2022). Co-occurring substance use disorder and anxiety-related disorders in adults: Epidemiology, pathogenesis, clinical manifestations, course, assessment, and diagnosis. *UpToDate*. Retrieved April 4, 2023, from https://www.uptodate.com/contents/co-occurring-substance-use-disorder-and-anxiety-related-disorders-in-adults-epidemiology-pathogenesis-clinical-manifestations-course-assessment-and-diagnosis

Baldwin, D. (2022). Generalized anxiety disorder in adults: Epidemiology, pathogenesis, clinical manifestations, course, assessment, and diagnosis. *UpToDate*. Retrieved April 4, 2023, from https://www.uptodate.com/contents/generalized-anxiety-disorder-in-adults-epidemiology-pathogenesis-clinical-manifestations-course-assessment-and-diagnosis

Chang, V. T. (2022). Approach to symptom assessment in palliative care. *UpToDate*. Retrieved April 18, 2022, from https://www.uptodate.com/contents/approach-to-symptom-assessment-in-palliative-care

Craske, M. (2021). Generalized anxiety disorder in adults: Cognitive-behavioral therapy and other psychotherapies. *UpToDate*. Retrieved April 10, 2023, from https://www.uptodate.com/contents/generalized-anxiety-disorder-in-adults-cognitive-behavioral-therapy-and-other-psychotherapies

Craske, M., & Bystritsky, A. (2021). Generalized anxiety disorder in adults: Management. *UpToDate*. Retrieved April 10, 2023, from https://www.uptodate.com/contents/generalized-anxiety-disorder-in-adults-management

Cuncic, A. (2020). *How do different cultures experience social anxiety disorder? Verywell Mind*. https://www.verywellmind.com/cultural-social-anxiety-disorder-3024706

McCabe, R. E., & Bui, E. (2021). Approach to treating specific phobia in adults. *UpToDate*. Retrieved April 10, 2023, from https://www.uptodate.com/contents/approach-to-treating-specific-phobia-in-adults

McCabe, R. E. (2021a). Agoraphobia in adults: Epidemiology, pathogenesis, clinical manifestations, course, and diagnosis. *UpToDate*. Retrieved April 21, 2022, from https://www.uptodate.com/contents/agoraphobia-in-adults-epidemiology-pathogenesis-clinical-manifestations-course-and-diagnosis

McCabe, R. E. (2021b). Specific phobia in adults: Epidemiology, clinical manifestations, course and diagnosis. *UpToDate*. Retrieved April 21, 2022, from https://www.uptodate.com/contents/specific-phobia-in-adults-epidemiology-clinical-manifestations-course-and-diagnosis

National Alliance on Mental Illness. (2022). *Anxiety disorders: Overview*. https://www.nami.org/About-Mental-Illness/Mental-Health-Conditions/Anxiety-Disorders

National Institute of Mental Health. (2023). Anxiety disorders. https://www.nimh.nih.gov/health/topics/anxiety-disorders

National Institute of Mental Health. (2022a). Obsessive-compulsive disorder. https://www.nimh.nih.gov/health/topics/obsessive-compulsive-disorder-ocd

National Institute of Mental Health. (2022b). Post-traumatic stress disorder. https://www.nimh.nih.gov/health/topics/post-traumatic-stress-disorder-ptsd

Nazir, M. A., AlSharief, M., Al-Ansari, A., El Akel, A., AlBishi, F., Khan, S., Alotabi, G., & AlRtroot, S. (2022). Generalized anxiety disorder and its relationship with dental anxiety among pregnant women in Dammam, Saudi Arabia. *International Journal of Dentistry, 2022*, 1578498. https://doi.org/10.1155/2022/1578498

Roy-Byrne, P. P. (2022). Panic disorder in adults: Epidemiology, clinical manifestations, and diagnosis. *UpToDate*. Retrieved May 5, 2022, from https://www.uptodate.com/contents/panic-disorder-in-adults-epidemiology-clinical-manifestations-and-diagnosis

Sareen, J. (2022). Posttraumatic stress disorder in adults: Epidemiology, pathophysiology, clinical manifestations, course, assessment, and diagnosis. *UpToDate*. Retrieved April 10, 2023, from https://www.uptodate.com/contents/posttraumatic-stress-disorder-in-adults-epidemiology-pathophysiology-clinical-manifestations-course-assessment-and-diagnosis

Simpson, H. B. (2022). Obsessive-compulsive disorder in adults: Epidemiology, pathogenesis, clinical manifestations, course, and diagnosis. *UpToDate*. Retrieved April 10, 2023, from https://www.uptodate.com/contents/obsessive-compulsive-disorder-in-adults-epidemiology-pathogenesis-clinical-manifestations-course-and-diagnosis

Fill in the Blank

Fill in the blank with the correct answer.

1. Free-floating anxiety occurs when the person is unable to _____ the anxiety to a_____.
2. _____ _____ _____ are behaviors the person is unaware of doing, and are aimed at relieving anxiety.
3. An excessive and persistent irrational fear of objects or situations that pose little threat of danger is referred to as a _____ _____.
4. Individuals with panic disorder often develop _____.
5. _____ are recurrent persistent and unwanted thoughts or images that cause intense anxiety for the person experiencing them.
6. Older adult clients receiving antihistamines or benzodiazepines should receive a _____ dosage rather than the recommended adult dosage.

Matching

Match the following terms to the most appropriate phrase.

1. _____ Mysophobia
2. _____ Hematophobia
3. _____ Ophidiophobia
4. _____ Cynophobia
5. _____ Claustrophobia
6. _____ Arachnophobia
7. _____ Trypanophobia
8. _____ Acrophobia

a. Fear of heights
b. Fear of snakes
c. Fear of spiders
d. Fear of confined spaces
e. Fear of injections
f. Fear of germs
g. Fear of blood
h. Fear of dogs

Multiple Choice

Select the best answer from the multiple-choice items.

1. Initially, which of the following nursing interventions would be the most important to implement when a client is experiencing a panic attack?
   a. Administer a dose of antianxiety medication.
   b. Provide a detailed explanation of what causes panic attacks.
   c. Assure the client you will remain until the panic attack subsides.
   d. Hug the client to show empathy for the distress they are experiencing.

2. A client with generalized anxiety disorder approaches the nurse and states they feel dizzy. Which of the following statements would be therapeutic for the nurse to make? *(Select all that apply)*
   a. "Don't worry, it is just one of the symptoms you can expect."
   b. "Stay right here. I will be back with some medication to help you."
   c. "I'll help you to your room so you can lie down and rest until you feel better."
   d. "Tell me what happened right before you felt dizzy."
   e. "Has this happened before in a similar situation?"

3. Which of the following symptoms would the nurse expect to observe in a client with a medical diagnosis of panic disorder?
   a. Hypotension
   b. Feelings of suffocation
   c. Constipation
   d. Logical thought processes

4. A college student with known social anxiety disorder receives an assignment that requires a class presentation. The student is so distraught over the assignment that they drop the class, even though it is required for their degree plan. What term would apply to this student?
   a. Free-floating anxiety
   b. Automatic relief behavior
   c. Uncued anxiety
   d. Anticipatory anxiety

5. Which of the following chart entries by the nurse would demonstrate progress in the client who experiences agoraphobia?
   a. Attends group therapy sessions four out of five times a week
   b. Conversing with two other clients during mealtime
   c. Participated in outing to park this afternoon
   d. Has showered and shampooed hair once today

6. Initially, which nursing intervention would receive the highest priority for the client with obsessive-compulsive disorder (OCD)?
   a. Confront the client about the uncommon nature of their behavior.
   b. Isolate the client to reduce proximity to others.
   c. Set limits on the client to conform to the unit schedule.
   d. Allow extra time for client to perform rituals.

7. Which client would require additional health teaching regarding the effects of a prescribed benzodiazepine medication? The client who:
   a. smokes two packs of cigarettes a day.
   b. drinks three cups of coffee each morning.
   c. is an internet stockbroker who jogs each day.
   d. works an average 50-hour week.

8. A client is being seen for increasing symptoms of panic attacks. The client asks the health care provider for "something for my nerves." Which of the following comments by the client should the nurse report to the provider?
   a. "The panic attacks happen most when I am in a room full of people."
   b. "None of my family seems to understand just how bad this feeling is."
   c. "I am happiest when I am breast-feeding my 2-month-old infant."
   d. "Sometimes I feel like I am going crazy and have to leave the room."

9. The nurse is doing client teaching for a client taking a newly prescribed antianxiety medication. Which statement by the client would alert the nurse to the need for further teaching?
   a. "I will continue taking the medication even if it makes me sleepy."
   b. "Maybe now I can enjoy an evening of wine and dinner with my wife."
   c. "I guess I won't feel better right away from taking this medication."
   d. "Hopefully, I will only need to take this for a short period of time."

10. Classifications of medications used to treat anxiety include: *(Select all that apply)*
    a. Barbiturates
    b. Benzodiazepines
    c. Beta Blockers
    d. Corticosteroids
    e. Antihistamines

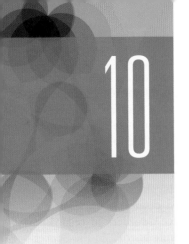

10 Mood Disorders

Introduction

Life involves everyday situations that trigger emotions. On one end of the emotional spectrum are feelings of sadness and loss. While most people feel a sense of sadness in response to disappointments such as not winning a ballgame or not receiving an anticipated job promotion, others also feel sadness during holidays or occasions on which a loss has occurred. Sadness is seen as a normal state of depression, often referred to as feeling "down" or "blue." For most people, this sadness is limited, and they are able to return to a usual state of functioning. On the other end of the emotional spectrum are feelings of happiness and joy. Elation is a feeling of well-being experienced because of success and during momentous occasions. The variance between happiness and sadness in most people is mild and congruent with the situation that triggers the feeling. However, the prolonged inability to maintain an emotional balance needs investigation.

Mood and Affect

Mood is an emotion that is prolonged and permeates the individual's entire psychological thinking. The feelings are changeable depending on the person's perception. For example, one individual might respond to a separation or divorce with deep feelings of sadness, regret, and failure, while another might feel a more contented feeling of relief and freedom. **Affect** describes the facial expression an individual displays in association with the mood (e.g., smiling when happy, grimacing when angry).

Alterations in mood can range from mild to severe. When the mood alterations are mild, the person may experience minor changes in daily routine with minimal impairment in functioning. One individual, for example, might be disappointed after the cancellation of a much-anticipated lunch date but view it as a simple change in plans, and another may feel sad for a time after the death of a pet but decide to replace the loss with another pet. Severe mood alterations, however, can cause significant impairment of the individual's ability to function. For example, the cancelled lunch date might be seen as personal rejection and a reason to become socially reclusive or the loss of a pet could be followed by despair and depression.

The prolonged inability to maintain a sense of emotional balance is cause for concern. A depressed mood is one in which sadness is intensified and continues longer than would normally be expected in a particular situation. In contrast, an excessive feeling of happiness or elation is seen in **euphoria**. This euphoric state can escalate to **mania**, a mood characterized by overactivity, extreme euphoria, impulsivity, and lowered inhibitions. Mania may lead to delusions or hallucinations.

Bipolar and related disorders are similar to psychotic and depressive disorders in regards to both symptoms and family history. In the depressive disorders, a common symptom of a sad and empty mood along with psychosomatic changes are present that can also be seen in the individual with a bipolar disorder. In bipolar and related disorders, there is a pattern of hyperactive behavior and alterations in speech and/or thoughts processes that can also be seen in the individual with a psychotic disorder. It is important to recognize that the individual with depressive symptoms is not always bipolar and the individual with bipolar symptoms is not always psychotic.

Depressive Disorders

Depression is described as a persistent and prolonged mood of sadness that extends beyond 2 weeks' duration or longer. In the depressive disorders, there is a distinctive change in an individual's affect and cognition, with the sadness being severe enough to interfere with the individual's functional activity. This state can occur in a single episode or in a recurring pattern over time. Depressive disorders are referred to as **unipolar**, indicating that the individual does not experience episodes of mania or hypomania. Specific types of depressive disorders include major depressive disorder and persistent depressive or dysthymic disorder. Risk factors for depression are listed in Box 10.1.

BOX 10.1

Risk Factors for Depression

- Family history of depression
- Prior episode of depression
- Being assigned female at birth
- Being in a postpartum period
- Chronic illness
- Chronic pain
- Having experienced a major loss
- History of experiencing abuse
- Having a substance use disorder

Major Depressive Disorder

Major depressive disorder occurs when an individual experiences a depressed mood or loss of interest in most activities for most of each day for a period of at least 2 weeks. This can occur as a single episode or recurrent depressive episodes. The persistence and severity of the symptoms during the major depressive episode help to differentiate it from that seen in other psychotic or delusional disorders. The depressive episode may have a precipitating circumstance, such as chronic pain, loss of a job, lack of a support system, financial difficulties, or conflict with a friend or loved one. People who are timid and anxious tend to have more difficulty adapting to loss and the increased pressures of life than people who are bold, confident, and easygoing. Recovery from the impact of these situations may precipitate depression in those with inadequate coping skills.

Depression that occurs without a precipitating event is often associated with decreased neurotransmitter availability in the brain and usually responds to antidepressant medication. An episode of major depression is usually severe enough to require treatment.

Just the Facts The average person with major depressive disorder experiences four episodes over a lifetime.

Signs and Symptoms

Indications of depression include feelings of hopelessness, guilt and self-blame, melancholy, fatigue, loss of appetite, weight changes, and a decreased libido or sex drive. In addition, an individual who suffers from major depression may experience crying episodes, irritability, excessive worry, anxiety, and increased somatic complaints (e.g., headaches, body pains, gastrointestinal disturbances). They may have lapses of memory, a lack of concentration, and difficulty making decisions. Even small tasks, such as dressing or brushing their teeth, may seem overwhelming, leading to decreased efficiency and productivity. For example, a parent who previously had no problem shopping for groceries to feed their family now is unable to make decisions in the supermarket. Instead of selecting items, they feel overwhelmed and leave the store with nothing. **Anergia**, a marked decrease in energy level, may make the individual depend on others for even basic needs.

Many individuals with depression experience sleep disturbances such as waking too early or having difficulty falling asleep. Others may wake in the middle of the night and be unable to return to sleep, while others may sleep for prolonged periods. They may require a longer time to complete basic tasks such as bathing and dressing. Hygiene is often neglected in response to the poor self-image and worthlessness they feel, or hygiene-related tasks may be too overwhelming to perform. Often **anhedonia**, or a lack of pleasure in things an individual previously enjoyed, accompanies the depressed state. This is illustrated by an individual who previously had enjoyed reading to children at the library and now avoids the sessions because they no longer feel worthy of the children's attention. The affect of the depressed individual is one of sadness and misery, with a lack of eye contact and apathy. Dwelling on exaggerated and perceived failures, they are unable to see strengths and successes. Recurring thoughts of death and suicide are common. Signs and symptoms for major depressive disorder are found in Box 10.2.

Incidence and Etiology

Depression is more common in females and those who have a familial tendency for the disorder. Adolescents between the ages of 12 and 17 and adults ages 18 to 25 have a higher incidence of major depression. Seventeen percent of adolescents in the United States had at least one major

---

BOX 10.2

Signs and Symptoms of Major Depressive Disorder

- Mood of worry, anxiety, hopelessness, and worthlessness
- Guilt and self-blame
- Crying episodes
- Fatigue, anergia
- Sleep disturbances
- Weight and appetite changes
- Decreased sex drive
- Poor concentration and memory lapse
- Difficulty making decisions
- Decreased productivity
- Irritability
- Extreme sadness with sad affect
- Physical complaints
- Anhedonia or decreased pleasure in things previously enjoyed
- Thoughts of death and suicide

CASE STUDY 10.1

"Bianca"

Bianca is 32 years old and has been working as a cashier for a local department store for the past 4 years. She is divorced with two young daughters, 6 and 9 years of age. Bianca is being seen at the clinic for evaluation. The nurse notes that Bianca has a sad affect with no eye contact, smeared make-up, and her hair is messy and uncombed. Bianca is teary-eyed and states, "My husband not only left me alone in this world but left me with all of the bills too. I just can't do this anymore!"

Digging Deeper

1. What data collected supports the health care provider's diagnosis of depression?

2. What leading questions might encourage Bianca to continue talking?

3. The health care provider prescribes the antidepressant medication escitalopram. What side effects may occur with this medication?

4. What reinforcing of client teaching should be done concerning this medication?

5. How will the nurse monitor the effectiveness of the medication at the next clinic visit?

---

depressive episode in 2020 (National Institute of Mental Health [NIMH], 2022c). Depression is seen in majority of individuals who attempt or die by suicide. A major depressive episode may develop over days or weeks and last for several months. Some may experience a single episode, while others have a recurrent pattern of symptoms. A major episode can occur at any age, although the average age of onset is the mid-20s. Studies show that approximately half of those experiencing a major depressive episode will have another.

Senior Focus
Depression is not a normal part of aging. Any signs of depression, in any individual regardless of age, need to be reported to the health care provider or registered nurse (RN).

There are various theories about the cause of depression. Perhaps the most common is related to decreased amounts of available neurotransmitters in the brain that lead to a chemical imbalance. This theory supports the successful use of antidepressants in the treatment process. In addition, genetic and biologic predisposition, substance/medication side effects, premenstrual dysphoria, viruses, endocrine disturbances (including thyroid), and psychosocial factors are all cited as possible causes.

Mind Jogger
What impact would the symptoms of major depression have on the individual's family, work performance, and social life?

Specific Nursing Interventions for a Suicidal Client

On admission, the client should be assessed for current risk factors that indicate suicide may be a possibility. Determine the content of any suicidal thoughts or ideations. If the client has a plan, this usually indicates that the client is more serious about committing suicide. Determine the lethality of the method. A more lethal method usually indicates increased likelihood of an attempt. It is also important to ask when the client intends to carry out the plan. The longer a client takes to carry out an attempt, the more time the client is willing to take to find another solution. If the client has decided on a location to do the act, determine how easy or difficult it will be to access this location.

Suicide precautions are usually initiated on admission to a mental health unit for those who are at risk of self-harm. These precautions may vary from one facility to another and often include levels of precaution. If the client has recently attempted suicide, continuous monitoring of the client with one-to-one observation may be indicated. Sharp and potentially dangerous items (e.g., scarves, belts, shoelaces, nail files, scissors, cell phone charging cords, etc.) are removed from the client's room and personal effects. A "no-harm" contract may be established with the client every shift and renewed at a specific time. The contract should include a statement that the client will not kill or injure themselves and will notify the staff when suicidal thoughts first occur. Random client checks are done to prevent the client from anticipating when the checks will happen. Clients often carry out incidents of self-harm during times when nurses are busiest, such as shift changes. Watch for "cheeking" behaviors in which the client holds medication in the pouch of the cheek to avoid swallowing it. The client can stockpile medication for use to overdose later.

It is especially important to spend time with the client who is considering suicide as the only option. By using active listening and being present, the nurse conveys a sense of caring and appreciation for the worth of the client who is unable to find that feeling within themselves.

Persistent Depressive Disorder (Dysthymia)

The individual with persistent depressive disorder, also called dysthymia, experiences a recurrent state of depression over a period of at least 2 years. Depressive symptoms become a part of the individual's day-to-day experience, never disappearing for more than 2 months at a time. The individual with persistent depressive disorder (dysthymia) has never had a major depressive episode and does not exhibit any symptoms of manic behavior. The symptoms of persistent depressive disorder (dysthymia) are less severe than those of major depression, but the disorder tends to be more chronic.

Common Signs and Symptoms

People with persistent depressive disorder (dysthymia) tend to exhibit symptoms of depression over a lifetime. Some individuals with chronic depression feel that their symptoms are unavoidable and untreatable and that nothing can be done to help their feelings. When the individual feels it is impossible to be rid of the feelings of depression, they may eventually give up trying to find a solution, even when presented with options. The feeling of having no hope for relief and a loss of control over the situation causes some individuals to behave in a helpless manner and overlook possible solutions. This is known as **learned helplessness**. They may seek options thought to be helpful but when the option is ineffective, it reinforces the initial feelings of helplessness. In an attempt

to cope with these continued feelings of despair, individuals with persistent depressive disorder may resort to substance use, spending sprees, sexual promiscuity, or acting-out behaviors to escape these feelings. They may use alcohol, nicotine, or drugs in an attempt to treat insomnia or anxiety. Signs and symptoms for persistent depressive disorder are found in Box 10.3.

Just the Facts The depressed person feels an ongoing sense that something considered essential for happiness is missing from their life.

Mind Jogger What life situations might cause an individual with dysthymia to be vulnerable? What can contribute to the individual being in a state of learned helplessness?

Incidence and Etiology

It is estimated that 2.5% of adults (about 6.46 million people) in the United States will experience persistent depressive disorder (dysthymia) in their lifetime and that it occurs two to three times more frequently in women than men (NIMH, 2022d). The disorder is more likely to occur in first-degree biologic relatives with depressive disorders.

Mind Jogger What might contribute to persistent depressive disorder (dysthymia) and depression occurring more commonly in women?

Postpartum Depression

Postpartum depression is seen in some people after the birth of their infant. Postpartum depression is different than the postpartum blues (lay term "baby blues") that some people experience after giving birth. Baby blues includes transitory feelings of sadness and crying that start about 2 to 3 days after delivery but do not last longer than 2 weeks and do not affect the person's ability to care for their infant. Symptoms of postpartum depression are the same as for other depressive disorders. It affects about 8 to 15% of those who are postpartum and can occur anytime from birth to 12 months after delivery (Viguera, 2021). Risk factors include having had a previous episode of depression (whether major depressive disorder or postpartum depression), a family history of depression, an unwanted or unplanned pregnancy, intimate partner violence, or a serious infant condition (infant born with a congenital malformation or premature) or death of the infant (miscarriage, stillbirth, or neonatal death). Treatment of postpartum depression is with antidepressants.

A rare disorder seen in the postpartum period is postpartum psychosis. Postpartum psychosis has a sudden onset and mimics bipolar disorder with delusions, hallucinations, severe agitation, hyperactivity, thoughts of suicide, and depression. Postpartum psychosis is a medical emergency and requires medical intervention.

Mind Jogger What factors related to the postpartum period might contribute to depression? How might this lead to a dangerous situation?

Seasonal Affective Disorder

Seasonal Affective Disorder, also called seasonal depression, is associated with decreased daylight hours. Symptoms usually start in late fall and last through the winter months. With a decrease in sunlight and weather prohibiting being outdoors, the individual has typical depression symptoms including sadness and lack of energy. This disorder is often treated with light therapy, psychotherapy, and sometimes antidepressants. It typically resolves during the spring months when there is increased sunlight, and the individual can go outdoors more.

Treatment of Depressive Disorders

Treatment of depressive disorders include a monotherapy (one treatment modality used) or a polytherapy (more than one treatment modality used) approach. Treatments include psychotherapy, pharmacology, and electroconvulsive therapy (ECT). Medications are used very successfully in managing depression and include antidepressants and mood-stabilizing medications, including some atypical antipsychotics. Other treatments are being researched and used with individuals with depression in addition to these methods.

Psychotherapy

Depending on the situation, the two most common psychotherapies are interpersonal therapy and cognitive behavioral therapy. Both have been demonstrated to be effective in the treatment of depression and dysthymia. Psychotherapy for the depressed individual involves assisting them in exploring how negative thoughts and feelings are affecting their behavior. Box 10.4 lists some topics that may be covered in psychotherapy. Once the individual understands the underlying thoughts and feelings, they can identify more effective ways of coping. The individual must be willing to explore and discuss painful thoughts for improvement to occur. Individual, group, and family psychotherapies may be needed. The health care provider determines the type of psychotherapy depending on the circumstances and

---

BOX 10.4

Psychotherapy Topics Related to Depression

- How to manage symptoms
- Trigger factors that contribute to or intensify the depression
- Coping strategies to manage the trigger factors
- Identifying negative beliefs and replacing them with positive ones
- Identify personal strengths and problem-solving skills
- Effective communication with others
- How to build or reinforce positive relationships
- Self-esteem evaluation and how to build self-esteem
- Learning to set and attain goals

Information modified from Hurley, K. (2020). *Persistent depressive disorder (dysthymia)*. Psycom. https://www.psycom.net/depression.central.dysthymia.html

severity of the depression. Support or self-help groups are very useful for long-term management of depression.

Electroconvulsive Therapy (ECT)

Electroconvulsive therapy (ECT) involves passing an electric current through the brain (see Chapter 4). The actual mechanism by which electroconvulsive therapy (ECT) works is not known. It is thought that changes in neurotransmitter systems lead to the expected mood elevation. Unfortunately, because of the many changes that occur during in the brain during electroconvulsive therapy (ECT), memory deficits may occur. Depending on whether unilateral or bilateral electroconvulsive therapy (ECT) is used, the individual may have either short-term or long-term memory deficits. Electroconvulsive therapy (ECT) is used in cases where the individual has experienced several episodes of severe depression and nothing else has worked. This type of depression is usually the result of a long period of events and losses that eventually lead to depression. When there is one incident that leads to depression, it is usually a more acute type of depression.

Pharmacologic

Psychotherapeutic medications are used very successfully in managing depression. As the medication becomes effective in restoring levels of neurotransmitters, the individual's mood and energy level usually improve as well. The medications can help them to be more accepting of other interventions, but when used alone without therapy, prove ineffective for long-term treatment. Although these medications can balance the brain chemistry to minimize the symptoms of the disorder, many individuals have to trial several different antidepressants before finding one that alleviates their symptoms.

Complementary and Alternative Medicine (CAM)

Some complementary and alternative medicines (CAMs) are used by individuals with depression. Regular exercise has been shown to help decrease depressive symptoms. Some herbs, such as St. John's wort or Ginkgo biloba, have been shown to have some effect on depression. However, they also have interactions with some medications and should be discussed with the health care provider. Acupuncture does not alleviate depressive symptoms but may help the individual in other ways that may improve their symptoms. Acupuncture has been reported to decrease pain, cause relaxation (both during and after the procedure), and help with stress relief. Increased stress and pain have been shown to increase depressive symptoms in many individuals. Massage and aromatherapy have benefits including helping the individual to relax.

Test Yourself
- ✔ What is the difference between mood and affect?
- ✔ Describe symptoms seen in depression.
- ✔ How is major depressive disorder similar to, and different from, Seasonal Affective Disorder?
- ✔ Name four treatment methods for depression.

Bipolar Disorder

Bipolar disorder is characterized by atypical and erratic shifts in mood, energy, activity, behavior, sleep, and cognition (Suppes, 2022). These episodes of alternate changes range from manic episodes (euphoric, excessively happy, high energy) to low depressive periods and may occur rapidly, be intermixed with periods of typical functioning, or occur simultaneously in a mixed episode. Since the individual exhibits both the low mood seen in depression in addition to the manic episodes, it is referred to as bipolar (having two poles or ends of the spectrum).

The rapid shifts in mood in a short period of time are referred to as **labile** (alternating from euphoria to dysphoria and irritability). The frequency of the mood swings between mania and depression is unpredictable and varies from person to person. The severity of the symptoms may also vary from mild to severe. If the individual has four or more episodes of mania or depression within a year, they are said to be **rapid cycling**.

Just the Facts Bipolar disorder typically begins with depression accompanied by at least one manic episode.

Signs and Symptoms

Although the disorder may not be recognized in its early onset, the first indications may be a state of mild to moderate mania called **hypomania** that lasts for a period of at least 4 days. The individual is unusually cheerful with excessive energy and the ability to keep going long after others are exhausted. The need for sleep may decrease to 3 or 4 hours. This level of acceleration may feel good to them, and they may deny anything is wrong. However, the elevated feeling or "high" does not stop at a controllable or comfortable level (National Alliance on Mental Illness [NAMI], 2022a) which leads to irritability, impaired judgment, or irrational thinking. Hypomania differs from mania in length, severity of symptoms, and level of impairment in daily life. The individual with hypomania does not experience psychotic symptoms of delusions or hallucinations.

In mania, the individual also shows the symptoms of hypomania but to a greater intensity. Symptoms of mania are severe, last for at least a week, and impair the individual's functioning in social, work, and daily activities. The changes in mood are obvious to others, but not usually severe enough to require hospitalization.

In addition to the symptoms of hypomania, in mania, the client has symptoms that involve mood, behavior, and altered thought processes. The individual with mania may be moody and irritable. Irresponsible and impulsive behavior are common. The individual tends to have lowered, or absent, inhibitions. For example, the individual may wander in public without clothes, dress in outfits that are uncharacteristically vibrant or extravagant, drive dangerously, or go on spending sprees. They will start and stop multiple projects without completing one before going on to the next. This is combined with a disregard for social boundaries, often causing the individual to offend others due to their lack of insight, which others see as insensitivity. It is common for the individual to spend large amounts of money on unneeded items (e.g., buying a new car when they do not have a job), gamble, or make senseless business deals. Use of drugs or alcohol is also common.

Altered thought processes that may be seen in mania include grandiosity, delusions of grandeur, and conversations that are not focused. The individual may exhibit **grandiosity**, which is larger-than-reality self-esteem or feelings. For example, the individual thinks they have more wealth or intelligence than they really do. To the observer, this sounds arrogant or boastful. This is different than **delusions of grandeur**, which are false or outrageous beliefs about oneself, for example, the individual states they discovered the cure for cancer or are the king of a great country. During this time, they may experience hallucinations or delusional thinking. They may demonstrate an increase in goal-directed activity but with increased irritability and moodiness. The individual usually talks incessantly with a flight of ideas (see Chapter 7) or jumps from one subject to another, and may state, "my mind is racing." The individual's attention is easily distracted by things in the environment that others deem insignificant. For example, they may say, "The lights in here are blue but in my room they are yellow."

Some of the first inhibitions the individual with mania may lose are those regarding sexual activity. A preoccupation with seductive thoughts often leads to an increase in sexual activity, and conversation is often focused on sexual topics. The individual may engage in sexual encounters multiple times a day or with multiple partners and may not be attentive to their own safety during these encounters. They may have unprotected or reckless sexual encounters with strangers. Masturbation is a common sexual activity for the client who is hospitalized.

> **Mind Jogger ❷**
> There are artists and actors who have created some of their best work while in a state of hypomania. What characteristics of the mood might account for this?

The lack of insight and excessive level of activity predisposes the individual to a dangerous and volatile psychotic state. This is a more severe form of mania and usually requires hospitalization. They may act in ways that are offensive or violate the rights of others. When their wishes are not fulfilled, their mood may shift from extreme euphoria to extreme aggressive irritability. During these interpersonal conflicts, the individual may perceive injustices where there is none or have **delusions of persecution** where they fully believe someone is planning to harm them or is conspiring against them. They typically have a flight of ideas which is a constant shift in attention from one thought to another. The individual

Signs and Symptoms of Hypomania/Mania

- Extreme euphoria
- Inflated self-esteem or grandiosity
- Talkative with rapid, racing speech (pressured speech)
- Flight of ideas
- Excessive energy
- Decreased need for sleep
- Easily distracted
- Extreme irritability and moodiness
- Reckless and impulsive behaviors
- Lack of judgment
- Increased motor activity
- Irresponsible buying sprees or business deals
- Sexual hyper-focus and activity
- Delusions of grandeur or persecution (mania)
- Auditory and visual hallucinations (mania)
- Exaggerated outfit, makeup, and accessories
- Lack of attention to hygiene

may speak in clang associations which are words that may be strung together in rhyming phrases or that have no connected meaning (i.e., "Hair is bare and bear is a scare, scare is a fair, fair is there, you are a pear…"). They project an expansive thought pattern of grandiosity with false beliefs of wealth, power, and identity. Auditory and visual hallucinations may occur during the height of the manic episode. They may dress in an uncharacteristically exaggerated manner, with bright colors, excessive jewelry, and excessive makeup. Hygiene is often neglected as the thought processes escalate and activity accelerates. Items such as magazine pictures, containers, and food may be collected and stockpiled as the hyperactivity absorbs the individual's time. Signs and symptoms for hypomania/mania are listed in Box 10.5.

Just the Facts During a state of mania, the individual has a continual mental flood of overly confident self-expectations that lead to frenzied and disorganized psychomotor activity.

Incidence and Etiology

It is estimated that 2.8% of the United States population (about 7 million people) have bipolar disorder (NAMI, 2022b). Women are at greater risk than men for developing manic episodes, which can occur at any time. The average age of onset for a first manic episode is in the early 20s, but it can be as early as adolescence and as late as age 50.

In many cases of bipolar disorder, there seems to be a genetic factor that is shown by the familial pattern of the illness. There are studies that show an increase in severity in future generations. Environmental factors are also cited as a cause, since not all cases have a family history of the disorder. Despite these theories, the exact cause of this condition is unknown. Evidence has linked bipolar symptoms to changes in the chemical neurotransmitters in the brain. Substance use disorder and stressful life events have also been linked to the episodes.

Just the Facts Bipolar disorders have a younger age of onset and shorter cycles than major depressive disorders.

Cyclothymic Disorder

Cyclothymic disorder is a chronic mood disturbance characterized by fluctuating periods of hypomanic symptoms and periods of depression. The symptoms of cyclothymic disorder are insufficient in number, severity, or duration to meet the criteria for a hypomanic or major depressive episode.

The symptoms of cyclothymia include recurrent episodes of hypomania and dysthymia. The signs and symptoms for cyclothymic disorder are found in Box 10.6. These alternating periods are recurrent, with short periods of more balanced mood that usually do not last longer than 2 months. Delusional thinking and hallucinations are not present. The individual's functioning is not severely impaired, and hospitalization is usually not necessary.

Cyclothymic disorder occurs equally in men and women and begins in adolescence or early adulthood. It is usually chronic with an insidious

Signs and Symptoms of Cyclothymic Disorder

- Recurrent episodes of hypomania and dysthymia
- States not as severe as in bipolar disorders
- Short periods or normalcy
- No psychotic symptoms
- Functioning not severely impaired

onset. Most people do not realize the disorder is present until many symptoms have existed over years. There is a greater risk for the individual with this disorder to develop bipolar disorder.

Test Yourself	✔ How does hypomania differ from mania? ✔ Name five symptoms that are seen in hypomania/mania. ✔ How is cyclothymic disorder different from bipolar disorder?

Pharmacologic Treatment of Mood Disorders

Depressive and bipolar disorders often require treatment with pharmacologic agents for the individual to return to a balanced state of functioning in their daily life. Medications that work for depression may also be effective for the client with bipolar disorder. There are many medications that have been proven to be effective, but not every medication is effective for everyone. This can cause the individual to start one medication only to find that it is ineffective in relieving their symptoms and that they must therefore start over with a different medication. This can be frustrating for the individual. Additionally, the individual needs to balance the effectiveness of the medication in relieving their symptoms with any side effects they may experience. For some individuals, the side effects are too great of an obstacle to continue the medication. In other individuals, once the medication provides therapeutic benefits and the symptoms are eliminated or minimized, they feel better and no longer see the need for the medication and therefore stop taking it. Once the therapeutic effects wear off, they have symptoms again.

Antidepressants

Antidepressants are used in the treatment of depression to elevate mood, increase physical activity and mental alertness, improve appetite and sleep, and restore interest or pleasure in usual activities and things previously enjoyed. Because the neurotransmitters involved in depression also affect these other body functions, they can be used to treat other types of disorders such as eating disorders and sleep dysfunction. As depression results from a decreased level of monoamine

neurotransmitter (norepinephrine, serotonin, or dopamine) that is insufficient to stimulate the receptors, most medications used to treat depression increase the amount of chemicals in the brain to help elevate mood. Research has demonstrated that by inhibiting the breakdown of the monoamines (by taking monoamine oxidase inhibitors) or by promoting their reuptake to increase their presence in the brain, mood can be effectively elevated. Antidepressants generally fall into three categories: **monoamine oxidase inhibitors (MAOIs)**, **tricyclic antidepressants (TCAs)**, and **serotonin-specific reuptake inhibitors (SSRIs)**. There are other classifications of medications that have also been effective in treating depression.

The effect of antidepressant medications on the state of depression is not immediate. Antidepressants must be taken continuously for several weeks before therapeutic effects are evident and the individual begins to feel better. This is because a continuous presence of the medication is needed in the brain for the level of the neurotransmitters to balance the deficit causing the depression. It is important that they continue to take the medication, even if it does not seem to be helping. All of these medications are effective, but some work better for certain types of depression. A withdrawn individual, for example, may benefit from a medication with stimulating effects, whereas another may benefit from one that has a calming effect. Dosage and medication used will depend on the type and severity of the condition and the age of the individual.

It is important to remember that these medications are not curative and cannot solve the problems underlying the individual's mental state. Those individuals with suicidal tendencies must be closely observed, because therapeutic levels of these medications can energize their ability to carry out a suicide plan. Antidepressant medication combined with therapy and counseling is usually the preferred approach to treating depression. Antidepressant agents, their chemical groups, and common side effects are listed in Table 10.1.

Monoamine Oxidase Inhibitors (MAOIs)

Early pharmacologic studies led to the development of a medication classification called monoamine oxidase inhibitors (MAOIs). Monoamine oxidase is an enzyme that metabolizes or inactivates the monoamine neurotransmitters. Specifically, monoamine oxidase inhibitors (MAOIs) work by preventing the breakdown of the neurotransmitter

TABLE 10.1	Antidepressant Medications	
Chemical Group	**Generic Name**	**Adverse Reactions and Side Effects**
Tricyclic antidepressants (TCAs)	Amitriptyline Amoxapine Desipramine Doxepin Imipramine Nortriptyline Protriptyline Trimipramine	Lethargy, sedation, blurred vision, dry eyes, dry mouth, cardiac arrhythmias, hypotension, ECG changes, constipation, urinary retention, photosensitivity, blood dyscrasias, nausea and vomiting, increased appetite and weight gain, changes in blood glucose
Heterocyclics	Bupropion Maprotiline Mirtazapine Trazodone	Agitation, headache, dry mouth, nausea, vomiting, change in appetite, weight gain or loss, photosensitivity, tremors, changes in blood sugar, seizures are possible, priapism, hypotension, tachycardia
Selective serotonin reuptake inhibitors (SSRIs)	Citalopram Fluoxetine Fluvoxamine Paroxetine Sertraline Escitalopram	Apathy, confusion, drowsiness, insomnia, weakness, agitation, anxiety, increased depression, cough, orthostatic hypotension, tachycardia, dry mouth, nausea, altered taste, ejaculatory delay, impotence, amenorrhea, photosensitivity, rash, pruritus, weight changes, tremors
Nonselective reuptake inhibitors (serotonin and norepinephrine) (SNRIs)	Venlafaxine Desvenlafaxine Duloxetine	Vivid dreams, anxiety, dizziness, headache, insomnia, nervousness, weakness, dry mouth, paresthesia, rhinitis, visual disturbances, altered taste, abdominal pain, nausea, vomiting, constipation, diarrhea, tachycardia, palpitations
Monoamine oxidase inhibitors (MAOIs)	Isocarboxazid Phenelzine Tranylcypromine	Dizziness, headache, orthostatic hypotension, constipation, nausea, arrhythmias, tachycardia May interact with numerous foods and medications to produce hypertensive crisis (severe hypertension, severe headache, fever, possible myocardial infarction or intracranial hemorrhage) (See Box 10.7)

monoamine, releasing monoamine neurotransmitters in the brain, blocking their reuptake into the presynaptic compartments, or mimicking the effects of the monoamines at the receptors. These medications can interact with numerous foods and other medications (Box 10.7) causing a hypertensive crisis. Foods to avoid contain tyramine, a precursor of norepinephrine.

Tricyclic Antidepressants (TCAs)

The tricyclic antidepressants (TCAs), named for their three-ring chemical structure, were developed in the 1950s. These medications work to correct the chemical imbalance of neurotransmitter concentrations in the synaptic cleft of the central nervous system (CNS) nerve cells. They work by inhibiting the reuptake of the neurotransmitters back into the presynaptic cells, which leads to higher concentration of the neurotransmitters available. Tricyclic antidepressants (TCAs) also affect other body chemicals and characteristically produce a number of adverse and potentially dangerous side effects, including cardiac arrhythmias. This factor requires that all individuals taking these agents be monitored closely.

Selective Serotonin Reuptake Inhibitors (SSRIs)

A new class of antidepressants that were designed to block the reuptake of serotonin, rather than norepinephrine, was developed in the 1980s. **Serotonin** is a potent vasoconstrictor thought to be involved in arousal, sleep, dreams, mood, appetite, and sensitivity to pain. The selective serotonin reuptake inhibitors (SSRIs) have relatively fewer side effects than the tricyclic antidepressants (TCAs), making them a safer and more desirable alternative. Figure 10.1 demonstrates the action of selective serotonin reuptake inhibitors (SSRIs) to selectively block the reuptake of serotonin into the presynaptic compartment of the nerve cell. This causes increased concentration of serotonin at nerve endings in the central nervous system (CNS). These medications have little or no effect on the cardiovascular system and fewer anticholinergic side effects.

Indications for Use

Antidepressant medications are used in the treatment of major depression, depression accompanied by anxiety, or depression related to another disorder

BOX 10.7

Foods and Medications to Avoid When Taking a Monoamine Oxidase Inhibitor (MAOI)

Note: These food and medication restrictions should also be continued for at least 2 weeks after discontinuing taking a monoamine oxidase inhibitor (MAOI).

FOODS

- Aged cheese (cheddar, Swiss, blue cheese, Parmesan, provolone, Romano)
- Alcoholic beverages (beer, especially tap or home-brewed; red wines)
- Beans or bean pods (snow, fava, soy)
- Dried or ripe fruits (raisins, avocados, bananas, figs)
- Caffeine-containing beverages
- Pickled/fermented items (caviar, kimchi, sauerkraut, pickled herring)
- Smoked and processed meats (hot dogs, bacon, salami, pepperoni, bologna, summer sausage, corned beef)
- Meat tenderizers
- Sauces (soy, miso, teriyaki)

Note: This is not a complete list of foods.
List adapted from Hall-Flavin, D. K. (2018). *MAOIs and diet: Is it necessary to restrict tyramine?* Mayo Clinic. https://www.mayoclinic.org/diseases-conditions/depression/expert-answers/maois/faq-20058035

MEDICATIONS

- Amphetamines
- Antiallergy or antihistamines containing ephedrine derivatives
- Antidepressants
- Antihypertensive medications
- Levodopa
- Meperidine

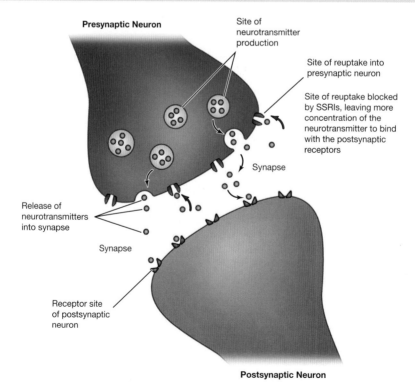

Figure 10.1 The release of serotonin from the presynaptic nerve ending into the synaptic cleft where the neurotransmitter is free to connect with the receptors of the next neuron. The neurotransmitter may be deactivated by chemical processes or be taken back into the presynaptic compartment (reuptake). Serotonin-specific reuptake inhibitors (SSRIs) block the site of reuptake so that more of the neurotransmitter is available at the receptor sites.

(for example alcohol use disorder, schizophrenia, or an intellectual disability). Antidepressants are also used in the treatment of other disorders including panic, dysthymia, bipolar, and obsessive-compulsive disorder (OCD). In children, antidepressants may be used in the treatment of attention deficit hyperactivity disorder (ADHD) and childhood enuresis. Chronic pain and bulimia are also treated with antidepressant medications. Bupropion is indicated for use with smoking cessation.

Contraindications

Antidepressants are contraindicated in individuals who are hypersensitive to the medication classification and those who are pregnant or lactating. Tricyclic antidepressants (TCAs) are also contraindicated in the acute recovery period following a myocardial infarction or in individuals with coronary artery disease. They should be used with caution in those individuals with a history of urinary retention or benign prostatic hypertrophy, glaucoma, asthma, or hepatic or renal disease. Dosages may need to be reduced in older adults. Individuals with Parkinson disease should not take serotonin-specific reuptake inhibitors (SSRIs).

Concurrent use of any other antidepressant (regardless of classification) with monoamine oxidase inhibitors (MAOIs) is contraindicated. Monoamine oxidase inhibitors (MAOIs) are further contraindicated in individuals with hepatic or renal insufficiency, a history of or existing cardiovascular disease, hypertension, severe headaches, or in children younger than 16 years. They should be used cautiously in individuals with a history of seizures, diabetes mellitus, suicidal tendencies, angina pectoris, or hyperthyroidism. There are many medication interactions that may occur with antidepressants. A health care provider or pharmacist should be consulted before combining an antidepressant with any other prescription or over-the-counter (OTC) medications.

Nursing Interventions for the Client Taking Antidepressant Medications

The nurse needs to monitor the client taking antidepressant medications for effectiveness of the medication and should monitor mood at frequent intervals. Criteria that may be used to monitor the effectiveness of antidepressants may include that the client: interacts and communicates with staff and others, demonstrates a more positive view of self, performs activities of daily living (ADLs), communicates feelings about their present situation,

Reinforcing Client and Family Teaching **10.1**

Important Information About Antidepressant Medications

- Take medication exactly as directed by the health care provider.
- Do not use more of the medication, do not use it more often, or do not use it for a longer period than ordered by the health care provider.
- Take the medication as directed consistently for several weeks to see a therapeutic effect.
- Take the medication with food or milk to avoid stomach upset.
- Keep regular health care provider appointments.
- Use caution when driving, operating dangerous equipment, or engaging in activities that require mental alertness and coordination.
- Do not mix medication with alcohol or take other central nervous system depressants.
- Report any side effects to the health care provider.
- Do not suddenly stop taking the medication—it must be withdrawn gradually.
- Take a missed dose as soon as possible—if several hours have lapsed or it is nearing time for the next dose, the dose should not be doubled to catch up.
- Avoid smoking when taking tricyclic antidepressants (TCAs)—smoking enhances the metabolism and increased dosage may be required.
- Wear protective sunscreen when outdoors when taking tricyclic antidepressants (TCAs).
- Rise slowly from a reclining position.

experiences normal sleep patterns and appetite, and participates in unit activities.

Observe for a sharp increase in mood, which may indicate the client has suicidal ideation. Monitor for hoarding of medications, cheeking, or other overdosing cues. The nurse also reinforces teaching related to antianxiety medications (see Reinforcing Client and Family Teaching 10.1).

The nurse should provide explanations of medication action and side effects. Monitor the client's blood pressure for orthostatic hypotension and advise them to change positions slowly. Also monitor for hypertensive crisis. Until the client's response to the medication is established, assist with ambulation, or instruct them to avoid activities requiring mental alertness such as driving a car. To help prevent gastrointestinal upset, administer with food or milk. Due to the drying effects of antidepressants, encourage the client to increase their fluid intake, offer hard candy or sugarless gum for dry mouth, discourage caffeinated beverages, and monitor for constipation.

CASE STUDY 10.2

"Bianca"

Recall Bianca from Case Study 10.1. Bianca has now been taking escitalopram 10 mg daily for 3 weeks. She was brought to the emergency department of the hospital this morning by her mother who states that her 9-year-old granddaughter called saying, "I can't wake Mommy up!" The grandmother hands the nurse an empty bottle of escitalopram. Bianca has an overwhelming odor of alcohol on her breath. The grand mother states that Bianca has recently been drinking heavily.

Digging Deeper

1. *What is the danger of mixing an antidepressant medication with alcohol?*

2. *After being stabilized in the emergency department, Bianca is admitted to the in-patient unit for observation and evaluation. What is Bianca's current nursing priority?*

3. *The health care provider has given orders to implement suicide precautions. What are some objects that should be removed from her room?*

4. *Once her room is made as safe as possible, the nurse plans to ask Bianca for a no-harm contract. What is the rationale for this intervention?*

5. *What might explain why this incident occurred now and not 3 weeks ago?*

The nurse also needs to monitor the client for side effects of antidepressant medications. Report any client side effects of abnormal bleeding, fever, hypertension, cardiac arrhythmias, changes in blood sugar levels, seizure activity, or severe headaches to the registered nurse (RN) and the health care provider.

Ketamine and Esketamine

Ketamine is a medication administered as an anesthetic. It also has analgesic and sedative properties. Esketamine is a component of ketamine. Ketamine and esketamine can also be used for treatment-resistant unipolar depression and suicidal ideation (Thase & Connolly, 2022). Ketamine and esketamine therapy are usually not a viable treatment option until other forms of therapy for depression have been tried and determined to not be effective at relieving the depression. Ketamine is usually given as an intravenous infusion while esketamine is administered as a nasal spray. Both forms require monitoring in a regulated setting prior to and after administration. Hallucinations in the immediate postadministrative period are common especially in an environment that has a lot of stimuli. The benefit of ketamine and esketamine is increased when used concurrently with psychotherapy and other forms of depression therapy.

Mood Stabilizers

Mood-stabilizing agents are the medications of choice to treat individuals with bipolar disorders. These medications may be used alone or in combination with selected atypical antipsychotics and are used along with psychotherapy to stabilize and control the initial extreme mood swings.

Lithium carbonate was the first medication to be labeled as a mood-stabilizer because of its combined antimanic and antidepressant properties. Today, the term mood stabilizer is currently used to describe psychotropic medications that reduce mood swings and the likelihood of subsequent episodes. In addition to lithium carbonate, anticonvulsants and second-generation antipsychotic medications are included in this category. It is important to note that lithium carbonate is used to treat both spectrums of mood shifts, whereas other medications in this category are primarily those that keep the manic episodes under control.

Lithium Carbonate

Lithium carbonate, commonly called lithium, is a naturally occurring metallic salt, much like sodium carbonate. It is used in the management of bipolar illness, both to treat manic episodes and to prevent the recurrence of these episodes. Lithium is more effective in treating highs or manic periods than in preventing lows or depressive periods.

Lithium is well absorbed from the gastrointestinal tract and may be given by capsule or concentrate. It has a peak blood level of 1 to 3 hours with a half-life of about 24 hours. Lithium is not metabolized by the body and is entirely excreted by the kidneys unchanged, so adequate renal functioning is necessary for its use. Most of a lithium dose is reabsorbed in the proximal renal tubules. The reabsorption of sodium and lithium is closely related, with any increase or decrease in dietary sodium intake affecting the levels of lithium in the blood plasma. A decrease in dietary sodium or loss through perspiration, vomiting, or diarrhea causes more lithium to be reabsorbed and increases the risk of lithium toxicity. Excessive intake of sodium causes an increase in the excretion of lithium and may lower the serum level to a nontherapeutic level. Therapeutic serum levels are 0.6 to 1.2 mEq/L and severe toxic reactions possible when levels reach 2 to 2.5 mEq/L. It is important to note that the therapeutic serum level of lithium is not much lower than a toxic serum level. Lithium dosage is determined based on both the clinical response and serum levels of the medication. Lithium blood levels should be monitored closely for therapeutic range. Acute lithium toxicity is manifested by increased tremors, headache, vomiting, and confusion.

Other Medications Used for Mood Stabilization

In recent years, more medications have become available for the treatment of bipolar illness. The wide use of anticonvulsants over lithium in treating acute mania and mood cycling is due to a wider therapeutic range and lack of renal toxicity. Atypical antipsychotics have also shown to be effective as mood stabilizing medications. There is not one medication that is effective for all individuals with symptoms of bipolar disorders. Mood-stabilizing agents, their chemical groups, and side effects are listed in Table 10.2.

Indications for Use

Mood-stabilizing agents are indicated for manic episodes associated with bipolar disorder and maintenance therapy to prevent or diminish future episodes. Lithium is also used in the treatment of migraine headaches and schizoaffective disorders. The action of anticonvulsants and calcium-channel blockers in the treatment of bipolar disorders is not clear; however, they have been used effectively to stabilize the manic episodes in bipolar disorders.

Contraindications

Mood stabilizers are contraindicated in individuals with hypersensitivity to the medication, cardiac

TABLE 10.2	**Mood-Stabilizing Medications**	
Chemical Group	**Generic Name**	**Adverse Reactions and Side Effects**
Antimanic	Lithium carbonate	Lethargy, drowsiness, headache, fatigue, dry mouth, metallic taste, nausea, vomiting, diarrhea, thirst, polyuria, leukocytosis, muscle weakness, fine tremors **Life threatening:** Arrhythmias, bradycardia, renal toxicity, epileptiform seizures, coma
Anticonvulsants	Carbamazepine[a] Clonazepam Divalproex, valproic acid Oxcarbazepine Lamotrigine Gabapentin[a]	Sedation, headache, nausea, vomiting, indigestion, diarrhea, diplopia, elevated liver enzymes, drowsiness, sore gums, increased appetite with weight gain, vertigo, ataxia, dry mouth, confusion, hallucinations, prolonged bleeding **Life threatening:** Heart failure, arrhythmias, blood dyscrasias, toxic hepatitis, respiratory depression
Calcium-channel blocker	Verapamil	Dizziness, headache, transient hypotension, constipation, nausea, elevated liver enzymes, prolonged bleeding time **Life threatening:** Heart failure, bradycardia, ventricular arrhythmias, AV block
Second-generation psychotropics (atypical antipsychotics)	Clozapine Olanzapine Quetiapine Risperidone Ziprasidone Aripiprazole	Sedation, weight gain, dry mouth, constipation, potential mental confusion, orthostatic hypotension, tachycardia, hypersalivation, nausea and vomiting, agranulocytosis, seizures, Parkinson-like symptoms (flat affect, stiff muscles, slowed movements), or internal feelings of restlessness or agitation (akathisia, see Chapter 11 under heading "Extrapyramidal Side Effects"), photosensitivity, rhinitis

Decreased dosages recommended for older adults.
[a]Not FDA approved for bipolar disorder but is used by many psychiatrists.

or renal disease, and sodium imbalance and in those who are pregnant or lactating. These agents should be used cautiously in older people and those with metabolic disorders, urinary retention, or seizure disorders.

Anticonvulsants and calcium-channel blockers should not be used in those who are hypersensitive to these medications, have a history of bone marrow suppression, or have taken a monoamine oxidase inhibitor (MAOI) within 14 days of therapy. They should be used with caution in older people, people who are pregnant or lactating, and those with hepatic or cardiac disease.

Nursing Interventions for the Client Taking Mood Stabilizing Medications

The nurse needs to monitor the client taking mood stabilizers for effectiveness of the medication. The nurse should monitor the client's mood at frequent intervals, draw lithium levels as ordered, monitor intake of 2,000 to 3,000 mL daily and monitor output. The nurse should ensure the client has an adequate sodium intake and provide salty foods if the client's activity results in heavy perspiration. Monitor the client for signs of toxicity in the client taking lithium which include muscle weakness, diplopia or blurred vision, severe diarrhea, persistent nausea and vomiting, tinnitus, and vertigo. Criteria that may be used to monitor the effectiveness of mood stabilizers may include that the client: maintains consistent therapeutic blood levels of lithium; participates in unit activities; maintains consistent dietary intake of sodium and fluids; and does not experience extreme mood swings.

The nurse also reinforces teaching related to mood stabilizing medications (see Reinforcing Client and Family Teaching 10.2). Important points to reinforce include that the client and caregivers verbalize importance of continuing medication therapy even if client is feeling well, keeping regular appointments with health care provider, and having medication levels drawn regularly. It is also important that the client and caregivers verbalize understanding of medication side effects and which symptoms to report to the health care provider.

The nurse should provide explanations of the medication's action and side effects. The nurse should monitor the client's blood pressure. Until the client's response to the medication is established, assist with ambulation, or instruct them to avoid activities requiring mental alertness such

---

Reinforcing Client and Family Teaching   10.2

Important Information About Mood Stabilizing Medications

- Use caution when operating a motor vehicle or dangerous machinery.
- Do not stop taking the medication abruptly as serious withdrawal symptoms can occur. It must be gradually decreased under the guidance of a health care provider
- Take the medication regularly, even when feeling well or if symptoms are absent.
- Report any side effects to the health care provider.
- Keep all health care provider appointments.
- Have regular blood samples taken (usually drawn 8 to 12 hours after last dose taken) if taking lithium.
- Take medication at the same time each day. If you miss a dose, do not double the next dose (toxicity could occur).
- Consult with the health care provider or pharmacist before taking any prescription or nonprescription medication with lithium.
- Report any extreme mood swings to the health care provider.
- When taking lithium, ensure a fluid intake of 8 to 10 8-ounce glasses of water each day. Maintain a consistent intake of dietary sodium each day, and increase intake if activity results in heavy perspiration.
- If you take a calcium-channel blocker, rise slowly from a sitting or reclining position.
- Side effects such as nausea, dry mouth, flatulence, dizziness, mild tremors, and insomnia should subside with continued treatment.

---

as driving a car. To help prevent gastrointestinal upset, administer with food or milk.

The nurse also needs to monitor the client for side effects of mood stabilizing medications. Report to the RN and the health care provider any indication of lithium toxicity including nausea, vomiting, and diarrhea. Side effects of cardiac arrhythmias, bradycardia, abnormal bleeding, fever, elevated liver enzymes, abnormal involuntary muscle movements or Parkinson-like symptoms should be reported immediately to the health care provider or the RN. Report any behavioral changes either mania or depression.

Test Yourself

- ✔ Name three categories of antidepressants
- ✔ Would a dehydrated individual who regularly takes lithium have a higher or lower serum lithium level?

Nursing Process and Care Plan *for the Client With a Mood Disorder*

When establishing a nurse–client relationship with the person experiencing a mood disorder, it is important to focus on the individual as a person and not the behaviors. The nurse should be empathetic to the client's current emotional state. These behaviors by the nurse help to establish and maintain a therapeutic relationship with the client. The nurse should realize that the client's mood will not resolve quickly and that outcomes may not occur for several days to weeks.

The nurse should allow for extra time when interacting with the client. The client with a depressive order may not walk or talk as fast as other clients and the nurse should not rush them or ask them to "hurry up" as the client mentally cannot process conversations at a typical pace and physically may not be able to do tasks quickly. The client with mania may perceive the nurse's lack of patience as a personal rejection and can become irritable and volatile. It is important to remember that because of the nature of mania, implementing nursing strategies may be difficult. Refrain from becoming emotionally reactive to the client's acting-out behaviors.

Assessment (Data Collection)

When working with a client with a mood disorder, collect data about mood and affect, thinking and perceptual ability, somatic complaints, sleep patterns (current and usual), changes in energy level, and the character of speech patterns. Mood and affect should be checked for congruency. For example, when observed crying, a client should report feeling sad or down. A client who says they are sad but is laughing is not showing this congruency. Because mood is a subjective experience, it is important to ask the client what feeling, or emotion, they are experiencing. Clients experiencing a manic episode will likely display a bright or happy affect, while those with depression will usually display a flat affect with a lack of eye contact.

Collect data on the client's thought and speech patterns. During mania, thought processes become faster and may become fragmented, leading to disorganized patterns of speech. The client may not be able to complete one thought process before the next one begins. Complaints of racing thoughts are also common, or there may be a preoccupation with delusional thinking. Monitor patterns of verbal speech. The tone of voice, pace at which thoughts

are processed and communicated, and the rate at which words are spoken are all relevant. Changes in the tone and rate can provide clues to mood and energy level. Clients in a manic state have very pressured or loud and forceful speech. Some clients may be unable to verbally communicate feelings but may be able to do so in drawings or written text.

The client may not be able to follow a conversation during a manic episode, so providing important information to the client or having them sign legal documents should not occur at this time. Any information that is presented should be given in one to two simple sentences at a time. Avoid multi-step or lengthy directions. Determine if the client understands what is being said. Observe behavioral clues for what the client may be thinking if they do not respond verbally.

Determine the client's level of orientation. In depressive states, thought processes are slowed. Concentration may be difficult for clients who are depressed or experiencing mania. Also provide short, simple directions for the client who is depressed and determine client's understanding.

Administer a depression screening tool such as the PHQ-9 (see Appendix A) as per facility policy. Ask the client if they have any thoughts of suicide (suicidal ideation) and if they have thought of or made a plan for committing suicide. Administer other screening tools per the facility policy. Ask the client about any somatic complaints. During depression, the tolerance for pain may decrease, giving rise to generalized body aches, headaches, and gastrointestinal disturbances.

Observe for clues that indicate increased or decreased sleep patterns. Individuals in a manic episode often go 2 to 3 days without sleep. Individuals with depression may have insomnia with difficulty falling asleep and staying asleep. Others may have hypersomnia and sleep for prolonged periods of time. Observe the client's energy level. Those with mania will usually report a drastic increase in energy, while those who are depressed usually report anergia or decreased energy levels.

Collect data on the client's appetite, recent eating patterns, and weight changes. Clients with depression may have little appetite or overeat as a coping tool. A loss of weight may be seen during a manic phase as the excessive activity minimizes the perceived need for food. The client does not take time to eat or is unable to remain seated long enough to eat. Determine the amount of assistance required for personal hygiene, dressing, and elimination needs. Both clients who are manic and clients who are depressed may lack attention to hygiene and bowel habits.

Nursing Care Focus

Once data have been collected, identify the individual needs of the client. The individual needs of the client who is depressed are very different from those of one experiencing a manic episode, but the focus of nursing care for either client follows Maslow's hierarchy, with safety, food, and sleep being priorities. For example, safety is a priority nursing care focus for both clients with depression and clients experiencing mania. For the client with depression, a nursing care focus might be "*Self-Harm Risk*, related to suicidal ideation" whereas in a client with mania it could be "*Self-Harm Risk*, related to reckless behaviors." Sleep needs may apply to both clients as well. In the client with depression, the nursing care focus regarding sleep could include "*Activity Intolerance*, related to anergia" but in the client who is experiencing mania it might be "*Sleep Deprivation* as evidenced by sleeping 2 hours per day."

The focus of nursing care for the client with a depressive disorder could include any of the following (depending upon data collected): Activity Intolerance, Bathing/Hygiene ADL Deficit, Chronic Low Self-Esteem, Coping Impairment, Depression, Fatigue, Orthostatic Hypotension, Psychosocial Needs, Safety, Self-Harm Risk, and Suicide Attempt Risk.

The focus of nursing care for the client with mania could include any of the following (depending upon data collected): Acute Confusion, ADL Deficit, Altered Body Image Perception, Dehydration, Fall Risk, Impulsivity, Injury Risk, Insomnia, Malnutrition Risk, Nonadherence, Risky Health Behavior, Safety, Self-Harm Risk, Sleep Deprivation, and Violence Risk.

Outcome Identification and Planning

Once the focus of nursing care has been identified, anticipated outcomes that are realistic in terms of the individual client should be formulated. Clients are often in a severe mood state when admitted to a psychiatric facility. Stabilization is necessary before the client is able to recognize and deal with the underlying issues. Careful consideration should be given to a realistic time frame in which the outcomes can be achieved. Box 10.8 lists some common desired outcomes for

the client with a depressive disorder and Box 10.9 lists common desired outcomes for the client in a state of mania.

BOX 10.8

Common Desired Outcomes for a Client With a Depressive Disorder

The client:
- Has increased energy level
- Identifies personal strengths
- Identifies positive coping skills they can use
- Expresses decreased feelings of self-blame and doubt
- Openly expresses feelings related to the loss
- Resumes sexual functioning with partner
- Interacts with individuals other than nursing or medical staff
- Participates in at least two unit activities per day
- Consumes at least 75% of each meal
- Has 4 to 6 hours of sleep before awakening but no more than 10 hours of sleep per day
- Reframes thoughts into positive statements
- Performs activities of daily living (ADLs) independently

BOX 10.9

Common Desired Outcomes for a Client in a State of Mania

The client:
- Demonstrates self-control and observes appropriate physical boundaries with others
- Demonstrates decreased agitation
- Verbalizes feelings in an appropriate manner
- Demonstrates decreased activity level
- Consumes at least 75% of each meal and nutritional supplements
- Performs activities of daily living (ADLs) independently
- Has 4 to 6 hours of uninterrupted sleep
- Demonstrates ability to complete simple tasks to completion
- Participates appropriately in unit activities
- Interacts appropriately with others
- Verbalizes realistic expectations of self
- Does not experience hallucinations or delusions

Nursing Care Focus

- Activity Intolerance, related to anergia

Goal

- The client is present for, and participates in, unit activities while awake.

Implementations for Activity Intolerance

The nurse should cluster care that is provided to the client and allow for rest periods between clusters. Assist the client with activities of daily living (ADLs) as needed but encourage them to be as independent as possible. Provide the client with extra time to complete activities of daily living (ADLs), eating, and completing tasks including taking medications. Encourage a regular bedtime routine for the client with decreased stimuli to help promote normal sleep patterns. Have the client refrain from consuming caffeinated beverages or sugary snacks that can cause the client's energy to rise and then drop causing fatigue. Encourage a balanced diet to provide energy. Encourage the client to participate in unit activities through a gradual increase in involvement. Start by having them sit in on the activity but do not force active participation. As the client's tolerance, and comfort level, increases, encourage the client to actively participate. Provide positive feedback as appropriate for participating in activities, interacting with others, progressing towards self-identified goals, or completing tasks. Administer antidepressant medications as ordered. Collaborate with occupational and/or recreational therapy members to have the client identify and participate in activities of interest to the client.

Evaluation of Goal/Desired Outcome

The client will:

- participate in two unit activities per day
- self-perform ADLs by discharge
- sleep 8 hours per night and one short nap during day

Nursing Care Focus

- Sleep Deprivation

Goal

- The client will sleep for 4 to 6 continuous hours each day.

Implementations for Sleep Deprivation

Provide a routine for the client that promotes sleep. This can be accomplished by having the client determine and stick to a regular sleep time. Thirty to 60 minutes prior to the set time, encourage a relaxation routine that includes eliminating stimuli such as turning off the television or shutting off phone or computer screens. Encourage the client to change into clothes appropriate for sleep, brush teeth, and perform a regular relaxation activity such as a self-foot massage or aromatherapy. A regular presleep routine helps the client's mind cue to a normal sleep pattern. Have the client refrain from caffeinated beverages or sugary snacks at least 2 hours before the set sleep time. Prior to the set time, have the client avoid activities that are energizing such as competitive games, exercise, and action movies. Administer mood stabilizing medications as ordered.

Evaluation of Goal/Desired Outcome

The client:

- maintains a regular sleep routine.
- sleeps for 4 to 6 continuous hours.

Nursing Care Focus

- Self-Harm Risk related to suicidal ideation

Goal

- The client does not attempt suicide.

Implementations for Self-Harm Risk

Provide a safe environment by removing potentially dangerous items and eliminating ligature points. Monitor the client for changes in their current depressive symptoms or for the development of new symptoms. Directly ask the client about any suicidal thoughts indicating a plan of how, when, or where they might harm or kill themselves. If the client identifies an immediate plan for self-harm, stay with them, do not leave them unobserved, and obtain an order for suicide watch. Do not promise a client that you will keep a secret—let them know that you will share information with the health care team as needed for their treatment and safety. Promising the client secrecy and then reporting observations to the RN or health care provider can harm or eliminate a therapeutic relationship between the nurse and the client. Observe the client for cheeking of medications or gathering of items that could be used to harm themselves. Monitor the client's energy level—as energy increases, the ability to carry out a plan for suicide increases. Assist in request for spiritual needs referral.

Evaluation of Goal/Desired Outcome

The client is without suicide attempts while hospitalized.

Nursing Care Focus

- Self-Harm Risk, related to impulsive behaviors

Goal

- The client will not engage in harmful behavior while admitted to the nursing unit.

Implementations for Self-Harm Risk

Nursing interventions are focused at maintaining a safe environment for the client in a state of mania and also for other clients on the nursing unit. Excessive environmental stimuli can further stimulate the client's mania. Dim lights as appropriate and lower or turn off televisions. Route other clients to a different part of the unit if needed. Observe the client frequently as harmful behaviors, including unprotected sexual activity with another client, can occur during brief periods of unsupervision. Monitor risk for accidents to self or others, including tripping over furniture or colliding with another client. The nurse should self-monitor their own anxiety level and convey messages with a neutral tone and lowered volume of voice. The nurse should refrain from becoming angry with clients who are hostile or behaving in an inappropriate manner. Avoid arguing with or being charmed by clients in a manic state. Convey a "matter-of-fact" or nonreactive attitude when the client displays exaggerated or sexually inappropriate behavior. Encourage noncompetitive activities to prevent escalating anxiety and anger. Monitor for escalation of behavior or mood that may lead to explosive behavior. Set and maintain limits such as unit rules and policies. All staff members should convey the same rules and policies to the client to avoid the client "playing" one staff member against another. Calmly restate the rules as needed. Spend time with the client—if the client is unable to sit, walk with them for short intervals. This conveys an unspoken message of acceptance to the client. The nurse should not let the client in a state of mania monopolize their time and attention; doing so negatively reinforces the behavior. Provide positive feedback when appropriate. Reinforce to the client that disrobes or acts out in a sexual manner that those behaviors are inappropriate and not allowed on the nursing unit. These behaviors may provoke another client who also has lowered inhibitions or impulsivity.

Evaluation of Goal/Desired Outcome

The client does not:

- engage in sexual activity with others while admitted.
- actively harm themselves or others.

CASE STUDY 10.3

"Byron"

Giulio_Fornasar/Shutterstock

Byron was admitted to the hospital while experiencing a manic episode. Over the past 4 days, he has become increasingly loud and animated. He describes himself as a diplomat assigned to gather information. He carries a number of calling cards in his shirt pocket that he states are his contacts. Today, the nurse is preparing to administer medication to another client and hears Byron asking very personal sexually oriented questions of a client sitting next to him. As the nurse approaches them, Byron says the conversation is private and he is collecting classified information.

Digging Deeper

1. What actions should the nurse take at this point?

2. What other symptoms can be anticipated in Byron's behavior?

3. What is the nurse's responsibility to the other clients?

4. Two days later, Byron approaches the nurse and says he has to leave because he has a meeting with other national leaders from around the world that evening. He goes on to say that since he has been elected head of the CIA, he has little time for trivial issues anymore. How should the nurse respond to this grandiose delusional thinking?

Cultural Considerations

Different Ways to Say "Depression"

While depression is seen worldwide, the term "depression" is not used worldwide. Worldwide terms for depressive symptoms also do not exist. This can create miscommunication with the client and also some depression assessment scales that use words such as "sadness," "depression," or "self-esteem" may not be accurate.

It is important to realize that some cultures view discussing depression (or other mental illness) as:

- inappropriate
- "airing one's dirty laundry"
- a sign of weakness
- having a great shame or negative stigma
- a natural part of life
- demonstrating a lack of faith/spirituality

Due to these views on depression, or mental illness overall, the individual may:

- not participate in the discussion or answer questions
- not seek treatment to avoid shame or gossip
- not willingly discuss their symptoms
- willingly accept their symptoms and not seek any kind of treatment
- only discuss their symptoms if asked direct questions but otherwise will not initiate a discussion about their symptoms
- not seek medical treatment but rather go to an imam, shaman, priest, or a traditional healer

Some cultures don't have an equivalent word for depression or believe in depression. Therefore, when they are asked about depression, they may not understand the nurse or answer if it is an unknown concept to them.

The table below gives examples of depression across cultures.

Cultural Focus	Words or Terms That May Be Used by the Client
Terms used instead of "depression"	*Nervios* (Hispanic American) The funk (African American) Soul loss (Native American) Heartbreak (Hopi) "Ghost Sickness" (Native American) Weakness of the nerves (Asian American) *Wacinko syndrome* (Oglala Sioux)
Terms for symptoms of depression	Melancholy Imbalance Down
No words or phrases for depression, but mental distress is expressed physically with terms the individual can identify (Asian American)	Feelings of inner pressure Discomfort Boredom Pain
Individual may not use terms "depression" or "sadness" but may use negative terms	"I am a burden" "I am a failure" "I can't do anything right"

Source: How minority cultures talk about depression. (2020). *GeneSight Blog.* https://genesight.com/blog/healthcare-provider/how-minority-cultures-talk-about-depression/

SUMMARY

- Alterations in mood levels affect every aspect of the individual's life, resulting in behaviors and issues that impact the individual and those around them.
- Mood is an emotion that is prolonged and permeates the individual's entire psychological thinking. Affect describes the facial expression an individual displays

in association with the mood (e.g., smiling when happy, grimacing when angry).

- Depression can occur as a single episode or in a recurring pattern. There may be a precipitating cause such as a loss, or it may occur without an identified reason.

- Depressive disorders include major depressive disorder, persistent depressive disorder (dysthymia), postpartum depression, and Seasonal Affective Disorder.
- Individuals with a depressive disorder do not exhibit any signs of euphoric states. Sadness and melancholy are present in all areas of their life with impaired functioning in personal, social, and work activities.
- An individual with persistent depressive disorder (dysthymia) exhibits a lower level of depression and demonstrates a recurring cycle of the depressed state over a 2-year period. They have feelings of hopelessness and despair and can exhibit behaviors or an attitude of learned helplessness.
- Bipolar disorders are characterized by shifts between mania and depression that produce dramatic behavior changes. Symptoms of mania are hyperactivity and decreased sleep, lowered inhibitions, irresponsible and impulsive behaviors, starting but not completing multiple tasks or projects, disregard for social boundaries, irritability and moodiness, and grandiosity. Psychotic symptoms of hallucinations and delusions may be present.
- During the manic phase, the individual's irrational thought processes, unrealistic inflated self-image, and irritability may lead to behaviors that pose safety risks, either to themselves or others.
- Cyclothymic disorder is characterized by mood disturbances. In cyclothymic disorder symptoms of hypomania and depression are present. However, the depressive symptoms are not as severe as in a major depressive episode.
- Treatment of mood disorders includes pharmacologic treatment, psychotherapy, electroconvulsive therapy (ECT), light therapy, and some complementary and alternative medicine (CAM).
- Psychotherapy for the client who is depressed involves assisting the client in exploring how negative thoughts and feelings are affecting their behavior and identifying more effective ways of coping.
- Most medications used to treat mood disorders increase the amount of chemicals or neurotransmitters in the brain that help to balance the moods. They are used to reduce the mood swings and the likelihood of subsequent episodes.
- The three common classifications of antidepressants include: monoamine oxidase inhibitors (MAOIs), tricyclic antidepressants (TCAs), and serotonin-specific reuptake inhibitors (SSRIs).
- Lithium is a common medication used to stabilize the mood of the individual with bipolar disorder. There are other classifications of medications that have also been effective in treating bipolar disorder including anticonvulsants, calcium-channel blockers, and second-generation psychotropics (atypical antipsychotics).
- Antidepressant medications must be taken continuously for several weeks before therapeutic effects are evident and the client notices an improvement in their mood. A continuous presence of the medication is needed in the brain for the level of the neurotransmitters to balance the deficit causing the depression.
- Clients taking antidepressants and mood stabilizers need information on food and medications to avoid and precautions to take (such as wearing sunscreen or reporting symptoms of an infection such as fever) that are specific to their medication.
- The client taking lithium needs blood levels drawn to help monitor therapeutic levels of the medication.
- Suicide or attempted suicide must be observed for in individuals who exhibit severe or chronic depression or in individuals who have an extreme mood elevation after starting antidepressants as therapeutic levels of antidepressants can energize their ability to carry out a suicide plan.
- Although medication therapy can level out the brain chemistry to minimize the highs and lows of bipolar disorder, many individuals do not adhere to treatment. This is in part related to the grandiose thinking in hypomania, which causes them to believe that they are fine and do not need medication. Once blood levels of the medication decline, a vicious cycle is begun. Maintenance of a continued state of mood stability will depend on adherence to the medication and follow-up treatment plan.
- Data Collection of the client with a mood disorder should include mood and affect, thinking and perceptual ability, somatic complaints, sleep disturbances, changes in energy level, and the character of speech patterns. Mood and affect should be monitored for congruency.
- Observe the client for current risk factors that indicate suicide may be a possibility. Determine the content of any suicidal thoughts or ideations. If the client has a plan, determine the lethality of the method.
- The client in a manic state can pose a safety threat to themselves and others. The nurse should monitor the client and intervene to protect the client or others as needed.
- As mania is reduced and excessive mood states are stabilized, the client can eat and sleep with less disturbance. The nurse should monitor the client's food intake and hours of sleep.
- Improved communication and social interaction result as thought processes become more rational and reality oriented.

BIBLIOGRAPHY

American Psychiatric Nurses Association. (2021). *APNA position paper: Electroconvulsive therapy*. Approved by the APNA Board of Directors. January 2011; Revised and approved July 2021. https://www.apna.org/news/electroconvulsive-therapy

Bains, N., & Abdijadid, S. (2021). Major depressive disorder. In *StatPearls [Internet]*. StatPearls Publishing. Retrieved May 16, 2022, from https://www.ncbi.nlm.nih.gov/books/NBK559078

Coryell, W. (2021a). *Bipolar disorders*. Merck Manual Professional Version. https://www.merckmanuals.com/professional/psychiatric-disorders/mood-disorders/bipolar-disorders

Coryell, W. (2021b). *Depressive disorders*. Merck Manual Professional Version. https://www.merckmanuals.com/professional/psychiatric-disorders/mood-disorders/depressive-disorders

Fleming, L. (2020). *Suicide assessment and precautions*. Elsevier Clinical Skills. https://www.elsevier.com/__data/assets/pdf_file/0008/1002311/Suicide-Assessment-and-Precautions-Skill-COVID-19-Toolkit_140420.pdf

Ionescu, D. F., Fu, D-J., Qiu, X., Lane, R., Lim, P., Kasper, S., Hough, D., Drevets, W. C., Manji, H., & Canuso, C. M. (2020). Esketamine nasal spray for rapid reduction of depressive symptoms in patients with major depressive disorder who have active suicide ideation with intent: Results of a Phase 3, double-blind, randomized study (ASPIRE II). *International Journal of Neuropsychopharmacology*, *24*(1), 22–31. https://doi.org/10.1093/ijnp/pyaa068

Janicak, P. G. (2021). Bipolar disorder in adults and lithium: Pharmacology, administration, and management of adverse effects. *UpToDate*. Retrieved May 16, 2022, from https://www.uptodate.com/contents/bipolar-disorder-in-adults-and-lithium-pharmacology-administration-and-management-of-adverse-effects

Kroenke, K., Spitzer, R. L., & Williams, J. B. W. (2001). The PHQ-9: validity of a brief depression severity measure. *Journal of General Internal Medicine*, *16*(9), 606–613. https://doi.org/10.1046/j.1525-1497.2001.016009606.x

Lyness, J. M. (2021). Unipolar depression in adults: Clinical features. *UpToDate*. Retrieved May 16, 2022, from https://www.uptodate.com/contents/unipolar-depression-in-adults-clinical-features

Lyness, J. M. (2022). Unipolar depression in adults: Assessment and diagnosis. *UpToDate*. Retrieved May 16, 2022, from https://www.uptodate.com/contents/unipolar-depression-in-adults-assessment-and-diagnosis

National Alliance on Mental Illness. (2022a). *Bipolar disorder*. https://www.nami.org/About-Mental-Illness/Mental-Health-Conditions/Bipolar-Disorder

National Alliance on Mental Illness. (2022b). *Mental health by the numbers*. https://www.nami.org/mhstats

National Institute of Mental Health. (2022a). *Bipolar disorder*. https://www.nimh.nih.gov/health/topics/bipolar-disorder

National Institute of Mental Health. (2022b). *Depression*. https://www.nimh.nih.gov/health/topics/depression

National Institute of Mental Health. (2022c). *Major depression*. https://www.nimh.nih.gov/health/statistics/major-depression

National Institute of Mental Health. (2022d). *Persistent depressive disorder (Dysthymic disorder)*. https://www.nimh.nih.gov/health/statistics/persistent-depressive-disorder-dysthymic-disorder

National Library of Medicine. (2022). *Antidepressants*. MedlinePlus. Retrieved May 16, 2022. https://medlineplus.gov/antidepressants.html

Rush, A. J. (2022). Unipolar major depression in adults: Choosing initial treatment. *UpToDate*. Retrieved January 6, 2023, from https://www.uptodate.com/contents/unipolar-major-depression-in-adults-choosing-initial-treatment

Suppes, T. (2022). Bipolar disorder in adults: Clinical features. *UpToDate*. Retrieved May 25, 2022, from https://www.uptodate.com/contents/bipolar-disorder-in-adults-clinical-features

Thase, M., & Connolly, R. (2022). Ketamine and esketamine for treating unipolar depression in adults: Administration, efficacy, and adverse effects. *UpToDate*. Retrieved May 16, 2022, from https://www.uptodate.com/contents/ketamine-and-esketamine-for-treating-unipolar-depression-in-adults-administration-efficacy-and-adverse-effects

Viguera, A. (2021). Postpartum unipolar major depression: Epidemiology, clinical features, assessment and diagnosis. *UpToDate*. Retrieved May 25, 2022, from https://www.uptodate.com/contents/postpartum-unipolar-major-depression-epidemiology-clinical-features-assessment-and-diagnosis

World Health Organization. (2021). *Depression*. https://www.who.int/news-room/fact-sheets/detail/depression

STUDENT WORKSHEET

Fill in the Blank

Fill in the blank with the correct answer.

1. _____ describes the facial expression an individual displays in association with the mood.
2. _____ disorder is a milder form of bipolar-related disorder characterized by recurrent symptoms of hypomania and dysthymia.
3. _____ is a recurrent state of depression over a period of at least 2 years.
4. Delusions of _____ occur during interpersonal conflicts where a perceived injustice is viewed as a threat of harm.
5. _____ is the most common mood-stabilizing medication used in the treatment of bipolar illness.
6. _____ therapy involves passing an electric current through the brain.
7. For clients on suicide precautions, the nurse should determine the _____ of the suicide plan.

Matching

Match the following terms to the most appropriate phrase.

1. _____ Euphoria	a. Being tired with decreased energy
2. _____ Anhedonia	b. Feeling that nothing will improve the symptoms and no longer trying solutions
3. _____ Clang association	c. Depressive episode without hypomania or mania
4. _____ Cheeking	d. Strings of words in rhyming phrases
5. _____ Anergia	e. Alternating from euphoria to dysphoria and irritability
6. _____ Learned helplessness	f. Lack of pleasure in previously enjoyed activities
7. _____ Rapid cycling	g. Holding medication in the mouth without swallowing
8. _____ Grandiosity	h. Four or more mood shifts within 1 year
9. _____ Labile	i. Thinking of self as excessively important
10. _____ Unipolar	j. Excessive feelings of happiness

Multiple Choice

Select the best answer from the multiple-choice items.

1. The nurse is monitoring a client with mania who is constantly pacing the hallway and unable to be seated when the other clients are eating. Which of the following nursing interventions would best meet the needs of the client at this time?
   a. Keep food at the nurse's station until the client asks for something to eat
   b. Allow the client to eat in a separate area to avoid distraction
   c. Provide finger sandwiches and juice for client during the activity
   d. Reinforce to the client the importance of nutrition in providing energy

2. Which of the following would be seen in the manic phase of bipolar disorder? *(Select all that apply)*
   a. Flashback of the traumatic event
   b. Sleeping for 8 to 10 hours at a time
   c. Speaking in clang association
   d. Dressing in a flamboyant or exaggerated manner
   e. Consuming 100% of all three meals

3. When caring for a client with a manic episode, what intervention would be appropriate?
   a. Tell the client to remain isolated until impulsive actions are controlled
   b. Allow the client to describe delusional thoughts as long as desired
   c. Walk alongside the client as long as pacing continues
   d. Reprimand the client for inappropriate sexual hand gestures

4. The nursing plan of care for a client with a diagnosis of major depressive disorder should include which of the following interventions?
   a. Group physical activity that will provide exercise and socialization
   b. Provide a structured schedule of activities that offers client participation
   c. No socializing activities unless the client asks to be included
   d. Encourage participation in competitive games of chess or ping pong

5. The nurse is caring for a client whose serum lithium carbonate level is 1.5 mEq/L. The nurse would expect the health care provider to:
   a. Order an additional dose to be given one time only.
   b. Increase the daily dosage of the medication.
   c. Order the next dose of the medication to be held.
   d. Stop the medication.

6. Which instruction would be included when providing information to the client taking a tricyclic antidepressant (TCA) medication?
   a. Take the medication with coffee or tea to enhance its effect.
   b. The medication can be discontinued after a few weeks of therapy.
   c. You can omit the morning dose of your medication if it makes you too sleepy.
   d. Wear a hat and long-sleeve shirt when you are outdoors in the sun.

7. The client for whom an MAOI is prescribed should be taught to avoid which of the following dietary items? *(Select all that apply)*
   a. Both tap and homebrewed beers
   b. Smoked or processed meat
   c. Fresh shrimp, salmon, trout
   d. Almonds, Brazil nuts, cashews
   e. Swiss, cheddar, parmesan cheese

8. A client states they used to enjoy taking their grandchildren to the park but this is no longer pleasurable. The client is describing feelings related to which symptom?
   a. Anhedonia
   b. Anergia
   c. Euphoria
   d. Negativism

9. A client who has been admitted after a suicide attempt from an overdose of antidepressant medication tells the nurse, "Why couldn't I just die? There is nothing left here for me." The most therapeutic response for the nurse is:
   a. "Why did you want to die?"
   b. "There is always a reason why things happen as they do."
   c. "What do you mean there is nothing left here for you?"
   d. "You are feeling as though life is meaningless right now?"

10. The nurse planning interventions for a client with major depressive disorder would give priority to which individual need?
   a. Social isolation
   b. Self-care deficit
   c. Low self-esteem
   d. Impaired relationship

11

Psychotic Disorders

Introduction to Psychotic Disorders

Psychosis refers to a set of symptoms that includes perceptual disturbances, disorganized thinking, and behavior alterations. Psychosis is not an illness. These symptoms demonstrate the disorganization that is present in the individual's mental processes and reflect the behavior, emotional response, and thought processes of the individual who has lost contact with reality. People usually associate the disturbances of "hearing voices" or other atypical behaviors with psychosis. Those who experience these symptoms also tend to withdraw from society.

There are a number of different situations in which the symptoms of psychosis are manifested. They may be seen in some medical conditions such as delirium, medication toxicity, dementia, mood disorders, and other delusional disorders (Box 11.1). In most situations, the symptoms are not present at all times. Psychotic disorders affect the mind and the individual's ability to think clearly and respond effectively to the world around them.

The major symptoms of psychotic disorders are delusions and hallucinations. Some individuals may experience this as a single psychotic event, such as that seen after an extremely stressful event, trauma, or illegal substance ingestion. The episode may last a few days and usually resolves within several weeks. In other situations, such as in schizophrenia, symptoms are gradual, even unnoticed, in the beginning and recur for the rest of the individual's life.

The most common and severe form of psychotic disorders is schizophrenia—a form of psychosis in which there are disorganized thoughts, perceptions, and atypical behaviors. The occurrence of schizophrenia is about 1%. About half of the clients admitted to mental units are diagnosed with schizophrenia. The cost of mental health care and social services related to schizophrenia in all age groups is significantly higher than that of other mental disorders.

Before discussing schizophrenia in depth and mentioning the other types of psychotic disorders, it is important to discuss the characteristic symptoms that are seen in psychosis.

Perceptual Disturbances

Hallucinations are false sensory perceptions that have no relation to reality and are not supported by actual environmental stimuli. When a hallucination occurs, the individual has the perception of seeing (visual), hearing (auditory), smelling (olfactory), feeling (tactile), or tasting (gustatory), although there is no stimulus present. Olfactory and gustatory misperceptions account for a small percentage of perceptual disturbances.

Although all of these may occur, auditory hallucinations are the most common. Most of these are in the form of voices or sounds that can only be heard by the one experiencing them. The voices may originate inside or outside the individual's head and may be talking to them or commenting on their behavior. The voices can be commanding, telling the individual to harm themselves or others. Those who experience the command hallucinations may react in panic or demonstrate violence toward themselves or others. It is important to ask the individual what the voices are saying. If the individual feels the voice is coming from someone they know and/or trust, the individual is more likely to follow the commands. Auditory hallucinations can be very frightening to the individual.

Mind Jogger Considering that the client hearing commanding voices is not in touch with reality, what is the best approach to communicating with them?

Visual hallucinations are less common but may involve seeing people or images that are not actually present. Feeling that something is crawling on the skin or moving inside the body parts are typical of tactile hallucinations. **Illusions** are experienced when sensory stimuli actually exist but are misinterpreted by the individual. For example, the individual may refer to spots on the floor as insects or to an electric cord as a snake.

BOX 11.1

Associated Causes of Psychosis

- Alcohol or other substance use
- Bipolar disorder
- Brain tumor
- Delirium
- Dementia
- Depression
- Epilepsy
- Huntington chorea
- Parkinson disease
- Stroke

Disorganized Thinking

In psychosis, the thought processes become confused and disrupted, leaving the individual with an inability to carry on a logical conversation. A **delusion** consists of fixed, false ideas or beliefs without appropriate external stimuli that are inconsistent with reality and that cannot be changed by reasoning. These thoughts usually involve a theme that is dominant in the mind. For example, the individual who thinks someone is trying to kill them will demonstrate this both verbally and behaviorally. The client might say, "I'm not taking this medication because you are trying to poison me," or "I'm not eating my food because the FBI put poison in it." Paranoid delusions are important to note as they may prevent the client from cooperating with the treatment plan. For example, if they fear being poisoned they may not eat meals or take medications. If the individual fears being a hostage they may resist going to a group home or leave a shelter and this may increase their risk of homelessness.

The content or theme of the delusions can include depressive, somatic, grandiose, or persecution. Box 11.2 lists the most common themes of delusions. There are also **delusions of reference,** which are false beliefs that the behavior of others in the environment is directed at them personally. For example, the individual may believe that something such as a newspaper article or television commercial is sending a special message to them. Content can also include a belief in **thought broadcasting**, in which the individual's thoughts can be heard by others. An example of this is a client stating, "I have a direct wire attached to the commander of intelligence to rule the underground." **Thought insertion** may also be claimed, in which the individual believes the thoughts of others can be inserted into their mind. A client stating, "Men from Mars are implanting seeds of destruction into the layers of my mental dirt," is demonstrating thought insertion. **Thought withdrawal** indicates a belief that others are robbing thoughts from one's brain. An example of this would be the client's statement of, "I wear this hat so they can't steal my ideas."

> **Just the Facts** The most common delusional themes are related to thoughts of persecution, religious ideas, or somatic reference.

A typical brain organizes and directs thought processes into spoken words, associations, or connections in a logical format. Content refers to the meaning of the words or conversation that is spoken. Individuals with disorganized thinking express the disorganization in the way they speak. They may be talking and suddenly change the course of the conversation to something with no logical connection to the original topic. The inability to organize and connect sudden changes in thought processes that are vague, unfocused, and illogical is exhibited by **loose associations** (sometimes called derailment), where the thoughts or ideas frequently jump from one topic to another that is unrelated. The individual will say a sentence such as, "This meat is tough, but I saw meat in the store and nails are keeping it together until the cows get home." Here there appears to be a central idea of "meat" but the thoughts are fragmented and loosely connected. **Word salad** is when the individual expresses random unconnected and disorganized thoughts, which indicates severe impairment. An example of this is the statement of, "You see I am living in the sky where it snowed yesterday with thunderous wires darting in and out of the highway. Brilliant colors keep the orchestra moving the ball down the railroad track toward the divine intellect of my intestines." In this example there are no thoughts that are loosely connected and the words or thoughts are mixed together randomly.

Alogia (sometimes called poverty of speech) is a decrease in the amount or speed of speech.

BOX 11.2

Common Delusional Themes

- Depressive (e.g., believing they have committed a terrible deed such as a terrorist attack)
- Erotomatic (e.g., believing a famous actress is madly in love with them)
- Grandiose (e.g., believing they are stronger than a superhero in a movie)
- Jealous (e.g., being very possessive for the attention of the nurse and believing they have an intimate relationship with them)
- Mixed (the individual has two or more delusional themes)
- Nihilistic (e.g., believing that their arm no longer exists)
- Persecutory (e.g., believing the mob is out to kill them)
- Reference (e.g., believing that a television ad is speaking directly to them to and the message has a personal meaning)
- Somatic (e.g., believing their body is disintegrating into another substance or infested with insects)

The individual with psychosis may not answer questions or may stop in the middle of a thought. The individual may make up new words and definitions (**neologisms**) that have special personal meaning such as, "The malitars are coming to get me." Clang associations may also be demonstrated with insignificant rhyming of words such as, "The sky is blue, so are you. Two plus two, much to do so to fear, far and near, let's have a beer." Also seen in psychosis is **echolalia,** in which the individual repeats another's speech word for word.

Behavior Alterations

Psychotic behavior is unpredictable. It may be described as agitated, aggressive, childlike, inappropriate, or made up. This behavior is an outward expression of the disorganized thinking. Wild, purposeless, agitated movements can be documented as "frenzied motor activity." The disorganized behavior can lead to an inability to perform activities of daily living or carry out goal-directed activity. The individual may appear very unkempt, dress inappropriately for the situation, wear multiple layers of clothing regardless of the environmental temperature, walk about naked, or remove clothing in public. The individual with psychosis has poor impulse control and therefore their behavior may also be sexually inappropriate, unpredictable, and include sudden explosive outbursts. They are unable to recognize what is considered by most as a norm of society. In psychosis the individual displays behavior that reflects their own personal thought process and is unaware of moral boundaries or social norms.

    Catatonic behaviors display a decreased reaction to environmental surroundings. Movements may be severely decreased or absent and accompanied by a **stupor** or lack of awareness and orientation. **Posturing** is seen when the individual is in a trance-like state with a rigid atypical posture, often held against gravity, and resists efforts to be moved for extended periods of time (e.g., in a "crucifix position"). An extreme form of posturing is termed **catalepsy**. **Waxy flexibility** occurs when the individual remains fixed in one position until someone changes it. An arm, leg, or other body part can be moved by another person and the body part will remain in that position until moved again.

    The individual with psychosis may demonstrate stereotyped repetitive, purposeless movements, such as rocking. They may also exhibit **mannerisms,** which are repetitive and goal-directed movements such as saluting or bowing. These behaviors involve excessive motor activity that is triggered by an internal, not external, stimulus. Another alteration in behavior seen in psychosis is **echopraxia** where another person's movements are imitated.

> **Test Yourself**
> ✔ Name three medical causes of psychosis.
> ✔ What is the difference between a hallucination and an illusion?
> ✔ Describe a delusion.
> ✔ Identify five examples of disorganized thinking seen in psychosis.
> ✔ Identify five examples of behavior alterations seen in psychosis.

Schizophrenia

Schizophrenia is a form of psychosis in which there are disorganized thoughts, perceptual alterations, inappropriate affect, and decreased emotional response as the connections to reality are broken. It is a chronic and disabling mental illness that causes the individual to withdraw into their made-up, self-perceived reality consisting of delusions, irrational thoughts, and misperceptions. The individual's ability to distinguish real from unreal becomes disordered. Although not all individuals with schizophrenia experience all the symptoms, the impact to their personal, family, and social life is severe. The word schizophrenia derives from Greek, meaning "split mind." This does not mean that their personality is divided as in multiple personality disorder. They retain their own, single, personality.

> **Just the Facts** The cost of mental health care and social services related to schizophrenia in all age groups is significantly higher than that of other mental disorders.

> **Just the Facts** About half of the clients admitted to mental health units are diagnosed with schizophrenia.

Signs and Symptoms

In the **prodromal phase**, the onset of symptoms of schizophrenia is insidious (subtle and seemingly

BOX 11.3

Behaviors Seen in the Prodromal Phase of Schizophrenia

- Easily distracted and inattentive to environment
- Memory impairment including trouble thinking clearly or concentrating
- Depressive, hopeless feelings
- Poor judgment or inability to interpret the environment correctly
- Illogical thought processing
- Impaired decision-making ability
- A decline in self-care or activities of daily living
- Difficulty in relating to others including being suspicious or uneasy around others

BOX 11.4

Symptoms of Schizophrenia

POSITIVE SYMPTOMS

- Delusions
- Word salad
- Clang associations
- Thought broadcasting
- Thought insertion
- Loose associations
- Neologism
- Hallucinations
- Illusions
- Depersonalization
- Unusual behavior
- Agitation
- Catatonia

NEGATIVE SYMPTOMS

- Blunt or flat affect
- Lack of energy (anergia)
- Failure to find pleasure in activities (anhedonia)
- Lack of motivation (avolition)
- Inability to initiate self-care skills
- Inability to interact with others
- Impoverished speech (alogia)
- Substance use
- Depression and suicidal acts
- Violent behavior

harmless), with the individual experiencing them for some time before the first full-blown psychotic episode occurs. The prodromal phase actually indicates the beginning of the illness (Box 11.3).

After the prodromal phase, the individual with schizophrenia has an ongoing progression of symptoms with periods of intense symptoms and periods where "things seem to get better." During the periods of intense symptoms, the individual may have increasing anxiety with inability to concentrate or complete goal-oriented tasks. There is a loss of connections, which destroys the ability to think and learn, so poor school or work performance may be seen. There may be an alternation between hyperactivity and inactivity. As the deterioration continues, the individual becomes more distracted and feels that something is happening or expresses fear of "losing my mind." The individual may misinterpret experiences that are happening in the environment, often becoming paranoid about being followed or poisoned. Delusions may center on imaginary people who appear and harass or ridicule the individual. Gradually the delusions and hallucinations become a part of each day with jumbled speech patterns and atypical behaviors. Social relationships deteriorate to the point that the individual is unable to function in a romantic, peer, or work relationship. Interest is lost in any type of goal setting or planning for the future. There tends to be an increase in the deterioration and dysfunction with each acute episode or relapse, meaning the individual never fully returns to their baseline state that was seen prior to the psychotic episode. A loss of self-confidence or self-esteem may be seen. The individual may use alcohol or recreational substances to self-manage their symptoms or as a coping mechanism for their feelings.

The symptoms of schizophrenia are primarily described as positive or negative. Positive symptoms are those typically thought of as symptoms of schizophrenia while negative symptoms are the absence or deficits of typical behaviors and affect. Negative symptoms are harder to treat than positive symptoms. Box 11.4 lists examples of positive and negative symptoms of schizophrenia.

 Mind Jogger People experiencing homelessness, without shelter or housing, feel a sense of isolation and rejection. What might contribute to the fact that those with psychotic disorders sometimes become part of this population?

Positive Symptoms

Positive symptoms are evidenced early in the progress of the disorder. These are usually demonstrated in the initial contact that the individual has with the health care system, which is usually a hospitalization for what is called acute schizophrenia.

These symptoms include alterations in thinking, perception, and behavior.

The delusional patterns seen in schizophrenia are distorted and often outlandish with no logical connections. In the case of psychosis, the behavior that occurs while thoughts are processed and spoken actually provides more information than the content of what is said. The fragmented and disorganized thought processes are demonstrated in speech patterns of word salad and derailed loose associations. These jumbled words can reflect the theme of what the individual is experiencing within their head. However, the theme reference and feelings can also be reflected in behavior. For example, the individual who has recurring delusions of persecution may demonstrate fear by constantly looking to the side or over a shoulder as if someone is lurking behind or following them.

Themes of persecution are the most commonly experienced delusions in individuals with schizophrenia. Clients experiencing delusions of persecution hold the false belief that someone is plotting to harm them. Often the individual believes this is being devised by very important people or alien powers (e.g., a client believes the CIA is sending signals through telephone wires or internet lines that will electrocute them). Beliefs such as these may hold some resemblance to life experiences, such as a young person who was abused as a child and believes their parent will electrocute them using

the light switches. Others are unrelated to previous experiences and have no realistic theme. For example, a client thinks there is a machine in their stomach that is timed to explode on New Year's Eve. The delusional thinking persists regardless of evidence that proves it inaccurate. Delusions of grandeur involve false beliefs that one is a very powerful and important person. These delusions often tend to have religious or governmental themes. For instance, a client may believe that they are a disciple sent by God to lead the world through the internet.

Perceptual alterations are positive symptoms. Auditory and visual hallucinations are the most common in those with schizophrenia. Hearing voices or sounds, both within the confines of the mind or externally, is perhaps the most familiar of these alterations. These individuals may respond to the voices, which often talk directly to them or make remarks about their actions. An example of this is an individual who thinks someone is talking to them from their shirt pocket and faces the wall as if wanting privacy, opens the flap of the pocket, and answers the voice.

Misperceptions of personal identity are also seen, with the inability to distinguish oneself from the realness of another. They are often confused about their bodily boundaries, feeling that parts of others are meshing with their own body parts. They may feel disconnected to their own body or depersonalize themselves. For example, they may

"Victoria"

altanaka/ Shutterstock

Victoria is a 20-year-old client on the mental health crisis unit. She was admitted after the police brought her to the hospital because she was not wearing clothes while at a local grocery store and "using made-up language." Victoria was first diagnosed with paranoid schizophrenia a year ago while a freshman student at the university. She has been living by herself in an apartment owned by her parents. She has a history of nonadherence with her antipsychotic medications as reported by her caseworker. Currently she is very delusional and refusing nursing care. She tells the nurse, "God told me to warn everybody that meteors are descending to the earth to get into the brains of all women and prevent the overpopulation of the outer planets." She drops to the floor with her arms over her head shouting, "Take cover, take cover—we are falling!" She crawls around on the floor and hides under the desk.

Digging Deeper

1. What type of theme does Victoria's delusional thought process indicate?

2. How would you describe the speech pattern of this client?

3. How can the nurse best approach Victoria about her behavior at this point?

CASE STUDY 11.1

view their blood vessels as worms floating through the air.

Unusual behavior can occur in many forms during psychosis. The individual may continuously wear items as "clothing" (such as an elaborate hat made out of tin foil or trash), assume strange positions (such as saluting a statue for hours), or demonstrate restless physical movements (such as jerking arms or legs while walking in circles). They may have behavior without purpose such as picking up trash items but not depositing them in a trashcan. Individuals with schizophrenia may demonstrate a negative response to directions or instructions by doing the opposite of what is asked of them. For example, when told to sit down and eat, they may get up and start pacing in the hall instead. Agitation is often relieved by pacing, with some individuals walking great distances without realizing how far they have gone.

Negative Symptoms

Negative symptoms develop slowly over time. They are reflected in the individual's inability to deal with the way their illness affects their life. The devastating effects result in isolation and withdrawal from the uncomfortable inability to interact with others in a meaningful way.

Affect is perhaps the most noticeable of these symptoms. The individual with schizophrenia typically has a blunted or flat affect that is expressionless and blank. The affect can also be inappropriate, such as smiling when the situation is sad. Other times, the individual may exhibit incongruous expressions such as giggling while mumbling to a water faucet in the bathroom. The behavior is often described as autistic, referring to a focus on an inner fantasy world while excluding the external environment.

The individual experiences **avolition**: lacking motivation to make decisions or initiate self-care such as hygiene and grooming. Dress becomes unkempt and inappropriate. Anergia or decreased energy and a passive lack of ambition are evident. **Anhedonia** is seen as little interest is shown in activities that were previously enjoyed. Speech may regress to brief phrases, a one-word response, or mutism. As the disorder takes over the individual's life, interrelating with others and maintaining relationships becomes strained or even impossible.

Substance use, suicide, and violence are common associated symptoms that accompany the effects of schizophrenia. The helpless feelings and isolated pattern of living can lead the individual to attempt suicide. Both psychoactive medications and illegal substances are used by individuals with schizophrenia. Alcohol, marijuana, cocaine, and other substances are used to offset the persevering symptoms of the illness. The use of these substances can contribute to violence toward others.

Mind Jogger ② Many individuals with schizophrenia who attempt suicide also have major depression. What factors might be contributing to this?

Test Yourself
✔ Describe the prodromal phase of schizophrenia.
✔ Describe the difference between positive and negative symptoms of schizophrenia.
✔ Identify three positive and three negative symptoms of schizophrenia.

Incidence and Etiology

Schizophrenia affects approximately 1% of the population. The onset typically occurs between late adolescence and mid-30s. There are instances where schizophrenia begins in childhood and a late-onset type that occurs after age 45. There is evidence that indicates that schizophrenia manifests differently in men than in women. For men, the average age of onset is between 18 and 25 years, and is between 25 and 30 years for women. Late onset is more common in women than in men. Women tend to experience less severe symptoms with fewer hospitalizations than men. This disorder is prevalent in all populations without bias as to race, gender, culture, or socioeconomic groups. There is a higher risk in those who have first-degree biologic relatives with the disorder. Most people who develop schizophrenia have the symptoms for the remainder of their lives (Fisher & Buchanan, 2022b).

Just the Facts ① Individuals with schizophrenia have higher rates of death by suicide than the general population. The risk is increased in the following groups: males who were diagnosed between the ages of 26–35 years, those with a history of drug use (but not alcohol use), those with a concurrent mood disorder diagnosis, or those with a previous history of suicide attempt (Zaheer et al., 2020).

There is no single cause of schizophrenia. A genetic factor is known to exist but the hereditary mechanism is not clear. An imbalance in the neurotransmitters dopamine and glutamate is thought to be a causative factor as well. Some studies show abnormalities in the brain structure of those with schizophrenia. All research efforts are being made to identify the genetic and contributing factors for the development of this mental illness. A history of environmental stressors, childhood trauma, and substance use disorder are also linked to individuals diagnosed with schizophrenia.

Subtypes of Schizophrenia

Along with the general diagnosis of schizophrenia, a further distinction is usually made based on the symptoms that are exhibited. The subtype can change during the course of the individual's illness.

Paranoid Type

Individuals with paranoid type schizophrenia experience prominent hallucinations and delusions. The hallucinations are often auditory in nature with delusions of being persecuted or followed. The delusions are usually very organized and focus on a theme. For example, the individual may think that everyone who wears black is sent by the devil to harm them. Everything the individual does is centered on this theme. Because this is threatening to them, they assume a defensive behavior toward anyone who is wearing black. This can endanger others if the delusion is severe.

Disorganized Type

Those with disorganized type schizophrenia exhibit disorganized and unintelligible speech, atypical behavior, and a flat affect. Delusions do not center on any particular theme but tend to be fragmented and varied in focus. Unusual mannerisms and posturing may prevent these individuals from eating, toileting, or attending to personal hygiene. They may demonstrate inappropriate laughter, be uncharacteristically silly, or even sit in an empty room laughing and acting theatrical even if they are alone in the room.

Catatonic Type

The catatonic type of schizophrenia is characterized by a severe decrease in motor activity and responsiveness to the environment. The individual may be mute and then suddenly start repeating words heard at an earlier time. They may make irregular motions with their arms while walking with rigid posture or make stereotyped movements that mimic the actions of others. When assuming a rigid, fixed posture for extended periods, these individuals usually have waxy flexibility and can be repositioned without a return to the previous pose. Catatonic type schizophrenia is rarely seen as a single subtype; it is often seen with other subtypes.

Undifferentiated Type

The individual with the undifferentiated subtype of schizophrenia exhibits a number of classic symptoms such as delusions, hallucinations, disorganized speech, atypical behavior, and blunted affect. The symptoms are not clearly defined to meet the criteria for any other subtype. The individual may exhibit the prominent symptoms but none that are specific to any one type of the disorder.

Residual Type

The individual with residual subtype of schizophrenia has experienced prominent psychotic symptoms with a previous diagnosis of schizophrenia, but no longer has the prominent symptoms. There is lingering evidence of unusual behavior, a blunted affect, some unrealistic thinking, or social withdrawal.

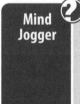

Mind Jogger Many individuals with schizophrenia are caught in a cycle that takes them from acute care management to a supervised milieu, and back to the community only to be readmitted with an acute exacerbation of the illness. Why do you think this pattern exists?

Disorders Related to Schizophrenia

In addition to schizophrenia there are other disorders that have symptoms of psychosis and are similar to schizophrenia. These disorders have an onset, duration, or causative factors that differentiate them from schizophrenia. Therefore, schizophrenia is classified as a spectrum. Some of the disorders in the schizophrenia spectrum and related psychotic disorders are detailed in Table 11.1.

Schizoaffective disorder is considered to be primarily a form of schizophrenia as the individual must have primary symptoms such as delusions, hallucinations, and disorganized behaviors. To be

TABLE 11.1	Schizophrenia Spectrum and Related Psychotic Disorders
Schizoaffective disorder	Active symptoms of schizophrenia occur together with a major mood disorder (major depressive or bipolar)
Schizophreniform disorder	Schizophrenic symptoms that last at least 1 month but less than 6 months (typically used as a preliminary diagnosis for schizophrenia)
Brief psychotic disorder	Short period of psychotic behavior that comes on suddenly, lasts less than a month, and is usually in response to a crisis or severely stressful event (e.g., catastrophic loss such as tornado, hurricane, or plane crash)
Delusional disorder	Delusional thoughts coinciding with life situations that could be true and last for at least 1 month
Psychotic disorder due to a medical condition	Active symptoms of schizophrenia that are a result of a medical condition that compromises brain function such as dementia, delirium, trauma, or brain tumor
Substance-induced psychotic disorder	Hallucinations and/or delusions that result from the direct use of, or withdrawal from, a substance such as alcohol, cocaine, or meth-amphetamine

given the diagnosis of schizoaffective, the individual must also at some time have demonstrated symptoms of major depression or mania. Schizoaffective disorder differs from a mood disorder in that, in schizoaffective disorder, the primary symptoms of schizophrenia are present for at least 2 weeks without any mood symptoms. This disorder tends to be chronic and disabling with some vacillating between a diagnosis of schizoaffective illness and schizophrenia.

Treatment of Psychotic Disorders

Most types of psychotic disorders are treated with a combined approach of medications and psychotherapy. The goal of treatment for the client with schizophrenia is to "minimize symptoms and functional impairments, minimize side effects of pharmacotherapy, avoid relapses, and promote recovery that allows self-determination, full integration into society, and pursuit of personal goals" (Stroup & Marder, 2022). Therapy sessions are done individually, in a group, or along with the family or support persons. For the individual with schizophrenia, psychotherapy includes cognitive-behavioral therapy and social skills training in addition to psychoeducational interventions with family members (Bustillo, 2022).

Family therapy is important to help promote medication adherence, a supportive environment, and to help the family or support persons with their feelings and reactions to caring for the member with a serious mental illness. There are many national groups that can provide support and information for both the individual with a psychotic disorder and their families or caregivers (Box 11.5).

Antipsychotic medications are the most common type of pharmacotherapy used. These medications do not provide a cure for the disorder,

but are used to help manage the problematic symptoms. Some individuals may require hospitalization for stabilization of their condition, while many can be managed as outpatients. Each individual responds to treatment differently with some improving quickly, and others taking weeks or months to receive symptom relief. Individuals with severe and disabling symptoms may need treatment indefinitely. Most individuals with schizophrenia need to take some type of medication along with supportive therapy for the rest of their lives.

Adherence to pharmacotherapy treatment is improved when used in conjunction with psychosocial treatment. Having a good relationship with a therapist or case manager, in addition to their mental health care provider, provides the support the individual needs to manage their illness on a day-to-day basis. Reasons for nonadherence to antipsychotic medications include not believing

---

BOX 11.5

Information Sources for Schizophrenia

- National Alliance on Mental Illness
  - https://www.nami.org/Home
  - text "NAMI" to 741741
  - 1-800-950-NAMI (6264)
- National Institute of Mental Health
  - https://www.nimh.nih.gov/health/topics/schizophrenia
  - https://www.nimh.nih.gov/health/find-help
- Mental Health Hotline
  - https://mentalhealthhotline.org/psychosis-hotline/
  - 1-866-903-3787
- National Library of Medicine
  - https://medlineplus.gov/schizophrenia.html
- American Psychological Association
  - https://www.apa.org/topics/schizophrenia

it is necessary, not remembering to take the medication at each scheduled time, or not liking the side effects. Difficulty with communication, access to care or a pharmacy, or developing relationships with the outside world add to isolation and medication nonadherence. A trained professional can often be the reminder and link to the individual's ability to manage their illness in a more effective way.

Antipsychotic Pharmacotherapy

Individuals with psychosis rarely have insight into the pathologic complexity of their symptoms and often do not realize they are ill. This lack of insight, both during periods of wellness and acute symptom exacerbation, is another dimension of the disabling nature of the psychotic disorders. Those with a psychotic disorder often mistakenly believe that because they are feeling better when taking medications that control the symptoms, they can stop taking them. This leads to acute exacerbations and hospitalization to restabilize the client.

Antipsychotic agents, sometimes referred to as neuroleptics, are used to treat serious mental illness such as bipolar affective disorder, major depressive disorder, and substance-induced psychosis, schizophrenia, and autism spectrum disorder. Because the symptoms of the psychoses are extremely uncomfortable for most individuals, the effects of antipsychotic medications are often a relief. They can reverse most or all symptoms in many individuals with a psychotic disorder. Early medications, such as chlorpromazine, produced remarkable reversal in symptoms and resulted in a dramatic decrease in the number of clients confined to mental institutions. This trend continues today, with shortened hospital stays and longer periods of functional living for many individuals whose symptoms are controlled with antipsychotic medication. However, since many individuals with a psychotic disorder lack insight into the complexity of their illness and need for continued treatment, adherence is generally inconsistent. This largely accounts for relapse and hospitalization to restabilize the individual and their medication treatment plan.

Typical antipsychotics, also known as traditional antipsychotics, block various dopamine receptors in the brain. Due to their varied chemical structures and strength, these agents are grouped into high, moderate, and low-potency

TABLE 11.2	Grouping of Typical Antipsychotic (Neuroleptic) Medications by Potency		
High Potency	**Moderate Potency**	**Low Potency**
Haloperidol	Loxapine	Thioridazine
Thiothixene	Molindone	Mesoridazine
Trifluoperazine	Perphenazine	Chlorprothixene
Fluphenazine	Droperidol	Chlorpromazine
Pimozide	Acetophenazine	Promazine
		Triflupromazine

classes, as shown in Table 11.2. The term potency indicates how much of the medication is required for it to be effective. The potency of the medication also influences the level and frequency of side effects experienced by the client. This accounts for the need for some individuals to receive higher dosages to achieve optimum clinical results. For example, a much larger dose of a low-potency medication (such as thioridazine) may be needed to produce the same level of symptom control from a lower dose of a high-potency medication (such as haloperidol). There is a significant difference in the side effects of the different medications. Low-potency agents cause more anticholinergic effects, whereas high-potency medications cause more extrapyramidal effects. Knowledge of the side effects enables the nurse to prepare the client for both the therapeutic benefits and potential adverse effects of the medication.

Later generation antipsychotic medications are classified as atypical because they do not fall into any particular chemical class. The newer agents have had a major impact on the reduction of negative symptoms of psychoses (such as flattened affect, verbal deficits, and diminished drive) with a reduced risk of extrapyramidal side effects. The reduction of negative symptoms is a desired outcome of antipsychotic therapy and is a tool used to measure progress of treatment. As a rule, the positive psychotic symptoms (hallucinations and delusions) are those that lead to the most atypical behavior. The positive symptoms are quite responsive to the typical antipsychotic medications. These medications also help to improve reasoning and decrease the ambivalent feelings and delusional thought processes. Reducing the inner stimuli the individual is experiencing allows the individual to devote more energy to external activity and interpersonal relationships.

TABLE 11.3	Antipsychotic Medication Agents	
Chemical Group	**Generic Name**	**Adverse Reactions and Side Effects**
Typical or Traditional Antipsychotic Medication Agents		
Phenothiazines	Chlorpromazine Fluphenazine Mesoridazine Perphenazine Prochlorperazine Promazine Thioridazine Trifluoperazine Triflupromazine[a]	Extrapyramidal reactions, tardive dyskinesia, sedation, pseudo parkinsonism, EEG changes, drowsiness, dizziness, blurred vision, dry mouth, constipation, increased appetite, urine retention, weight gain, mild photosensitivity **Life threatening:** seizures, neuroleptic malignant syndrome, blood dyscrasias
Butyrophenone	Haloperidol Pimozide[b]	Severe extrapyramidal reactions, tardive dyskinesia, sedation, drowsiness, lethargy, headache, insomnia, confusion, vertigo, tachycardia, hypotension, blurred vision, dry mouth, anorexia, nausea, constipation, diarrhea, dyspepsia, urine retention, rash
Dibenzoxazepine Dihydroindolone Thioxanthene	Loxapine Molindone Thiothixene Chlorprothixene	Extrapyramidal reactions, sedation, drowsiness, numbness, tardive dyskinesia, pseudo parkinsonism, dizziness, tachycardia, orthostatic hypotension, blurred vision, dry mouth, constipation, urine retention, weight gain, rash **Life threatening:** neuroleptic malignant syndrome, blood dyscrasias
Atypical Antipsychotic Medication Agents		
Benzisoxazole Partial dopamine agonist	Risperidone Aripiprazole[c]	Somnolence, extrapyramidal symptoms, headache, insomnia, agitation, anxiety, tardive dyskinesia, arthralgia, aggressiveness, tachycardia, rhinitis, constipation, nausea, vomiting, dyspepsia, cough, rash, dry skin, photosensitivity **Life threatening:** neuroleptic malignant syndrome, prolonged QT interval
Dibenzodiazepine Dibenzothiazepine Lurasidone Thienobenzodiazepine	Clozapine Quetiapine Latuda Olanzapine Ziprasidone Paliperidone palmitate[d]	Extrapyramidal symptoms, dystonia, orthostatic hypotension, increased QT intervals, tachycardia, increased risk of myocarditis, abdominal pain, nausea, dry mouth, constipation, hypersalivation, urinary retention, face edema, myalgia, photosensitivity, agitation, dyspnea, fungal dermatitis, weight gain **Life threatening:** agranulocytosis, neuroleptic malignant syndrome, cardiomyopathy, heart failure

[a]Available in long-acting injectable form—Fluphenazine.
[b]Available in long-acting injectable form—Haloperidol.
[c]Available in long-acting injectable form—Risperidone, aripiprazole (once monthly).
[d]Available in long-acting injectable form—Olanzapine, paliperidone palmitate.

Antipsychotic agents are listed in Table 11.3, including categories, adverse reactions, and side effects. Several long-acting injectable (LAI) antipsychotics are now available in the United States, primarily used as a strategy for treating individuals with schizophrenia who are nonadherant with taking their antipsychotic medication. The long-acting injectables (LAIs) are administered by injection at 2- to 4-week intervals. In addition to inhibition of postsynaptic receptors of the neurotransmitters, these medications also have properties that affect the cholinergic, histamine, and alpha-1-adrenergic receptors. This allows them to be used as antiemetics and in treating neurologic conditions such as intractable hiccups and tics (Tourette syndrome).

Smoking lowers the blood levels of antipsychotic medications including haloperidol, chlorpromazine, olanzapine, and clozapine due to nicotine increasing the metabolism of antipsychotic medications. The client who regularly uses nicotine may need a higher than normal dosage to compensate for this. Some medications, such as allopurinol, may be used in conjunction with antipsychotic agents to help improve symptom control.

Extrapyramidal Side Effects (Drug-Induced Movement Disorders)

Antipsychotic agents are capable of producing numerous side effects. The lower-potency medications tend to produce the anticholinergic effects such as dry mouth, urine retention, constipation, and blurred vision. They also produce the antiadrenergic actions including hypotension. The higher potency medications can produce severe extrapyramidal side effects. **Extrapyramidal side effects**, also called drug-induced movement disorders, are

"Victoria"

Recall Victoria from Case Study 11.1. Victoria was discharged 3 weeks ago from the step down mental health unit. Today, her mother brings her to the mental health clinic and reports Victoria has stopped taking her medications again. Her mother also reports that Victoria now believes there is a scientific meteor in her colon that is clipping off pieces of her internal organs to ship to the FBI. Victoria is curled in a chair across the room and yells, "I'm not sick anymore and I don't need that poison!"

Victoria tells the nurse that she is fine and that it is actually her mother who is "wacko!" She has agreed to come with her mother today so she will quit nagging her about the medicine. She also states, "That stuff makes me dizzy and my mouth dries up like a bone. I can feel them clipping in my colon and I have diarrhea big time!" Victoria's mother shows you the bottle of quetiapine that was prescribed at the time of discharge from acute care.

Digging Deeper

1. How would you describe Victoria's present behavior?

2. What is the best nursing approach to begin a therapeutic relationship with Victoria?

3. How might her reported symptoms be related to her medication?

4. What nursing interventions might be planned to help Victoria?

CASE STUDY 11.2

---

side effects of antipsychotic medications and include the inability to sit still, involuntary muscle contractions (such as repeated arm jerking), tremors, and involuntary facial movements. These are seen because the antipsychotic medication blocks the neurotransmitter dopamine, which causes irritation of the pyramidal tracts of the central nervous system (CNS) that coordinates involuntary movements. These reactions are much more devastating than anticholinergic and antiadrenergic side effects and contribute to the nonadherence of medication treatment. The nonadherence to medication treatment leads to relapse and return of symptoms with readmission to acute hospitalization. The health care provider can make dosage adjustments or prescribe medications that counteract these effects if they occur and are recognized early. Extrapyramidal side effects are described in Box 11.6.

Test Yourself

✔ What primary neurotransmitter do typical (traditional) antipsychotics block?

✔ Which client would most benefit from a long-acting injectable (LAI) antipsychotic medication?

✔ What effect does smoking (nicotine) have on antipsychotic medication?

✔ Describe extrapyramidal side effects (drug-induced movement disorders) and give four examples.

BOX 11.6

Extrapyramidal Side Effects (Drug-Induced Movement Disorders)

- **Akathisia**—motor restlessness, inability to sit still.
- **Dystonia**—rigidity in muscles that control posture, gait, or eye movement.
- **Tardive dyskinesia**—late-appearing and irreversible movements of the mouth and face that include lip-smacking and grinding of teeth, protruding tongue movements. A mask-like facial appearance, tremors, shuffling gait, cogwheel rigidity, pill-rolling, and stooped posture are common indications that long-term use of these medications has occurred.
- **Drug-induced parkinsonism**—symptoms that mimic parkinsonism such as tremors, rigidity, akinesia, or absence of movement with diminished mental state.
- **Neuroleptic malignant syndrome**—a potentially fatal reaction most often seen with the high-potency antipsychotic agents. This response typically has an onset from 3 to 9 days after treatment is initiated. Symptoms include muscular rigidity, tremors, inability to speak, altered level of consciousness, hyperthermia, autonomic dysfunction (hypertension, tachycardia, tachypnea, diaphoresis), and elevated white blood cell count. Although neuroleptic malignant syndrome occurs in a very low percentage of clients taking these medications, the need for early recognition and immediate medical intervention is imperative.

Water Intoxication

Associated with psychotic disorders is the potential for individuals to overhydrate by drinking excessive liquids, sometimes as much as 10 to 15 L a day. They are seen constantly carrying a cup or container with frequent trips to the water fountain or requests for something to drink. Some have been observed drinking from the toilet bowl or sink. The continued intake of fluid may result in **water intoxication** or a psychosis-induced metabolic state of fluid overload that can lead to cerebral edema and other potentially lethal situations. It is thought that a possible cause of this overload is related to the effects of antipsychotic medications on the pituitary gland, which produces antidiuretic hormone (ADH) and thereby inhibits the excretion of water.

Indications for Use

All antipsychotic medications are used in the treatment of acute and chronic psychoses, mania, and dementia-induced psychosis. The phenothiazines and haloperidol are also indicated in the treatment of intractable hiccups and control of tics and vocal disturbances. In addition, the phenothiazines may be used as antiemetics.

Contraindications

Antipsychotic agents are contraindicated in clients with hypersensitivity; coma or severe depression; liver, renal, or cardiac insufficiency; blood dyscrasias; and Parkinson disease. They should be used with caution in older clients; those with diabetes mellitus, chronic pulmonary disease, or prostatic hypertrophy; and in clients who are pregnant or lactating.

Nursing Interventions for the Client Taking Antipsychotic Medications

The nurse needs to monitor the client for effectiveness of the antipsychotics by monitoring for decreased symptoms of psychosis. The nurse should use therapeutic communication skills to determine the client's thought processes. Ask the client if they are having any hallucinations or hearing voices. Listen to the content of the client's speech and observe for any positive or negative symptoms of schizophrenia.

Observe the client to see if they are cheeking, or hiding medications in their mouth but not swallowing them. Clients with paranoid delusions may think they are being poisoned and may not fully swallow their medication. In cases where the client refuses to take medications and are a harm to themselves or others, injectable medications may be used. If the client refuses medications, document their reasons why and use exact client quotes. Also inquire about the client's perception of the need to take the medications even if they are feeling "well."

Prior to discharge the nurse should inquire about the client's schedule for taking their medication and if they have a system in place to help remind them such as an alarm on a watch or phone, a check-off list, or a friend or relative enlisted to help remind them. Reinforce the importance of consistent adherence with medication therapy. Promoting adherence to antipsychotics can be done by simplifying medication routines as much as possible with fewer medications, fewer pills, and fewer doses per day. Actively engaging clients in their medication treatment planning is called shared decision making. Shared decision making has been shown to increase medication adherence.

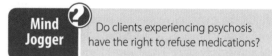

Mind Jogger Do clients experiencing psychosis have the right to refuse medications?

Monitor the client for extrapyramidal side effects of antipsychotic medication therapy using the Abnormal Involuntary Movement Scale (AIMS) assessment scale. The AIMS assessment tool and procedure are found in Appendix B. The nurse should observe the client during all interactions for observable signs of extrapyramidal side effects such as lip-smacking, protruding tongue movements, pill-rolling, or an inability to sit still.

Observe the client for anticholinergic effects of medications including reports of dry mouth, urinary retention, constipation, or blurred vision. Document the client's reported symptoms and report them to the registered nurse (RN) and the health care provider. Provide sugarless candy, gum, or frequent sips of liquid to combat dry mouth. Encourage frequent oral hygiene. Observe elimination pattern for difficulty urinating or constipation. Monitor intake and output. Observe for any excessive water intake or thirst behaviors.

Since hypotension is a potential side effect of antipsychotic medications, the nurse should instruct the client to slowly stand or get out of bed and to avoid activities that require mental alertness until the client's response to the medication is known. The nurse should also do blood pressures before and after standing and lying to determine any orthostatic hypotension.

Reinforcing Client and Family Teaching

 11.1

Important Information About Antipsychotic Medications

- Take medication only as directed—discuss effects of nonadherence and the return of symptoms when medications are discontinued.
- Side effects may occur—discuss interventions to help relieve them.
- Report any signs and symptoms of tardive dyskinesia to the health care provider.
- Take medication with food or milk to decrease stomach irritation.
- Avoid taking antipsychotic medication within 1 hour of taking antacids or antidiarrheals (may decrease effectiveness of antipsychotic medication).
- Several days to several weeks of medication therapy may be needed before full effects of treatment are achieved.
- Keep scheduled appointments with the health care provider and follow through with laboratory testing.
- Use caution when operating motor vehicles or machines that require coordination and mental alertness as drowsiness may occur with medication.
- Avoid direct exposure to sunlight, or use a sunscreen when in the sun.
- Avoid vigorous exercise and overheating while taking the medication.
- Phenothiazines may turn urine pinkish red, red, or reddish brown (is harmless and may be expected).
- Do not stop taking medication abruptly without checking with the health care provider.
- Avoid alcoholic beverages while taking the medications (will potentiate central nervous system action).
- Avoid orthostatic hypotension by rising slowly from a sitting or reclining position.
- Antipsychotics such as clozapine, risperidone, paliperidone, iloperidone can cause orthostatic hypotension and associated tachycardia. These effects are most pronounced during the first days of treatment and occur most frequently with clozapine and iloperidone.
- Anticholinergic side effects include tachycardia, dry mouth, urinary hesitancy, constipation, visual changes, and cognitive impairment. Anticholinergic effects are seen with clozapine, chlorpromazine, olanzapine, and, to a lesser extent, with quetiapine, iloperidone, and loxapine. These side effects tend to be worse in older patients.

It is essential that the client and responsible family or support members receive information about antipsychotic medications and the potential for adverse effects. At the same time, the importance of continuous adherence to the treatment must be stressed. The nurse also reinforces teaching related to antipsychotic medications (see Reinforcing Client and Family Teaching 11.1). Important points to reinforce include that the client and caregivers verbalize the importance of continuing medication therapy even if client is feeling "well" and keeping regular appointments with the health care provider. Initially the health care provider may order medication levels drawn regularly. Inform the client and caregivers of the need for these blood medication levels as the dosage may be changed depending on the values. It is also important that they verbalize understanding of medication side effects and which symptoms to report to the health care provider.

Criteria that may be used to evaluate the effectiveness of antipsychotic agents in the client are listed in Box 11.7.

Antiparkinsonian Medications

Antiparkinsonian medications are used to relieve the medication-induced extrapyramidal symptoms

BOX 11.7

Anticipated Outcomes for the Client Taking Antipsychotic Medications

The client:
- Has symptoms that are reduced to minimal occurrence
- Controls and refrains from violent behaviors
- Learns to use appropriate outlets for anger and frustration
- Identifies and seeks help when symptoms are overwhelming
- Takes medications as directed
- Experiences reduced incidence of psychotic symptoms and behaviors
- Seeks help when beginning to feel behavior is out of control
- Experiences minimal side effects
- Adheres to therapeutic medication regimen
- Participates in planning care and long-term medication adherence
- Expresses understanding of relationship between psychotic symptoms, medication adherence, and behavior
- Verbalizes an understanding of prescribed medication regimen and potential side effects

associated with the antipsychotic medication agents. The two most commonly used are benztropine and trihexyphenidyl. These medications are synthetic anticholinergic agents that resemble both atropine and diphenhydramine in their chemical structure. The dosage is determined by the severity of symptoms.

The main contraindications to antiparkinsonian medications are hypersensitivity to the medication, narrow-angle glaucoma, myasthenia gravis, urinary retention, peptic ulcer disease, and prostatic hypertrophy. These medications must be used with caution in older adults because of significant side effects including urinary retention, visual disturbances, palpitations, and increased intraocular pressure.

Antipsychotic Medications and the Older Client

For older clients who have dementia-related aggression, distressing repetitive behaviors, delusions, hallucinations, or agitation, the use of antipsychotic medications may be used to reduce and managing the incidence of these symptoms. Federal law limits the use of antipsychotic medications for residents in long-term care facilities, and the guidelines specify that these medications can only be used for specific diagnoses and when behavioral and environmental measures are unsuccessful in managing symptoms. Specific monitoring must also be done. Research data on the safety and response of the older client to antipsychotic medications are limited, further suggesting a cautious approach to the use of these medications.

TABLE 11.4	Age-Related Physiologic Changes and Medications in Older Clients
Physiologic Change	**Medication Risk**
Higher body fat-to-lean ratio	Increased risk of cumulative effects
Less serum albumin and protein-bound medication	More free medication in bloodstream
Less total body water	Dehydration increases the concentration of medication in body
Decreased liver metabolism	Clearance of medication is delayed or slowed
Decreased renal elimination	Slowed elimination of medication from system

less total body water, fewer brain cells, and slower liver metabolism and renal clearance than young adults, they need a lower dosage to produce a therapeutic effect. The higher fat composition of tissue increases retention of the medication, resulting in effects that persist longer, sometimes even after the medication is discontinued. Because older clients have less protein to bind with the medication, more is free to circulate. A slowed metabolic rate and renal excretion time allow the medication to remain in the body longer. Table 11.4 shows these physiologic changes and their risks to older clients when administering an antipsychotic agent.

All of these factors highlight the importance of monitoring the response to and recognizing the adverse effects of antipsychotic agents in the older client. It is considered extremely important that all alternative approaches be considered before the use of the medications and that, if used, treatment is discontinued if the individual is adversely affected by the medication.

Senior Focus In the older adult, the half-life of a medication tends to increase by as much as five to six times, increasing the risk of toxicity. The effects accumulate slowly and may not be apparent for days or weeks after the initiation of the medication (Ruscin & Linnebur, 2021).

Senior Focus In the older client, always consider whether a new symptom or behavior may be related to medication therapy.

Test Yourself
✔ Name six nursing interventions for the client taking antipsychotic medications.
✔ Describe anticholinergic effects seen with antipsychotic medications.
✔ Describe the role of antiparkinsonian medications in the treatment of psychosis.
✔ Identify five physiologic changes in the older client that can cause a medication risk.

The impact of age-related physiologic changes on antipsychotic medication therapy accounts for many of the serious side effects that occur in older adults. Many antipsychotic medications, either by themselves or in interaction with other medications, can cause the very symptoms they are prescribed to treat, such as agitation or delusions. Because older adults have a higher body fat-to-lean ratio, less serum albumin,

Nursing Process and Care Plan *for the Client With a Psychotic Disorder*

It is important to remember that the client with a psychotic disorder is experiencing their own form of reality that seems real to them. The nurse should show acceptance of the client as a person and focus on the psychotic behaviors. The nurse should maintain a calm attitude with matter-of-fact response to reinforce reality.

Challenging the client's delusions can cause them to become defensive or aggressive. The client experiencing hallucinations can be a safety risk to themselves or others. The client who is hearing voices may be commanded by the voices to harm themselves or others. For these reasons, the nursing care plan must always focus on safety.

The client with psychosis may not be able to effectively communicate their needs or their alterations in perceptions. The nurse must use observation skills in addition to therapeutic communication skills to determine the plan of care.

Assessment (Data Collection)

Data collection will include information regarding any previous incidence of mental illness or psychotic episodes. Because the individual with psychosis may not always be a reliable source of information, be sure to consult family members or other individuals familiar with the client. Data are most often compiled according to the nature of the symptoms such as perceptual disturbances, thought processes, speech, behavior, mood, and self-care activities.

When the client is experiencing perceptual disturbances, such as hallucinations or illusions, it is important to collect data regarding the type of disturbance the client is experiencing. This includes determining the specific sense that is affected, if there were any precipitating factors or events, and the client's feelings while thought alterations are evident. If the client is demonstrating disorganized thinking or delusions, it is important to look for a central theme and determine content. If the delusion is persecution oriented, determine the nature of the threat and whether there is a risk for violence to themselves, staff, or other clients as a result. Observe speech patterns associated with the delusions. Delusional thinking is characterized by speech in which the individual jumps from one unrelated subject to

another. When documenting speech, be sure to use direct quotes from the client to illustrate the type of speech alteration observed.

Just the Facts The manner in which speech is manifested along with the accompanying behavior will usually provide more information about the delusion than the content.

Note the affect and emotional tone of the client and whether they are appropriate in relation to the present situation. Apathy or a lack of interest in the environment and flatness of affect are characteristic signs of schizophrenia. Redirect the client if they exhibit inappropriate behavior or language.

Observe the client's behavior patterns, activity, sleep habits, and interactions with other clients. Monitor their appearance, hygiene, and ability to perform self-care activities. Monitor percent of meals eaten and for any signs of increased water intake. Weigh the client weekly as some medications can cause weight gain.

Observe for posturing or other psychomotor disturbances such as those seen in catatonia. For clients who are on antipsychotics, observe for extrapyramidal side effects (drug-induced movement disorders). It is very important for the nurse to determine any suicidal intent or recent attempts that may have been made.

Nursing Care Focus

After careful review of the data, the focus of nursing care can be determined. Safety is always a priority focus of nursing care for the client with psychosis. Multidisciplinary approaches to treatment are usually selected on their ability to reduce and control the symptoms. Nursing care should be planned to focus on symptomatic relief as well, with careful attention to the physical, emotional, and social needs imposed by impaired mental functioning. Focus of nursing care for the client with schizophrenia could include any of the following (depending upon data collected): Altered Health Maintenance, Bathing/Hygiene Activities of Daily Living (ADL) Deficit, Chronic Confusion, Chronic Low Self-Esteem, Coping Impairment, Injury Risk, Nonadherence, Safety, Psychosocial Needs, or Violence Risk.

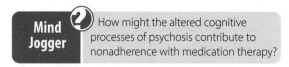

Mind Jogger ② How might the altered cognitive processes of psychosis contribute to nonadherence with medication therapy?

Outcome Identification and Planning

The anticipated outcomes for the client with schizophrenia will depend on the level of functioning demonstrated by the client. This will depend on the severity of symptoms and the effectiveness of antipsychotic medication therapy or other therapeutic approaches. It is important that the goals and time frame for improvement be realistic. With each psychotic episode experienced, the client's baseline functioning may be reduced, so it is not realistic for outcomes and timelines from prior hospitalizations to be used. Box 11.8 lists common desired outcomes for the client in a state of psychosis.

BOX 11.8

Common Desired Outcomes for a Client With a Psychotic Disorder

The client:

- develops reality-based ways to communicate and meet self-needs
- remains oriented to self and the environment
- interacts appropriately with others
- performs self-care and hygiene with minimal prompting
- demonstrates increased trust of others
- exhibits increased ability to associate behavior with misperceived environmental stimuli
- participates in unit activities with appropriate behavior
- identifies realistic self-expectations and perceptions
- experiences reduced incidence of hallucinations
- cooperates with staff in taking medications

Nursing Care Focus

- Safety, related to altered thought processes

Goal

- The client does not injure self or others.

Implementations for Promoting Safety

Nursing interventions for the psychotic client related to safety are accomplished through the administration of medications, observing for situations that have the potential for violence, and observing the client's symptoms. Reassure the client that the environment is safe. This is reinforced by explaining unit routines and procedures. The client is less likely to feel threatened if they feel they are safe and they know what to expect. Do not make promises you cannot keep as this leads to mistrust which can lead to violence.

Selecting appropriate interventions that the client can tolerate requires careful planning. It is important to encourage clients to maximize their ability to function and be realistic about their capabilities. Understanding the client's ability to focus, process, and follow instructions provides direction for the selection of nursing interventions. It is important to consider the holistic picture of the client, including physiologic, emotional, cultural, and spiritual needs.

Set and maintain limits with expectations on unsafe or inappropriate behavior and provide explanations. For example, instead of telling the client "Don't curse," say "While you are here, the rule is no cursing." This helps the client understand social norms and self-correct their behavior. It is important to observe the client for escalating behavior and intervene before an "out-of-control" situation occurs. Provide positive feedback for appropriate behaviors. This helps the client recognize behaviors that should be continued and positive social norms. Do not set limits to punish the client.

In some instances, when other interventions do not work and the client is at risk of harming themselves or others, a temporary restraint with a time-out in seclusion may be imposed to allow the client to regain self-control. When this situation occurs, nurses must use every measure to show respect for the client, reassuring the client of the temporary nature of these restrictions. Nutritional, hygiene, and toileting needs should be met in accordance with unit policies.

Provide a safe environment by removing unsafe objects and diffusing potentially violent situations before they escalate. If the client identifies a specific person or situation that voices are telling them to hurt, separate the client from that person or situation (such as anyone wearing black). Avoid abrupt touching of the client, which can be perceived as threatening. To help avoid confrontations, use a neutral tone and lowered volume of voice.

Maintain a reality-based approach when communicating with the client. Clients experiencing delusions tend to be mistrusting and suspicious, making them resistant to taking medications and accepting information. Avoiding a confrontation or argumentative approach while also not reinforcing the delusional belief helps to reinforce reality.

Provide a nonstimulating environment that reduces external stimuli. Some clients experiencing psychosis are unable to filter stimuli while self-controlling their behavior at the same time, and may become aggressive with excessive stimuli. Dimming lights, turning down the volume on television sets, or having the client interact with smaller groups help to decrease stimuli. Encourage participation in social interaction with others while recognizing that a group activity may be threatening to the client with paranoia.

Evaluation of Goal/Desired Outcome

- The client is free from harm during hospitalization.

Nursing Care Focus

- Chronic confusion, related to nonreality-based thinking

Goal

- The client will make reality-based statements.

Implementations for Decreasing Confusion

Provide reality orientation during the daily routine, giving the date, day of the week, and location. A whiteboard by the nurses' desk can be used to reinforce this information. The nurse should always introduce themselves, explain that they are a nurse, and identify the unit or facility where they are during initial interactions with the client.

The nurse should make direct statements that shed doubt on the illogical thinking of the client. Acknowledge the perceptual or thinking alteration as being real to the client while reinforcing reality (e.g., "I understand that the voices must be frightening to you, but I do not hear them."), which helps the client to recognize symptoms as part of the illness. Encourage client to verbalize feelings of anxiety, frustration, or those associated with altered thoughts and behaviors.

The nurse should monitor for behavioral clues that indicate hallucinations or delusions such as staring at an inanimate object, whispering, inappropriate giggling, or facial or hand gestures. Ask the client direct questions including "Are you hearing voices?" "What are they telling you?" and "Do you recognize the voices?" These are important to determine the client's thoughts. Document exactly what the client states and use direct quotes as much as possible. Documentation helps monitor if altered thought processes are increasing, decreasing, or staying about the same. The nurse should interact with the client on the basis of real things and not focus on the delusions. Do not joke about or belittle the client's beliefs, as they are not funny to the client, and the client may not understand the attempt at humor.

Provide prepackaged foods for clients who are paranoid. Clients are more likely to eat foods they can open themselves than food already prepared. Foods such as casseroles, mashed potatoes, meats, and gravy should be avoided during times of increased paranoia. Instead, items such as cheese slices, potato chips, crackers, milk, and complete nutritional prepackaged drinks can be offered as supplemental foods. Some units keep snacks, fruit, and nutritional drinks in an area that is accessible to clients.

Recreational or art therapy is beneficial for the client as it aids them in concentrating on tasks instead of responding to voices or delusions. Engage them in real activities or interactions instead of watching television or movies. Avoid competitive games. Engage in simple topics of conversation as it is easier for the client to talk about basic things such as the weather or what they had for their last meal.

Initially do not give choices; rather, give the client short directions such as, "It is time to go to the cafeteria." Long explanations can add to their confusion. When offering choices, minimize the options to avoid creating confusion. For example, ask the client, "Do you want apple or orange juice?" instead of naming all juices available. The nurse should avoid asking open-ended question such as, "What kind of juice do you want?"

Provide periods of decreased stimulation and unstructured time. Decreased stimuli decreases the chances of the client misinterpreting the cause. Providing these break periods helps the client from becoming overstimulated and gives them time to process their thoughts. The client also has a decreased ability to cope with the excess stimuli. Monitor number of hours the client sleeps each 24-hour period. Decreased sleep can increase disorganized thought processes.

Administer medications as prescribed. Monitor the client during administration to ensure swallowing of medications. Document any refusal of medications or client's statements regarding medications.

When monitoring the effectiveness of planned interventions, the nurse should look for signs that indicate improved functioning of the client. It is anticipated that adherence with medication therapy will diminish the positive symptoms of psychosis the client experiences. Hopefully, this is accompanied by an increase in the client's understanding of actual and real events that precipitate the perceptual and delusional alterations. This is demonstrated as the client is able to identify these factors and practice diversional techniques to avoid the anxiety that encourages the psychotic behavior.

Communication with staff and other clients in an appropriate and reality-based conversation is evidence of improved thinking processes. A decrease in atypical and inappropriate behavior will occur as thoughts and perceptions decrease the need for their use. Reduced suspiciousness is evidenced by increased willingness to trust staff and other clients. This is a slow process for a client who has lived with a world of perceived threats and injustice. Any small gain should be viewed as progress. Adherence with taking medications and increased food intake are also evidence that the client has decreased fear of poisoning by ingested substances.

Involvement in unit activities is a demonstration of the client's willingness to engage in the company of others. This also may be seen in the client who follows a task to completion such as in occupational therapy, clearing tables in the dining area, or taking a shower and dressing without assistance.

Evaluation of Goal/Desired Outcome

The client:

- demonstrates a decrease in altered thought processes.
- interacts with others during unit activities and focus on a task.
- communicates their needs.
- sleeps for 4 to 6 continuous hours.
- demonstrates adherence to medication treatment.

"Carmen"

Carmen has been living in an apartment since her discharge from acute care. Since she also has diabetes and takes daily insulin injections, Carmen has been assigned home health visits three times a week to make sure she is taking her medications and appropriately managing living in an independent setting.

On this day, the LPN/LVN arrives to visit Carmen, who does not answer the doorbell. The nurse hears voices from inside the apartment indicating Carmen is at home. The nurse tries to open the door, finds it unlocked, and notices Carmen standing on top of the couch talking to the ceiling fan. Carmen does not acknowledge that anyone has entered the room. The nurse calls out Carmen's name softly and states who they are and the reason why they are there. Carmen suddenly spins around, faces the nurse, and says, "They are telling me the insulin will poison me and I am slowly being destroyed by maggots from my food. They tell me to destroy all the food. Don't come near me."

Digging Deeper

1. What data should the nurse collect?

2. How would the nurse best approach Carmen to get her attention?

3. What steps should the nurse take at this point?

CASE STUDY 11.3

Cultural Considerations

Cultural Reactions to Caregiving

People with psychotic disorders often require a family member to act as a caregiver. The caregiver's physical and mental health can be negatively impacted from giving care to a family member with a mental illness. Factors that contribute to the caregiver's wellbeing or distress include cultural values, the caregiver's coping style, social support available to the caregiver, and the seriousness of the illness. Reactions to caregiving were very similar across cultures.

Caregiving is perceived as "the right thing to do" regardless of culture. In some cultures, caregiving is expected and engrained into the culture to the extent that providing care to a family member is done without question, and to not provide care is seen as a rejection or abandonment of the individual. Regardless of ethnic background, stigma remains one of the greatest barriers to families and caregivers.

Common Reactions to Caregiving Seen (Regardless of Culture):

- Chronic sorrow
- Guilt
- Caregivers who felt stigmatized had poorer self-care, increasing the risk of caregiver depressive symptoms
- Older caregivers at higher risk for depressive symptoms and malnutrition
- Caregivers with more active coping strategies or more support perceived caregiving as less of a burden
- Women experience a greater sense of burden and frustration than men
- Depressive symptoms higher in caregivers who are younger or have lower levels of education or those caring for an individual with more severe symptoms of mental illness

- Caregiver workshops are an effective way to decrease levels of depressive symptoms
- Receiving social support can reduce the negative effects of caregiving
- Caregivers often cope with their own suffering by seeking solace in religion

Specific Cultural Beliefs Regarding Caregiving

- In cultures that focus on the nuclear family model, caregiving is often done because of a crisis situation. The caregiver may not have had prior exposure to caregiving (American, East European).
- The manner which filial piety (allegiance to parents) is expressed is changing in some cultures. Instead of providing care first-hand, paying for care is seen as a positive activity (Chinese).
- Familism, or family obligation, dictates that the needs of the family take priority over the needs of individual family members (Vietnamese).
- The use of institutional services is discouraged and care is provided in the home (Vietnamese, Traditional Confucianism).
- The oldest child, or daughter, or daughter-in-law is given the responsibility of caregiving (Japanese, Chinese).
- Caregivers can be kinship relationships and not necessarily immediate family members (African American).
- Caregivers with a high sense of obligation were less likely to perceive positive support from available helpers (Chinese, Japanese, Korean).
- An individual with a mental illness is thought to bring shame to their family, relatives, and ancestors. To maintain their reputation, families may hide the individual's mental illness (Vietnamese).
- Religion may place an importance on alleviating the suffering of others (Buddhism).

Sources: Bui, Q. N., Han, M., Diwan, S., & Dao, T. (2018). Vietnamese-American family caregivers of persons with mental illness: Exploring caregiving experience in cultural context. *Transcultural Psychiatry, 55*(6), 846–865. https://doi.org/10.1177/1363461518793185; Business Bliss Consultants FZE. (2018). Literature review of caregivers stress and coping. https://nursinganswers.net/litreviews/literature-review-of-caregivers-stress-and-coping-nursing-essay.php; Knight, B. G., & Sayegh, P. (2009). Cultural values and caregiving: The updated sociocultural stress and coping model. *The Journals of Gerontology: Series B, 65B*(1), 5–13. https://doi.org/10.1093/geronb/gbp096; Pharr, J. R., Francis, C. D., Terry, C., & Clark, M. C. (2014). Culture, caregiving, and health: Exploring the influence of culture on family caregiver experiences. International Scholarly Research Notices. https://doi.org/10.1155/2014/689826; Young, L., Murata, L., McPherson, C., Jacob, J. D., & Vandyk, A. D. (2019). Exploring the experiences of parent caregivers of adult children with schizophrenia: A systematic review. *Archives of Psychiatric Nursing, 33*(1), 93–103. https://doi.org/10.1016/j.apnu.2018.08.005; Wong, Y. L. I., Kong, D., Tu, L., & Frasso, R. (2018). "My bitterness is deeper than the ocean": Understanding internalized stigma from the perspectives of persons with schizophrenia and their family caregivers. *International Journal of Mental Health Systems, 12*(14). https://doi.org/10.1186/s13033-018-0192-4

SUMMARY

- Psychosis is when a severe disarray is evident in the mental processes of thinking, perceiving, and behaving. Behavior is directly linked to perceptions and thoughts about environmental stimuli and changes when these processes are distorted and disorganized.
- The characteristic symptoms of psychosis reveal a loss of touch with reality and those things that give life meaning. Loss of the ability to communicate meaningfully with others leads to a deterioration of relationships and contact with society.
- Hallucinations are false sensory perceptions that have no relevance to reality and are not supported by actual environmental stimuli. The individual has the perception of seeing, hearing, smelling, feeling, or tasting although there is no stimulus present. Auditory or hearing hallucinations are the most common. "Voices" may originate inside or outside the individual's head and may talk to the individual about their behavior. Some voices are commanding, telling them to harm themselves or others and can be very frightening to the individual.
- Illusions are experienced when sensory stimuli actually exist but are misinterpreted by the individual, such as thinking an electrical cord is a snake.
- Delusions are thought processes that are confused and disrupted, leaving the individual unable to carry on a conversation. The content or theme of the delusions include depressive, somatic, grandiose, persecutory, reference, jealous, erotomatic, or mixed.
- Behavior alterations seen in psychotic disorders are unpredictable, and can be described as agitated, aggressive, childlike, inappropriate, or made up. The disorganized action most often leads to an inability to perform activities of daily living or to carry out goal-directed activity.
- Schizophrenia is the most common psychotic disorder. A prodromal period often precedes the actual first psychotic event, during which the individual may begin experiencing inability to concentrate and finish things. Thoughts may become distorted and speech patterns reflect a jumble of misplaced words.
- Positive symptoms of schizophrenia are evidenced early in the progress of the disorder and include alterations in thinking, perception, and behavior. The delusional thoughts are distorted and often there is no logical connection. The fragmented and disorganized thought processes are demonstrated in speech patterns of word salad and derailed loose associations.
- Negative symptoms of schizophrenia develop slowly over time and include a blunted or flat affect that is expressionless and blank. The individual's responses are often inappropriate to the mood of the real world around them. Behavior may be described as autistic, referring to a focus on an inner fantasy world which excludes the external environment.
- Subtypes of schizophrenia include paranoid, disorganized, catatonic, undifferentiated, and residual types.
- Psychotic disorders related to schizophrenia include schizoaffective disorder, schizophreniform disorder, brief psychotic disorder, delusional disorder, psychotic disorder due to a medical condition, and substance-induced psychotic disorder.
- Schizoaffective disorder is characterized by a combined presence of schizophrenic symptoms and those of a mood disorder (bipolar disorder or major depressive disorder). The variance from a mood disorder lies in the presence of the primary symptoms of schizophrenia for at least 2 weeks without any mood symptoms.
- Treatment of the client with schizophrenia centers on reduction and control of the debilitating symptoms. A combined approach of antipsychotic medication therapy and psychotherapy is the most common approach. Management of positive symptoms by medication therapy may be limited by side effects and nonadherence.
- Antipsychotic medications aid in reducing or reversing the delusions, hallucinations, and disorganized behaviors common to the disorders.
- The incidence of antipsychotic adverse side effects and a lack of insight into the need for continued treatment both contribute to the nonadherence seen in many clients with psychosis who require antipsychotic medications to stabilize their illness.
- The potency of an antipsychotic medication will influence the level and frequency of side effects experienced by the client.
- The Abnormal Involuntary Movement Scale (AIMS) assessment tool (Appendix B) can be used to monitor the extrapyramidal side effects of antipsychotic agents.
- Antiparkinsonian or anticholinergic agents are used to decrease the extrapyramidal side effects exhibited in those taking antipsychotic agents.
- Antipsychotic medications are used with caution in the older client because of age-related physiologic changes. The medication effects persist longer and remain in the body longer. Careful monitoring is mandated to avoid the adverse consequences of their use.

BIBLIOGRAPHY

Bustillo, J. (2022). Psychosocial interventions for schizophrenia. *UpToDate*. Retrieved June 27, 2022, from https://www.uptodate.com/contents/psychosocial-interventions-for-schizophrenia

Chokhawala, K., & Stevens, L. (2022). Antipsychotic medications. In: *StatPearls [Internet]*. StatPearls Publishing. Retrieved July 5, 2022, from https://www.ncbi.nlm.nih.gov/books/NBK519503

Coffey, M. J. (2021). Catatonia in adults: Epidemiology, clinical features, assessment, and diagnosis. *UpToDate*. Retrieved July 5, 2022, from https://www.uptodate.com/contents/catatonia-in-adults-epidemiology-clinical-features-assessment-and-diagnosis

D'Souza, D., & Hooten, W. M. (2022). Extrapyramidal symptoms. In: *StatPearls [Internet]*. StatPearls Publishing. Retrieved July 5, 2022, from https://www.ncbi.nlm.nih.gov/books/NBK534115

Fisher, B. A., & Buchanan, R. W. (2022a). Schizophrenia in adults: Clinical manifestations, course, assessment, and diagnosis. *UpToDate*. Retrieved January 7, 2023, from https://www.uptodate.com/contents/schizophrenia-in-adults-clinical-manifestations-course-assessment-and-diagnosis

Fisher, B. A., & Buchanan, R. W. (2022b). Schizophrenia in adults: Epidemiology and pathogenesis. *UpToDate*. Retrieved January 7, 2023, from https://www.uptodate.com/contents/schizophrenia-in-adults-epidemiology-and-pathogenesis

Harvey, P. D., Strassnig, M. T., & Silberstein, J. (2019). Prediction of disability in schizophrenia: Symptoms, cognition, and self-assessment. *Journal of Experimental Psychopathology*, *10*(3). https://doi.org/10.1177/2043808719865693

Lauriello, J., & Campbell, A. R. (2022). Pharmacotherapy for schizophrenia: Long-acting injectable antipsychotic drugs. *UpToDate*. Retrieved July 5, 2022, from https://www.uptodate.com/contents/pharmacotherapy-for-schizophrenia-long-acting-injectable-antipsychotic-drugs

Lintunen, J., Lähteenvuo, M., Tiihonen, J., Tanskanen, A., & Taipale, H. (2021). Adenosine modulators and calcium channel blockers as add-on treatment for schizophrenia. *NPJ Schizophrenia*, *7*(1). https://doi.org/10.1038/s41537-020-00135-y

Musco, S., Ruekert, L., Myers, J., Anderson, D., Welling, M., & Cunningham, E. A. (2019). Characteristics of patients experiencing extrapyramidal symptoms or other movement disorders related to dopamine receptor blocking agent therapy. *Journal of Clinical Psychopharmacology*, *39*(4), 336–343. https://doi.org/10.1097/JCP.0000000000001061

National Alliance on Mental Illness. (2022). *Psychosis*. https://nami.org/About-Mental-Illness/Mental-Health-Conditions/Psychosis

National Institute of Mental Health. (2022). *Schizophrenia*. https://www.nimh.nih.gov/health/topics/schizophrenia

Ruscin, J. M., & Linnebur, S. A. (2021). *Pharmacokinetics in older adults*. Merck Manual Professional Version. https://www.merckmanuals.com/professional/geriatrics/drug-therapy-in-older-adults/pharmacokinetics-in-older-adults

Stroup, T. S., & Marder, S. (2022). Schizophrenia in adults: Maintenance therapy and side effect management. *UpToDate*. Retrieved June 27, 2022, from https://www.uptodate.com/contents/schizophrenia-in-adults-maintenance-therapy-and-side-effect-management

Tamminga, C. (2022). *Schizophrenia*. Merck Manual Professional Version. https://www.merckmanuals.com/professional/psychiatric-disorders/schizophrenia-and-related-disorders/schizophrenia

Upasen, R., & Saengpanya, W. (2021). Compassion fatigue among family caregivers of schizophrenic patients. *Journal of Population and Social Studies*, *30*, 1–17. https://so03.tci-thaijo.org/index.php/jpss/article/view/254870

Wijdicks, E. F. M. (2022). Neuroleptic malignant syndrome. *UpToDate*. Retrieved July 5, 2022, from https://www.uptodate.com/contents/neuroleptic-malignant-syndrome

Zaheer, J., Olfson, M., Mallia, E., Lam, J. S. H., de Oliveira, C., Rudoler, D., Carvalho, A. F., Jacob, B. J., Juda, A., & Kurdyak, P. (2020). Predictors of suicide at time of diagnosis in schizophrenia spectrum disorder: A 20-year total population study in Ontario, Canada. *Schizophrenia Research*, *222*, 382–388. https://doi.org/10.1016/j.schres.2020.04.025

STUDENT WORKSHEET

Fill in the Blank

Fill in the blank with the correct answer.

1. Low-potency antipsychotic medications cause more _____ side effects, whereas high-potency antipsychotic medications cause more _____ side effects.
2. Extrapyramidal reactions are monitored by the _____ assessment scale.
3. _____ are perceptual disturbances in which the individual misinterprets sensory stimuli that actually exist.
4. A psychosis-induced metabolic state of overhydration in the schizophrenic client is referred to as _____ _____.
5. Delusions of _____ centralize on false beliefs that the individual is very powerful and important.
6. The individual with schizophrenia typically has a _____ affect that is expressionless and blank.

Matching

Match the following terms to the most appropriate phrase.

1. _____ Avolition
2. _____ Derailment
3. _____ Clang associations
4. _____ Thought broadcasting
5. _____ Word salad
6. _____ Waxy flexibility
7. _____ Delusion of reference

a. Individual remains in one position until changed by another person.
b. "I know all the judges can hear what I am thinking."
c. Lack of motivation to make decisions or do self-care.
d. "Our bowl is loud star to a wet red noodle carried by the military in excess of the earth."
e. "Take the pill up the hill winter kill."
f. "Tom Brokaw is telling me I hold the key to security in outer space."
g. Loose associations that are off track or not connected to each other.

Multiple Choice

Select the best answer from the multiple-choice items.

1. The nurse is caring for a client who states, "The radio is sending signals to my intellectual processes to inflict damage on myself." How would the nurse document this delusional pattern?
   a. Experiencing auditory hallucinations
   b. Having delusions of persecution
   c. Having delusions of grandeur
   d. Speaking in loose associations

2. Which of the following statements best describes poverty of speech?
   a. A jumble of unconnected and disorganized thoughts
   b. Insignificant rhyming of words
   c. Thoughts of others can be inserted in one's mind
   d. Decrease in amount or speed with which an individual talks

3. A client approaches the nurse and states, "This little elf keeps following me with a leash, and it really is getting on my nerves." Which of the following would be the most appropriate response for the nurse to make at this time?
   a. "I understand seeing the elf is frustrating to you, but no one else sees it."
   b. "Why don't you just tell the elf to sit down and leave you alone?"
   c. "You are only making that up in your mind."
   d. "That is silly. There is no one following you."

4. The nurse observes protruding tongue movements and pill-rolling motions in a client taking the medication haloperidol. These observations would be recognized as:
   a. Signs of extrapyramidal side effects to the medication
   b. Normal response to long-term use of the medication
   c. Part of the illness and unrelated to the medication
   d. Indications an increased dosage may be needed

5. The nurse is providing client teaching to a client for whom the antipsychotic agent risperidone has been prescribed. Which statement by the client would indicate a need for further teaching?
   a. "I need to take the medication when I eat so it doesn't upset my stomach."
   b. "It may be a week or two before I feel really good."
   c. "I can still go riding on my bike in the afternoon like I usually do."
   d. "I better sit on the edge of the bed awhile before I get up in the morning."

6. The client has been regularly taking the medication haloperidol. Which finding reported to the health care provider would result in the medication benztropine also being ordered?
   a. Increased delusional thinking
   b. Intractable hiccups
   c. Diminished drive and apathy
   d. Protruding tongue movements

7. Which of the following would be considered a positive symptom of schizophrenia? *(Select all that apply)*
   a. Presents with a blunted affect
   b. Describing atypical thoughts
   c. Expresses indications of avolition
   d. Having auditory hallucinations
   e. Disheveled and unkempt appearance

8. Which nursing intervention would be important to include in the plan of care of a client taking haloperidol?
   a. Adding extra salt to prepared foods or beverages
   b. Offering sugar-free hard candy or frequent liquids
   c. Having the client rinse their mouth after taking the medication
   d. Observing for grayish discoloration of tongue

9. The nurse is planning care for a client who has been newly diagnosed with paranoid schizophrenia. Which of the following perceptual changes should the nurse anticipate?
   a. Client does not notice nor respond to changes in the environment
   b. Client recognizes that they are not responding normally to stimuli
   c. Client accepts and understands the irrational nature of their ideations
   d. Client frequently misinterprets social and environmental stimuli

10. A client with paranoid schizophrenia believes their medications are tainted with poisonous substances and refuses to take them. Which action should the nurse take?
   a. Matter-of-fact reinforcement of the need to take the medication
   b. Ask the client what the medication is tainted with
   c. Ask the client why they think the medication is tainted
   d. Withhold the medication and try again later

12 Personality Disorders

LEARNING OBJECTIVES

After learning the content in this chapter, the student will be able to:

1. Describe the difference between personality traits and personality disorders.
2. Identify and group 10 personality disorders.
3. Describe the main behavioral characteristics for each group.
4. Describe characteristic behaviors of each personality disorder.
5. Identify coexisting mental health conditions that may be seen in the individual with a personality disorder.
6. Describe the treatment options available for the individual with a personality disorder.
7. Describe the nursing process for the client with a personality disorder.

KEY TERMS

entitlement

ideas of reference

magical thinking

narcissism

passive-aggressive

personality disorders

personality traits

self-mutilation

splitting

Introduction

Each individual is born with a set of traits, temperament, and patterns of behavior that helps make up their distinctive personality. These inborn qualities are further shaped by the individual's family and peers, interactions with others, and life experiences. Distinguishing aspects of personality are demonstrated in the individual's thoughts, feelings, and attitudes regarding themselves and the world around them. Behavior characteristics are demonstrated in the person's thinking processes, emotional reactivity, interpersonal relationships, and self-control.

Personality traits are persistent ways in which an individual views and relates to other people and to society as a whole. These traits include the way the individual controls their behavior including how they emotionally respond to situations, how they think about themselves or others, and how they relate to other people. People with healthy personalities are able to adapt to life stressors and form interpersonal relationships. Some personality traits are seen as negative. These negative traits tend to be more extreme for the individual with a personality disorder, creating difficulty in their personal and social relationships as well as functioning in regular day-to-day activities.

Personality disorders are deeply ingrained, persistent, inflexible, and maladaptive patterns of behavior that are in conflict with a cultural norm. Unless they become frustrated with their life pattern or relationships, most individuals with a personality disorder are oblivious to their problem. The atypical behavior is usually frustrating or aggravating to those around them, which leads to difficulties in relationships. Most individuals with a personality disorder have demonstrated their uncommon personality characteristics and symptoms by adolescence or early adult life.

Unlike in other mental disorders that have varying intensity of symptoms, the symptoms seen in personality disorders tend to be consistent and constant. The individual rarely seeks treatment because of their inability to identify the problem or denial that a problem actually exists. When treatment is obtained, adherence to the treatment plan is often inconsistent and therefore less successful.

Individuals with personality disorders tend to share some common characteristics that define them as having inflexible and maladaptive behaviors. Because behavior is the result of the way an individual perceives and thinks about the world around them, these characteristics tend to permeate their personal and social lives. The individual tends to view their life in terms of all good or all bad with little understanding that something or someone can have both qualities. In some of the personality disorders, there are characteristics of behaving in an arrogant and self-indulgent manner, with the inability to delay satisfaction of their needs to allow for the wishes or needs of another person. Many of the personality disorders have roots in the way the individual was raised.

Some individuals display **passive-aggressive** behaviors, in which they indirectly and subtly act on hostile feelings by displaying a passive and pleasant affect, but act based on underlying pessimism and bitterness. These behaviors may take the form of self-destructive acts meant to manipulate another person into conforming to the individual's wishes. The individual may project faults onto others to avoid dealing with their own feelings of inadequacy or incompetence. For example, an individual displaying passive-aggressive behavior might avoid deadlines, such as through procrastination or other delay strategies, in order to sabotage the efforts of others. If the passive manipulation fails, the individual may respond with angry emotional outbursts.

There are 10 generally recognized personality disorders, each having a particular set of behaviors and symptoms. They are often grouped by their main behavioral characteristics (Fig. 12.1). In the first group, the behaviors come across as aloof or eccentric, while those in the second group are seen as dramatic, emotional, or erratic. The behaviors seen in the third group are described as anxious or fearful. Psychiatrists will often call these "Cluster A," "Cluster B," and "Cluster C" disorders.

> **Test Yourself**
> ✔ Name and group 10 personality disorders.
> ✔ What are the main behavioral characteristics for each group?

Personality Disorders Characterized by Aloof or Eccentric Behaviors

This group includes paranoid, schizoid, and schizotypal personality disorders. Individuals with these disorders tend to be described as aloof or distant, or exhibit eccentric behaviors.

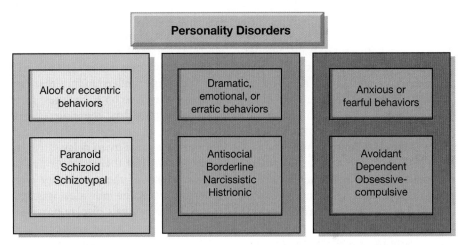

Figure 12.1 Personality disorders grouped according to the particular behavioral characteristics exhibited.

Paranoid Personality Disorder

Paranoid personality disorder is characterized by an individual interpreting the actions of others as intentionally trying to harm, mistreat, or demean them. There is an ongoing mistrust or suspicion of others and their motives for interacting with the individual. This distrust occurs even though there is no obvious reason for their suspicions.

Signs and Symptoms

Individuals with paranoid personality disorders are often viewed as being cold and aloof. Their suspicious nature leads them to be watchful, resentful, and guarded in their interactions with others. They are unable to believe that others can be good to them. A compliment might be perceived as a ploy to secure something in return. A well-intended act of kindness may be viewed as a scheme or an attempt to trick them. There is a reluctance to share personal information with others for fear that it will be used against them later. Angry or hostile outbursts are perceived as necessary to defend against what they interpret as the disloyalty and deceit of others. They are unable to accept constructive criticism, but at the same time are critical of others. Grudges are maintained with no hint of forgiveness for a perceived insult or injustice.

Individuals with paranoid personality disorder usually have a long history of inability to achieve closeness in interpersonal relationships. Many jealous accusations of infidelity and indiscretion are made toward partners or spouses. They attempt to maintain control of the relationship by confronting the partner with demanding questions concerning places they have gone or their intent for going (e.g., vehicle mileage may

be monitored to support the perceived disloyalty). This suspicion is further seen in their projection of blame for their own faults onto others. Their need to counterattack for a perceived injustice often leads to lawsuits against those blamed for the action. Their rigid, inflexible nature prevents any type of mutual agreement to resolve a problem. Although they tend to work better independently, those with paranoid personality disorder are often quite efficient and dedicated to their employment situation. Their interests are often in areas such as electronics, physics, and inventive ideas. Box 12.1 lists common symptoms seen in an individual with a paranoid personality disorder.

> **BOX 12.1**
>
> ### Symptoms of Paranoid Personality Disorder
>
> - Cold and aloof manner
> - Rigid and inflexible
> - Doubts about loyalty and honesty of others
> - Watchful and guarded
> - Resentful, accusing, and argumentative
> - Inability to tolerate criticism
> - Mistrustful and unable to confide in others
> - Feelings that others are out to deceive them
> - Angry or hostile outbursts
> - Maintenance of grudges against others
> - Controlling relationships
> - Extreme jealousy
> - Projection of faults to others
> - Inability to perceive self as a problem

Schizoid Personality Disorder

Individuals with schizoid personality disorder are withdrawn, detached from others or what is going on around them, and demonstrate a lack of ability or desire to form close relationships. They don't tend to show emotions and are therefore often viewed as not caring about other people or what is going on around them.

Signs and Symptoms

Because they are usually absorbed in their own feelings and thoughts, individuals with this personality disorder tend to be indifferent to, or may not enjoy, close relationships and intimacy. They are viewed as being "loners" or "reclusive," and usually choose to pursue solitary activities and interests. The individual with this personality disorder derives little pleasure from things that are widely considered to be soothing and sensuous such as music, romance, or beauty. Sexual experiences are usually not desired. Their facial expression or affect is usually bland and unresponsive to positive emotions in others. Emotions such as elation or anger are seldom felt or displayed and they are indifferent to praise or criticism. Delusional thinking can be precipitated by stressful events. Box 12.2 lists common symptoms seen in an individual with a schizoid personality disorder.

Those individuals with schizoid personality disorder are often described as daydreaming, fantasizing, and without purposeful goals. They are usually oblivious to how their behavior is perceived by others. Working situations that require social interaction are usually avoided. However, they may do well in an employment setting where interaction is not necessary and they can work alone, such as at a night job or in a lab. Their interests are often in the areas of mechanics or art. Most individuals with schizoid personality disorder do not seek treatment, as their behavior does not bother them and they do not see it as a problem.

BOX 12.2

Symptoms of Schizoid Personality Disorder

- Withdrawal and seclusion
- Emotional indifference
- Avoidance of close relationships and intimacy
- Preference for solitary activities
- No interest in pleasurable experiences
- Decreased interest in sexual experiences
- Bland facial expression
- Daydreaming
- Social avoidance

Schizotypal Personality Disorder

Individuals with schizotypal personality disorder also tend to have discomfort with close relationships and social interactions. In addition to being secluded and withdrawn from social situations, they exhibit uncommon patterns of thinking and communicating. They may be described as being "strange" in the way they speak or dress.

Just the Facts — While schizoid and schizotypal personality disorders sound like schizophrenia and have some similar behaviors at times, they are not the same disorder.

Signs and Symptoms

The thinking patterns and opinions of individuals with schizotypal personality disorder are irrational and often have paranoid undertones. These individuals will often display **magical thinking**, or the belief that their thoughts, words, or actions can cause or prevent an occurrence in another person, usually by extraordinary means. For example, they may say they can forecast the future or read the minds of others. **Ideas of reference** are seen, in which the individual believes that everyday occurrences have a special and significant personal meaning. For example, the individual may think a news headline was written specifically for them or that the host of a game show is speaking directly and only to them. Perceptual distortions and illusions are common. Emotions are rigid and inflexible, with limited ability to respond to feelings and expressions of others. Dress habits and mannerisms may be eccentric or unusual.

Increased fear and anxiety are experienced in social situations. This results in a diminished ability to form interpersonal relationships. Those with schizotypal personality disorder are often unhappy about not having social friends and relationships but are unable to overcome their social challenges and suspiciousness of others. Psychotic behavior may occur in brief episodes of minutes to hours. It is believed that this disorder is a mild form of schizophrenia but without the continuous thought alterations. Box 12.3 lists common symptoms seen in an individual with a schizotypal personality disorder.

BOX 12.3

Symptoms of Schizotypal Personality Disorder

- Idiosyncratic thinking and beliefs
- Paranoia and suspiciousness
- Magical thinking
- Ideas of reference
- Perceptual distortions, illusions
- Inflexible emotions
- Eccentric dress habits
- Social isolation
- Remorse over lack of social relationships

Just the Facts

In schizoid personality disorder the individual has an overall disinterest in social relationships, whereas the individual with schizotypal personality disorder has an intense discomfort with close relationships—not a lack of interest in them.

In schizotypal personality disorder, the individual has atypical thoughts and behaviors (such as magical thinking) that are not seen in schizoid personality disorder.

Schizotypal personality disorder typically is apparent during childhood and adolescence. Their unconventional behavior is often the target of ridicule by other children, leading to early social isolation. There is an increased rate seen in those with a first-degree biologic relative with schizophrenia. Treatment is usually sought for coexisting symptoms of anxiety or depression rather than for the symptoms of the personality disorder itself.

Test Yourself

- ✔ How might the individual with paranoid personality disorder act when a coworker gives them a compliment?
- ✔ What are two differences between schizoid and schizotypal personality disorders?
- ✔ What symptoms are seen in both schizotypal personality disorder and schizophrenia?

Personality Disorders Characterized by Dramatic, Emotional, or Erratic Behaviors

This group includes antisocial, borderline, narcissistic, and histrionic personality disorders. Individuals with these disorders tend to be described as dramatic or emotional, or display erratic behaviors.

Antisocial Personality Disorder

Individuals with antisocial personality disorder exhibit a persistent pattern of disregard and

---

TheVisualsYouNeed/Shutterstock

CASE STUDY 12.1

"Raylin"

Raylin is at the college health clinic today for overwhelming feelings of anxiety and panic. She is seated in the far end of the waiting area with a hooded sweatshirt covering her head, her arms folded, and legs crossed with visible shaking noted. As the nurse enters the waiting area and calls her name, Raylin suddenly gets up and runs to the exit door shouting, "Don't hurt me, don't hurt me!"

Digging Deeper

1. *How should the nurse approach this situation?*

2. *What characteristics of a personality disorder are suggested by Raylin's behavior?*

3. *How would feelings of paranoia affect anxiety?*

overstepping on the rights of others, in addition to a consistent disregard for laws, rules, and social norms. A false sense of privilege is demonstrated by indifference to the laws of society and humanity. Initially, the individual comes across as very charming and full of charisma. However, they often behave in a way that appears selfish or lacking conscience to others. Lying and stealing are common, along with a failure to accept or follow through with responsibilities of everyday living, parenting, or work-related tasks. An individual with this personality disorder was previously called a sociopath. A childhood and early adolescence marred with abuse and neglect add to the risk of developing antisocial behaviors in adulthood. The disorder tends to be chronic and one of the most difficult to treat.

Signs and Symptoms

Individuals with this disorder are suspicious and feel betrayed by the world. Thinking that humans are basically evil and out to undermine them, the individual acts impulsively and recklessly to avoid being sabotaged. Vandalism, fighting, explosive anger, and verbal assault are common. Clients with antisocial personality disorder that are hospitalized, whether in a mental health setting or a medical setting, are at risk for harming other clients or staff. Therefore, safety is a priority in the care of this client.

They frequently have a history of school expulsion, truancy, and delinquency. Their interactions with others are often dishonest or deceitful and may involve harming individuals or animals. These actions are done without care for the rights of others or how others may be impacted or feel. An example would be obtaining bank information of a family and emptying the bank account to buy a car. When confronted with the behavior, their response might be, "Who cares? They can just work for more money." Their way of thinking may be described as cold, arrogant, and ruthless, with insensitivity to the feelings of others. An example might be coercing a relative to change their will and leave them all their valuables while leaving other family members with nothing. Their behavior results in continued and frequent encounters with law enforcement officials. Despite the continued conflict with the law, these individuals do not feel remorse or responsibility for the consequences of their behavior or the individuals they have hurt. In their mind, getting caught is seen as a failure

BOX 12.4

Symptoms of Antisocial Personality Disorder

- Suspiciousness of others
- Impulsive and reckless behavior
- Vandalism, fighting
- Explosive anger
- Deceitfulness and dishonesty
- Lying
- Coldness and insensitivity
- Arrogance
- Violation of rights of others
- Lack of remorse or guilt
- Manipulation
- Projection of blame
- Irresponsibility
- Use of alias names
- Charm and scheming
- Recklessness
- Sexual promiscuity and exploit
- Dysphoria

to achieve success. Rarely do they benefit from incarceration or treatment programs. Projection of blame to others is typical as they try to rationalize and minimize their vengeful actions. Box 12.4 lists common symptoms seen in an individual with an antisocial personality disorder.

Individuals with antisocial personality disorder may use alias names, relocate, or change jobs in an attempt to avoid recognition by law enforcement or other regulatory agencies. Little regard is given to dependent or financial responsibilities. They often display superficial charm, smooth conversation skills, and excessive self-assurance as they manipulate others for their personal gain and pleasure. There is a reckless disregard for the safety of others as seen in careless driving, actions that put others in danger, or destruction of property. Exploitive relationships with a lack of concern for partners are common. Unable to tolerate boredom, the individual with antisocial personality disorder may become dysphoric and may look for something stimulating such as sex, alcohol, gambling, or other compulsive self-indulgence activities to compensate for this feeling. Substance use is common, as it helps with feelings of irritability.

Mind Jogger What character(s) in a movie or book would you identify as having antisocial personality disorder?

Incidence and Etiology

Most individuals with antisocial personality disorder have a history of behavioral problems starting before the age of 15. Situations of child abuse, unstable parenting, and inconsistent parental discipline may increase the chances of developing antisocial personality disorder. There is a higher incidence among the prison population and those who have a history of substance use disorder. There tends to be a familial pattern, with it occurring more often in those who have first-degree biologic relatives with antisocial personality disorder. The disorder tends to be chronic but may become less evident as the person ages.

Borderline Personality Disorder

Individuals diagnosed with borderline personality disorder have a persistent pattern of unstable interpersonal relationships, insecure self-image, and mood swings. They often behave impulsively and have intense outbursts of anger. Anger is often preceded by anxiety with a recurrent emotional swing between anxiety, sadness, and anger.

Signs and Symptoms

Individuals with borderline personality disorder often feel a chronic sense of emptiness and abandonment accompanied by continued anxiety and efforts to avoid the perceived rejection. The fear often leads to dependent behavior with rapid attachment to a nurturing partner. Individuals with borderline personality disorder quickly become overinvolved and attached in the relationship, but soon feel threatened that the partner will leave. Without warning, they may suddenly view the caring partner as evil and cruel, pushing them away to avoid future rejection. While rallying between the labile emotional states of self-admiration and self-dislike, the individual with this disorder becomes confused about self-identity. There are intense episodes of dysphoria and irritable moods that may last hours or days. The quick change from clingy and dependent extremes to angry outbursts in a short period of time is typically referred to as a "Jekyll and Hyde" characteristic. This is very frustrating to those who try to befriend them and impairs most of the individual's relationships.

Along with the mood change, the individual usually demonstrates an extreme view, or **splitting**, of their relationship to the world. Things are seen as all or none, black or white, love or hate, with no neutral ground. For example, the loss of a partner might mean to them, "I am a bad person." When a relationship ends, the individual with borderline personality disorder believes it proves their feelings of worthlessness. Dissociation may occur to escape the feeling of being alone. At times, there may be brief episodes of paranoia and

CASE STUDY 12.2

"Ed"

Ed, a 28-year-old, was admitted to the psychiatric unit yesterday under a court order. He has been arrested many times during his adolescent years. His most recent arrest was for driving under the influence of drugs and assault of a police officer. Because this is not his first substance-related offense, he is court-ordered to receive treatment for substance use disorder and anger management.

Ed is charming and good-looking. His manner is convincing as he freely gives polite compliments and makes friendly gestures. Today he tells you that his girlfriend, Maggie, has "gone off the deep end" and that he "dumped her" because she was acting "weird and freaking out." He tells you that he thinks you are attractive and would like to take you out. He asks for your phone number so he can call you when he is discharged. Although you inform him you cannot give him this information, he is persistent. When confronted with his manipulative behavior, Ed becomes enraged and says, "I guess you wouldn't recognize a good thing if you saw it. You're a horrible nurse!"

Kues/Shutterstock

Digging Deeper

1. How should the nurse respond to this situation?

2. Why is limit-setting so important in dealing with Ed's behavior?

3. What safety issues would the nurse anticipate for Ed and for other patients on the unit?

4. What are the chances that Ed will benefit from the treatment process?

hallucinations because their ability to maintain a state of reality is unstable. This is often the time when repeated threats of suicide or self-mutilation are exhibited. **Self-mutilation** is an intentional act of inflicting bodily injury to oneself without intent to die as a result of the injury. It demonstrates an outward focus of control over inner pain and serves to restore the individual's sense of realism and value. Self-injury stimulates a release of endorphins that leads to the release of inner tension. This reinforces and feeds the repetitive pattern of the self-injurious behaviors. The physical pain of the self-injury serves as a coping mechanism that distracts from, and allows, the individual to avoid dealing with the emotional pain. Some of the acts are self-stimulating such as head-banging or cheek-chewing. Other actions may be more intermittent but habitual such as burning and cutting various body sites (Box 12.5), or skin picking the body using fingernails, tweezers, pins, teeth, or other instruments. These behaviors bring a distorted sense of emotional relief to the individual. Although ashamed of their actions, they feel a compelling need to continue the behavior. They may also engage in impulsive behaviors that have the potential for self-destruction such as substance use, gambling, sexual promiscuity, reckless activity, or excessive eating patterns.

Mind Jogger How could self-mutilation be used as a manipulative behavior?

Individuals with borderline personality disorder may demonstrate caring for others, but with an expectation for self-gain. Rarely do they experience any positive emotions of happiness or well-being. If their wishes are ignored, the display of acting-out behaviors demonstrates their inability to delay satisfaction of their needs. These

---

BOX 12.6

Symptoms of Borderline Personality Disorder

- Unstable relationships
- Insecure self-image
- Mood swings
- Dissociation
- Impulsive outbursts of anger
- Chronic sense of abandonment
- Clingy, dependent, manipulative behavior
- Splitting
- "Jekyll and Hyde" characteristic
- Self-mutilating behaviors
- Suicidal threats and gestures
- Inability to delay gratification of needs

---

behaviors are usually in the form of emotional outbursts, impulsive anger, and sarcasm directed at others. They are easily enraged if authority figures do not provide instant response to their wishes. This behavior often tends to undermine their successes because they often quit before a goal is achieved. Multiple employment losses, broken relationships, and unfinished education are common. Box 12.6 lists common symptoms seen in an individual with a borderline personality disorder.

Just the Facts Individuals with borderline personality disorder may engage in additional self-destruction by repeatedly becoming involved in no-win relationships with others who are emotionally unstable or abusive.

Borderline personality disorder is more common in those with a family history of the disorder. There seems to be more instability during the early adult years, with some stabilization of moods seen by the 30- to 40-year-old age-group. The incidence of suicide in this group is the highest during young adulthood.

The exact cause of this condition is not known. It is believed that perhaps instances of parental neglect, separation from the primary caregiver, and child abuse may contribute to development of the disorder. An infant who is suddenly removed from the emotional attachment figure learns that a comfortable trusting relationship is followed by anxiety when that person is no longer available. Trust is lost and the separation is viewed as abandonment. Once the security and comfort of the

---

BOX 12.5

Cutting: What to Look For

- Small, straight cuts
- Frequent injuries with unconvincing explanations
- Low self-esteem
- History of relationship problems
- Isolated and loner tendency
- Razor or knife in bag or purse
- Blood stains on clothing
- Clothing with long sleeves in warm weather

good relationship changes to anxiety in a bad situation, the child learns to see "all good" and "all bad." There is continued difficulty in being able to recognize that these two conditions can occur in the same person. This leads to splitting, in which the individual reacts to people in either a very positive or very negative way.

> **Test Yourself**
> ✔ What would be a priority nursing goal when a client with antisocial personality disorder is admitted to the unit?
> ✔ Identify five self-mutilating behaviors.
> ✔ Give an example of splitting.

Narcissistic Personality Disorder

The term **narcissism** is from a Greek word, meaning "excessive love and attention given to one's own self-image." The individual with narcissistic personality disorder has a continued need for lavish attention and admiration with little regard for the feelings of others. Other people may be used unfairly to satisfy the individual's desires.

Signs and Symptoms

Individuals with narcissistic personality disorder have an exaggerated and grandiose sense of importance. This is exhibited as arrogance and claims of **entitlement,** where they believe others owe them because of their superiority. For example, when shopping for services or merchandise they will ask to see the manager or owner of the establishment instead of a "regular employee," indicating their internally-viewed sense of importance. Any personal achievement is over-exaggerated with demands for praise and approval. They tend to perceive themselves to be superior to others; for example, they may feel they are more powerful, beautiful, and successful than most people and believe they can only be understood by those who are on the same level. They may talk at length about themselves, not realizing that others are not showing an interest in the conversation. Box 12.7 lists common symptoms seen in an individual with a narcissistic personality disorder.

Although individuals with narcissistic personality disorder perceive a superior self-worth, they have an underlying feeling of inferiority and envy of others. They may inwardly resent and dislike those who are awarded more respect or attention and are usually highly sensitive to failure, which results in feelings of insecurity. The overinflation of the self is often overcompensation for their low self-esteem. Because of their extreme sensitivity to criticism, individuals with narcissistic personality disorder may experience

CASE STUDY 12.3

"Maggie"

Bricolage/Shutterstock

Maggie was brought to the emergency department by her mother, who checked on her and found her lying on the bathroom floor bleeding from her arms. She has been seen several times in the past for self-mutilation. She tells the nurse she cut her forearms 28 times with a kitchen knife. She had just discovered that her live-in boyfriend of 2 years had moved out. Her history reveals many broken relationships and four previous suicide attempts, including two overdoses, walking in front of a fast-moving vehicle, and a gunshot wound to her left leg. Before the present incident, she says she telephoned her boyfriend, Ed, who abruptly hung up on her. Her mother tells the nurse that she doesn't understand why this is so upsetting to Maggie. She says that 2 months ago Maggie told Ed to "get lost." In between episodes of crying, Maggie tells the nurse, "I must have done something bad for him to do this. If I were a good person he would still be there." Maggie is now demonstrating symptoms of borderline personality disorder and depression. She has been admitted for suicidal observation.

Digging Deeper

1. *How does Maggie's behavior demonstrate her underlying sense of insecurity?*

2. *How is "splitting" evident in her behavior?*

3. *How should the nurse respond to Maggie's last statement?*

4. *What nursing interventions are important to implement at this time?*

Symptoms of Narcissistic Personality Disorder

- Grandiose sense of self-importance
- Intense need for admiration and approval
- Lack of empathy for others
- Exploitation of others for own needs
- Sense of entitlement
- Demand for the best of everything
- Overexaggerated sense of power, beauty, success
- Underlying feelings of inferiority
- Hypersensitivity to criticism
- Anxiety
- Social withdrawal
- Poor insight into behavior and how it affects others
- Arrogance

Symptoms of Histrionic Personality Disorder

- Attention-seeking behavior
- Extreme egocentricity
- Overdramatic and exaggerated behavior
- Shallow, superficial relationships
- Provocative sexual behavior
- Melodramatic but vague speech
- Manipulation
- Unmet dependency needs

humiliation, intense anxiety, and shame if reprimanded or disappointed. The need for admiration increases to overcome these feelings of being "bad" if they are not receiving attention. They do not have insight into their behavior and unrealistic thinking. Social withdrawal and mood alterations are common during periods of frustration and anxiety.

Mind Jogger How are narcissistic attitudes affected by social media?

Although there is a tendency for adolescents to have a narcissistic view of themselves as they search for their identity, this does not mean that narcissistic personality disorder exists. It is only when the narcissistic traits become inflexible and maladaptive enough to cause dysfunction in the individual's life that a disorder may be diagnosed. Those who develop the disorder rarely seek treatment and often blame the negative results of their behavior on society. Narcissistic personality disorder is more common in men than women and usually has an onset during early adulthood.

Histrionic Personality Disorder

The individual with histrionic personality disorder displays a pattern of egocentric and excessive emotion in a demanding manner to gain personal attention. Individuals with this disorder are uncomfortable in situations where priorities are not focused on them.

Signs and Symptoms

Individuals with this disorder exhibit reactions that are overdramatic in proportion to the situation and may seem fake or exaggerated in their behavior. By creating a scene that gets the attention of others, they usually receive sympathy or affectionate gestures in return. As a result, they may develop attachments easily but tend to be superficial and easily dissatisfied with the relationship. They may also demonstrate unexpected sexual advances in their interactions with others. They often describe their relationships in detail as involving more intimacy than is actually present. A casual acquaintance may be introduced as a best friend or a wonderful, dear person. Provocative dress and mannerisms are often used to draw attention. Speech tends to be melodramatic with numerous hand gestures but is vague and lacking in content. The behavior is a manipulative ploy to satisfy underlying needs of dependency and protection. Individuals with this personality disorder may be easily influenced by others and overly trusting of those perceived as able to solve all their problems. Box 12.8 lists common symptoms seen in an individual with a histrionic personality disorder.

There is a strong association between the disorder and dissociative symptoms. It is also common for these individuals to demonstrate other behaviors such as somatization, manipulative behavior, sexual promiscuity, and self-indulgence. Only when the histrionic traits of the individual become maladaptive and impair functioning is it considered a disorder.

Test Yourself
✔ How is narcissism expressed?
✔ How might the individual with histrionic personality disorder describe a coworker they just started working with?

Personality Disorders Characterized by Anxious or Fearful Behaviors

This group includes avoidant, dependent, and obsessive-compulsive personality disorders. Individuals with these disorders tend to be described as anxious or fearful.

Avoidant Personality Disorder

The individual with avoidant personality disorder is typically shy and very sensitive to negative comments from others. Feelings of inadequacy and intense discomfort are felt in social situations that involve people other than family. They tend not to have any close relationships outside of their family circle, but would like to, and tend to be upset about their lack of relationships.

Signs and Symptoms

Because of their extreme fear of ridicule or disapproval, individuals with this disorder tend to avoid events or situations that involve interaction with others. Educational and work-related opportunities may be rejected out of fear that criticism may follow. They are afraid that others might become aware of their self-doubt and tend to withdraw from relationships if there is a chance these feelings might be exposed. Intense anxiety is experienced when in a group of people. This feeling is linked to those of inferiority and incompetence. Any indication of disapproval will prevent the individual from becoming involved, though they may be encouraged and offered support by others in the group. There is a perception of rejection even when it does not exist. Unless

individuals with avoidant personality disorder are certain of being liked, there is usually an unwillingness to trust the environment. Although they desire to have intimate interpersonal relationships, this guardedness often prevents them from doing so. Shyness and fear of new situations exhibited in childhood tend to increase by adolescence in individuals with this disorder. There is some evidence that it decreases with age. The avoidant behaviors are often associated with social phobia. Box 12.9 lists common symptoms seen in an individual with an avoidant personality disorder.

Just the Facts Dwelling on perceived inadequacies and previous mistakes, the individual with avoidant personality disorder tends to view themselves as inferior in all aspects of life.

Dependent Personality Disorder

Individuals with dependent personality disorder demonstrate a consistent and extreme need to be cared for that leads to a reliance on others. At the same time, they perceive themselves as helpless and incompetent. If one relationship ends, there is immediately a pressing need to begin a new one.

Signs and Symptoms

Those with dependent personality disorder have difficulty making decisions that affect everyday life unless prompted and reassured by others. They relinquish control and priority for their own needs to someone else. Feelings of insecurity and doubt prevent them from making self-care decisions. They may not be able to select items to wear, requiring another to choose their daily attire. Although they may disagree with those caring for them, they do not express these feelings for fear of upsetting the other person. It is not uncommon for them to demonstrate acting-out behaviors to show their inability to make a decision or know what to do in a given situation. They require this constant advice, guidance, and reassurance and are easily hurt by criticism and disapproval.

The individual who has dependent personality disorder will search at length to find relationships where the dependent support will continue. Because of the extreme anxiety experienced when someone is not present to make decisions for them, a replacement figure is needed if a relationship

---

BOX 12.9

Symptoms of Avoidant Personality Disorder

- Extreme shyness
- Hypersensitivity to rejection or negative comments
- Feelings of social inadequacy
- Social withdrawal/isolation
- Self-doubt
- Fear of criticism or embarrassment
- Intense anxiety in social settings
- Feelings of inferiority
- Low self-esteem
- Lack of trust in others
- Lack of close friends
- Fear of intimate relationships
- Reluctance to take risks or try new things

Symptoms of Dependent Personality Disorder

- Inability to make decisions without approval from others
- Extreme reliance on others
- Insecurity and self-doubt
- Extreme fear of being alone
- Excessive anxiety
- Feelings of helplessness and incompetence
- Constant need for reassurance
- Self-sacrificing behavior
- Relinquishment of control to others
- Submissive behavior

ends. Independent or self-initiated involvement in activities is not an option for individuals with this disorder. There is an increased incidence of abuse and surrender that is tolerated in these relationships. Because the individual is so afraid of being alone, the abuse is endured even when help is offered to leave the situation. Their passive nature and fear of abandonment overrides any expression of unmet personal needs. It is one of the most frequently reported personality disorders. Age and cultural factors can contribute to the behavior or can lead to a misdiagnosis. For example, in some cultures, women are expected to be subservient to men. The distinction between what is considered respectful and what is excessive relative to one's culture must be made. Children and adolescents who experience chronic physical illnesses or separation anxiety disorder have an increased risk of developing this personality disorder. Box 12.10 lists common symptoms seen in an individual with a dependent personality disorder.

Mind Jogger ❷ How would the individual with dependent personality disorder react when experiencing "empty-nest" syndrome (the syndrome experienced by a parent when all of their children have grown and no longer live at home)?

Test Yourself
✔ How might the individual with avoidant personality disorder feel about their close relationships?
✔ How might the individual with dependent personality disorder perceive themselves?

Obsessive-Compulsive Personality Disorder

Individuals with obsessive-compulsive personality disorder are conscientious, highly organized, and preoccupied with order and perfection. They are usually dependable but want rigid control and lack the flexibility to allow for compromise. Obsessive-compulsive personality disorder is not the same as obsessive-compulsive disorder (OCD) (Chapter 9). In obsessive-compulsive disorder (OCD) the individual has obsessions (reoccurrence of persistent thoughts that cause them anxiety) and compulsions (repetitive behaviors they engage in to reduce the anxiety), whereas in obsessive-compulsive personality disorder the individual is highly focused on perfectionism and detail. Individuals with obsessive-compulsive disorder (OCD) are usually very aware of their obsessions and compulsions and how those can affect others. In obsessive-compulsive personality disorder, the individual is not self-aware of their behavior, and this can impact their relationships with others.

Signs and Symptoms

Individuals with obsessive-compulsive personality disorder pay excessive attention to details and rules to the point that tasks are left unfinished. For example, a manager is so concerned that specific rules of order be maintained during a meeting that nothing is accomplished. Compulsive individuals tend to insist that their way is the only right way to do things and have a desire to be in charge of situations. As a result, they have difficulty delegating to others, preferring to do the task their way so it is done right. If tasks are assigned, lengthy detailed instructions are given. They are highly critical of others and of themselves if mistakes are made or deviations made from the instructions. It is difficult for individuals with this disorder to feel satisfaction for their accomplishments. They experience high anxiety levels if deadlines or prioritizing are expected of them. If they must rely on others they feel a sense of isolation and helplessness.

Miserly spending and hoarding are often seen, motivated by a refusal to waste or throw away items that "might be needed" at some future time. It is common for items such as magazines or paper sacks to be saved and arranged precisely in piles with all corners exactly in line to perfection. There is an inability to discard items that are worthless or no longer functional. Their need to keep things is often an annoyance to those around them. Individuals with obsessive-compulsive personality

BOX 12.11

Symptoms of Obsessive-Compulsive Personality Disorder

- Preoccupation with orderliness
- Rigidness and controlling behavior
- Focus on details
- Unrealistic expectations, inflexibility
- Missed deadlines
- Inability to relax
- Rigid moral and ethical standards
- Hoarding of items
- Inability to delegate
- Stubbornness
- Miserliness with material things
- Shallow display of emotions

disorder rarely take time off from work for leisure activities or vacation, believing that to do so is a waste of time. Relationships are often more serious and shallow. They believe that public display of emotion or affection is foolish and typically exhibit a limited ability to express feelings or intimacy toward another. Box 12.11 lists common symptoms seen in an individual with an obsessive-compulsive personality disorder.

> **Just the Facts** The person who has an unconscious feeling of powerlessness may attempt to achieve self-control by controlling others.

Individuals with this disorder are often employed in situations such as research where precision and detail are required. They rarely seek treatment because to do so would require change. Any diversion from their rigid nature is highly threatening to them.

Treatment of Personality Disorders

In order for the individual with a personality disorder to be treated, they must first have some type of understanding that their behavior is causing them distress. In most of the personality disorders, the individual does not see their behaviors as the problem and usually seeks treatment for a secondary cause such as depression, anxiety, relationship counseling (at the request of the partner), or substance use disorder. This is often difficult because most individuals with a personality disorder lack

insight to their behavior and how it affects them or others and resist change. If the individual is admitted for an associated mental disorder such as anxiety, depression, substance use, or other mood disorders, they may adhere to treatment for that problem while avoiding the personality symptoms completely. Many individuals with a personality disorder also have trouble trusting others, which leads to difficulty in their social relationships. This factor often prevents them from forming a therapeutic relationship with a health care provider. Their ineptness in social interactions also leads to a poor self-image and feeling of personal despair.

> **Just the Facts** No-harm contracts, journals, and behavior logs can help the individual who self-mutilates or engages in cutting to track their thoughts and behavior patterns. This can prove beneficial by encouraging them to explore ways of regaining self-control.

Various types of psychotherapy are used, including cognitive-behavioral therapy and individual, group, and family approaches. The type used for any given client will depend on the underlying issue and behaviors being identified or addressed. Since many of these individuals have deeply ingrained beliefs and attitudes, they may not feel the need to change their behavior and may resist suggestions that their behavior is an issue and needs self-reflection or changing. Behavioral change done by the individual may revert to the previous pattern of behavior. Reducing environmental stress is often the first step in treatment.

A combination of psychotherapy and medication is the preferred approach to treatment of personality disorders. Medications do not treat the personality disorder or eliminate the behaviors. Medications are used in personality disorders to treat symptoms that cause the individual distress, such as anxiety or depression, which can be treated with antianxiety and antidepressant agents. Thinking errors may improve some with antipsychotic medications such as risperidone and olanzapine.

> **Just the Facts** There are no medications that treat personality disorders. Medications used in treatment only address the co-occurring symptoms such as anxiety.

Typically, treatment also involves family members and friends of the client. Often, the actions of those most closely associated with the individual may affect the behavior issues and are useful in the treatment process. Treating personality disorders is a prolonged process and requires diligent patience and understanding on the part of the therapist and/or family members and friends.

Senior Focus
Medications are used with caution in the older client because of potential side effects and medication interactions. In addition, other medical problems may be affected by these medications. Focus should be on identifying recent stressors that may intensify current behavior problems.

Test Yourself
✔ How might the individual with obsessive-compulsive personality disorder behave when participating in a group project?
✔ What medications are used to treat co-occurring symptoms that may be seen in personality disorders?

Nursing Process and Care Plan *for the Client With a Personality Disorder*

Providing nursing care for individuals with personality disorders is very challenging. The nurse must identify personal feelings about the client's behaviors and maintain a continuous awareness to provide appropriate interventions. Since personality and its associated behaviors are set in the individual early in their life, change of the maladaptive behaviors will take time, if they change at all. Safety is a priority for individuals with a personality disorder.

Assessment (Data Collection)

It is not often that a client is admitted with a personality disorder as a primary cause for treatment. Treatment may be sought by the individual or family members when the maladaptive personality behaviors become problematic and disrupt their life. Other disorders such as depression, maladaptive substance use, or suicide attempt may be the stated reason for admission. It is important to first develop a trusting relationship by using an empathetic and nonjudgmental approach.

Clients with personality disorders are often unaware of how their behaviors affect others. Ask questions that will provide information on their perspective. Use direct questions to find out what events or behaviors led to the admission. Have them describe their current living situation and how they feel about it. Determine their social relationships including who they are close to, who they trust, how they feel about those relationships.

The client with a personality disorder has developed individualized ways of coping. It is important to acknowledge the unique individual that the client is and determine how they cope. This will assist the nurse in determining a focus of nursing care and individualized implementations for the client. Inquire about how the client usually copes with problems and what problem-solving techniques they use. It is important to inquire about the client's culture and how that impacts their communication and coping. Determine if the client uses any substances to help their coping, the type of substance, and the frequency with which they use them. Note any scars or cuts that may indicate self-mutilating behaviors. Inquire about what type of situations occur prior to the self-destructive behavior.

Ongoing data collection regarding coping skills should look at the client's tolerance for frustration, any type of impulsive behavior, their ability to delay gratification, ability to follow unit rules, and any socially unacceptable behavior.

Determine the client's level of anxiety. The client may not be able to verbalize their anxiety so it is important to note any resistance to questioning or indication of impulsive reaction to requested information. Look for inconsistencies between what is said and mannerisms or behavior. Observe nonverbal behavior for signs of anxiety.

Some clients with personality disorders have altered thought processes. Note any ideas of reference or magical thinking. Observe for their affect and note if it is appropriate, flattened, or indifferent. Observe their thought processes for content and clarity, all or none thinking, or narcissistic behaviors or statements.

Determine any risks for safety. Ask if suicidal thoughts have occurred and verify whether a plan has been made. Determine if the client is at risk for cutting or other self-harm behaviors. If old scars from previous cutting or burning events are noted, ask the client what events or feelings led to the cutting. Manipulative behavior may include encouraging other clients to disobey or encouraging others in altercations. It may also include the individual trying to obtain sexual favors from other patients on the unit.

Because clients with personality disorders tend to behave in a way that may be seen as irritating and demanding, it is important for the nurse to recognize and deal with their own feelings toward such clients. The client with a personality disorder can be manipulative and conniving with nurses and other clients. It is important to view the situation objectively. Therapeutic intervention can only occur if self-awareness allows the nurse to project an appropriate attitude of caring and concern for the well-being of the client.

Nursing Care Focus

The specific focus of care depends upon the data collected. Since the client may be admitted with a different diagnosis than the personality disorder, it is important to prioritize the focus of nursing care based upon data collected and take physical needs into consideration. A focus of nursing care may be applicable for more than one personality disorder because many share similar symptoms and problems. However, in several of the personality disorders the individual is at risk for harming themselves or others; therefore, Safety must always be considered as a nursing care focus.

The focus of nursing care for the client with a personality disorder can include: Altered Skin Integrity Risk, Chronic Anxiety, Chronic Low Self-Esteem, Coping Impairment, Fear, Impulsivity, Injury Risk, Risky Health Behavior, Safety, Self-Harm Risk, or Violence Risk.

Outcome Identification and Planning

The nurse should recognize that outcomes for the client with a personality disorder are long-term in nature. Since the maladaptive personality behaviors have been present for much of the client's life, they will not change short-term. Parts of their behavior will never change, but the client may be able to learn more adaptive coping styles and more effective communication strategies. Box 12.12 lists common desired outcomes for a client with a personality disorder.

Changes do not occur quickly and are often not recognizable during the brief treatment

---

BOX 12.12

Common Desired Outcomes for a Client With a Personality Disorder

The client:
- expresses thoughts and feelings appropriately
- increases interaction with others
- exhibits decreased hostility and anger
- participates in unit activities
- conforms to unit rules
- gains control over impulses
- decreases manipulative behaviors
- manages anxiety without acting-out behaviors
- refrains from harming self or others
- identifies precipitating factors of anxiety
- refrains from using splitting or clinging behaviors
- claims ownership of own feelings and thoughts
- verbalizes positive qualities about self
- makes independent decisions about self-care

---

period. The nurse's ability to set boundaries and maintain a therapeutic approach to the behaviors is often one indicator of progress. Short-term outcomes that involve interaction with other clients and impulse control can be evaluated within the confined milieu. The client's behavior following discharge will demonstrate whether actual improvement has occurred. Regardless of efforts expended by the mental health team, the potential for improvement is limited by the deeply ingrained patterns of pervasive behaviors that have developed over time. Unlike an acute medical problem, the maladaptive personality traits are usually hidden to those who exhibit them. They cannot solve the problem because they are unable to identify the reason for the problem.

Nursing Care Focus

- Violence Risk

Goal

- The client refrains from hostile or violent behavior that is directed at others.

Implementations for Promoting a Violence-Free Environment

Ensure that the environment is safe for all clients and staff. Remove objects that may be used as a weapon. Clients with a history of violence may feel that they are entitled to the weapon "to protect themselves." A search of the client and/or their belongings may be needed. Be aware of objects that may not seem like a weapon but could be used as one, such as a ball point pen.

Remind the client that staff is there to ensure it is a safe environment for everyone and will intervene if the client is not able to control their behavior. Explain all unit rules and enforce them fairly and consistently. Be aware that aggression tends to increase when limits or rules are enforced. All staff members need to be consistent and act as a team with enforcing set rules and limits. Manipulative clients will attempt to divide staff or "get permission" from one staff member, especially if the staff member is distracted. Maintain alertness to manipulative behaviors of clients. Do not make exceptions or show favoritism. Communicate problems with manipulative clients to other team members.

If the client becomes hostile, the nurse must refrain from becoming argumentative or defensive and should not take it personally. Anger is a common reaction when limits are enforced and the client does not get their way or is unable to manipulate staff.

Approach clients from the front and speak clearly. This is especially true for the client with paranoia. If the client becomes hostile it may necessary to remove other clients from the vicinity, but do not isolate staff members. Observe and intervene before escalation of behavior occurs. Use time-out for curbing acting-out behavior if client is resistant to redirection.

Require the client to take responsibility for their own behavior. Identify inappropriate behavior and discuss possible alternative behavior with the client. Discuss with the client how their behavior affects others and assist to explore alternative actions. Be aware that clients with a history of manipulation may state that they are willing to change or not harm others but actually will not change.

Evaluation of Goal/Desired Outcome

The client:

- does not engage in violent behavior during hospitalization.
- does not harm others during hospitalization.

Nursing Care Focus

- Self-Harm Risk

Goal

- The client will be free from self-harm during hospitalization.

Implementations for Promoting Safety

Prevention is the first step to helping protect the client from self-harm. Provide a safe environment by removing all objects that can be used for self-injury. Obvious items include eating utensils, cigarettes, and sharp objects such as safety pins. Keep track of all needles used on the unit. Other objects to be monitored include items such as keys, pens, and their internal mechanisms (such as springs or caps that are removable). Items used in recreational therapy such as scissors (even blunt edged ones) need close supervision. Items such as twigs, toothbrushes, and handles from paintbrushes should be confiscated as they can be sharpened for a cutting edge.

Observe the client for self-harm urges or attempts to hide from staff. The client's room should be close to the nurses' desk where the client can be easily observed. Avoid placing the client in a room far away from the nurses' desk.

Be consistent with setting and maintaining limits. Observe for self-harm behaviors when limits are being enforced. If cutting or other self-harm behaviors are noted, encourage the client to discuss events and feelings that occurred just prior to the event. This can help the client to become aware of the connection between the events or feelings and their desire to harm themselves. Encourage the client to identify alternate ways of coping when these events or feelings reoccur. Provide honest and positive feedback to the client when they refrain from hurting themselves. A nonharm contract may be useful for some clients to help them refrain from cutting or other self-harm behaviors. A nonharm contract may be ineffective for the client who is manipulative.

Evaluation of Goal/Desired Outcome

- The client does not harm self during hospitalization.

Cultural Considerations

Personality Disorders and Cultural Ideas of Gender

Since personality disorders are not generally seen for treatment, one question that often arises is "Are some personality disorders seen more often in one gender as compared to another?" Since the rate of personality disorders in the general population is determined based upon those individuals who seek treatment or are admitted for another condition (such as depression or an eating disorder), the actual prevalence rate in the general population is an estimate.

Some personality disorders may be thought of as more typically seen in women such as borderline, histrionic, and dependent, while others are thought to be more typically seen in men such as antisocial or paranoid (Holthausen & Habel, 2018). This may be in part due to cultural stereotypes of men being more aggressive and impulsive, while women might be seen as more emotional and dependent upon others for providing for them. However, this may lead to some personality disorders being overlooked when the behavior does not fit a gendered stereotype.

Cultural views on expected behaviors differ throughout the world. These can include showing submission to another gender, ability to speak to or touch another gender, decision making responsibilities, demonstrating emotions in facial expressions or words, verbal communication (loud vs. soft voice), hand gestures during communication (minimal vs. grandiose hand waving), and handling conflict (avoid or openly confront). This makes observing the individual's behavior through the individual's cultural view very important.

Source: Holthausen, B. S., & Habel, U. (2018). Sex differences in personality disorders. *Current Psychiatry Reports, 20*, 107. https://doi.org/10.1007/s11920-018-0975-y

SUMMARY

- Personality disorders are defined by personality traits and characteristics that are deeply embedded, inflexible, and maladaptive. Although the feelings that accompany the disorder cause misery, the individual usually does not recognize the problem and sees the behavior as normal.
- Failure to identify the problem limits the success of treatment programs and interventions. Most individuals with personality disorders endure a lifetime of unsuccessful attempts to secure stability in their personal and social relationships and encounters.
- Three groups of personality disorders are generally recognized. Regardless of the disorder, commonalities exist between the groups.
- Paranoid, schizoid, and schizotypal personality disorders are in the group that exhibit aloof or eccentric behaviors.
- Paranoid personality disorder is a persistent pattern of suspicion and mistrust in which the actions or motives of others are seen as intentionally threatening or humiliating. Although the suspicious is unfounded, the individual may become hostile and attack without warning.
- Individuals with schizoid personality disorder are withdrawn and secluded, demonstrating an emotional indifference toward social relationships.
- In addition to being secluded and withdrawn from social situations, individuals with schizotypal personality disorder exhibit unusual patterns of thinking and communicating.

- Schizoid and schizotypal personality disorders are not the same as schizophrenia.
- Antisocial, borderline, histrionic, and narcissistic personality disorders are in the group that exhibit dramatic, emotional, or erratic behaviors.
- Individuals with antisocial personality disorder exhibit a persistent pattern of disregard and infringement on the rights of others in a society. A false sense of privileged revenge against others is demonstrated by their basic indifference to the laws of society and humanity. They have a lack of remorse in regards to their effects their actions have on others and are seen as callous.
- Individuals with borderline personality disorder have a persistent pattern of unstable interpersonal relationships, insecure self-image, and mood swings. Impulsiveness, intense outbursts of anger, splitting, and self-mutilation are seen in this personality disorder.
- Splitting describes the way an individual with borderline personality disorder views the world where things are seen in terms of black and white, all or none, love or hate, with no neutral ground.
- A pattern of self-mutilation or self-injury tends to restore the individual's sense of realism and value, demonstrating an outward focus of control over inner pain.
- Narcissistic personality disorder is exhibited by a continued need for lavish attention and admiration with little regard for the feelings of others. Other people may be used unfairly to satisfy the individual's desires.

- The individual with histrionic personality disorder displays a pattern of egocentric and excessive emotion in a demanding manner to gain personal attention.
- Avoidant, dependent, and obsessive-compulsive personality disorders are in the group that exhibit anxious or fearful behaviors.
- The individual with avoidant personality disorder is typically shy and very sensitive to negative comments from others, with feelings of inadequacy and intense discomfort in social situations that involve people other than family. They exhibit an intense fear of criticism or embarrassment, adding to feelings of inferiority and low self-esteem.
- Individuals with dependent personality disorder demonstrate a consistent and extreme need to be cared for that leads to a reliance on others. Viewing themselves as helpless, incompetent, and unable to make decisions; they have a profound insecurity and sense of self-doubt with an extreme fear of being alone.
- Those with obsessive-compulsive personality disorder are conscientious, highly organized, and preoccupied with order and perfection. They are usually dependable, but insist on rigid control and are inflexible without room for compromise.
- Obsessive-compulsive personality disorder is not the same as obsessive-compulsive disorder (OCD).
- Most clients receive treatment for their personality disorder in connection with care received for another disorder, mainly depression, anxiety, and substance use disorder. In many cases, the individual may have engaged in self-destructive behaviors that bring them to the attention of the health care system.
- There are no medications to treat a personality disorder. Medications used are to help the secondary conditions such as depression or anxiety.
- Manipulative, annoying, and disruptive behaviors exhibited by the client can lead to frustration and irritation by the treatment team. Although the maladaptive behaviors are obvious to nurses and others, the individuals with these disorders are often oblivious to the impact their actions have on those around them.
- It is important that boundaries and limits be set and strictly enforced for behavior. Nurses must have an awareness of their own feelings and be alert for the manipulative efforts of the client.
- A therapeutic climate includes the nurse being accepting and nonjudgmental as attempts are made to evoke change in the client who is resistant to the treatment strategies.
- Efforts to implement therapeutic interventions are limited by the individual's deeply ingrained and pervasive patterns of thoughts and behaviors that have developed over time. Improvement can only occur if the client's self-awareness allows them to identify the reason for the problem.

BIBLIOGRAPHY

Caligor, E., & Petrini, M. J. (2021a). Narcissistic personality disorder: Epidemiology, pathogenesis, clinical manifestations, course, assessment, and diagnosis. *UpToDate*. Retrieved July 28, 2022, from https://www.uptodate.com/contents/narcissistic-personality-disorder-epidemiology-pathogenesis-clinical-manifestations-course-assessment-and-diagnosis

Caligor, E., & Petrini, M. J. (2021b). Treatment of narcissistic personality disorder. *UpToDate*. Retrieved July 28, 2022, from https://www.uptodate.com/contents/treatment-of-narcissistic-personality-disorder

Mental Health America. (2022). *Borderline personality disorder (BPD)*. https://www.mhanational.org/conditions/borderline-personality-disorder

Mitra, P., & Fluyau, D. (2022). Narcissistic personality disorder. In: *StatPearls [Internet]*. StatPearls Publishing. Retrieved August 1, 2022, from https://www.ncbi.nlm.nih.gov/books/NBK556001

National Alliance on Mental Illness. (2022). *Borderline personality disorder*. https://www.nami.org/About-Mental-Illness/Mental-Health-Conditions/Borderline-Personality-Disorder

National Institute of Mental Health. (2022). *Borderline personality disorder*. https://www.nimh.nih.gov/health/topics/borderline-personality-disorder

Nelson, K. J. (2021). Pharmacotherapy for personality disorders. *UpToDate*. Retrieved July 28, 2022, from https://www.uptodate.com/contents/pharmacotherapy-for-personality-disorders

Paris, J. (2019). Suicidality in borderline personality disorder. *Medicina*, 55(6), 223. https://doi.org/10.3390/medicina55060223

Skodol, A. (2022a). Borderline personality disorder: Epidemiology, pathogenesis, clinical features, course, assessment, and diagnosis. *UpToDate*. Retrieved July 28, 2022, from https://www.uptodate.com/contents/borderline-personality-disorder-epidemiology-pathogenesis-clinical-features-course-assessment-and-diagnosis

Skodol, A. (2022b). Overview of personality disorders. *UpToDate*. Retrieved July 28, 2022, from https://www.uptodate.com/contents/overview-of-personality-disorders

Zimmerman, M. (2021). *Overview of personality disorders*. Merck Manual Professional Version. https://www.merckmanuals.com/professional/psychiatric-disorders/personality-disorders/overview-of-personality-disorders

STUDENT WORKSHEET

Fill in the Blank

Fill in the blank with the correct answer.

1. _____ _____ are persistent ways in which an individual views and relates to other people and to society as a whole.
2. Magical thinking and ideas of reference are seen in _____ personality disorder.
3. There are no _____ that treat personality disorders.
4. Those who exhibit a sense of _____ feel that others owe them because of their superior and powerful status.
5. _____ is an intentional act of inflicting bodily injury to oneself that demonstrates an outward focus of control over inner pain.
6. A persistent pattern of disregard and infringement on the rights of others is characteristic of _____ personality disorder.

Matching

Match the following terms to the most appropriate phrase.

1. _____ Personality traits
2. _____ Splitting
3. _____ Narcissism
4. _____ Dependency
5. _____ Projection
6. _____ Acting-out behavior
7. _____ "Jekyll and Hyde" characteristic
8. _____ Antisocial
9. _____ Avoidance

a. Defense mechanism in which faults are attributed to others
b. Individual who disregards the rights of others without remorse
c. Withdrawal related to extreme self-doubt and fear of disapproval
d. Aggressive response to underlying negative feelings
e. Extreme view of all good or all bad
f. Persistent ways of viewing and relating to the world
g. Perceived state of helplessness leading to extreme reliance on others
h. Extreme mood shift from clingy dependent behavior to angry outbursts
i. Grandiose sense of self-importance

Multiple Choice

Select the best answer from the multiple-choice items.

1. A client has been admitted with self-inflicted burns to their abdomen. While the nurse is doing wound care, the client states, "I deserve to be in pain." Which of the following best describes the underlying feelings in this statement?
   a. Arrogance
   b. Worthlessness
   c. Suspicion
   d. Egocentricity

2. The nurse notes that a client is monopolizing most of the conversation during breakfast. They are loud and criticizing other clients. What is the appropriate intervention for the nurse to do?
   a. Reprimand them for their inappropriate behavior
   b. Administer medication to calm them down
   c. Put them in seclusion until they can control their actions
   d. Redirect and reinforce limits on their behavior

3. Which of the following statements is true regarding clients with personality disorders? *(Select all that apply)*
   a. They are aware that they have a behavior problem.
   b. Their manipulative patterns often render treatment ineffective.
   c. They have a sincere motivation to change behaviors.
   d. They recognize how their behavior affects others.
   e. They will be treated with medications to minimize the pathologic behaviors.

4. Which of the following behaviors would be interpreted as a form of self-destruction?
   a. Avoiding close relationships and intimacy
   b. Involvement in no-win relationships
   c. Eccentric dress habits and mannerisms
   d. Exaggerated sense of importance

5. An individual who loudly demands to see the manager of a restaurant when they are not seated immediately upon their arrival is displaying which behavior?
   a. Projection
   b. Splitting
   c. Entitlement
   d. Ambivalence

6. What would indicate that the client with a history of cutting is improving? The client:
   a. Tells their roommate when they have urges to cut.
   b. The client states they no longer have any urge to cut.
   c. Notifies a staff member when their discomfort is increasing.
   d. Retreats to their room after another client called them "worthless."

7. A client approaches a staff member with multiple requests and states "I want the charge nurse to fix these now!" What is the best response of the staff nurse at this time?
   a. Explain to the client what requests they will address.
   b. Remind the client that they need to take their requests to their assigned staff member.
   c. Instruct the client to return to the activity room and tell them they cannot leave that area.
   d. Have the client go to their room and think about their behavior.

8. An individual is crying, banging on the counter, and loudly calling out for help in order to attract the attention of a cashier. This behavior is typically seen in which personality disorder?
   a. Schizotypal
   b. Histrionic
   c. Dependent
   d. Obsessive-compulsive

9. Which of the following correctly describes the individual with a narcissistic personality disorder?
   a. Has a profound insecurity, sense of self-doubt, and a fear of being alone
   b. Rigid and controlling with unrealistic expectations and standards
   c. Exhibits unusual patterns of thinking and communicating
   d. May use other people unfairly to satisfy a selfish need for lavish attention

10. Which of the following would be characteristics common to all personality disorders?
   a. Inflexible and maladaptive behaviors
   b. Odd or eccentric behaviors
   c. Cold, aloof, and suspicious tendencies
   d. Ideas of reference displayed in everyday occurrences

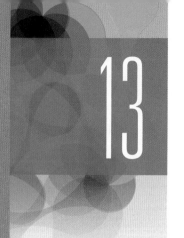

13

Somatic Symptom and Related Disorders

Somatic Disorders

The term used when the individual's concerns and physical symptoms are experienced as a result of significant psychological stress is **somatization** (soma = Greek for "body"). Somatic disorders are those which are characterized by somatization. In somatic disorders, the physical symptoms suggest that a medical condition exists, but often the diagnostic findings do not support a medical diagnosis to explain the symptoms.

The individual with a somatic disorder is not consciously aware of the psychological factors underlying the disorder and does not intentionally continue the symptoms. The symptoms are an involuntary expression of psychological conflict, and the individual is not in voluntary control of the symptoms. Therefore, the somatization that occurs with these disorders is considered a defense mechanism. The somatic symptoms provide a psychological or **primary gain** as the anxiety is relieved and focus is diverted to the physical problem. **Secondary gain** comes from the subsequent attention the person receives from a health care provider or family member. Other defense mechanisms that are used by individuals with this disorder include repression of trauma or conflict, denial that psychological factors exist, and displacement of anxiety and conflict to body symptoms.

> **Just the Facts** Somatic disorders are characterized by disturbances in sensory or motor functioning, while dissociative disorders (see Chapter 14) affect the sense of identity or memory.

Types of Somatic Disorders

Somatic disorders include somatic symptom disorder, illness anxiety disorder (previously called hypochondriasis), and conversion disorder. A condition that is included in somatic disorders, but differs from the others, is factitious disorder. A **factitious disorder** is one where the individual intentionally falsifies, simulates, or creates medical symptoms as though there is an illness when in fact, there is not one, for the sole purpose of primary gain. Factitious disorder is included with somatic disorders because the symptoms appear somatic in nature. The individual may or may not recognize their reason for the somatic symptoms in factitious disorder.

These disorders share the common feature of physical symptoms that suggest a medical condition is the cause, but typically, the clinical findings do not support the existence of a medical issue. The symptoms are severe enough to cause significant distress and dysfunction for the individual in their daily life. The autonomic nervous system response to stress may be associated with an increased awareness of physiologic symptoms such as acceleration of the heart rate, muscle tension, or increased gastrointestinal motility. These symptoms may initially seem to indicate a medical problem for which the individual seeks treatment. The individual is more commonly seen in primary care and medical settings rather than in mental health settings. The somatic disorders are described on the basis of these medically unexplained somatic symptoms plus the emphasis the individual places on the thoughts and feelings. Additionally, the impact the symptoms have on their daily life or functioning must be excessive or atypical to the symptoms.

Individuals with a somatic disorder often have long histories of medical and unnecessary surgical treatments by several different health care providers. This fact, in addition to the somatic nature of the symptoms over which the person has no control, tends to complicate the process of distinguishing the symptoms from actual medical problems. The individual tends to perceive the presence of an illness or injury despite reassurance to the contrary by the health care provider. The impact of the perceived problem can include excessive absences for symptoms or health care visits in addition to impairing job or school performance, finances, and family and social relationships.

Somatic Symptom Disorder

A **somatic symptom disorder** is characterized by one or more somatic symptoms that do not have a medical cause, are disturbing to the individual, and cause disruption in their daily functioning. Individuals typically have multiple somatic symptoms although one—most commonly pain—may be more severe than others. Symptoms may be described specifically, such as localized pain (e.g., abdominal or back pain), or nonspecifically, such as "hurting all over" or fatigue. Typically, these symptoms are not explained or supported by medical testing but continue to cause significant distress for the client. The client's behaviors and distress over the symptoms are often disproportionate as compared to the lack of a diagnosed medical condition.

The client often goes from one health care provider to another seeking a medical diagnosis for their symptoms. Any reassurance from the health care provider that the symptoms are not serious does not give the individual peace of mind and the somatic symptoms continue to exist. Often the person will seek out another health care provider for a resolution to their symptoms. This in turn leads to a series of repeated diagnostic tests and x-ray studies in an attempt to rationalize a medical problem. Clients with somatic symptom disorder also risk the potential hazard of concurrent medical treatments (such as duplicate medications or medication interactions) when seeing several different providers.

Signs and Symptoms

A somatic symptom is considered valid if it has a cause and requires medical treatment (such as medication). In somatic symptom disorder, there are one or more somatic symptoms that cannot be completely explained by medical findings. The individual's description of the somatic symptoms and recurrent thoughts and feelings related to the somatic symptoms are often disproportionate to the objective findings by the medical staff or the medical diagnosis given. Symptoms of persistent moderate to severe levels of anxiety and depression are commonly seen in addition to the somatic symptoms. The individual may or may not have an underlying medical condition, but if the client's concern and behavior indicate excessive mental distress over the symptoms, a diagnosis by the health care provider of somatic symptom disorder may be made.

> **Just the Facts** Chronic pain, regardless of the source, can lead to depression.

The somatic subjective symptoms cannot be controlled by the person and are perceived as real by the person experiencing them. As long as the focus is on the somatic concerns, the origin of the anxiety is not addressed. The primary gain for the individual with somatic symptom disorder is the overshadowing of anxiety by the somatic symptoms, while the secondary gain is often the attention the person receives in response to the symptoms. The individual receives gains from

---

BOX 13.1

Signs and Symptoms of Somatic Symptom Disorder

- Somatic symptoms are those that suggest physical illness or injury, but are unexplained by medical findings
- Recurring somatic symptoms usually continue for several years (may include pain)
- Excessive worry or anxiety over physical health symptoms that is disruptive to the person's life
- Exaggerated belief in the severity of their symptoms and health
- Excessive time is devoted to investigating their health symptoms
- Anxiety and depression

---

both the health care provider–client relationship and personal relationships as they receive attention, empathy, emotional support, and assistance with health care visits or daily tasks. The individual is not aware of these gains and does not consciously seek them out. They may become upset when they feel their symptoms are not being addressed or may interpret the health care provider's unwillingness to perform more tests as "uncaring." Signs and symptoms for somatic symptom disorder are found in Box 13.1.

Incidence and Etiology

The percentage of the United States population affected by somatic symptom disorder is less than 1%. It is seen much more prominently in women than men. Commonly, the individual with somatic symptom disorder also has a medical diagnosis of anxiety, post-traumatic stress disorder (PTSD), or depression. The somatic symptoms may increase the symptoms or severity of the diagnosed conditions. Somatic symptom disorder tends to run in families along with coexisting diagnoses such as anxiety, depression, or substance use. Familial patterns of behavior are often learned and replicated by children and adolescents, especially when those behaviors receive the attention of others. This imitation, as well as differences in the perception and expression of pain, may be factors in the generational tendency.

> **Mind Jogger** How might the secondary gain received by a parent with somatic symptom disorder encourage a child to imitate the behavior?

Illness Anxiety Disorder

Individuals with **illness anxiety disorder** (previously called hypochondriasis) may or may not have a medical condition, but they do have increased body sensations and are extremely anxious about the possibility of an existing serious undiagnosed illness. The individual devotes a great deal of time and energy to researching the health concerns. People with this disorder experience considerable distress over their presumed and undiagnosed health issues and are not readily reassured if no medical problem is found.

Signs and Symptoms

The individual with illness anxiety disorder is preoccupied with the possibility of having or acquiring a serious illness despite reassurance to the contrary. Somatic symptoms are usually absent or of mild intensity. A thorough medical examination usually fails to support the medical condition for which the person has sought medical attention, or if a diagnosable condition exists, the person's concern and anxiety are disproportionate to the disorder itself. The person's distress related to fears and worry about the suspected medical diagnosis is evident. If a physical symptom is present, it usually is a normal physiologic sensation (e.g., positional dizziness or food-related indigestion).

Individuals with this disorder tend to become alarmed and overconcerned when reading or hearing about someone having a health-related problem such as cancer or a contagious illness. Attempts by medical personnel to reassure the individual or suggested home remedies for minor symptoms or concerns do not alleviate their anxiety and fears. They are very aware of their own personal bodily sensations and often misinterpret them as a sign of a serious medical issue. The overconcern and worry about health issues consume the individual's everyday life and become a central theme for their identity and conversation with others. They spend time doing detailed research on their suspected illness and seek continued support and reassurance from family and friends. They may join social media groups related to the perceived illness. Family gatherings and community activities may be avoided as the fear of becoming ill intensifies. The individual often consults multiple health care providers for the same problem and feel they are not taken seriously if negative test results do not support their suspected condition. Signs and symptoms for illness anxiety disorder are found in Box 13.2.

Incidence and Etiology

The actual etiology of illness anxiety disorder is not known. It is suggested that, like in other somatic disorders, the overindulgence in self-concern fulfills a need to satisfy strong dependency needs. The prevalence of this disorder is less than 1% and tends to be similar in men and women, with the peak incidence in the late 30s for men, and late 40s for women. The disorder tends to be chronic in nature, with a pattern that reflects a heightened awareness of body functions with an obsessive preoccupation that a problem exists. Because of the underlying psychological need for dependency, only a few people can associate the somatic symptoms with their mental state. Depression is common as the individual continues to believe their fears and refuses to accept reassurance to the contrary.

Just the Facts

Individuals with somatic disorders who are overconcerned about their symptoms may become dependent on analgesic or antianxiety medication. A pattern of repeat health care provider office and emergency room visits, prescriptions from several providers, and having prescriptions filled at various pharmacies ensures a constant supply of medication.

Mind Jogger ② Clients who repeatedly access the health care system searching for answers often undergo many diagnostic tests and exploratory surgeries. What risks could this pose for the client?

Conversion Disorder

A **conversion disorder** (sometimes called functional neurologic symptom disorder) exists when an individual exhibits symptoms that indicate a sensory or neurologic impairment; however, the impairment is not supported by results of diagnostic testing. Usually, a related stress or trauma factor occurs concurrently with the onset of the symptoms. The somatic symptom is a substitution for a conflict that causes great mental anguish for the individual. The conflict is not apparent initially. Because the symptoms essentially involve voluntary motor or sensory functioning, they are considered **pseudoneurologic**, or false neurologic, disturbances. Examples of this might be a person who loses functional use of their dominant arm and hand before a piano recital they do not want to perform or a parent going blind after witnessing their child being murdered.

Just the Facts ① Family stress and physical or sexual abuse are thought to be the most common causes of conversion disorders in children and adolescents.

Signs and Symptoms

The conversion symptoms are a way to divert attention away from the underlying conflict that causes the individual mental anguish. The transfer of this anxiety to a loss of physical functioning serves as a primary gain for the client. The changes in social, work-related, or family circumstances that result from the temporary disability may provide the secondary gain of avoiding unpleasant tasks or responsibilities along with the accompanying attention the person receives. Individuals with conversion disorder often exhibit an attitude of *la belle indifference,* which is demonstrating little anxiety or concern over the implications of the symptoms.

Motor symptoms may include impaired coordination or balance, paralysis of a limb, inability to speak, difficulty swallowing, or urinary retention. Sensory deficits may involve a loss of pain sensation, visual or hearing malfunction, and hallucinations. Occasionally, episodes of abnormal generalized shaking with apparent loss of consciousness that resemble a seizure may occur, or episodes of unconsciousness that are similar to syncope. Unlike a pathologic seizure, a conversion or **psychogenic** (nonepileptic) seizure will vary from one incident to the other without a distinct pattern of activity and may resemble a seizure that has been described to the individual.

The symptoms seen in conversion disorder differ from actual neurologic deficits in that the

"Jerry"

Jerry is a 30-year-old heavy equipment operator. His wife, Angela, has been a homemaker and mother to their three children for the past 12 years. Now that the children are all in school, Angela has decided to fulfill a lifelong dream and enroll in college classes to become a nurse. She has asked Jerry to help her with the children so she can have more time to study. She feels that once she is a nurse, she can supplement the family income. Three months after Angela begins her classes, Jerry develops severe back pain that requires him to take a leave of absence from work. He undergoes extensive imaging studies, but no medical reason is found for the pain. He states that the analgesics and muscle relaxants just don't seem to help. He requests a referral to a large medical clinic 400 miles from his present location, stating that the local doctors don't seem to want to help him. He also states that he cannot help with caring for the children or household chores because of his back pain. Two months later, Jerry takes a leave of absence from his job and Angela must become the family support. She drops her classes and finds a job as a receptionist for a local insurance agency.

Digging Deeper

1. What underlying psychological conflict may be causing Jerry's symptoms?

2. What are the primary and secondary gains?

CASE STUDY 13.1

BOX 13.3

Signs and Symptoms of Conversion Disorder

- Sensory or neurologic impairment that is not supported by diagnostic testing
- Lack of conscious control over the symptoms
- Loss of balance or paralysis of body part
- Loss of swallowing, speaking, seeing, or hearing
- Loss of pain or touch sensation
- Impaired functioning in social or work-related areas caused by symptoms
- Exhibiting *la belle indifference*
- Inconsistent seizures or convulsion-like behaviors
- Lack of physical change or disability in affected body part
- Functional ability and symptoms inconsistent with usual neurologic disorders

individual's description of the problem does not suggest a dysfunction of the typical nerve pathway. Typically, the symptoms do not lead to any physical changes or disabilities, as are seen in neurologic disorders. There may be an inability to perform a particular movement, but other functions of the body part may be intact. Sometimes the individual will inadvertently move the extremity described as dysfunctional when their attention is temporarily directed away. Although a limb is described as nonfunctional, the neurologic reflexes are intact. Signs and symptoms for conversion disorder are found in Box 13.3.

Mind Jogger ❓ What symptoms usually seen in a pathologic or epileptic seizure might be missing in a conversion, or psychogenic, seizure?

Incidence and Etiology

Conversion disorder may begin at any age but tends to develop during adolescence or early adulthood. The disorder is more commonly found in women. It does not seem to run in families. Childhood abuse, emotional or sexual, is a common finding in the history of an individual with conversion disorder. The incidence varies based upon the population studied and ranges from less than 1% to 5% and is more common in individuals from low-income socioeconomic backgrounds (Peeling & Muzio, 2021).

Adolescents with this disorder often have overprotective parents with a subconscious need to see their child as "ill." The symptoms then become the focus of the family's attention and lifestyle. Conversion disorder tends to be of short-term duration, with most clients recovering in 2 to 4 weeks without reoccurrence.

Factitious Disorder

The term "factitious" stems from a Latin word that means artificial or false. Factitious disorder is where the individual is falsifying having symptoms or an illness for primary gain. This disorder is seen in one of two forms: factitious disorder imposed on self (the common lay term used for this is Munchausen syndrome) or factitious disorder imposed on another (the common lay term used for this is Munchausen syndrome by proxy). When factitious disorder is imposed upon a child, it is often termed "medical child abuse." The primary characteristic of both forms of factitious disorder is the falsification of medical or psychological signs and symptoms of an illness.

Signs and Symptoms

Individuals with factitious disorder deliberately falsify signs and symptoms of illness for the primary purpose of assuming the sick role or the attention they receive from being the caregiver of the "ill" person. They may describe a false history of illness or surgeries and may present falsified lab reports or other documents. The individual may even present "evidence" of a symptom to support their claim, such as putting blood in their urine. The description of symptoms is vague and stereotyped. Absence of typical symptoms that would usually be seen in people presenting with the same medical issue is common (e.g., absence of bacteria in urine with symptoms typical of bladder infection). The symptoms may be intentionally induced in oneself or another. Examples might include exposure to an infectious agent, ingestion of a harmful or toxic substance, or ingestion of excessive medication that guarantees a hospital admission or explorative surgery. The inconsistencies between the client's subjective symptoms, atypical presentation, and the objective findings raise doubts about the legitimacy of the illness. Detailed knowledge of a textbook description of the illness or unusual use of medical terminology by a nonmedical person also indicates the possibility of a factitious disorder. There is usually a long history of frequent health care provider, urgent care, or emergency department visits, along with numerous hospital admissions.

BOX 13.4

Signs and Symptoms of Factitious Disorder

- Deliberate falsification of physical or mental symptoms primarily to assume the sick role
- Inconsistencies between history and findings on objective examination
- Symptoms that are more severe than those seen in others with same "condition/illness"
- Contradicting self when reporting symptoms or medical history
- Extensive knowledge of medical terminology and medical testing procedures
- Being indifferent, or eager, when given plan of care that involves in-depth diagnostic testing and admission
- Symptoms that change once treatment has begun
- Reluctance to have the current health care provider consult prior providers or mental health provider
- Evidence of self-induced physical signs
- Evidence of multiple surgical scars

Adapted from Cleveland Clinic. (2020). *Munchausen Syndrome (Factitious disorder imposed on self).* https://my.clevelandclinic.org/health/diseases/9833-munchausen-syndrome-factitious-disorder-imposed-on-self

The deception is caused by the person's deep-seated emotional need to be seen as ill or injured that provides them with the attention they desire. Although aware of their actions, the person may be unaware of the underlying motivation for the behavior. They resent and reject referrals to mental health professionals. Because the repeated false symptoms tend to build strained health care provider–client relationships, the presence of a real medical condition may be overlooked. Social and family relationships also become disturbed as the focus is constantly drawn to the person's physical well-being. Signs and symptoms for factitious disorder are found in Box 13.4.

Factitious disorder differs from malingering. In factitious disorder, the individual intentionally creates symptoms to remain in the role of client. In **malingering**, the individual is intentionally being deceptive regarding their symptoms or an illness to avoid a situation such as work or incarceration or to gain something such as opioids or disability benefits.

Incidence and Etiology

The incidence of factitious disorder is estimated to be less than 1%. The true rate of this disorder is unknown due to individual's deception, as they often have multiple health care providers, and present to different settings and facilities for their symptoms. A common presentation is arrival at the health care provider's office and hospitals reporting symptoms such as persistent skin rashes or wounds that do not heal, unexplained blood disorders such as anemia and hematuria, or neurologic problems such as numbness of a body part or reported seizures that have only been witnessed by the person reporting them.

Individuals with factious disorder are often women 20 to 40 years of age, who are working in the medical field with a knowledge of how diseases might be acquired or have access to the means with which to accomplish the intended falsification of symptoms. It is thought that a history of abuse, abandonment, or a history of frequent childhood illnesses, especially those requiring hospitalization, may contribute to an individual developing factious disorder. Personality disorder is a common medical codiagnosis.

Treatment of Somatic Disorders

Treatment for somatic disorders consists of both a medical and a mental health approach. Often the primary health care provider is the one who coordinates the care with consultation from a mental health care provider. Scheduling regular outpatient appointments for routine checks is helpful instead of waiting for active symptoms to appear. The client then does not need a symptom to receive clinical attention.

Relaxation training along with cognitive-behavioral therapy (CBT), psychoeducation, short-term psychotherapy, problem solving therapy, antidepressants, and exercise plans have been shown to be effective in the treatment of these disorders. Not all clients with a somatic disorder are willing to receive treatment and may refuse to see or consult with health care providers who indicate this is a mental health issue and not a medical one. Because these disorders tend to reoccur, it is important to recognize that the symptoms can reappear if psychological defenses and coping strategies fail.

For conversion disorder, the first treatment option by the health care provider is education about the diagnosis. This can result in almost immediate recovery for about half of the clients; however, a recurrence is possible (Stone, 2022). The health care provider will evaluate and treat any coexisting depression or anxiety, as these conditions can worsen conversion symptoms. Physical therapy may be needed for the client with a conversion disorder to maintain the functioning of the affected body part.

In factitious disorder, the standard treatment is psychotherapy. Many clients with factitious disorder, however, do not follow up with mental health care providers. Since clients with factitious disorder often have a coexisting diagnosis of anxiety, depression, or a personality or psychotic disorder, they should also receive the standard treatment for those disorders as well.

Test Yourself	✔ How does factitious disorder differ from illness anxiety disorder? ✔ Describe *la belle indifference*. ✔ How do actual seizures differ from psychogenic seizures?

Nursing Process and Care Plan *for the Client With a Somatic Disorder*

Because the somatic disorders are associated with physical symptoms, the client is often first seen by a health care provider for the subjective symptoms. Before a somatic determination is made, physical examination and diagnostic testing are necessary to determine any underlying medical condition for which the individual may need to be treated. It is of major importance that nursing observations and data collection contain information that will be of help in this process. It is challenging for health care professionals to recognize that the client with somatic symptom disorder or illness anxiety disorder is unaware of possible underlying psychological issues and is unable to consciously control the symptoms. In factitious disorder, the false illness behavior is conscious and intentional, but is considered to have an unconscious psychogenic origin.

Assessment (Data Collection)

It is important for the nurse to first create an accepting, safe, and supportive atmosphere that allows open communication with the client and their family. This accepting environment encourages the client to express feelings and needs more honestly. The nurse should focus on the whole person, including psychological, social, and family factors, in addition to the physical symptoms.

A careful data collection of reported physical symptoms and the accompanying behavior should be made, taking into consideration any statements made by the client, thoughts and feelings about the symptoms, and the way they are expressed. Note any preoccupation with the symptoms and any inconsistency between what is being described and what is observed in the client. Inquire about the client's thoughts and expectations about the symptoms.

Elicit any pattern of repeatedly reported symptoms by taking a history of current and past health status. Because most clients with somatic symptoms are frequent users of both outpatient and inpatient health care services, it is important to include a history of previous symptoms, hospital admissions, surgeries, and current medications along with a medication history. Document the type and amount of medications the client is taking.

It is important to note the client's attitude toward the symptoms and how they may view any limitations caused by them, including occupational, recreational, and social activity limitations. It should also be noted whether the client is aware of events surrounding the onset of symptoms. In addition, the client's level of stress or anxiety and previous coping skills should be noted. Questions should be asked to determine whether the symptoms have imposed any limitations related to their lifestyle and whether the client's role has changed within the family system. Any behavior that indicates an increased dependency need, such as repeatedly turning on a call light for assistance, should also be noted and documented.

The health care provider may have the client complete a PHQ-9. This is a 9-item self-administered questionnaire that is designed to both screen for and monitor somatic symptoms (Appendix A).

Just the Facts	Secondary gains may be determined by asking questions concerning any previous work or activity the client is now unable to perform as a result of the symptoms. The nurse can also ask in what way the client's life has been altered by the symptoms.

Nursing Care Focus

Planning care for the client with a somatic disorder must consider that the client is often frustrated and angered by the implication that the symptoms are psychological. The focus of nursing care,

CASE STUDY 13.2

"Angelica"

Krakenimages.com/ Shutterstock

Angelica has a history of chest pain that radiates to her arms and unrelenting back pain. She has been to four different health care providers attempting to find an answer to her repeated bouts of chest and back pain. Despite an extensive diagnostic work-up by a cardiologist that revealed no cardiovascular abnormalities or problems, Angelica is convinced that she has angina. She believes it is only a matter of time before she has a major heart attack. Last week, her employer stated her leave of absence has lapsed and she must either return to work or lose her job. Rather than face having to work every day, Angelica decided to quit her job and tells her spouse that she is afraid to overwork her heart by going to work every day. Angelica refuses to go to family gatherings or outings with their friends, stating she will get too tired and start having chest pain. Today, Angelica comes into the emergency department stating, "I know I am having a heart attack. The pain is in my chest, then goes down my arms and back. What do I have to do to get someone to listen to me?" During data collection, Angelica tells the nurse there have recently been a lot of layoffs where she worked and that her department was in the process of reorganization before she quit because of her cardiac problems.

Digging Deeper

1. *What data should the nurse gather related to the symptoms Angelica is experiencing?*

2. *What underlying feelings may be contributing to Angelica's anxiety and somatic symptoms?*

3. *What secondary gain does Angelica receive from the physical symptoms?*

---

once a medical condition has been ruled out, is on the client and their behaviors, not on the symptoms. The focus of nursing care for the client with a somatic disorder may include the following: Chronic Anxiety, Denial, Chronic Pain, Coping Impairment, Altered Body Image Perception, or Insomnia.

Outcome Identification and Planning

Once the focus of nursing care has been identified for the individual client situation, planning will include realistic outcomes during treatment. The overall goal for the client with a somatic disorder is to reduce health anxiety and the behaviors related to the symptoms, rather than eliminating the symptoms entirely. Goals related to improving occupational and interpersonal functioning are important.

The client will need to address the unrecognized anxiety before the somatic symptoms are resolved. Recognition of the cause of their symptoms is an ongoing and time-consuming process, so goals need to be realistic in terms of the time it will take to achieve them. Focusing on the somatic symptoms as an outcome should be avoided as the symptoms provide distraction from the underlying cause of the disorder. Box 13.5 lists some common desired outcomes for the client with a somatic disorder.

BOX 13.5

Common Desired Outcomes for a Client With a Somatic Disorder

The client:
- expresses feelings of anxiety and positive means of coping with the anxiety
- acknowledges understanding and perception of present health problem
- discusses present health problem with health care provider and family
- acknowledges that physical pain may be associated with psychological stress
- participates in development of a plan for effective pain control
- participates in a graduated exercise plan
- expresses positive feelings about self
- identifies positive coping strategies to use
- performs self-care needs independently and willingly
- verbalizes understanding of psychological factors associated with alteration in physical functioning
- reports a decrease in sleep-related problems
- participates in social activities and interaction
- reduces statements that demand a focus on self and physical symptoms

Nursing Care Focus

- Altered Health Maintenance, related to preoccupation with perceived illness

Goal

- The client will exhibit a decrease in somatic concerns.

Implementations for Improving Health Maintenance

Establishing a trusting relationship with clients experiencing a somatic disorder is the first step in helping them to improve their health maintenance. Reassure the client that their concerns about symptoms and illness have been heard and will receive appropriate attention. It's important that the client feels their concerns are understood and not dismissed as "all in their head." A safe and supportive environment helps to lower their anxiety to a level that allows expression of underlying feelings. Respond to the client with understanding and patience. It is important for the nurse to identify and come to terms with any anger or negative feelings related to clients with a somatic disorder. This ensures that the nurse is non-biased in their interactions with the client.

To assist the client in improving health maintenance, the nurse should avoid confronting the client concerning the psychological defense nature of their symptoms and minimize time and attention given to physical symptoms. To help the client shift their focus from somatic symptoms, the nurse should help the client to use words rather than physical means to express feelings. One way to do this is to encourage the client to keep a diary of daily happenings and feelings, along with physical symptoms. Give the client positive feedback when they take responsibility for situations related to them or verbalize their feelings instead of making a somatic reference. Since the client is used to focusing on somatic symptoms for attention, the nurse should schedule uninterrupted one-on-one time with the client. Help the client to identify positive diversion activities that they enjoy. Help the client to identify positive coping mechanisms to utilize when stressed or anxious rather than focusing on somatic symptoms.

Evaluation of Goal/Desired Outcome

The client will:

- identify two positive coping strategies to use instead of focusing on a somatic symptom.
- keep a diary of their interactions, feelings, and physical symptoms.
- identify two diversion activities they can perform instead of focusing on their somatic symptoms.

Nursing Care Focus

- Activities of Daily Living (ADL) Deficit, related to perceived loss of function or paralysis of body part

Goal

- The client will return to a functional state in self-care activities.

Implementations for Improving Activities of Daily Living (ADL) Functioning

It is important to let the client with a conversion disorder know that although their body is not working properly, they can improve as there is no structural damage. However, avoid giving false reassurance such as "There is nothing to worry about," or nontherapeutic statements such as "It's only in your mind."

The nurse should encourage the client to discuss their life history, recent emotional events, and fears. If the client is reluctant to talk about these topics, encourage journaling as a substitution. Have the client participate in diversionary activities that they enjoy. The nurse should help the client explore and practice coping strategies such as progressive relaxation, breathing exercises, and problem-focused coping strategies.

Compare an affected limb to the unaffected one and perform neurologic checks including temperature, color, pulse, and capillary refill. Perform range of motion to an affected limb to help preserve function. Assist the client with physical or occupational therapy exercises as prescribed. These implementations help monitor the affected site and prevent any harm from lack of use.

Encourage the client to perform activities of daily living (ADLs) as much and as independently as possible. Provide only minimal assistance and intervene only if the client is at risk for injuring themselves. The nurse should minimize attention given to the client's impairment and the supervision of the client's activities of daily living (ADLs). Point out to the client their strengths and abilities that are observed.

Evaluation of Goal/Desired Outcome

- The client will perform activities of daily living (ADLs) independently.

CASE STUDY 13.3

"Angelica" (continued)

9 nong/ Shutterstock

Remember Angelica from Case Study 13.2. She has been admitted to the medical unit as an inpatient for observation and cardiac monitoring. She has been given a sedative for her anxiety.

Digging Deeper

1. What nursing interventions are important in addressing Angelica's reported symptoms?

2. What is the best approach to her physical concerns?

3. What information will be important to document?

Cultural Considerations

"Tell Me How You Feel"

Cultures express somatic symptoms in different forms, terms, and illnesses. Expressions that may be different from a North American and European viewpoint include:

- Placing an emphasis on the body
  - China, Japan, Papua New Guinea, aboriginal Australia, and West Africa.
- Emphasizing somatic symptoms rather than emotional states
  - Many Chinese idiom expressions involve body parts (examples include "to have one's heart in one's mouth", "shock the heart", "drop the gallbladder").

- Having a term that does not have an English translation.
  - "seselelame," which might translate to "feel-feel-inside-the-body" used in West Africa
- Having culture-bound syndromes that are somatic idioms of distress.
  - neurasthenia (literally meaning "weakness of nerves") seen in China
  - "Hwa-byung" (fire or anger illness) seen in Korea
- Using more somatic expressions when relating distressing experiences (Korea)
- Common to many of these cultures is a focus on harmony and holism.

Sources: Choi, E., Chentsova-Dutton, Y., & Parrott, W. G. (2016). The effectiveness of somatization in communicating distress in Korean and American cultural contexts. *Frontiers in Psychology, 7*, 383. https://doi.org/10.3389/fpsyg.2016.00383; Ma-Kellams, C. (2014). Cross-cultural differences in somatic awareness and interoceptive accuracy: A review of the literature and directions for future research. *Frontiers in Psychology, 5*, 1379. https://doi.org/10.3389/fpsyg.2014.01379

S U M M A R Y

- Somatic disorders are characterized by the transfer of anxiety or psychological conflict into somatic (physical) symptoms with atypical focus placed on their symptoms. Typically seen in medical nonmental health settings, individuals with these disorders may or may not have a diagnosed medical condition.

- The individual with a somatic disorder is not consciously aware of the psychological implications of their disorder. The symptoms are involuntary and are not consciously controlled.
- Somatic symptoms provide a psychological or primary gain as the anxiety is relieved and focus is

diverted to the physical problem. Secondary gain comes from the subsequent attention the individual receives from a provider or family members.

- Somatic symptom disorder is characterized by one or more somatic symptoms that have no medical cause, are disturbing to the individual, and cause disruption in their daily functioning. Unexplained by medical testing, the symptoms continue to cause significant distress for the individual. The disproportionate distress caused by the atypical thoughts, feelings, or behaviors related to the symptoms is the primary factor in the health care provider's diagnosis of this condition.

- Illness anxiety disorder is characterized by an excessive fear or preoccupation with having a serious illness that is based on a misinterpretation of somatic signs and symptoms. Excessive time and energy are used by the individual in researching the suspected health concern. Despite medical testing and reassurance that a disease does not exist, the individual continues to experience fear and distress over the symptoms. Access to health care for verification of their fears results in a pattern of changing health care providers in an attempt to find one who will confirm their perceived illness.

- Conversion disorder consists of a sensory or neurologic impairment that is not supported by diagnostic testing. There is a lack of conscious control over the symptoms. Individuals with this disorder may exhibit an attitude of *la belle indifference*, where they demonstrate little anxiety or concern over the implications of their symptoms.

- In factitious disorder, the key feature is the deliberate falsification of medical or psychological signs and symptoms, or the induction of an injury or disease to oneself or another without obvious external benefits. The deceitful behavior is done with the primary purpose of assuming the sick role. The individuals with this disorder invest much time and many resources through unnecessary medical visits, laboratory testing, and hospital stays.

- Treatment of somatic disorders includes anxiety reducing techniques such as relaxation training, cognitive-behavioral therapy (CBT), psychoeducation, short-term psychotherapy, problem solving therapy, antidepressants, and exercise.

- The goal of treatment is to develop a trusting relationship with the client and family that will foster an understanding of somatization. Interventions are planned to help the person acknowledge the anxiety issues and their connection to the somatic symptoms. Once this occurs, the resolution of the symptoms will hopefully follow as more effective coping strategies are employed.

- Somatic disorders tend to reoccur. If the underlying emotional conflict is confronted and resolved, the reoccurrence tends not to happen.

BIBLIOGRAPHY

Carnahan, K. T., & Jha, A. (2022). Factitious disorder. In *StatPearls [Internet]*. StatPearls Publishing. Retrieved May 27, 2022, from https://www.ncbi.nlm.nih.gov/books/NBK557547

Dimsdale, J. E. (2020a). *Factitious disorder imposed on another*. Merck Manual Professional Version. https://www.merckmanuals.com/professional/psychiatric-disorders/somatic-symptom-and-related-disorders/factitious-disorder-imposed-on-another

Dimsdale, J. E. (2020b). *Factitious disorder imposed on self*. Merck Manual Professional Version. https://www.merckmanuals.com/professional/psychiatric-disorders/somatic-symptom-and-related-disorders/factitious-disorder-imposed-on-self

French, J. H., & Hameed, S. (2022). Illness anxiety disorder. In *StatPearls [Internet]*. StatPearls Publishing. Retrieved May 27, 2022, from https://www.ncbi.nlm.nih.gov/books/NBK554399/

Gokarakonda, S. B., & Kumar, N. (2022). La belle indifférence. In *StatPearls [Internet]*. StatPearls Publishing. Retrieved May 27, 2022, from https://www.ncbi.nlm.nih.gov/books/NBK560842/

Irwin, M. R., & Bursch, B. (2021). Factitious disorder imposed on self (Munchausen syndrome). *UpToDate*. Retrieved May 27, 2022, from https://www.uptodate.com/contents/factitious-disorder-imposed-on-self-munchausen-syndrome

Levenson, J. L. (2020). Illness anxiety disorder: Epidemiology, clinical presentation, assessment, and diagnosis. *UpToDate*. Retrieved May 27, 2022, from https://www.uptodate.com/contents/illness-anxiety-disorder-epidemiology-clinical-presentation-assessment-and-diagnosis

Levenson, J. L. (2021a). Somatic symptom disorder: Assessment and diagnosis. *UpToDate*. Retrieved May 27, 2022, from https://www.uptodate.com/contents/somatic-symptom-disorder-assessment-and-diagnosis

Levenson, J. L. (2021b). Somatic symptom disorder: Epidemiology and clinical presentation. *UpToDate*. Retrieved May 27, 2022, from https://www.uptodate.com/contents/somatic-symptom-disorder-epidemiology-and-clinical-presentation

Peeling, J. L., & Muzio, M. R. (2021). Conversion disorder. In *StatPearls [Internet]*. StatPearls Publishing.

Retrieved May 27, 2022, from https://www.ncbi.nlm.nih.gov/books/NBK551567

Roesler, T. A., & Jenny, C. (2020). Medical child abuse (Munchausen syndrome by proxy). *UpToDate*. Retrieved May 27, 2022, from https://www.uptodate.com/contents/medical-child-abuse-munchausen-syndrome-by-proxy

Stone, J. (2022). Conversion disorder in adults: Treatment. *UpToDate*. Retrieved June 23, 2022, from https://www.uptodate.com/contents/conversion-disorder-in-adults-treatment

Stone. J., & Sharpe, M. (2021). Conversion disorder in adults: Epidemiology, pathogenesis, and prognosis. *UpToDate*. Retrieved May 27, 2022, from https://www.uptodate.com/contents/conversion-disorder-in-adults-epidemiology-pathogenesis-and-prognosis

Stone. J., & Sharpe, M. (2021a). Conversion disorder in adults: Clinical features, assessment, and comorbidity. *UpToDate*. Retrieved May 27, 2022, from https://www.uptodate.com/contents/conversion-disorder-in-adults-clinical-features-assessment-and-comorbidity

Todd, S. E. (2014). *Factitious disorder imposed on self (Munchausen's syndrome)*. Medscape. http://emedicine.medscape.com/article/291304-overview

STUDENT WORKSHEET

Fill in the Blank

Fill in the blank with the correct answer.

1. _____ is when the individual's concerns and physical symptoms are experienced as a result of significant psychological stress.
2. The attention the person with a somatic disorder receives from providers and family in response to the symptoms is referred to as _____ _____.
3. In a conversion disorder, the transfer of anxiety into a loss of physical functioning serves as a _____ _____ as the emotional conflict is avoided and relieved.
4. The lack of concern or anxiety over the implications of functional loss in the person with a conversion disorder is known as _____ _____ *indifference*.
5. A nonepileptic or nonpathologic seizure is called a _____ seizure.

Matching

Match the following terms to the most appropriate phrase.

1. _____ Factitious disorder
2. _____ Conversion disorder
3. _____ Malingering
4. _____ Illness anxiety disorder
5. _____ Somatic symptom disorder

a. Intentionally being deceptive regarding one's symptoms or an illness to avoid a situation or to gain something
b. Fear of having a serious illness based on a misinterpretation of somatic symptoms
c. Characterized by one or more somatic symptoms that do not have a medical cause but are disturbing to the individual and cause disruption in their daily functioning
d. Sensory or neurologic impairment not supported by medical testing
e. Intentionally falsifying, simulating, or creating medical symptoms as though there is an illness when in fact, there is not one, for the sole purpose of primary gain

Multiple Choice

Select the best answer from the multiple-choice items.

1. A client with illness anxiety disorder would most likely make which statement?
   a. "I don't eat much because I will have diarrhea if I do."
   b. "I can't understand why no one can find out what is wrong with me."
   c. "I know I have colon cancer just like my dad."
   d. "I just don't have the energy I used to."

2. A client was functioning without difficulty until today when they suddenly developed numbness in their right arm. No apparent reason is found for the paralysis. Which of the following is correct regarding this somatic disorder?
   a. The cause is related to actual neurologic dysfunction.
   b. The symptoms represent a primary gain for the client.
   c. The client is aware that the cause of the paralysis is emotional.
   d. The client will be greatly concerned by the inability to use their arm.

3. Which intervention is appropriate for the client with a somatic symptom disorder? *(Select all that apply)*
   a. Providing diversion from the sick role to other more productive activities
   b. Supportive interventions that focus on dependency needs
   c. Confronting the client about their underlying feelings of anxiety
   d. Observing for inconsistency between the client statements and client behavior
   e. Focusing on details of the somatic symptoms

4. A client has been repeatedly seen in the clinic for severe lower back pain that radiates down their left leg. Prescription medication has not relieved the pain and diagnostic testing does not indicate a medical cause. What would be a therapeutic nursing intervention for this client? *(Select all that apply)*
   a. Acknowledge that their symptoms are real to them.
   b. Refocus the client on other concerns and problems.
   c. Confront the client with normal diagnostic findings.
   d. Document the client's pain medication on the communication board by their bedside.
   e. Have the client keep a detailed record of the leg pain.

5. Which statement made by the client would be seen in factitious disorder?
   a. "I don't know why the doctor wants to do more tests; I just want to go home."
   b. "I really need the pain medication so I can go back to work."
   c. "I would like the doctor to run more tests; I don't mind staying in the hospital."
   d. "I don't know why my heart is beating so fast all the time."

6. Which of the following is true regarding a client with a somatic disorder?
   a. The client has an awareness of the psychological factors underlying their symptoms.
   b. The client's anxiety and feelings are effectively resolved.
   c. The client's anxiety is relieved as focus is diverted to a physical problem.
   d. The client acknowledges that a disease may not exist.

7. Which of the following poses the most significant mental health risk to the client experiencing chronic pain?
   a. Sleep disturbances
   b. Depressed mood
   c. *La belle indifference*
   d. Lack of attention

8. During a routine clinic visit, a client tells the nurse they suddenly experienced an inability to use their left arm. They are unable to initiate movement upon command. Which of the following observations would alert the nurse to a possible conversion disorder?
   a. The client rotates their left wrist for nurse to take radial pulse.
   b. The client's spouse demonstrates serious concern over the symptoms.
   c. The client extends their right arm for the nurse to take blood pressure.
   d. The client states their friend had the same problem.

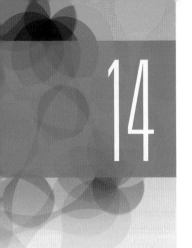

14 Dissociative Disorders

Dissociation

Dissociation is the mechanism that allows an individual's mind to separate certain memories, most often of unpleasant situations or traumatic events, from conscious awareness. These separated parts are repressed (kept in the unconscious) and may re-emerge at any time. Repression, a common defense mechanism, may keep painful thoughts and memories buried until a situation is encountered that is similar to the original trauma. The individual cannot prevent or control the reoccurrence of these thoughts. However, because the unconscious mind also contains learned behaviors, they can go on "automatic pilot" to carry on with routine activities of daily living such as driving a car, parenting, reading, or cooking.

All people have occasional periods of dissociation. For example, while driving a car, they suddenly realize that they don't remember what has happened during the commute. Or, while listening to someone talk, they realize that they did not hear part or all of what the person said. In these examples of dissociation, the individual's everyday activities are not disrupted, and this is sometimes called normative dissociation. It is nonpathologic. It is similar to the absorption that an individual may experience when watching a movie or deeply engrossed in reading a book. In these cases, the absorption (or dissociation) is even pleasurable.

> **Just the Facts** Dissociation, or the "not me," is used unconsciously to minimize or avoid certain events or experiences to decrease the anxiety that accompanies them.

The dissociative disorders are characterized by disturbances in conscious awareness, memory, identity, or view of oneself in relation to the environment. Oftentimes these disorders occur as a response to severe or long-term trauma or abuse. This is because the brain is believed to process and store traumatic events in a different, more distant, way than it handles and maintains everyday or pleasant memories. The mental disturbance may be sudden or gradual; it may be intermittent or chronic. This disorganization causes significant interference with the person's general functioning, social relationships, and work environment. The disruption of functioning is characterized by a dissociation, or interruption, in the ability to recognize personal information such as identity, background, and family history. The person's cultural background plays an important part in regards to what symptoms are seen.

Types of Dissociative Disorders

There are three types of dissociative disorders commonly seen. These are dissociative amnesia (which includes dissociative fugue), dissociative identity disorder, and depersonalization/derealization disorder. These disorders are often seen after an individual has experienced some type of trauma; therefore, the individual may also have a medical diagnosis of post-traumatic stress disorder (PTSD), borderline personality disorder, depression, or anxiety.

Dissociative Amnesia

Dissociative amnesia is characterized by an inability to remember important personal information, usually of a traumatic or stressful nature. This lack of recall includes a loss of information beyond ordinary forgetfulness. The void may cover the entire scope of the person's life or may be confined to certain details related to the traumatic event itself. The four different types of dissociative amnesia are listed in Box 14.1.

Signs and Symptoms

Localized amnesia usually occurs within a few hours following the traumatic incident. This acute form is more common in response to events such as war combat, natural disasters, or severe trauma. For example, a mother who experiences the activity of a tornado may not remember the hours immediately following the storm that has destroyed her home and taken the life of her child. The mother retains an overall understanding of who she is but forgets fragments of the experience.

> **BOX 14.1**
>
> ### Types of Dissociative Amnesia
>
> - Localized amnesia: Usually occurs within hours after incident
> - Selective amnesia: Retention of overall identity, but fragments are forgotten
> - Generalized amnesia: Inability to recall any aspect of one's life
> - Continuous amnesia: Inability to recall any aspect of identity, both past and present

BOX 14.2

Common Signs and Symptoms of Dissociative Amnesia

- Inability to recall portions or all of memory or identity inconsistent with normal forgetting
- Depression
- Anxiety
- Depersonalization
- Trance state
- Loss of sensation
- Impaired social and occupational relationships
- Suicidal gestures or acts

In **selective amnesia**, a person retains memory of some portions of the event, but not all details are remembered. The woman whose home was destroyed by the tornado may remember the storm but not that her child was killed by flying debris. A person with **generalized amnesia** is unable to recall any aspect of their life. **Continuous amnesia** encompasses a period up to and including the present that is lost from conscious recollection. Common signs and symptoms of dissociative amnesia are found in Box 14.2.

 Just the Facts The person with amnesia usually appears alert and may give no indication to observers that anything is wrong.

Incidence and Etiology

Dissociative amnesia can occur in any age group from children to adults. The main manifestation is a gap in memory for past events that may cover minutes or years. There has been a recent increase in incidence, perhaps because of more awareness and newer therapeutic approaches that address traumatic childhood memories. An individual can have more than one episode of amnesia in their lifetime. Some individuals claim amnesia symptoms to avoid accountability for personal actions.

Dissociative amnesia is not part of dementia. In dementia there are gaps in the individual's memory that may return and then disappear again. However, in dementia there is a progressive degeneration of the individual's memory, thinking, reasoning ability, and ability to perform daily tasks. This degeneration of cognitive functions is not seen in dissociative amnesia.

 Just the Facts Using the mental mechanism of dissociation can change an individual's ability to look at themselves and their actions objectively and prevent them from making positive changes in their behavior. Providing a safe and nondemanding environment encourages the client to reconnect with the feelings and perhaps painful events that underlie the mental escape of dissociation.

"Elizabeth"

Elizabeth is a 23-year-old married mother of 2-year-old twin boys. Despite her ability to state her first name, she is unable to recall her last name or that she is married and has a family. Her spouse states that 3 weeks prior to the onset of the symptoms, "Elizabeth was in a bad car accident. The other vehicle was thrown into the path of a semi-truck and the mother and two children in it were killed on impact. After the accident she was treated for minor cuts and released from the local hospital."

Now, several weeks after the accident, Elizabeth is unable to recall any details of the accident or recognize her spouse or the twins as being familiar to her. She has been spending most of her days laying on the couch and has not attempted to care for the boys or to interact with them since the accident. Her spouse is afraid she will never "come back to them."

Digging Deeper

1. How are Elizabeth's symptoms characteristic of localized amnesia?

2. What is the best way to approach Elizabeth?

3. How can the nurse help Elizabeth's spouse cope with the present situation?

CASE STUDY 14.1

Mind Jogger ❓ What approach would the nurse use to initiate a therapeutic relationship with the client who is experiencing amnesia?

Dissociative Amnesia With Dissociative Fugue

Dissociative amnesia with **dissociative fugue** is demonstrated by the inability to recall some or all of a person's past or identity, accompanied by the sudden and unexpected travel of the person away from home or place of employment. The person often assumes a new identity in the new geographic location. Travel may include simple short trips for a few hours or days, or more extensive travel across many miles over a period of weeks or months. The person usually does not demonstrate outward indications of a psychological problem and adapts to a new social setting without being noticed. Box 14.3 lists common signs and symptoms seen in dissociative fugue.

Signs and Symptoms

Although people with dissociative fugue forget their name, family, and where they live, they seem to remember things unrelated to their identity, such as how to drive a car or how to read. When they suddenly return to their former self, they are unable to remember the time of the altered identity or the fugue itself. This escape from their identity is usually caused by a traumatic event that has resulted in severe psychological stress, none of which they are able to remember. Most cases of fugue are seen in adults and occur during times of disaster or periods of environmental or personal chaos when there is an actual threat of death, injury, or loss. It is important to recognize that this type of dissociation may also occur in people who

---

BOX 14.3

Common Signs and Symptoms of Dissociative Amnesia With Dissociative Fugue

- Inability to recall some or all of one's past or identity
- Sudden travel away from home
- Assumption of new identity
- Mood swings
- Anxiety
- Grief
- Shame or guilt
- Suicidal behaviors

---

are trying to avoid a legal, financial, or unwanted personal situation. This is referred to as **malingered fugue** and is especially relevant in forensic or criminal activity.

Most cases of the disorder are brief—hours or days—with most people experiencing full recovery. A person typically recovers abruptly from dissociative fugue in a state of disorientation and dismay with no recollection of what happened during the time they were in the fugue state or how they got to the unfamiliar place. They may be picked up and questioned by law enforcement authorities. Some resistant amnesia can persist for an extended period of time. The extent and length of the fugue may result in a loss of employment or severely disrupt marriage and family relationships.

Test Yourself
✔ Define dissociation.
✔ Name the four types of amnesia.
✔ How might dissociative fugue be similar to, or confused with, malingering?

Incidence and Etiology

Less than 0.5% of the population is diagnosed with dissociative fugue. However, its prevalence may increase during times of extremely stressful events. These can include the impact of war and combat, events such as a terrorist attack, or natural disasters such as severe hurricanes, earthquakes, or tornadoes.

Dissociative Identity Disorder

In **dissociative identity disorder** (formerly known as multiple personality disorder), two or more distinct identities or personalities are present in the same person. These identities alternate in assuming control of the person's behavior. In addition, there is an inability to recall important personal information that cannot be explained as simple forgetfulness. People with this disorder are unable to connect various aspects of their identity with the past and the present, resulting in fragmentation of the original personality. It is believed that people with severe sexual, physical, or psychological abuse during childhood are predisposed to the development of this disorder. The child who endures severe stress may be unable to integrate all of their experiences into one cohesive identity. An intolerable traumatic event at a time when the psychological defenses are inadequate to deal with

"Art"

Art is a 47-year-old division dean of a university extended campus location. He is married and the father of two teenage children. He has been active in campus and community affairs, including assisting with productions of the local amateur theater. Art is scheduled to board an 8:15 AM flight to meet a professional colleague in a city 300 miles from his hometown. At 9:00 AM the day after his intended arrival, the colleague notifies the university and Art's wife that Art did not arrive on his scheduled flight. When his wife checks with the airport, she is told that her husband never boarded the flight. Art's car is found at the airport with the keys locked inside.

Several months pass, and investigators have uncovered no clues as to Art's whereabouts or what may have occurred in his disappearance. One day, Art walks into his office at the university accompanied by an unfamiliar woman whom he introduces as his wife. It is apparent to the office personnel that he does not recognize them or his previous position in the division office. He states that a young man saw him at a restaurant in a neighboring state and told him about his real identity. Art states he has no recollection of the institution or his family. He is admitted for treatment in a state of severe anxiety with suicidal ideation.

Digging Deeper

1. What symptoms indicate that Art is experiencing a dissociative state?

2. What type of dissociative disorder do Art's symptoms suggest?

3. How should the nurse approach Art when discussing past traumatic events?

CASE STUDY 14.2

---

the anxiety may result in dissociation of the event and feelings associated with the memory, resulting in the split of the personal identity.

Signs and Symptoms

The dissociated part of the personality takes on characteristics of its own. This subpersonality learns to deal with feelings and emotions that could overwhelm the primary personality. Each personality character may appear as if it has a distinct personal history, self-concept, identity, and name with its own memories, behavior patterns, and social relationships that are evident when that personality is in control (Box 14.4). These behavior patterns may include aggression,

---

BOX 14.4

Fragmented Personality States of Awareness Seen in Dissociative Identity Disorder

- Original personality is usually unaware of the alternate personalities.
- Alternate states are aware of the original one and have varying awareness of each other.
- Alternate personality states often display traits that are foreign to the original personality, such as a giddy, extroverted personality in a person who is naturally very shy.

---

sexual promiscuity, pleasure seeking, or childlike fearfulness. Only one personality is manifested at a time, with one of them usually being dominant during the course of the illness. Psychiatrists refer to this main personality as the "host" person. This primary or host personality usually assumes the person's given name and is passive, dependent, self-blaming, and depressed; it is often the personality that seeks treatment. The host is unaware of the other states during their dominance, but the others may be aware of each other to some extent. The alternate identities usually emerge in a pattern and are often in conflict and critical of the others. The changing of one personality to the other usually occurs very abruptly and is referred to as the **switching process**. This switch is most often triggered by psychosocial stress and may be preceded by behaviors such as rapid eye blinking, facial changes, changes in voice and persona, or a sudden break in the continuity of thought processes. The number of identities can range from as few as two to as many as 100. Box 14.5 lists the common signs and symptoms of dissociative identity disorder.

Persons with this disorder experience memory gaps for both recent and remote memory. The passive aspects of the personality tend to have less recall, whereas the more hostile and controlling states retain a more complete memory. Sometimes an identity that is not in control will introduce auditory or visual hallucinations to gain control of the conscious state, such as a voice that criticizes the present identity for something they are doing.

Mind Jogger How would a person with dissociative identity disorder differ from one who has a personality disorder?

Incidence and Etiology

Dissociative identity disorder is very rare and the prevalence ranges from 0.5% to 2% of the population having this disorder. It is diagnosed more frequently in adult women. Women tend to have more identities than men. The disorder tends to run a lengthy and chronic course from symptom recognition to diagnosis, with the average onset during the early school years. The disorder is less pronounced after age 40. People with this disorder often report a history of severe physical and sexual abuse, particularly during childhood. There is some question that these memories may be distorted, especially if the trauma occurred during periods when imaginary and fantasy play is considered normal. Many times, however, the abuse is validated by actual evidence such as scars from the trauma.

Depersonalization Disorder

Depersonalization is a persistent and repetitious feeling of being detached from one's mental thoughts or body. The person with this disorder has a feeling of not recognizing themselves or is unsure about their personal information and identity. The person may sense that their body is imaginary, in an altered state, or disappearing. They may say that it is like they are watching a movie of themselves.

Just the Facts Individuals with depersonalization report feeling like robots or being an outside observer of their body and thoughts, yet fully aware they are really not detached or living in a dream.

Signs and Symptoms

People who have this disorder are socially dysfunctional because of the intensity imposed by the feelings of detachment. In **derealization**, the person perceives the external environment as unreal or changing. They may see other people as mechanical but be able to recognize the illogical nature of these feelings. There may also be accompanying anxiety, panic, depression, or obsessive and somatic complaints. The person may perceive an unusual change in the size or shape of objects, or people may seem unfamiliar and mechanical. People with this disorder may not seek treatment until adolescence or early adulthood, although symptoms may have been present since childhood. The condition tends to be chronic with recurrent brief episodes related to traumatic or stressful events in the person's life. The episodes or feelings of detachment may occur periodically or continuously. Signs and symptoms for depersonalization/derealization disorder are listed in Box 14.6.

Incidence and Etiology

The prevalence of depersonalization as a chronic disorder is unknown. It is estimated that perhaps half of all adults may have experienced a single brief episode of depersonalization, usually precipitated by severe stress or life-threatening situational experience. This feeling can also occur with sleep deprivation or after taking certain mind-altering drugs such as marijuana, hallucinogens, ecstasy, or PCP.

> **Just the Facts**
>
> The individual experiencing depersonalization retains insight and is aware that the experience is not real, but rather a feeling of being unreal. The ability to recognize this distinction differentiates it from being a psychotic episode.

> **Test Yourself**
>
> ✔ Which individuals might be predisposed to dissociative identity disorder?
> ✔ What is the difference between depersonalization and derealization?
> ✔ What can be a causative factor for depersonalization/derealization disorder?

Treatment of Dissociative Disorders

Many people with dissociative disorders achieve complete recovery without treatment. Treatment is sought only if the disorder persists, causes the person considerable anguish, or disrupt the individual's everyday activities. Diagnostic testing must be done to determine if there are any coexisting mental health conditions or substance use disorder involved. Antianxiety medications and antidepressants may be useful for symptoms of anxiety or depression associated with these disorders.

Various types of psychotherapy are the usual approach to the dissociative states. Cognitive behavioral therapy can allow the person to talk and identify the underlying negative thoughts associated with the traumatic events. Understanding that these thoughts determine resulting behavior can aid the individual in realizing that changing the way one thinks about a situation can also lead to a more positive behavior outcome. Some therapists use hypnosis to aid in recollection of events and feelings associated with repressed trauma. Other forms of therapy include creative art processes to facilitate expression of feelings and thoughts. All types of psychotherapy are intended to help the person work through the trauma that triggered and resulted in the dissociative symptoms.

Nursing Process and Care Plan *for the Client With Dissociation*

Nurses are faced with a challenging and frustrating task of accepting the client's dissociative behavior while trying to understand the complex nature of the dissociative states. Providing a safe and trusting environment with acceptance and support assists the client to develop a sense of power and self-control. The client must also come to understand the relationship between the dissociative state and the anxiety they feel when they remember past trauma or the anxiety caused by being unable to recall parts of their personality or events experienced.

In dissociative identity disorder, progress centers on the client's acknowledgment of the existence of more than one personality and how these various states function as protection from the anxiety related to traumatic memories. It is also important to note the client's progress toward the ultimate goal of integrating all personalities into a single personality.

Assessment (Data Collection)

During the data intake process, any physical condition that could produce the symptoms of amnesia and dissociation must be ruled out by the health care provider. Collect data from the client regarding any past or current symptoms of a head injury, epilepsy, brain disease, medication side effects, or substance use disorder. The health care provider will also rule out any psychotic disorders such as schizophrenia, determine any significant childhood or adult trauma, and perform psychological tests to evaluate the authenticity of the client's symptoms.

Collect data on the client's level of orientation or disorientation, level of anxiety, statements regarding amnesia, any symptoms of depression, and the extent to which functioning in the social and work environment is affected. It is important for the nurse to describe the client's behavior and verbalized statements because clients with dissociative disorders can present ambiguous pictures or personalities to various staff members.

Nursing Care Focus

From the data collected, identify the individual needs of the client. A client with dissociative amnesia or depersonalization may have more anxiety than the client with dissociative identity disorder. Safety is an important focus of nursing care in the client with dissociative identity disorder as a different personality may pose a harm risk to themselves or to others. The focus of nursing care for the client with dissociation could include any of the following (depending upon data collected): Acute Anxiety, Acute Confusion, ADL Deficit, Altered Body Image Perception, Memory Impairment, or others as identified.

Outcome Identification and Planning

Outcomes for the client with a dissociative disorder vary based upon the symptoms seen, the distress the symptoms cause the client, and the impact the symptoms have on their day-to-day functioning. Also, the time frame in which a realistic expectation can be anticipated for symptom resolution differs with the type of dissociative disorder. In some clients, the timeline is days and for others it may be years. For example, a client with localized amnesia may be able to recall the events within a few hours to a few days and then work on the anxiety caused by the event, whereas the client with dissociative identity disorder has an ultimate goal of integrating the fragmented personalities into one identity which may take years. Box 14.7 lists common desired outcomes for the client with dissociation.

Nursing Care Focus

- Acute anxiety, related to inability to recall stressful events

---

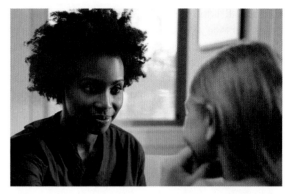

Figure 14.1 The nurse uses a variety of techniques to build a therapeutic relationship with a client.

Goal

- The client will verbalize their anxiety related to the event is at an acceptable level.

Implementations for Managing Anxiety

The nurse must first establish a trusting and supportive therapeutic relationship with the client (Fig. 14.1). It is important to use active listening and communication techniques that encourage verbalization of feelings, conflicts, and information regarding the traumatic events that led to the current dissociative state. This process assists the client to develop personal insight and an awareness and understanding of the self and behaviors that are related to the event. The nurse assists the client to develop alternative plans for coping with their anxiety.

It is important to note, and share with the client, the progress the client has made toward identifying and demonstrating a more adaptive response to stressful stimuli. This step is helpful in decreasing the dissociative response. Clients need encouragement and support to achieve control over their anxiety and previous dissociative response to those situations that trigger the symptoms. People with these disorders are overwhelmed with fear of not knowing or being out of control.

Nursing interventions for managing anxiety focus on recognizing anxiety triggers, reducing anxiety to a manageable level as identified by the client, and promoting positive coping skills. Encourage the client to keep a daily journal of thoughts and feelings. This will help them to identify situations or stimuli that might be a trigger for the anxiety. Assist the client to identify environmental stressors that trigger the dissociative symptoms. When the client identifies that they are feeling anxious, have them also identify any physical symptoms they may

---

BOX 14.7

Common Desired Outcomes for a Client With a Dissociative Disorder

The client:
- Associates memory deficit with past stressful events.
- Recovers memory deficits.
- Identifies improved coping mechanisms to deal with stressful events.
- Verbalizes reality-based perception of environmental stimuli in stressful situations.
- Verbalizes understanding of multipersonality states and the need to consolidate all the personalities into one.
- Performs self-care activities independently.
- Verbalizes feelings and identifies positive and effective ways of managing fear and anxiety.
- Demonstrates self-control over behaviors toward self and others.

be having. This helps them to be aware of their response and how a trigger may make them feel.

Assist the client in developing effective coping skills. For example, if the client notices in their journal that every time they see fire that their heart races and their palms sweat, the nurse can have them practice breathing or grounding exercises that can help lower their heart rate. The nurse can also use therapeutic questions to have the client discuss what it is about fire that causes these symptoms.

Evaluation of Goal/Desired Outcome

The client will:

- report that their anxiety is at an acceptable level for them.
- identify two coping mechanisms they can use when feeling anxious.

Nursing Care Focus

- Memory Impairment related to inability to recall details of stressful event.

Goal

- The client will recall details of the event without becoming overwhelmed.

Implementations for Improving Memory

The nurse's first implementation is to establish a trusting and nonjudgmental relationship with the client. This allows the client to recall information at their own pace instead of feeling pressured. Using therapeutic communication, inquire about previous life events that were both pleasurable and stressful. Explore previous coping strategies the client used in both types of situations. The nurse can have the client utilize previous positive coping strategies to help them with the current situation.

Decrease anxiety-producing stimuli that are identified by the client. Use stimuli that stimulate pleasant memories and pleasurable feelings for the client. This assists the client to remember past experiences without the risk of precipitating increased trauma. Help the client to understand that periods of increased anxiety are to be expected as details are remembered and will decrease as coping strategies are utilized.

The nurse should avoid flooding the client with details of the traumatic event. The client may be overwhelmed with all the details that they are not prepared to work through. Flooding may cause the client to regress further into the dissociative state that is serving to protect them from the emotional pain.

Evaluation of Goal/Desired Outcome

- The client recalls details of the traumatic event.

"Phillip"

Monkey Business Images/ Shutterstock

Phillip has just arrived in his hometown after recovering from shrapnel wounds received during military action. He is brought to the emergency room after he was found wandering on a boat dock incoherent and bleeding from his wrists. When asked his name, it is obvious that he has no recollection of his identity or what he was doing on the pier. However, when asked about recent events in his life, he states he attended class at the high school the day before. When Phillip's family is located, they tell the nurse that Phillip is 26 years old and has not attended high school in 8 years. Once his lacerations are treated, Phillip is admitted to the mental health unit with a diagnosis of dissociative generalized amnesia.

Digging Deeper

1. What feelings may be responsible for Phillip's attempted suicidal acts?

2. Why is it important to obtain information from the family about Phillip's likes, dislikes, activities, or hobbies?

3. What is the purpose of reintroducing things and people from his past that represent pleasant experiences for him?

4. Why is it important not to flood Phillip with information about his recent war injury?

CASE STUDY 14.3

Cultural Considerations

Two Different Viewpoints

There are two ways to view dissociation. One is from the Western/psychiatric viewpoint which sees it as a psychological issue, which is triggered by a traumatic event or after taking a drug. The second way is from an anthropologic standpoint that views dissociation as a way for the individual to express themselves in a culturally appropriate manner or as part of a religious, spiritual, or healing ritual.

In the anthropologic view, the individual can even "suspend" their normal self, or social norms, and express new or forbidden feelings and behaviors. An example of this would be a sudden expression of spirit possession where the individual calls another person derogatory names or expresses dissatisfaction with their environment. Because of the spirit possession, the individual wasn't in control of what was said and therefore cannot be held accountable but was able to vocalize what couldn't be said directly. Another example would be a possession trance that is attributed to the influence of a spirit, power, or a deity. Dissociation in some religious rituals may even be viewed as a positive experience. In these anthropologic examples, dissociation is not related to trauma or a biologic imbalance and may not be viewed as a negative or anxious experience by the individual.

Sources: Seligman, R., & Kirmayer, L. J. (2008). Dissociative experience and cultural neuroscience: narrative, metaphor and mechanism. *Cult Med Psychiatry*, *32*(1), 31–64. https://www.ncbi.nlm.nih.gov/pmc/articles/PMC5156567/#; Minow, L. R. (2020). Dissociation as an alternative state of consciousness? A call for a holistic view of dissociation in psychiatry. *[anthro]metronom*. https://www.anthrometronom.com/post/dissociation-as-an-alternative-state-of-consciousness; Lewis-Fernández, R., Martínez-Taboas, A., Sar, V., Patel, S., & Boatin, A. (2007). The Cross-Cultural Assessment of Dissociation. In: Wilson, J. P., & Tang, C. S. K. (Eds.), *Cross-Cultural Assessment of Psychological Trauma and PTSD. International and Cultural Psychology Series*. Springer. https://doi.org/10.1007/978-0-387-70990-1; Somer, E. (2006). Culture-bound dissociation: A comparative analysis. *Psychiatric Clinics of North America*, 213–226. https://www.academia.edu/3342113/Culture_Bound_Dissociation_A_Comparative_Analysis

SUMMARY

- The dissociative disorders are characterized by an interruption from the conscious acquaintance with identity, personal background, and family history. These disorders are most often seen in people who have experienced severe trauma or abuse.
- Dissociation is the mechanism that allows the mind to separate these traumatic memories from the conscious awareness. These repressed memories can resurface at any time, usually triggered by environmental factors. The recall of these thoughts cannot be controlled or prevented by the client when they are occurring.
- Dissociative amnesia is a localized amnesia that occurs shortly after an incident where the person retains an overall understanding of who they are but forgets pieces of the identity picture.
- When dissociative amnesia is accompanied by sudden travel away from home or place of employment with the establishment of a new identity, it is referred to as a dissociative fugue. The person functions in this new location without drawing any attention to the false identity. When the fugue is terminated, the person may return home with no recollection of the events before or during the fugue.
- Dissociative identity disorder is when two or more distinct identities or personalities are present in the same person and alternately assume control of the person's behavior. Treatment of dissociative identity disorder may be extensive and focuses on reintegration of the personalities into the original personality.
- Depersonalization occurs with a persistent and repetitious feeling of being detached from one's mental thoughts or body.
- Treatment of dissociative disorders involves psychotherapy to help the individual recapture the feelings and thoughts associated with the trauma toward understanding how these are connected to their current behavior and symptoms.
- Before beginning any treatment, the nurse must first establish a trusting and supportive therapeutic relationship with the client.

BIBLIOGRAPHY

Foote, B. (2022). Dissociative identity disorder: Epidemiology, pathogenesis, clinical manifestations, course, assessment, and diagnosis. *UpToDate*. Retrieved May 27, 2022, from https://www.uptodate.com/contents/dissociative-identity-disorder-epidemiology-pathogenesis-clinical-manifestations-course-assessment-and-diagnosis

Loewenstein, R. L. (2018). Dissociative amnesia: Epidemiology, pathogenesis, clinical manifestations, course, and diagnosis. *UpToDate*. Retrieved May 27, 2022, from https://www.uptodate.com/contents/dissociative-amnesia-epidemiology-pathogenesis-clinical-manifestations-course-and-diagnosis

Mitra, P., & Jain, A. (2022). Dissociative identity disorder. In: *StatPearls [Internet]*. StatPearls Publishing. Retrieved June 2, 2022, from https://www.ncbi.nlm.nih.gov/books/NBK568768/

National Alliance of Mental Illness. (2022). *Dissociative disorders*. https://www.nami.org/About-Mental-Illness/Mental-Health-Conditions/Dissociative-Disorders

Pietkiewicz, I. J., Bańbura-Nowak, A., Tomalski, R., & Boon, S. (2021). Revisiting false-positive and imitated dissociative identity disorder. *Frontiers in Psychology, 12*, 637929. https://doi.org/10.3389/fpsyg.2021.637929

Simeon, D. (2019). Depersonalization/derealization disorder: Epidemiology, pathogenesis, clinical manifestations, course, and diagnosis. *UpToDate*. Retrieved May 27, 2022, from https://www.uptodate.com/contents/depersonalization-derealization-disorder-epidemiology-pathogenesis-clinical-manifestations-course-and-diagnosis

Spiegel, D. (2021a). *Depersonalization/derealization disorder*. Merck Manual Professional Version. https://www.merckmanuals.com/professional/psychiatric-disorders/dissociative-disorders/depersonalization-derealization-disorder

Spiegel, D. (2021b). *Dissociative amnesia*. Merck Manual Professional Version. https://www.merckmanuals.com/professional/psychiatric-disorders/dissociative-disorders/dissociative-amnesia

STUDENT WORKSHEET

Fill in the Blank

Fill in the blank with the correct answer.

1. _____ is the mechanism that allows an individual's mind to separate certain memories, most often of unpleasant situations or traumatic events, from conscious awareness.
2. When certain memories are removed from conscious awareness, the separated parts are _____ in the unconscious and may resurface at any time.
3. In dissociative identity disorder, the main personality is referred to as the primary, or _____.
4. The changing of one personality or the _____ process in dissociative identity disorder usually occurs very abruptly and is most often triggered by psychosocial stress.
5. A persistent and repetitious feeling of being detached from one's mental thoughts or body is referred to as _____ disorder.

Matching

Match the following terms to the most appropriate phrase.

1. _____ Fugue
2. _____ Localized amnesia
3. _____ Malingered fugue
4. _____ Depersonalization
5. _____ Derealization

a. Acute inability to recall personal information shortly after a traumatic event
b. Persistent feeling of being detached from one's mind or body
c. Seeing the external environment as unreal or changing
d. Sudden travel from one's home setting accompanied by the inability to recall one's past
e. Inability to recall one's past accompanied by unexpected travel to avoid unwanted situation

Multiple Choice

Select the best answer from the multiple-choice items.

1. A woman who claims to be the client's biologic sister visits him in his home. She tells him that he has a family in another location. When she asks him why he doesn't come home, he replies, "I'm sorry, but I don't know who you are." The client is demonstrating symptoms of:
   a. Derealization
   b. Malingering
   c. Dissociative fugue
   d. Depersonalization

2. Alice has been admitted to the psychiatric unit with a diagnosis of dissociative identity disorder. The nurse observes that during interaction with other clients, Alice is laughing and quite talkative. When the nurse approaches Alice to administer her medications, Alice slumps her shoulders as she looks away with tears in her eyes and says in a childlike voice, "Are you going to hurt me?" What is the nurse's best response in this situation?
   a. "You were laughing a minute ago. What happened to Alice?"
   b. "These medications are to help Alice feel better."
   c. "I'll come back later when you feel better."
   d. "Why do you think I am going to hurt you?"

3. The client has dissociative amnesia. What is an appropriate expected outcome for this client?
   a. Client will discuss past experiences that occurred at time of amnesia
   b. Client will verbalize thought processes that are not detached
   c. Client will demonstrate an understanding of the role of each personality
   d. Client will function independently in all self-care activities

4. The nurse is addressing past memory deficits with a client who has a dissociative disorder. To avoid flooding the client, what it is important for the nurse to do?
   a. Instruct the client to focus on the current stress factors
   b. Reorient the client to time, place, and person at each contact
   c. Observe for cues that the client is ready to revisit the traumatic incident
   d. Include details of the traumatic events surrounding the memory loss in the first session

5. A client tells the nurse a rather confusing story of recent events surrounding her symptoms of amnesia. What is the most therapeutic response made by the nurse?
   a. "You must be very angry that it is difficult for you to remember this."
   b. "You seem to overreact each time you try to talk about this."
   c. "Let me see if I correctly understand what you are telling me."
   d. "We will try this again when you can tell the story like it happened."

6. A client states she is married and has three children but cannot recall that she recently had an infant who died from sudden infant death syndrome. The nurse would recognize this as:
   a. Localized amnesia
   b. Selective amnesia
   c. Generalized amnesia
   d. Continuous amnesia

7. Which of the following would be true of the primary or host personality in the person with dissociative identity disorder?
   a. Usually dominant and critical of the others
   b. Often in conflict with other personality states
   c. Is aware of all alternate personalities
   d. Demonstrates a passive, dependent, and self-blaming personality

8. A client describes recurring feelings that they are "out of their body" and sees themselves as fragmented with disconnected body parts. What would this client likely demonstrate?
   a. Inability to recall all or most of past identity
   b. Being oriented to person
   c. Sudden and unexpected travel
   d. Alternate personality states

6. Which of the following are symptoms of derealization? *(Select all that apply)*
   a. Perceiving the external environment as unreal or unchanging
   b. Seeing other people as robots
   c. Recognizing the distorted thoughts as illogical
   d. Seeing an unusual change in the size of objects
   e. Being unsure of their identity

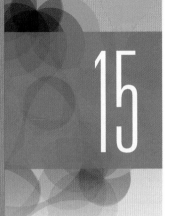

15 Substance Use and Addiction

LEARNING OBJECTIVES

After learning the content in this chapter, the student will be able to:

1. Define terminology related to substance use disorder and addiction.
2. Describe the four phases of substance dependency.
3. Describe factors that contribute to substance use disorder and addiction.
4. Identify 10 classes of substances commonly used and misused.
5. Describe substances from each class and effects seen on the individual using them.
6. Describe substance use disorder among health care workers and the nurse's role in reporting an impaired nurse.
7. Describe treatment for the client toward long-term sobriety.
8. Describe the nursing process for the client with substance use disorder.

KEY TERMS

addiction
blackout
codependent
craving
delirium tremens
detoxification
enabling
inhalants
intoxication
opiates
opioids
relapse
substance
substance use disorder
tolerance
Wernicke–Korsakoff syndrome
withdrawal

Substance Use Disorder and Addiction

The term **substance** is used in reference to any drug, medication, or toxin that shares the potential for misuse. In 2020, 15.4% of the U.S. population (approximately 38.7 million persons) aged 18 or older had a substance use disorder. Of those individuals, 71% used alcohol, 44% used illicit drugs, and almost 16% used both alcohol and illicit drugs (Substance Abuse and Mental Health Services Administration [SAMHSA], 2022). Illicit drug, alcohol, and tobacco use impacts not only hospitalizations and treatment/recovery programs but also the criminal justice system, unemployment, and lost work due to substance use disorder. When discussing substances, it is important to define and discuss the topics of intoxication, substance use disorder, addiction, tolerance, withdrawal, and codependency.

Intoxication

Intoxication is the state where an individual's physical or mental status is affected or diminished due to the consumption of a substance such as alcohol or drugs. The person that is intoxicated has a change in their physiologic and mental status and may be aggressive, have a labile (changing) mood, exhibit impaired thinking, judgment, and functioning that is unrelated to any other medical condition. The most common changes that occur with intoxication involve disturbances in the areas of perception, sleep–wake cycle, attention, concentration, thinking, judgment, psychomotor activity, and interpersonal relationships. The person who is intoxicated may have a flushed appearance, have red or blood-shot eyes, have an increased heart rate or elevated blood pressure, and may be nauseated or vomit. Some symptoms are drug specific and others may be indicative of the use of several drugs.

Substance Use Disorder

Substance use disorder is a maladaptive pattern of substance use that demonstrates physiologic, cognitive, and behavioral indications that the person continues to use the drug despite the adverse substance-related problems they may be experiencing. There is evidence of compulsive drug-seeking behaviors. Substances can change the energy use and activity in the brain, alter the shape of brain cells, and change the function of

the signals and networks within the central nervous system (CNS). This underlying change triggers the brain's reward system with an intense **craving**, or strong desire to use the substance for the reward of the intense feelings the substance produces. This extreme desire for the substance often is pursued even if other aspects of the person's life are neglected.

Substance use disorder results in repeated absences from work, school, or home activities with repeated poor performance in these areas because of hangover effects. The incidence of substance use disorder includes excess of substance use over repeated episodes, such as when the person becomes inebriated on a weekend or at a particular event. There tends to be an increase in encounters with disciplinary authorities as a result of substance-related behaviors, such as arrests for disorderly conduct, public intoxication, driving while intoxicated, suspension or expulsion from school, or involvement of child protective services. Despite the persistent negative personal and interpersonal problems that result from repetitious use of the substance, the person does not abstain from continued use.

The pattern of compulsive use is demonstrated as larger amounts of the substance are taken over a more extensive period than was intended. The person may indicate a desire or attempt to decrease the substance use but is unsuccessful in these efforts. Much time and energy is devoted to planning activities necessary to obtain the substance. What once may have been valued and enjoyable time spent with work, family, friends, and colleagues is instead focused on substance use. Even though the person may have recurrent physiologic and psychological ill effects from substance usage, it continues. As psychological dependence develops, the person feels they cannot function without continued use of that substance. This inability to refrain from using the substance even when the harmful effects are known is the key symptom of substance use disorder.

Addiction

Addiction is a physiologic and psychological dependence on a substance to the extent that withdrawal symptoms are experienced when the substance is discontinued. Addiction is accompanied by maladaptive behaviors and relationships. It is important to know that addiction, regardless of the substance, is seen in all cultures, educational levels, and socioeconomic status. The nurse must avoid making assumptions about the likelihood of a client having an addiction based on their background. For example, the nurse should not assume that a wealthy professional cannot experience addiction or that someone from a low-income background is more likely to experience addiction.

Tolerance develops as the brain and body adapt to repeated doses of the substance with a declining effect as it is taken repetitively over time. This results in the need to use greater amounts of the substance to obtain the same effect. The tolerance may vary depending on the substance involved and its effect on the body. Substantial levels of tolerance may develop with heavy substance use that would be lethal to a person who does not use that substance. For example, in people who smoke cigarettes, smoking 2 to 3 packs per day indicates a tolerance to nicotine that would produce toxic effects in someone who does not smoke. High blood levels of a substance without obvious symptoms of intoxication often signifies tolerance.

Substance use disorder and addiction impact the health care system in the form of treatment, detoxification, and rehabilitation programs. Hospitalizations related to associated medical issues such as overdose or infections occur. Society is affected by drug-related criminal behaviors that involve both the participation in usage or sale of drugs and the violence associated with the drug industry. The arrest and incarceration of individuals involved in drug-related crimes has risen steadily over the past several decades. In addition, there is the cost of lost jobs and wages from absences or poor performance. Child abuse and neglect can occur because of substance use and addiction. Deaths attributed to drug use enlarges this picture to include not only financial losses but also the loss of human lives.

 Mind Jogger What are the extended personal costs of substance use disorder and addiction?

Test Yourself
✔ Describe the difference between substance use disorder and addiction.
✔ Describe the difference between intoxication and tolerance.

Withdrawal

Withdrawal occurs as the blood or tissue concentrations of a substance declines in a person who has developed a tolerance for the substance. Specific withdrawal symptoms and time of onset vary depending upon the substance. Withdrawal symptoms range from mild to severe, even including death, depending upon the substance and level of tolerance that has developed. Once these symptoms occur, the person often seeks relief by reingesting the substance. The signs and symptoms of withdrawal develop within several hours to a few days after drug cessation and vary with the substance involved.

It must be noted that tolerance and withdrawal are not unique to substance addiction, as these features of physical dependence can be normal responses to prescribed medications that affect the CNS. With some substances, marijuana for example, there are no physical symptoms of tolerance or withdrawal, although the substance severely impairs the functional ability of the individual.

 Just the Facts The presence of withdrawal symptoms poses a higher risk for medical problems and relapse rate.

 Just the Facts Short-acting substances tend to have a higher potential for withdrawal than do those substances with a longer duration of action. The duration of the withdrawal period tends to parallel the half-life of the substance (in other words, the longer the action of the drug, the longer the withdrawal period).

Codependence

People who are **codependent** tend to feel a responsibility for the person with a substance use disorder's problem and internalize a form of guilt for the behavior of that person. As a result, they continue to do everything possible to sustain the relationship and are unable to recognize the detrimental effects of the codependency on their own physical and mental health. Codependent people deny their own needs while living and doing for another what they need to do for themselves. People in this situation learn to tolerate and excuse the maladaptive behavior. This tolerance results in adjustment to the circumstances and the appearance of normalcy to the outsider.

This pattern of either consciously or unconsciously helping the maladaptive behavior to continue is referred to as **enabling**. The person who is enabling this behavior commonly makes excuses or lies to others about behaviors related to the substance use. They may also cover up financial and legal problems out of a false sense of responsibility. Social events may be avoided because of shame or fear of ramifications related to the substance use, such as questioning or abusive language and actions. People who demonstrate enabling behaviors are often passive, silently complying with the choices and decisions of the user even though they may not agree with them. The codependent person learns to make allowances for the person who uses in order to make life easier for all members of the family. This behavior allows the person who uses substances to maintain a perceived sense of control over their dependency and provides a false permission for the addiction to continue. People who enable substance use are caught in a cycle of thinking they are helpless to change the situation because to stop these actions would bring greater disaster. This becomes a cyclical pattern as making allowances for the disruptive behavior enables the person who uses to continue their behavior without consequences. These learned patterns of behavior can cause the codependent person to feel they are expected to support the behavior regardless of their own personal costs, such as work absences or limiting outside relationships. This can lead to feelings of "being trapped" in this dysfunctional situation.

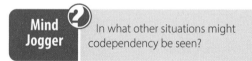

Mind Jogger In what other situations might codependency be seen?

Phases of Substance Dependency

Substance use and dependency is a progressive process from the first use of a substance to decline. Most people who become substance dependent do not intend to develop a dependency. They often start with a need to belong, to escape, or to experiment, and are often unaware of the substance's potential for overuse and addiction. Substance dependency is a progressive and predictable continuum of symptoms that increase in severity and frequency. The characteristic warning signs of substance dependency are described in Table 15.1.

There are four phases that occur from the first use of a substance to dependency (Fig. 15.1). In Phase 1, beginning with the first use, the person

TABLE 15.1	Warning Signs of Substance Dependency
Early	Uses substance to relax in social situation
	Avoids situations where drugs/alcohol will not be available
	Is preoccupied with substances and their usage
	Has occasional blackouts (periods where the person cannot remember drug use)
	Experiences personality change during substance use
Problem Use and Dependency	Shows increase in tolerance
	Denies substance problem—hides substance use from others
	May switch to other chemical use
	Neglects and loses friends
	Blames others for problems—projection
	Has increased craving
	May have aggressive behaviors with substance use
	Has physical withdrawal symptoms when use is interrupted
	Consumes unpredictable amounts of substance
	Neglects nutritional needs
Chronic	Shows irreversible physical damage (liver, brain, and other medical problems)
	Has decreased tolerance
	Has severe withdrawal symptoms
	Feels persistent remorse
	Has substance-related arrests
	Has delirium tremens (DTs)
	Hallucinates
	Has seizures
	Death may occur

experiences a mood of euphoria or "high" and learns that the substance can provide a temporary escape or altered emotional state each time it is used. The individual learns to control the effects by regulating the amount of substance and prioritizing the opportunities to use it.

During Phase 2, the person experiences hangover effects and starts to feel guilty for behaviors related to use of the substance. A need for the drug may develop, leading to tolerance and increased use to obtain the same effect. The person's friends and companions may change to a group who approve of and indulge in similar drug-related behaviors.

As the person enters Phase 3, a dependent lifestyle begins, with periods in which control over substance use is lost. The person can no longer predict the outcome and begins to engage in behaviors that compromise their values. As the substance assumes control, insight is lost and a revolving cycle begins in which the drug use becomes the priority.

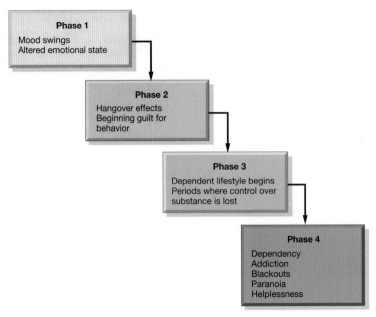

Figure 15.1 Phases of substance dependency.

Lastly, in Phase 4, the person demonstrates dependency or addiction with periods of blackout, paranoia, and helplessness. **Blackout** is a form of amnesia for events that occurred during the drinking period (e.g., client does not remember conversations or activities engaged in during the time of drinking). Engaging in the acquisition of the substance is no longer seen as a social activity, but as survival.

Classes of Substances

The classes of substances used and misused are listed in Box 15.1. The class listed as "Synthetic Drugs" includes those substances that can cause an intoxication response from an unknown chemical such as those found in bath salts. Prescription and over-the-counter medications are grouped into their respective class. Medications that have potential for misuse are seen in Box 15.2.

CASE STUDY 15.1

"Keshaun"

Keshaun is being admitted to a substance use treatment facility after police arrested him for driving under the influence (DUI). This was his third DUI in the past 2 months. During the intake interview he states this is his second admission to the treatment facility. When you ask Keshaun about his alcohol use, he states that he started drinking alcohol to feel good at parties.

When gathering data about his drinking history, Keshaun tells you that his father was "a heavy drinker but wasn't a mean drunk." Keshaun states he started drinking alcohol when he was 15 years old. That was the year he started a new school. His father was upset that Keshaun didn't have many friends so he tried fitting in with different groups at school to please his parents. Keshaun found it easier to fit in at parties when he drank and liked how alcohol made him feel relaxed and popular.

Digging Deeper

1. What phase of substance dependency would you identify Keshaun as being in? Describe why you picked that phase.

2. What are some of the reasons that Keshaun used, or currently uses, alcohol?

3. How might Keshaun react when facing a stressful situation without using alcohol?

Substance Classifications

- Alcohol
- Caffeine
- Cannabis
- Hallucinogens (includes PCP)
- Inhalants
- Nicotine
- Opiates
- Synthetic drugs
- Sedatives, hypnotics, or anxiolytics
- Stimulants (amphetamines, methamphetamines, cocaine)

Exposure to toxins and other chemical substances can result in a mental disorder as well. Toxic substances that may cause substance-related illness include those listed in Box 15.3. Volatile substances such as gasoline and paint, if used for the purpose of intoxication, are referred to as **inhalants**. The most common symptom associated with these toxic substances is alterations in cognitive functioning or mood, which usually resolve over a period of weeks or months once exposure is terminated.

Causes of Substance Use and Addiction

Much research has been done regarding causes or potential influences on a person's life that lead to substance use or addiction. Often, it is not one single cause or factor, but a combination of several. Most common influences for substance use and addiction are genetics, psychosocial and environmental influences, and personality.

Medications With Potential for Misuse

These classifications include, but are not limited to:

- Analgesics (esp. opioids)
- Anesthetics
- Antianxiety
- Benzodiazepines
- Muscle relaxants
- Over-the-counter medications such as sleep aids, antihistamines, decongestants, weight-loss agents, gastrointestinal aids, and pain-relief medications
- Stimulants (including those prescribed for Attention Deficit Hyperactivity Disorder)

Toxins and Other Chemical Substances

- Heavy metals (lead, aluminum, iron)
- Pesticides
- Nerve gases
- Carbon dioxide
- Ethylene glycol (antifreeze)

Mental illness can also be a causative factor for substance use by some individuals. For example, some individuals with psychosis may use cannabis or nicotine to help minimize symptoms such as anxiety, stress, and insomnia. There are other mental health conditions that the individual initially may cope with by using substances that may lead to substance use. Examples of these conditions include post-traumatic stress disorder (PTSD) and social anxiety.

Genetics and Family Influences

Social learning involves the effects of modeling, imitative, and identification behaviors that begin at an early age. Children of parents with substance use disorder are at a greater risk for substance use and addiction because of both genetic and environmental factors. There is an apparent link between heredity and substance use, and this is especially true for alcohol use disorder. Research also shows that the younger a person is when substance usage begins, the greater the probability that it will progress to excessive use and addiction. Chaotic home environments and association with peers who engage in maladaptive substance use behaviors also increase the likelihood that this will occur. This scenario is often accompanied by weak parent–child attachment with ineffective parenting and hostile, troubled relationships. There is some evidence that genetics may determine the variances in the doses necessary to produce intoxication in different people.

Mind Jogger In what way does a strong solid family system aid in reducing the risk of adolescent substance use?

Peer Pressure

Adolescence is a time when new things are exciting and the pressure to conform to one's peers is at its highest. Teenagers may get involved with substances for various reasons and experimentation is common. They often do not see the connection between their present actions and the consequences these actions may impose. Teenagers with a family history of substance use disorder, those who are depressed or have low self-esteem, and those who feel like misfits are at particular risk for developing substance use disorder. Adolescents tend to perceive the substance-using behavior on the part of family, peers, and community as an endorsement of drug usage.

Environmental Stress Factors

Stressful situations increase the need for coping strategies to manage the resultant anxiety. This is often the reason a person may use to justify their repeated use of the substance. Stress is cited as a major factor in the initiation and continued use of alcohol and other substances. Stress and poor coping skills are identified as significant factors when a person relapses and returns to a pattern of self-destructive behaviors and substance use.

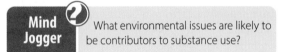

Mind Jogger   What environmental issues are likely to be contributors to substance use?

Personality Characteristics

A dependent personality is seen in some people with substance use disorder. The need to depend on an external force to provide a sense of self is reflected in the form of poor self-esteem and an inability to define values and boundaries for behavior. Box 15.4 lists some internal and external factors that help define one's sense of self. Conformity and blending into the social drug culture contribute to the substance taking control of the person's existence. The person may use the substance in order to fulfill a need for affection and power. Most people who engage in excessive use of substances have difficulty expressing feelings and may release these explosively as the substance diminishes their ability to control them. Feelings of emotional isolation and a low frustration tolerance further drive the need to borrow a feeling of strength and security from an external substance.

BOX 15.4

Determinants of Sense of Self

EXTERNAL CONTROL
- Primary motivation is acceptance by others
- Will compromise values under peer pressure
- Depends on external source of strength (other people, drugs, activities)

INTERNAL CONTROL
- Acts on clearly defined self-chosen beliefs and convictions
- Accepts responsibility for decisions and consequences of those choices
- Recognizes and is willing to act on the need for change

Test Yourself
- ✔ Describe the four phases of substance dependency.
- ✔ List 10 classes of substances frequently used and misused.
- ✔ Identify four factors that can lead to substance use disorder.

Substances Used and Misused

As mentioned, all 10 classes listed in Box 15.1 can be involved in substance misuse or addiction. Substance use can range from mild to severe depending on the number of signs that are present (Box 15.5). Mild is usually indicated by two or three symptoms, moderate by four to five symptoms, and severe by six or more symptoms. Each substance causes symptoms of intoxication and withdrawal. Alcohol, amphetamines,

BOX 15.5

Signs of Substance Use Disorder
- Denial of the drug problem
- Tolerance and withdrawal from continued use of a substance
- Strong urge or desire to use drug despite negative consequences or craving of the substance
- Substance is taken in larger amounts over longer period than was intended
- Unsuccessful attempts and inability to control substance use
- Much time is spent in pursuit of obtaining the substance
- Important activities are given up because of substance use

BOX 15.6

Conditions Related to Substance Use

- Delirium
- Amnesic disorder
- Psychotic disorder, with delusions
- Psychotic disorder, with hallucinations
- Mood disorder
- Anxiety disorder
- Sexual dysfunction
- Sleep disorder

cocaine, inhalants, cannabis, and hallucinogens all have the potential of causing psychoactive symptoms. The substances can also cause conditions that are seen in mental health disorders as well (Box 15.6).

Alcohol

Alcohol is commonly used in most cultures. It is the cause of considerable associated physiologic problems and sometimes death. The use of alcohol is associated with a significant increase in the risk of accidents, violence, and suicide. An increase in absenteeism from work, job-related accidents, and decreased employee productivity are commonly linked to alcohol. There is a strong familial pattern of alcohol-related problems, with approximately half of occurrences thought to be genetically linked.

The majority of adults in the United States have used alcohol to some degree, but most people are able to moderate their drinking and avoid related problems. Fifty percent of Americans aged 12 years and older reported using alcohol in the past month people and almost 16% of adults 18 to 25 years old have an alcohol use disorder (SAMHSA, 2022). Alcohol is associated with nearly one-third of traffic related deaths (National Highway Traffic Safety Administration, 2022).

Chronic use of alcohol can affect nearly every body system and may result in liver cirrhosis or failure, esophageal varices, heart enlargement, and cancer of the pancreas, stomach, and esophagus. Chronic use can also result in an encephalopathy and psychosis known as **Wernicke–Korsakoff syndrome**. This is a nutritional disease of the nervous system found in those with alcohol use disorder, caused primarily by thiamine and niacin deficiency. Significant cerebral deterioration and actual brain cell death occur with chronic and permanent impairment.

With Wernicke encephalopathy and Korsakoff psychosis, there is progressive memory loss and disorientation with emotional lability and apathy, weakness, and fatigue.

Withdrawal from alcohol can cause anxiety, tremors, seizures, and hallucinations. Chronic alcohol users who stop drinking are at risk for alcohol-induced delirium, or **delirium tremens** (DTs), a state of profound confusion and delusions along with all of the usual symptoms of alcohol withdrawal. The episode generally ends after several days of insomnia and rigorous activity when the individual falls into a deep sleep. On awakening, they are coherent but without memory of the events during the delirium. The delirium may last from 2 to 5 days, during which there is a 5% to 15% fatality rate (Rahman & Paul, 2021).

Individuals with a severe alcohol addiction may consume common substances containing alcohol to satisfy their craving such as liquid cough or cold preparations and mouthwash. In desperation, they may even consume substances such as cologne, aftershave, or rubbing alcohol, all of which can cause severe organ damage or death.

Just the Facts The development of seizure activity during delirium tremens (DTs) is a life-threatening situation and must be considered a medical emergency.

Mind Jogger What are some effects chronic alcohol use has on the body?

Cannabis (Marijuana)

Cannabis, or marijuana, is derived from the cannabis plant and is used widely in the form of rolled cigarettes, but it may also be taken orally or mixed in tea or food. Many states have legalized cannabis for medicinal or recreational purposes. Specialty stores may sell cannabis in the form of gummy products and other edibles in addition to the dried form. While the state may have legalized the substance, many professions and jobs (such as nursing and heavy equipment operators) still prohibit their employees from using cannabis for safety reasons.

The essential features include a high feeling followed by euphoria, inappropriate laughter, grandiosity, lethargy, impaired short-term memory, delayed mental processing, impaired judgment, distorted sensory perceptions, and impaired motor function. There may be accompanying anxiety, dysphoria, or social withdrawal as the use increases. Within 2 hours after marijuana use, there is conjunctival redness, increased appetite, dry mouth, and increased heart rate. The effects of cannabis usually last 3 to 4 hours. Because the drug is fat soluble, the effects may be detected in the urine for 7 to 10 days and up to 4 weeks in those who engage in heavy use.

Cannabis is often used along with other substances. It can also be mixed and smoked with opioids, phencyclidine (PCP), or hallucinogenic drugs. In people who use high doses, regular use commonly results in depression, anxiety, and irritability, with psychoactive effects similar to those of the hallucinogens. High use can also result in severe anxiety or panic attacks, as well as episodes of paranoid delusional thinking or depersonalization. Chronic cannabis use is associated with weight gain, sinusitis, pharyngitis, and persistent cough. Although there is an increase in respiratory illnesses among people who smoke marijuana frequently, the actual carcinogenic effects of cannabis or risk for lung cancer have not yet been determined. It is known that marijuana affects brain development, and with heavy use, its effects on thinking and memory may be permanent.

Caffeine

Caffeine is found in many different sources including coffee, carbonated soft drinks, tea, over-the-counter pain relievers, cold remedies, antidrowsiness aids, and weight-loss agents. Chocolate and cocoa have a lower caffeine content than the other sources listed. There is no link between the intake of caffeine and a clinical picture that meets the criteria for substance dependence or substance use disorder. However, it is mentioned here because excessive use or misuse can cause harm, especially if combined with other stimulants or alcohol.

Energy drinks containing caffeine are used widely by teens and young adults. Many of these drinks contain up to 500 mg of caffeine per 24 ounces. Some of these drinks also contain guarana which is an additional source of caffeine. A popular trend is to mix energy drinks with alcohol. However, this is dangerous since the person is often unaware of how intoxicated they actually are (Centers for Disease Control and Prevention, 2022).

> **Just the Facts**
>
> The average consumption of caffeine in the United States is approximately 500 mg/day. Intake in excess of 10 grams can cause grand mal seizures, respiratory failure, and death.

Mild sensory alterations, such as ringing in the ears or flashing lights, have been reported by those who are heavy users. Physical symptoms from excessive intake may include anxiety, agitation, restlessness, sweating, flushed face, and diarrhea. Cardiac arrhythmias and gastrointestinal discomfort have also been reported.

Hallucinogens

Hallucinogens are usually taken orally, although injection does occur. Tolerance to the euphoric and psychedelic effects of these substances develops rather quickly, but there is no clear documented evidence regarding a withdrawal pattern. However, most users continue to use hallucinogens despite knowledge of the adverse effects, such as memory impairment, panic reactions, or flashback episodes or "bad trips" that may occur during drug intoxication.

PCP is commonly used several times a week by those with dependence on the substance. Those who use PCP often demonstrate dangerous behaviors because of lack of insight and judgment under the influence of the drug. Aggressive behaviors, such as fighting, are a particular problem with PCP use. The drug can be taken orally, injected, or smoked. PCP is the most commonly misused hallucinogen.

Under the influence of a hallucinogenic drug, the person may display mood swings, fearfulness, anxiety, and feelings of going insane or dying. Many of these drugs have stimulant effects similar to those of amphetamine intoxication. The perceptual disturbances and impaired judgment seen in toxic episodes or flashbacks may result in fatal accidents such as users believing they can fly and subsequently jumping from a building or bridge. Associated physiologic changes include increases in blood glucose and cortisol hormones.

Psychologic effects of PCP may include inability to control emotions, anxiety, rage, aggression, panic, flashbacks, and disorganized thinking. Medical problems such as hyperthermia, hypertension, and seizures can compound the picture with recurrent PCP use. Other indicators of use may be nystagmus (involuntary motion of the eyes that is rhythmic and the pattern is side-to-side, up and down, or circular), hypertension, hepatitis, or human immunodeficiency virus (HIV) disease. Evidence of needle tracks may also be present. Those with substance intoxication may exhibit delirium, psychotic symptoms, catatonic posturing, or coma. Younger people who use PCP may experience more intense emotional states as a result of the drug effects.

> **Just the Facts** Fresh needle marks look like punctures or bruising along a vein. Old needle track marks appear as darkened pigmented lines that follow along a vein path.

Inhalants

Most drug compounds containing nitrous oxide that are inhaled can produce psychoactive effects. Tolerance is reported with heavy use, although withdrawal patterns that meet the criteria for an assigned disorder have not been documented. Because inhalants are inexpensive, legal, and easily accessible, they tend to be used over a longer time. This may result in the person spending more time recuperating and giving up important social, occupational, or recreational activities. Substance use often continues despite the person's awareness of both physical and psychologic problems caused by the chemicals.

Behavioral or psychological changes include confusion, belligerence, aggression, apathy, and impaired judgment and social functioning. Hallucinations, delusional thinking, and perceptual changes may develop during periods of confusion and intoxication. These changes are usually accompanied by dizziness, visual disturbances, unsteady gait, tremors, and euphoria. Higher doses can lead to lethargy, slowed psychomotor response, muscle weakness, and stupor. People who use inhalants usually have an odor of paint or solvent on their breath or clothing with a residual "glue-sniffer's rash" evident around the nose and mouth. There may be redness of the eyes, respiratory distress, coughing, sinus discharge, headache, weakness, and abdominal pain with nausea or vomiting. Inhalants can cause permanent damage to both the central and the peripheral nervous system. Death can occur from cardiac arrhythmias or respiratory failure, commonly referred to as "sudden sniffing death." Box 15.7 provides interventions for the person who is inhaling or huffing.

> **BOX 15.7**
>
> ### Interventions for the Person Who Is Inhaling or Huffing
>
> - Use a calm approach—do not excite or argue with the person (can become aggressive)
> - Try to determine what substance was used (aerosol cans, bags, rags, etc. can provide clues)
> - Keep person calm in a well-ventilated environment (may have respiratory difficulty)
> - Avoid stimulation (can cause hallucinations or violence)
> - Get help for the user as quickly as possible!

> **Just the Facts** "Sudden sniffing death syndrome" can occur with the use of inhalants, on the first incident or any time. Death is the result of acute cardiac arrhythmias, hypoxia, or electrolyte imbalances as the inhaled substance sensitizes the heart muscle to the body's own adrenaline, leading to a fatal heart rhythm disturbance.

During adolescence, the use of inhalants may first be noticed because of school-related problems such as truancy, a drop in grades, or dropping out of school. Most adolescents use inhalants under the influence of peer pressure in a group setting. However, heavy usage tends to be a solitary pattern.

Nicotine

Although not considered a misused substance by most people who use it, nicotine is known to have addictive and dependent properties. The health dangers related to cigarette smoking are well publicized with warning labels related to these health hazards printed on all tobacco products. Nicotine dependence can develop with use of all forms of tobacco (cigarettes, cigars, chewing tobacco, snuff, pipes, and vaping). The nicotine content of tobacco, added to the repetitive nature of its use, contributes to its ability to produce rapid dependence. Tolerance to nicotine is demonstrated by a more intense effect the first time it is used without producing adverse effects such as dizziness or nausea.

The most common signs of chronic nicotine use include strong tobacco and ash odors on the individual's clothes and breath, cough, excessive skin wrinkling, and chronic pulmonary disease. Tobacco use markedly increases the risk of lung, oral, and other cancers and increases the risk for cardiovascular and cerebrovascular conditions.

Nicotine withdrawal symptoms are experienced within 24 hours of cessation or reduction in usage. Symptoms include a depressed mood, insomnia, irritability, frustration, anxiety, decreased concentration, restlessness, bradycardia, and increased appetite with weight gain. These symptoms usually peak in intensity between the first and fourth days with considerable improvement by 3 to 4 weeks. The hunger and weight gain may persist for 6 months or more. Some medications are used during smoking cessation programs along with nicotine patches and/or nicotine gum.

Nicotine use usually begins in adolescence, and almost all of those who continue to smoke use it daily. People often use nicotine to relieve or avoid symptoms of withdrawal early in the morning or after prolonged periods where use of the substance is not permitted.

Opioids

The term **opioids** refers to all natural, synthetic, and semisynthetic forms of the substance while **opiates** refers to the substance that naturally occurs from opium and its three forms, which are heroin, morphine, and codeine. Synthetic opioids are not naturally occurring; they must be made (synthesized), but affect the brain like the naturally found opiates do. Examples of synthetic opioids include fentanyl and methadone. Opiate medications, such as codeine or morphine, are regularly prescribed treatments and are contained in analgesics, anesthetics, antidiarrheal agents, and cough suppressants. Heroin is synthesized from morphine, a natural substance extracted from the seed pod of the Asian opium poppy plant. It usually appears as a white or brown powder or as a black sticky substance, known as "black tar heroin." Heroin may be injected or snorted.

> **Just the Facts**
> Opiates refers only to the three forms of the substance (heroin, morphine, and codeine) from the natural plant matter opium.
> Opioids refers to all natural, synthetic, and semisynthetic forms of the opium substance and is a broader term.

Two commonly prescribed semisynthetic opioids are oxycodone and hydrocodone. Like morphine, oxycodone is generally prescribed as an analgesic. Hydrocodone is effective as a cough suppressant and analgesic. All oxycodone products are Schedule II medications. They are used orally, crushed and sniffed, or dissolved and injected. Hydrocodone is usually prescribed for pain relief in combination with acetaminophen but can also combined with aspirin, ibuprofen, and antihistamines. There is a prohibited automatic refill of these products. The hydrocodone products are the most frequently prescribed drug agents for pain in the United States. Despite this medicinal advantage, these are among the most misused prescription medications and are associated with drug trafficking, diversion, and addiction. Law enforcement documentation of diversion by theft, doctor shopping, fraudulent prescriptions, phony "called-in" prescriptions, and internet fraud is widespread. Misuse of prescription opioid pain medications may lead to subsequent heroin use as they both attach to the same receptors in the brain.

Opioid dependence is evident by compulsive, prolonged self-administration of these substances for no legitimate medical reason. The medications are usually purchased through illegal channels or by falsely reporting medical conditions or acquiring multiple prescriptions from different health care providers. Health care professionals with opioid dependence may resort to drug diversion in their place of employment or to prescription forgery to obtain the medication (see the section "Substance Use by Health Care Professionals" in this chapter).

With opioid intoxication there is an initial high followed by apathy, depressed mood, inability to coordinate motor functioning, and impaired judgment. These changes are accompanied by drowsiness, slurred speech, inattention, memory lapses, and pupil constriction. Severe intoxication can lead to respiratory depression, unconsciousness, and death. Opioid dependence is commonly associated with a history of drug-related crimes and unprofessional conduct among health professionals who have access to controlled medications. Periods of depression are common after repeated use of the drug.

Family members of people with opioid dependence typically have an increased incidence of other substance-related disorders related to the observing and modeling of the substance use as a coping style. They may also have an increased incidence of antisocial personality disorder. Those with antisocial personality disorder often show a disregard for accepted social behaviors and blame others for their troubles. This may lead them to initially use substances as a coping behavior and a reason to rationalize their behavior.

Synthetic Drugs

Substances that are used or misused can include synthetic drugs. Two main types of synthetic drugs are bath salts and K2 (also known as Spice). Bath salts are composed of synthetic cathinones, which are related to the substance found in the khat plant that grows in East Africa and Southern Arabia. The leaves of the khat plant can be chewed to produce a stimulant-like effect. In the United States synthetic cathinones are sold as bath products or even as plant food or jewelry cleaners under the disclaimer "not for human consumption." Synthetic cathinones are chemically similar to amphetamines and produce similar symptoms. However, severe reactions including permanent psychosis and death have been associated with synthetic drugs, and their effects as a stimulant are not always predictable.

K2, or Spice, is a synthetic cannabinoid. It is made up of dried, shredded plant material and herbs or spices, which is then usually sprayed with cannabinoids. Cannabinoids are the psychoactive part of cannabis/marijuana. As with bath salts, the effects are unpredictable and can have permanent psychomotor reactions or death.

Sedatives, Hypnotics, or Anxiolytics

Sedative, hypnotic, and anxiolytic medications include the benzodiazepines, carbamates, barbiturates, and other sedative agents. All prescription sleeping medications and antianxiety medications also fall into these categories. These agents are all depressants and are particularly lethal when mixed with alcohol. These medications are available both by prescription and on the illegal street market. The medications with a rapid onset are more likely to be misused by those who obtain them by prescription.

Craving during use or after a period of abstinence is a typical feature of this category of medications. Significant levels of tolerance can develop to any of the sedative, hypnotic, or anxiolytic agents. The clinical picture is usually one of maladaptive behavioral and psychological changes such as mood lability, impaired judgment and functioning, and inappropriate sexual or aggressive behavior. Other indicators may be slurred speech, unsteady gait, nystagmus, and impaired mobility or coordination. Physiologic effects may include tachycardia, tachypnea, hypertension, hyperthermia, diaphoresis, tremors, insomnia, anxiety, and nausea.

Dependence and misuse of these agents is often associated with harmful use of other substances such as alcohol, cannabis, cocaine, heroin, methadone, or amphetamines. The sedatives may be used to counteract the adverse effects of the other substances. Those who misuse these agents regularly are usually in search of the original feeling of euphoria and take increased doses trying to achieve this end. Accidental overdose and acute respiratory arrest that result in death are not uncommon.

Most people take these medications as directed by their health care provider for legitimate medical reasons with no intent of misuse but some acknowledge using them illicitly. Those who originally obtained the prescription for medical reasons and have continued to increase doses often justify the continued use by claiming the original symptoms. They often go to multiple health care providers (called "doctor shopping") in different locations to acquire the prescriptions to continue their use.

Stimulants

The amphetamine and amphetamine-type stimulants include both those sold on the illegal market and those that may be obtained by prescription for the treatment of obesity, attention deficit hyperactivity disorder (ADHD), and narcolepsy. Most of the effects of these medications are similar to those of cocaine, although the risk for inducing cardiac arrhythmias and seizures is lower. The three main subcategories are cocaine, amphetamines, and methamphetamines.

Crack cocaine is a common form of cocaine. It is easily vaporized and inhaled, making the onset of effects particularly rapid. Cocaine, in any form, has extremely potent euphoric effects, which increases the potential for dependence after the drug has been used for a very short time. An early sign of dependence is that the person is unable to resist using the drug when it is available. Because of the 30- to 50-minute half-life of the drug, the drug must be used frequently to maintain the high. This short effect and the craving for more leads those

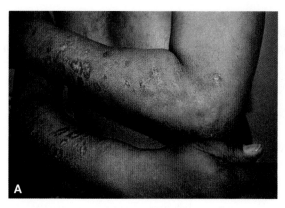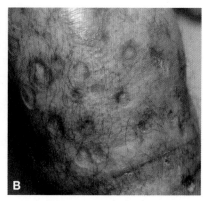

Figure 15.2 Scars from "skin popping," or injecting illicit drugs just below the skin. (Image sources [left to right]: Hobbs, M. M., & Cornelissen, C. N. [2019]. *Lippincott illustrated reviews: Microbiology.* Wolters Kluwer Health, Inc; Scott Robert Perry/Shutterstock.)

who use the drug to spend thousands of dollars in a short time, with extreme personal and financial consequences. Most people with dependence have signs of tolerance and withdrawal at some point. Common mental and physical complications of chronic cocaine use are paranoid ideation, anxiety, and weight loss. There may be rambling speech, headache, ringing in the ears, and hallucinations. Tactile hallucinations are reported as feeling like something is crawling under the individual's skin and is commonly referred to as "coke bugs."

Amphetamines are prescription stimulant medications used to treat certain conditions such as narcolepsy, some forms of depression, obesity, and ADHD and are the most commonly misused prescription stimulants. They are often used by high school and college students as a means to keep them awake in school or for test preparation. The medications are typically crushed and snorted or dissolved in water and injected.

Figure 15.2 shows examples of scars from "skin popping" (injecting illicit drugs just below skin and not into a vein).

The withdrawal symptoms of amphetamines are likely to enhance craving and the likelihood of reusing the substance. Because of its powerful effects on the CNS, it is common to see erratic and aggressive behaviors. Mood changes such as depression with suicidal ideation, irritability, anhedonia, emotional swings, and inattentiveness are also seen. The substance takes over the person's life to the point of social isolation.

Methamphetamine is also a stimulant but is an illegal substance that has no medicinal value. It is a powerful chemical substance similar to the neurotransmitter dopamine. Because of this similarity,

methamphetamine can change the function of any neuron that contains dopamine. It can also affect neurons that contain the neurotransmitters serotonin and norepinephrine. Methamphetamine is able to trick the neurons into taking it up just like they would dopamine. For this reason, the person feels an initial "high" that eventually stops and ends in a surge of unpleasant feelings called a "crash." This leads the person to use more of the drug with less and less chance of obtaining the pleasurable feeling.

The psychoactive effects of most amphetamines and methamphetamines last longer than those of cocaine, and the stimulating effects on the autonomic nervous system may be more potent. The person may develop mood changes, weight loss, and malnutrition. Chronic use produces a psychosis that resembles schizophrenia with paranoia, picking at the skin, delusions, and hallucinations. Violent and erratic behavior is frequently seen among those who engage in chronic use. It is common for people who use amphetamine to also use alcohol and benzodiazepine antianxiety drug agents to calm the jittery feelings caused by the stimulant.

Table 15.2 summarizes symptoms of intoxication and withdrawal that can be seen in the 10 classes of substances discussed.

Substance Use by Health Care Professionals

People who work in the health care professions work in a fast-paced, stressful, and demanding environment. The decision to use alcohol or

TABLE 15.2 Information on Substance Use and Withdrawal

Intoxication	Withdrawal	Substance-Related Information
Alcohol		
• Difficulty focusing with glazed appearance of eyes • Loosened inhibitions • Manner may be passive, argumentative, or emotional • Memory impairment • Odor on breath or clothes • Poor concentration • Slurred speech • Stupor • Uncoordinated and unsteady gait	**Common** • Agitation • Diaphoresis • Insomnia • Irritability • Nausea and vomiting • Tremors ("the shakes") **Severe** • Delirium tremens (DTs)—can last 3–4 days • Hallucinations • Seizures—occur 1–2 days after stopping alcohol and can occur even if no other symptoms seen	• Alcohol equivalents: 1-oz spirits = 5-oz wine = 12-oz beer • Legal level of intoxication is 0.08–0.10% in most states • Withdrawal may occur several hours to several days after alcohol ingestion stops or blood alcohol level decreases
Marijuana/Cannabis		
• Anxiety • Conjunctival redness • Distorted sensory perception and sense of time • Dry mouth • Euphoria and inappropriate laughter • Impaired judgment and coordination • Increased appetite • Lack of motivation • Memory impairment • Nervousness/paranoia • Sleepiness	• Anger • Anxiety • Decreased appetite • Depression • Irritability • Sleep disturbances	• Many states have legalized usage for medicinal or recreational purposes • May be used to aid relief of chronic pain • Teens who smoke tobacco are eight times more likely to use marijuana • Withdrawal symptoms occur within 1 week of stopping
Caffeine		
• Diuresis • Insomnia • Nervousness • Restlessness • Tachycardia	• Decreased alertness and difficulty concentrating • Drowsiness • Fatigue • Headache • Irritability • Withdrawal peaks at 1–2 days and lasts 2–9 days	• Caffeine combined with aspirin or acetaminophen used for migraine relief • May improve short-term memory in some • May worsen pre-existing anxiety, bipolar, or cardiac conditions
Hallucinogens		
• Body temperature altered • Diaphoresis • Dilated pupils • Hallucinations • Images seen, sounds heard, or sensations felt that all seem real but do not actually exist (distorted sensory perceptions) • Mood and behavior changes • Nausea • Panic or paranoia • Perceptual disturbances and impaired judgment (may cause accidents or attempts to fly from high places) • Psychosis • Sleep disturbance • Tachycardia	• Hallucinogens do not create a physical addiction, but prolonged use can cause flashbacks with persisting perception disorder days or even months after an LSD "trip" • Diarrhea and chills may occur after abruptly stopping after prolonged use	• Classic hallucinogens: LSD, mescaline, psilocybin (found in certain mushrooms) • Dissociative hallucinogens: PCP, ketamine, and dextromethorphan • Many forms are tasteless, colorless, and odorless—undetectable in beverages, and may be administered to person without their knowledge • Referred to as a "trip" • Unpleasant experience referred to as a "bad trip" • With PCP there can be unpredictable behavior, violence and inability to control emotions, anxiety, rage, aggression, panic

(continued)

TABLE 15.2 Information on Substance Use and Withdrawal (*Continued*)

Intoxication	Withdrawal	Substance-Related Information
Inhalants		
• Aggression • Blurred vision • Coughing • Dyspnea • Euphoria • Impaired thinking • Loss of consciousness • Muscle weakness • Poor coordination • Rash around nose or mouth • Runny nose, watery eyes, conjunctival irritation • Slurred speech • Tremors	Physical withdrawal symptoms not as common but may include: • Agitation • Hand tremors • Insomnia • Nausea and vomiting • Seizures • Sweating • Tachycardia	• Lungs allow rapid absorption with rapidly peaking blood levels that penetrate the brain • Many people who use inhalants have serious respiratory problems and permanent brain damage • May be painted on hands, fingernails, or wrist bands to allow continued use • Sniffed directly from open or pressurized container, huffed from a rag soaked in substance, or filled balloon held to the face
Nicotine		
• Cough • Dizziness • Nausea • Tobacco odor on breath, clothes, hair	• Anxiety • Depressed mood • Difficult concentration • Increased appetite with weight gain • Insomnia • Irritability and frustration	• Excessive skin wrinkling • Risk of cardiovascular disease including hypertension • Risk of cerebrovascular disease • Risk of lung/oral cancer
Opioids: Morphine, codeine, oxycodone, hydrocodone, hydromorphone		
• Constricted pupils that are nonreactive to light • Drowsiness • Lethargy • Memory and attention impairment • Respiratory depression • Slurred speech	• Chills • Cramps • Craving substance • Depression • Diarrhea • Diaphoresis • Increased sensitivity to pain • Panic attacks • Suicidal ideations • Tremors • Vomiting	• Death from overdose • Easily misused and addictive • Scars from injecting are called track marks • Sharing needles can cause transmission of HIV, Hepatitis B and C • Withdrawal symptoms can last from 48–72 hours
Opioids: Heroin		
• Bradycardia • Decreased sensitivity to pain • Decreased respirations • Depression • Drowsiness and mental lethargy • Eyes are red or glassy • Mood swings • Nausea/vomiting • "Rush" is accompanied by warm flushing of skin, dry mouth, and heavy feelings in extremities • Severe itching	• Anxiety or panic attack • Chills • Depression • Diarrhea • Excessive sweating • Irregular heart rhythm • Muscle and bone pain • Restlessness and leg movements • Vomiting	• Derived from morphine • Is a depressant • Particularly addictive because of rapid entry across blood–brain barrier • Death from overdose can occur • Withdrawal symptoms may occur within a few hours after last use or when dosage is reduced • Withdrawal can last 2–3 days and some symptoms may remain as long as 30–60 days

TABLE 15.2	Information on Substance Use and Withdrawal *(Continued)*	
Intoxication	**Withdrawal**	**Substance-Related Information**

Synthetic Drugs

Bath Salts (Synthetic cathinone)

• Agitation	• Anxiety	• Chemically similar to amphetamines and cocaine
• Delirium	• Depression	• Can cause death
• Hallucinations	• Intense and uncontrollable drug craving	• Permanent psychosis with delusions and flash-
• Hypertension	• Paranoia	backs have occurred
• Increased friendliness	• Sleep disturbance	
• Increased sex drive	• Tremors	
• Panic attacks		
• Paranoia		
• Tachycardia		
• Violent behavior		

K2 Spice (Synthetic cannabinoid)

• Agitation	• Anxiety	• Contains dried, shredded plant material, herbs,
• Altered perception	• Cravings	and usually sprayed with cannabinoids (the
• Elevated mood	• Diarrhea	psychoactive part of marijuana)
• Hallucinations	• Lethargy	• High can last from 1 to 8 hours
• Hypertension	• Nausea	• Effects are unpredictable and severe
• Palpitations	• Hungry but unable to keep food down	• May be smoked or used in vaping
• Paranoia	• Violent temper	
• Seizures	• Withdrawal period can last up to 3 days	
• Vomiting		

Sedatives, Hypnotics, or Anxiolytics

• Bradycardia and decreased respiratory rate	• Anxiety	• Includes barbiturates, benzodiazepines,
• Flat affect	• Hallucinations	flunitrazepam (utilized as party or "date rape"
• Impaired attention, memory, and thinking	• Hand tremors	drug), GHB, paraldehyde, chloral hydrate,
• Incoordination	• Insomnia	meprobamate, zaleplon, and zolpidem
• Labile mood	• Nausea/vomiting	• GHB is an odorless, colorless liquid or white
• Nystagmus	• Psychomotor agitation	powder
• Sleepiness or stupor	• Seizures	
• Slurred speech	• Sweating	
	• Tachycardia	

Stimulants: Amphetamines

• Anxiety	• Amphetamines not typically physically addictive	• Addiction is hard to break
• Eyes bloodshot	but if stopped abruptly may have symptoms of	• Can cause heart attack and stroke
• Dilated pupils	withdrawal	• Causes intense highs
• Euphoria	• Anxiety	• Includes MDMA, Ecstasy, and speed
• Hyperactivity	• Depression	• Weight loss common
• Hypertension	• Extreme fatigue	
• Nausea	• Sleep disturbances	
• Restlessness	• Suicidal ideation	
• Sleep disturbance		
• Tachycardia		

(continued)

TABLE 15.2	Information on Substance Use and Withdrawal *(Continued)*	
Intoxication	**Withdrawal**	**Substance-Related Information**
Stimulants: Methamphetamine		
• Aggressive and violent behavior • Amnesia • Apathy • Delusions • Dilation of pupils • Dramatic weight loss • Euphoria • Hallucinations • Hyper-excitability • Hypertension • Hyperthermia • Mood changes • Nausea • Sleep disturbance • Tachycardia	• Deep depression • Inability to feel pleasure • Drug craving • Fatigue • Increased appetite • Suicidal thoughts	• Anhedonia with use • Causes severe dental problems referred to as "meth mouth" • Decreased appetite with extreme weight loss • Does not cause physical dependency but does create a severe psychological addiction • Methamphetamine can cause extensive long-term damage to dopamine receptors in the brain • Synthetic stimulant that produces an intense high known as a "flash" that lasts for only a few minutes
Stimulants: Cocaine		
• Anxiety • Cardiac arrhythmias • Dilated pupils • Headache • Hypertension • Nosebleed • Rambling speech • Restlessness • Ringing in ears • Tachycardia • Tachypnea • Violent behavior	• Anxiety • Fatigue • Mood swings • Increased appetite • Irritability • Delusions • Drug craving • Withdrawal is referred to as a "crash" or "come down"	• Can cause seizures, heart attack and death • Depression occurs as elevated mood fades • Gives temporary illusion of enhanced power and energy • Increasing difficulty to abstain from use, with need for frequent dosing for "high" (short half-life) • "Coke bugs" (tactile hallucinations)

another substances as a means of coping with the pressure is prevalent within the health care industry. The easy accessibility of sedative, hypnotic, anxiolytic, and opioid medications to those who work in health care professions has also contributed to the number of impaired health care workers. Most of them do not start using a substance with the intention of engaging in chronic use or developing a dependency. However, once the cycle of misuse or drug diversion begins, the individual is often powerless to control the need for the substance and dependence takes over.

Professional ethics and practice standards of these groups and a personal set of values are the reasons why most people in the health-related fields refrain from ever engaging in harmful substance use. Most health care workers are able to provide care that includes medication administration without misusing substances. However, some health care workers cite physical exertion, family demands, emotional strain of caregiving, or the false belief that the substance can enhance performance to rationalize their drug diversion.

Substance use among health care workers is usually noted first by coworkers. In most states, it is an ethical and legal mandate of the Nurse Practice Act for a licensed nurse to report an impaired nurse to the regulatory division of the Board of Nursing. An obligation to protect the client from unsafe nursing actions is a responsibility concurrent with licensure to practice nursing. Table 15.3 provides some indicators that a nurse may be impaired or engaging in drug diversion along with reporting guidelines. To address the numbers of health care workers who fail in keeping these standards, many states have formed professional help groups for impaired health professionals. These groups work closely with professional licensing boards to develop guidelines by which the individual may seek and receive treatment. There are very strict and specific compliance rules and regulations governing

TABLE 15.3	The Impaired Nurse or Health Care Provider	
Clues—Drug-Related Problems		**When to Report**
Alcohol		
Moody and irritable		At least two people witness smell of alcohol on breath, hair, or clothing
Unkempt appearance		A positive blood alcohol level
Numerous excuses for behavior		Displays a pattern of poor nursing judgment or repeated medication
Smell of alcohol on breath or hair		errors
Excessive use of mouth fresheners		Slurred speech, falling asleep, or staggering while on duty
Social isolation		Charge of driving under the influence (DUI) while driving to work or on
Slurred speech, motor incoordination		duty (home health)
Bloodshot eyes		
Flushed face		
Substances Including Medications		
Changes jobs frequently		Positive urine drug screen result for which a legitimate prescription
Repeated tardiness to work		cannot be produced
Pinpoint pupils		Falling asleep at work, staggering gait, or slurred speech
Rapid mood swings or changes in performance		Forgetfulness, poor performance, frequent errors
Social isolation		Drug diversion evidence
Frequent breaks or use of bathroom		Giving medications to clients without a health care provider's order
Repeatedly volunteers for extra shifts, overtime		Signing out medications to discharged or deceased clients
Offers to give medications for other nurses		
Consistently signs out for vial or ampule of controlled medications so wasting is necessary		
Discrepancies in signing for controlled substances and on medication record		
Clients report ineffective pain medication		
Always wears clothing with long sleeves		
Befriends health care providers who may prescribe medications		
Multiple family problems		

For further information please refer to National Council of State Boards of Nursing. (2018). A Nurse's Guide to Substance Use Disorder in Nursing. From https://www.ncsbn.org/public-files/ SUD_Brochure_2014.pdf

the status of the license to practice in these situations. The stipulations as to whether the individual may or may not return to practice varies with the situation. The license may be suspended and reinstated once the requirements for treatment have been proven, or the license may be revoked. The regulations and consequences are set by the individual's state board of nursing.

Treatment of Substance-Related Disorders

Substance use disorder is a disease of serious consequences and adverse effects that do not seem to deter the person using substances from a compulsive craving and seeking of the substance. Many engage in chronic use with relapses common even after long periods of abstinence. The **relapse**, or return to using the substance after apparent recovery, is a factor in the approach to treatment-based programs. Although this cycle is a complex problem,

treatment can enable the individual to change their behavior and assume a more wholesome lifestyle.

Ultimately, the long-term goal of treatment programs is for the individual to attain complete abstinence. The incidence of successful recovery increases with longer lengths of time an individual remains in treatment; therefore, it becomes critical to find a treatment that is suited for each individual client.

Intensive multidisciplinary efforts are needed to assist the client in order for the treatment to be effective. Incentives must be established to encourage sobriety and behavior changes during the treatment process. Short-term goals of reducing substance use, decreasing the negative medical and social effects of substance use, and helping the individual find meaningful employment with a more productive life are the integral ingredients in reaching abstinence. Whether treatment is voluntary or court ordered, the chronic nature of the disorder and potential for relapse limit the chance that a single short-term treatment plan

CASE STUDY 15.2

"Judy and Patrick"

Judy is a licensed nurse who works the day shift in an oncology center. Patrick, a registered nurse who lives across the street from her, works the night shift on the same unit. He often works with only one night off and fills in for other nurses who want time off. His wife stays home with their five children, three of whom are under the age of 6 years. Judy has noticed that for the past few weeks, Patrick has been less social and more distant when she tries to talk to him. He seems so tired and sluggish; sometimes his speech is even slurred in the morning during shift report. There have been several times that Judy has asked him to complete charting that he leaves undone. She is concerned that maybe he is working too much and mentions the change in behavior to the unit supervisor.

The unit supervisor asks Judy if she has been giving more unit doses of injectable morphine to the clients. She states that the unit supply of morphine has been refilled almost daily for the past few weeks. Judy states that the majority of the clients with increasing doses are on patient-controlled analgesia (PCA) pumps and that she is administering about the same number of single injections each day. When they check the sign-out register for controlled medications, they note that most of the injectable doses are being given during the night shift. Some of the doses are signed out for clients who have PCA pumps who would not be receiving routine single doses of the drug.

Digging Deeper

1. *What are the indicators for a problem in this situation?*

2. *What symptoms does Patrick demonstrate that may explain the increased need for stock refills?*

3. *What factors may have led to Patrick's situation?*

4. *What legal responsibilities does Judy have?*

---

will be enough. In addition, coexisting medical and mental illnesses together with individual-specific social, marital, and family issues complicate the overall picture. This is the reason for ongoing multiple support methods and therapy to help the individual during the rough spots in this long road to recovery.

A combined approach of behavioral therapies together with medications and other services has proven the most effective in substance use treatment programs. A continuum of interventions that emphasize life changes often use the Twelve Step recovery program such as that used in Alcoholics and Narcotics Anonymous.

Detoxification

Detoxification is the first phase of dependency treatment and consists of immediate withdrawal from the physical and psychological effects of the drug that usually last from 3 to 5 days. For those individuals who are severely physically dependent on a substance, the withdrawal can produce life-threatening symptoms that include delirium, seizure activity, and coma. Unsupervised, the withdrawal from drug dependence can result in death.

For example, if street drugs are used to self-medicate the withdrawal symptoms, the result may be a lethal drug interaction and overdose. To provide a safe withdrawal, the supervised use of appropriate medications can help by aiding to restore normal brain functioning, diminish cravings, and minimize or counteract the withdrawal symptoms during the treatment process. Medications are currently available for detoxification of clients with opioid, nicotine, cocaine, methamphetamine, and marijuana addiction. Psychoactive medications such as antidepressants, antianxiety agents, mood stabilizers, and antipsychotic medications may be crucial to the treatment of those with a coexisting mental health disorder. The specific medications used will vary depending on the individual needs and severity of the individual's mental health disorder.

Planned interventions during the acute withdrawal state are directed toward controlling the symptoms of withdrawal without over sedating the client. Benzodiazepines are usually the medication of choice for alcohol detoxification, starting with a relatively large dose with daily reductions until withdrawal is complete. Multivitamin therapy and thiamine replacement therapy are used to prevent

"Keshaun" (continued)

fizkes/
Shutterstock

Recall the case of Keshaun, who started drinking when he was 15 to help him fit in with his peers. While you talk to him, he remembers being admitted to the local hospital on several occasions and has experienced withdrawal symptoms when he was unable to have his daily alcoholic drink. He says he has had several experiences where he went to a bar with some friends but couldn't recall the events that had happened after leaving the bar.

Keshaun states that he wants to stay sober this time and is willing to attend daily Twelve Step meetings after discharge from the facility. Part of the discharge plan includes goals and interventions the client sets for themselves for after discharge. You help Keshaun to frame these goals in a specific, measurable, and realistic format, much like nursing outcomes.

Digging Deeper

1. *What are some of the indications of a physical dependence on alcohol?*

2. *What are some of the ways that a client will often react when confronted with the behaviors they are exhibiting?*

3. *Write 2 goals you think Keshaun might come up with. Remember to make them specific, measurable, and realistic.*

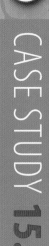
CASE STUDY 15.3

neuropathy and encephalopathy from chronic alcohol use (Wernicke–Korsakoff syndrome), because those who engage in chronic alcohol use are usually deficient in thiamine and niacin.

Disulfiram is a long-term alcohol use disorder treatment that inhibits alcohol ingestion by producing severe adverse effects if alcohol is ingested. The client should be advised to avoid hidden sources of alcohol such as artificial food flavorings or mouthwash that contains alcohol. During withdrawal, anticonvulsants may be ordered if seizure activity is not controlled by the benzodiazepines. Antiemetic agents may also be used to control symptoms of nausea and vomiting.

Opioid withdrawal symptoms can be minimized with clonidine in a detoxification setting. This agent lowers blood pressure, so it is essential to monitor vital signs closely during the withdrawal period. This approach is not as effective as using an opioid substitute, but the benefit is that it is nonaddicting and can keep the client opioid free so that other therapies can be initiated. Methadone is typically the opioid substitute used in heroin withdrawal maintenance programs. It is a chemical relative of heroin and is taken once daily by mouth to prevent symptoms of heroin withdrawal and to reduce craving for the drug. The daily dose is titrated over 2 weeks to a maintenance dose. The client may be in a maintenance program for up to 2 to 4 years. A longer-acting medication called orlaam can be taken three times

weekly and is used in some situations. In addition, the regimen for opiate withdrawal may include a muscle relaxant, antianxiety agent, and an anticholinergic for abdominal cramping.

Treatment Programs

Both inpatient and outpatient programs are available for substance use treatment. Once detoxification has taken place, continued treatment may be provided by medical and nonmedical services. Length of stay in residence facilities is dependent on the needs of the individual with the average being 6 to 12 months. Outpatient programs are designed to follow up the more intensive inpatient treatment. Cognitive-behavioral therapy is used in treatment centers for alcohol, marijuana, cocaine, and methamphetamine use. Both individual and group therapy are utilized to assist the client in identifying and understanding their maladaptive patterns of thinking and drug-seeking behaviors. A core element in the approach of therapy is to help the individual to anticipate the reality of relapse and ways to cope with desire for the drug. They are taught ways to avoid situations where relapse is more likely and to engage in new social support systems that are drug free.

Realizing that addiction is a complex problem that has severe effects on the entire life of the individual offers some insight into the difficulty seen in their ability to maintain abstinence.

Incentives and multiple means of encouragement must be provided as the client takes steps toward a more positive and productive lifestyle. Individual and family education groups, relapse prevention groups, follow-up drug testing, and Twelve Step programs (see Box 15.8) are some of the approaches for continued support during the recovery process. Reversing the addictive behaviors is difficult and relapse is common, but recovery and abstinence remains the ultimate goal.

BOX 15.8

Alcoholics Anonymous, Al-Anon, Narcotics Anonymous: Hope and Help for People Who Use Substances and Their Families

- Alcoholics Anonymous (AA) is an international fellowship of people who have a drinking problem. Anyone may attend open AA meetings, but only those with a drinking problem may attend closed meetings.
  - Members share their experiences, provide anonymity to each other, and meet together to attain and maintain sobriety. AA is a program of total abstinence. Members stay away from one drink, 1 day at a time. Sobriety is maintained through sharing experience, strength, and hope through meetings and the Twelve Steps for recovery from alcoholism.
- Purpose of Al-Anon is to help families and friends of people with alcohol use disorder recover from the effects of living with the problem of drinking of a relative or friend. Alateen is a recovery program for young people and is sponsored by Al-Anon members. The only requirement for membership in these groups is that there be a problem of alcoholism in a relative or friend.
- Narcotics Anonymous (NA) was started from the AA concept for those for whom drugs have become a major problem. Membership is open to all people with drug addictions, regardless of the particular drug or combination of drugs used. When this group was formed, the word "addiction" was substituted for "alcohol" to reflect the disease concept of addiction. One of the keys to the success of this group is the therapeutic value of people with addictions working with other people with addictions, sharing their successes, and challenges in overcoming active addiction. The Twelve Steps and Twelve Traditions of NA are the core principles of the recovery program.

Websites:
- https://www.aa.org
- https://al-anon.org
- https://www.na.org

Nursing Process and Care Plan *for the Client With a Substance Use Disorder*

It is important for the nurse to remember that any client they encounter may be using or misusing substances. This could include a pediatric client hospitalized for appendicitis, a postpartum client who delivered their first child, or a client who is post myocardial-infarction (heart attack). Each one of these clients may use a substance to the extent that they may experience withdrawal symptoms during their hospitalizations. Clients with substance use issues must be monitored for withdrawal symptoms, and safety should always be a priority. While the client is experiencing withdrawal or under the influence of a substance, the nurse should not attempt to discuss the client's feelings, treatment plan, or substance use.

Assessment (Data Collection)

When gathering data on the client with a substance use disorder, remember that underneath the surface of denial and rationalization are the feelings of fear, insecurity, anxiety, and low self-esteem. Some individuals may present voluntarily for treatment, whereas others are required to undergo treatment subsequent to a substance-related arrest.

The assessment interview should be directed toward identifying the type of substance the individual has been using, the amount and frequency of use, the last time substance was used, the method of ingestion, and the length of time the substance has been used. Many clients use more than one substance and may be willing to admit to one substance but deny using others, even when toxicology screens are positive. It is also important to obtain a description of any attempts to decrease or discontinue using the substance and any previous treatment.

Remember that most people with substance use disorders underreport the amount they ingest. The CAGE questionnaire is often used to screen for alcohol dependency. CAGE is an acronym that includes the following questions:

1. Have you ever felt you should **C**ut down on your drinking?
2. Have people **A**nnoyed you by criticizing your drinking?
3. Have you ever felt **G**uilty about your drinking?
4. Have you ever had a drink first thing in the morning (**E**ye-opener) to steady your nerves or get rid of a hangover?

A positive answer to two or more of these questions indicates that the client has an alcohol use disorder. This information is reported to the registered nurse and the health care provider.

Just the Facts	Since it was first introduced, the CAGE questionnaire has also been adapted to apply to other substances and is referred to the CAGE-AID questionnaire.

Also take note of any suicidal ideation or intent, along with the presence and character of any withdrawal symptoms. Withdrawal may be an issue, especially if the individual enters the hospital for another medical reason other than substance use. Knowledge of withdrawal symptoms for various substances can help you recognize and report their occurrence.

Try to identify the client's motivation for treatment as it is crucial to the outcome. Reason for admission is often a determining factor in the client's willingness to comply with the terms of the treatment contract. If the client is seeking relief from the substance-related problems with a sincere recognition of the problem, an expectation of success is more realistic than if the client has been admitted involuntarily or for another medical reason not pertaining to the substance-related problem.

Mind Jogger	How might someone with a substance use disorder employ a false attitude of sincerity and willingness to change as a way to get discharged?

Nurse–client interactions during the initial interview help to establish a trusting therapeutic relationship. The nurse should convey a manner that demonstrates the client is accepted and respected as an individual and not devalued for their addiction. Long-term recovery is often marked by periods of relapse with reoccurrence of substance using behavior after a significant period of abstinence. The nurse should refrain from judging the client or referring to this episode as failure. The nurse acts as a role model to demonstrate more effective problem-solving and coping skills. Active listening is used to reinforce that the client has an identity independent from the substance and to offer concern and support for the efforts to gain control over their life.

Collection of data that provides baseline physical and emotional information is done on admission. Box 15.9 lists data that should be collected.

BOX 15.9

Admission Data Collection on the Client With a Substance Use Disorder

NERVOUS SYSTEM

- Orientation
- Level of consciousness (LOC)
- Coordination, gait
- Short- and long-term memory (any difficulty following commands)
- Signs of depression or anxiety
- Tremors or decreased reflexes
- Pupils (constricted or dilated)

CARDIOVASCULAR AND RESPIRATORY

- Vital signs
- Peripheral pulses
- Dyspnea on exertion
- Abnormal breath sounds (a client with alcohol use disorder is susceptible to aspiration while intoxicated)
- Arrhythmias
- Fatigue
- Peripheral edema

GASTROINTESTINAL

- Nausea or vomiting
- Changes in weight or appetite
- Time of last meal
- Signs of malnourishment
- General nutritional status
- Ascites
- Color and consistency of stool

INTEGUMENTARY

- Location, size, and characteristics of any skin lesions
- Needle tracks or scarring on arms, legs, fingers, toes, under the tongue, or between gums and lips
- Complexion (ruddy or pale, petechiae)
- Skin color including jaundice or bruising

EMOTIONAL BEHAVIOR

- Affect
- Rate of speech
- Suspiciousness, anger, agitation
- Occurrence of hallucinations, blackouts
- History of violent episodes
- Support system: Is anyone present with the client? How do they interact with each other? Are they willing to be involved in the treatment of the client?

kurhan/
Shutterstock

CASE STUDY 15.4

"Frank"

Frank is a mechanic who is currently unemployed and has been admitted for evaluation and treatment of polysubstance use with opiate and alcohol dependency. Following a motor vehicle accident while "wiped out" on cocaine and alcohol. Frank is voluntarily admitting himself for detoxification. He has been using heroin, cocaine, and alcohol constantly for the past week. He is unable to remember where he has been or how long it has been since his last meal. He states he spends $200 to $300 a day on drugs and drinks at least a six pack of beer daily. He admits to doing many "bad things" to acquire the drugs. He is divorced and has not seen his three children in more than 2 years.

Digging Deeper

1. How would the nurse approach Frank on admission?

2. What questions would be important to ask Frank?

Frank states the last time he injected heroin and cocaine was 24 hours ago, shortly after which the accident occurred. He has had two previous admissions to treatment programs, but has not been successful in maintaining his abstinence.

The nurse assesses Frank's affect as appropriate and his mood as anxious and dysphoric. He remains isolated in his room with the curtains drawn. He states he is having some abdominal cramping and his legs are "knotting." He denies craving at this time but says his skin feels like it is "crawling."

1. The health care provider orders methadone tablets for the next 72 hours. What is the rationale for giving this medication? What other medications might be used instead?

2. How does Frank's behavior indicate symptoms of withdrawal?

3. What other nursing interventions are important for Frank during the detoxification process?

4. Frank tells the nurse, "I have nothing to live for anymore." How should the nurse respond?

Nursing Care Focus

Once the assessment data has been collected, a nursing care focus is determined. The focus will be different if the client is in withdrawal or if they are stable and admitted to a substance treatment center. Regardless of the facility and sobriety status, the client's safety is always a priority. Some clients will continue to seek a substance to use in order to counteract the side effects of acute withdrawal. Others may seek, obtain, and use the substance while undergoing a treatment program.

Outcome Identification and Planning

During the acute stage of withdrawal, the client needs physical and psychological support to return to a more stable state of health. The detoxification is usually accomplished within 7 days, depending on whether it is a short-acting or long-acting substance and the time needed for it to be eliminated from the body. Once the substance is out of the system, the client may experience sleeping and eating difficulties along with varied levels of irritability and anxiety. Remember that the without the substance, the client with a substance use disorder is a person who is hungry, angry, lonely, and tired, whose mind and body will want the substance. Short-term outcomes are that the client no longer exhibits any signs or symptoms of substance intoxication or withdrawal and has sustained no injuries during the detoxification period.

One barrier to long-term treatment success and sobriety is the client's use of denial. Denial is used by the client who has issues with the use of substances or is addicted to them. The individual uses denial to continue their use of the substance and as a self-protective mechanism during treatment. Since denial is a coping mechanism the individual has used for many years, it is a long-term coping strategy that takes continuous work by the individual to unlearn and change. Box 15.10 lists

BOX 15.10

Common Desired Outcomes for a Client With a Substance Use Disorder

During withdrawal the client will:
- Be free from harm during hospitalization.
- Exhibit a stable fluid and electrolyte balance.
- Demonstrate a restful sleep pattern.
- Exhibit decreased anxiety and increased relaxation.
- Exhibit stable vital signs.
- Be seizure free.

The client working on continued sobriety will:
- Identify the substance as a problem and take ownership of the problem.
- Identify changes in lifestyle that are necessary.
- Acknowledge responsibility for their own behavior and recognize the association between the substance and personal problems.
- Verbalize understanding of substance use and dependence as an illness requiring continued treatment and support.
- Identify alternative coping mechanisms to use in response to stress instead of the substance.
- Demonstrate increased feelings of self-worth by verbalizing positive statements about self.
- Verbalize understanding of illness and the recovery process.
- Demonstrate willingness to participate in a group recovery treatment program.

common desired outcomes for the client experiencing withdrawal and those for the client working on continued sobriety.

Nursing Care Focus

- Injury Risk

Goal

- The client will be safe and free from injury throughout hospitalization.

Implementations for Preventing Injury

The client who is withdrawing is at risk for injury that may be physical, neurologic, or self-inflicted in nature. Provide a quiet and safe environment. Consider placing them in a room near the nurses' station or where the staff can observe them closely. It may be necessary to assign a staff member to remain with the client at all times during the withdrawal period. Remove hazardous articles and furnishings. For example, provide only an electric shaver as the client may be shaking and risk cutting themselves with a bladed razor.

The client may experience a seizure during the withdrawal period. Seizure precautions should be started (padded side rails up, airway at bedside, etc.) upon admission. To help minimize the risk for seizures, the nurse should decrease environmental stimulation (avoid bright lights, TVs, electronic screens, visitors). Cluster care provided to the client to allow for rest periods and overstimulating them. Monitor vital signs, sleep pattern, and neurologic signs every 1 to 2 hours during the first 3 to 4 days of withdrawal, then as needed. Administer medications as prescribed.

During withdrawal, the client may be confused or experience hallucinations. Reorient as necessary to person, time, place, and situation as indicated when the client is confused or disoriented. Talk to the client in simple, direct, concrete language. Avoid lengthy interactions; keep your voice soft; speak clearly. Reassure the client that the bugs, snakes, and so on are not really there. Tell the client that you know these sights appear real to them, and acknowledge the client's fears, but leave no doubt about hallucinations not being real. Utilize a floor mattress if they attempt to climb out of bed.

During withdrawal the client may have a metabolic imbalance. Assess for hypoglycemia, electrolyte imbalance, respiratory depression, or arrhythmias. IV infusions may be ordered to help with fluid and electrolyte balance during withdrawal.

Clients may have suicidal ideation during this time. Report any statements the client makes about harming themselves. Ensure the client's room does not have any ligature points (hooks or furnishings that they can use to strangulate themselves on). Clients may be unaware of their surroundings and may need supervision.

Evaluation of Goal/Desired Outcome

The client will:

- not have a seizure while withdrawing.
- not harm themselves during a hallucination.
- not fall while withdrawing.
- not attempt suicide during hospitalization.

Nursing Care Focus

- Denial

Goal

- The client does not use denial to rationalize their behavior.

Implementations for Reducing Denial

The nurse should always maintain a nonjudgmental attitude. Do not criticize the client's use of a substance. The client will use denial with statements such as "I'm not an alcoholic because I have a job and a house. Only homeless people are alcoholics." Or "I can control my drinking." Or "I only use on weekends not during the week." The nurse should not argue but should dispel these statements with factual ones. Provide the client with factual information about substance use in a matter-of-fact manner.

The client will use denial by focusing on external problems (such as relationship or employment) but not associate the external problem in relation to their substance use. They will identify the troubles they are experiencing as being the fault of someone else and that they feel they are really the victim. The nurse should encourage the client to identify problems and the behaviors that led to those problems rather than letting the client focus on blaming others. It is important for the client to identify their role in their problems.

Do not allow the client to focus on circumstances that are out of their control. For example, the client states, "I have to work overtime because the company needs to make a profit," or "I'm stressed about all the crime in the city." Instead, redirect the client's focus to their own problems and to what they can do about them.

Provide the client with honest, positive reinforcement. This is especially important when they identify and expresses feelings or show insight into their behaviors and the consequences of their behaviors, including consequences related to their substance use (such as a driving while intoxicated arrest). Encourage the client to participate in unit and treatment activities. Give positive feedback when the client meets goals during treatment.

Evaluation of Goal/Desired Outcome

The client:

- admits they have a substance use problem.
- accepts responsibility for their behavior.
- accepts the consequences of their behavior.

CASE STUDY 15.5

Marcos Mesa Sam Wordley/Shutterstock

"Tom"

Tom is admitted for detoxification after his arrest for driving while intoxicated. He has been drinking for the past 3 days, with his last drink taken 12 hours ago. The following day, Tom is hollering and anxious because, he says, "There are black bugs all over this bed!"

Digging Deeper

1. How should the nurse respond to Tom's comment?

2. While doing a physical assessment of Tom, the nurse notes adventitious breath sounds. What action should the nurse take?

3. Tom's wife, Anna, tells the nurse she shouldn't have gone to her mother's earlier in the week because he did not want her to go. She says he wouldn't have been drinking if she had stayed home. How would the nurse describe this behavior?

4. How should the nurse respond to Anna?

5. How can involvement in an Alcoholics Anonymous treatment program benefit Tom?

6. What is essential to Tom's success at sobriety?

Cultural Considerations

Religious Use of Substances

Some religions around the world use substances as part of ceremonies. When the substance is part of a religious ceremony or ritual, it is for the specific purpose of connecting to the spiritual world or to obtain a significant vision. There are also religions that have a strong belief against the use of substances. The table below summarizes some religions that use, or prohibit the use of, substances. It is important for the nurse to document the client's religion and religious use of substances that the client identifies as using.

Religion	Substance	Purpose
Native American Church	Peyote	Heal, teach, and connect with God
Rastafarianism	Alcohol	Encouraged to avoid
	Cannabis	To increase spiritual awareness
Hinduism	Cannabis	To promote spiritual experiences
	Illegal drug use	Disapproved of
	Soma (a drink)	Used in worship
Islam	Alcohol and illegal drugs	Opposed to using
	Tobacco	Strongly discouraged
Seventh-Day Adventist	Alcohol, illegal drugs, and tobacco	Encouraged to abstain
Mormon (Church of Jesus Christ of Latter-Day Saints)	Alcohol, caffeine, illegal drugs, and tobacco	Opposed to using

Reference: Thomas, S. (2022). *Drug use in religions.* Recovery.org https://recovery.org/religions/

SUMMARY

- Substances that are used or misused are grouped into 10 categories. Substances can be prescription or over-the-counter medications, or illicit drugs. They can also include toxins, volatile substances such as gasoline or antifreeze, and other chemicals used with the intent of intoxication.
- Various theories exist regarding why substance use and dependence occurs, including genetics, observational learning of maladaptive coping behaviors, and the urge to conform to the group.
- The characteristic feature of substance use disorder is the behavioral, cognitive, and physiologic indications that the individual continues to use the substance regardless of the negative effects it imposes on their daily life. There is also an intense craving for the substance leading to substance-seeking behaviors.
- Addiction is a physiologic and psychological dependence on alcohol or other drugs that affect the central nervous system (CNS) in such a way that withdrawal symptoms are experienced when the substance is discontinued.

- All of the substances mentioned in this chapter have potential to be addictive.
- Treatment for substance-related disorders is twofold, beginning with detoxification and withdrawal from usage, followed by therapy. Therapeutic techniques may be part of an inpatient or residence program, or through an outpatient program. The ultimate goal of treatment is complete abstinence, which is difficult due to the chronic nature of addiction.
- The first step in recovery is for the individual to admit that a problem exists. Success is often dependent on involvement in a recovery group such as Alcoholics Anonymous, where participants support each other in their continuing efforts of abstinence.
- Relapse is common in the long-term treatment process. Cognitive and behavioral changes along with lifestyle alterations that encourage a substance-free existence are necessary.
- Acceptance of the responsibility to remain in treatment long enough for a positive recovery is ultimately a choice the client has to make.

BIBLIOGRAPHY

Alcoholics Anonymous. (2023). *The Twelve Steps.* https://www.aa.org/the-twelve-steps

Centers for Disease Control and Prevention. (2022). *Alcohol and caffeine.* Division of Population Health, National Center for Chronic Disease Prevention and Health Promotion. https://www.cdc.gov/alcohol/fact-sheets/caffeine-and-alcohol.htm#

Hartwell, K., & Brady, K. (2021). Determining appropriate levels of care for treatment of substance use disorders. *UpToDate.* Retrieved September 21, 2022, from https://www.uptodate.com/contents/determining-appropriate-levels-of-care-for-treatment-of-substance-use-disorders

Hoffman, R. S., & Weinhouse, G. L. (2021). Management of moderate and severe alcohol withdrawal syndromes. *UpToDate.* Retrieved September 21, 2022, from https://www.uptodate.com/contents/management-of-moderate-and-severe-alcohol-withdrawal-syndromes

National Council of State Boards of Nursing. (2022). *Substance use disorder in nursing.* https://www.ncsbn.org/nursing-regulation/practice/substance-use-disorder/substance-use-in-nursing.page

National Council of State Boards of Nursing. (2018). *A nurse's guide to substance use disorder in nursing.* https://www.ncsbn.org/public-files/SUD_Brochure_2014.pdf

National Highway Traffic Safety Administration. (2022). *Traffic safety facts annual report tables.* United States Department of Transportation. https://cdan.nhtsa.gov/tsftables/tsfar.htm

National Institute on Alcohol Abuse and Alcoholism. (2022). https://www.niaaa.nih.gov

National Institute on Drug Abuse. (2021a). *Cocaine DrugFacts.* National Institute on Drug Abuse; National Institutes of Health; U.S. Department of Health and Human Services. https://nida.nih.gov/publications/drugfacts/cocaine

National Institute on Drug Abuse. (2021b). *Heroin DrugFacts.* National Institute on Drug Abuse; National Institutes of Health; U.S. Department of Health and Human Services. https://nida.nih.gov/publications/drugfacts/heroin

National Institute on Drug Abuse. (2020a). *Inhalants DrugFacts.* National Institute on Drug Abuse; National Institutes of Health; U.S. Department of Health and Human Services. https://nida.nih.gov/publications/drugfacts/inhalants

National Institute on Drug Abuse. (2020b). *Synthetic Cannabinoids (K2/Spice) DrugFacts.* National Institute on Drug Abuse; National Institutes of Health; U.S. Department of Health and Human Services. https://nida.nih.gov/publications/drugfacts/synthetic-cannabinoids-k2spice

National Institute on Drug Abuse. (2019). *Cannabis (Marijuana) DrugFacts.* National Institute on Drug Abuse; National Institutes of Health; U.S. Department of Health and Human Services. https://nida.nih.gov/publications/drugfacts/cannabis-marijuana

Rahman, A., & Paul, M. (2021). Delirium Tremens. In *StatPearls.* StatPearls Publishing. Retrieved September 20, 2022, from https://www.ncbi.nlm.nih.gov/books/NBK482134/

Rigotti, N. A. (2022). Patterns of tobacco use. *UpToDate.* Retrieved September 21, 2022, from https://www.uptodate.com/contents/patterns-of-tobacco-use

Substance Abuse and Mental Health Services Administration. (2022). *The National Survey on Drug Use and Health: 2020.* https://www.samhsa.gov/data/sites/default/files/reports/rpt37924/2020NSDUH-NationalSlides072522.pdf

United States Drug Enforcement Administration. (2022). *Drug fact sheets.* U.S. Department of Justice. https://www.dea.gov/factsheets

Vera, M. (2022). *5 alcohol withdrawal nursing care plans.* Nurseslabs. https://nurseslabs.com/5-alcohol-withdrawal-nursing-care-plans/

Fill in the Blank

Fill in the blank with the correct answer.

1. A _____ is used in reference to any drug, medication, or toxin that has the potential for misuse.
2. _____ is a pattern of either consciously or unconsciously helping the maladaptive behavior to continue.
3. _____ is a physiologic or psychological dependence on a substance in which withdrawal symptoms are experienced if substance is discontinued.
4. The first phase of treatment is _____ or immediate withdrawal from the effects of drug use that usually lasts from 3 to 5 days.
5. A state of profound confusion and delusions along with all of the usual symptoms of alcohol withdrawal is _____ _____.
6. A nutritional disease of the nervous system caused by a thiamin and niacin deficiency found primarily in people with alcohol use disorder is _____-_____ _____.

Matching

Match the following terms to the most appropriate phrase.

1. _____ Shakes	a. Form of amnesia for events during drinking period
2. _____ Denial	b. Early symptom of alcohol withdrawal
3. _____ Thiamine	c. Strong inner drive to use a substance
4. _____ Codependence	d. Reversible behavior pattern caused by recent substance use
5. _____ Withdrawal	e. Overly responsible behavior
6. _____ Tolerance	f. Develops as brain adapts to repeated use of substance with declining effects
7. _____ Intoxication	g. Marked symptoms of "crashing" following intense period of substance use
8. _____ Nystagmus	h. Vitamin used in treatment of alcohol dependence
9. _____ Blackout	i. Constant involuntary movement of eyeball
10. _____ Craving	j. Not admitting to having a substance use problem

Multiple Choice

Select the best answer from the multiple-choice items.

1. The nurse is taking hourly vital signs on a client in acute alcohol withdrawal. The client's blood pressure and pulse were recorded as 132/68, 78 at 2200; 138/72, 84 at 1400; 148/86, 90 at 0200; and 160/94, 100 at 0400. Which of the following actions would the nurse initiate?
   a. Increase fluid intake to 3,000 cc in the next 12 hours
   b. Initiate interventions for fall precautions
   c. Obtain a clean catch urine specimen
   d. Notify the health care provider

2. A client is admitted to the psychiatric unit with a blood alcohol level of 0.03%. They are disoriented with slurred speech and a staggering gait. The nurse would correctly infer that this client:
   a. Has symptoms of intoxication
   b. Has developed a tolerance to alcohol
   c. Is experiencing alcohol withdrawal
   d. Is probably using more than one substance

3. The client tells the nurse they are not "an alcoholic" and only drink "two or three beers" with their coworker every day after work and maybe one or two drinks at home and says, "I can handle it. I've never missed work because of it." The coping mechanism being used is:
   a. Denial
   b. Projection
   c. Displacement
   d. Rationalization

4. While the nurse is collecting data on a client being admitted for treatment of alcohol dependency, the client says, "I suppose you think I am just another drunk." The nurse's best response to this statement would be:
   a. "I care for many people who have the same problem you do."
   b. "Why do you think you are a drunk?"
   c. "At least you are being honest about it."
   d. "I am most concerned that you receive treatment for your problem."

5. A licensed nurse is admitted for treatment of prescription drug dependency. Which attitude by the nursing staff would be considered an enabling behavior?
   a. Helping the client to identify the issues in the nursing environment as a result and not the cause of their drug habit
   b. Agreeing that the staff shortages and increasing pressures at work may have led to the drug-using behaviors
   c. Supporting the client as they acknowledge that this treatment is required by the State Board of Nursing
   d. Encouraging the client to participate in a drug-related support group

6. The nurse is collecting data on a client who has been admitted from the emergency department after several days of inhaling spray paint. What symptoms would the nurse see in this client?
   a. Dilated pupils, masklike facial appearance, nystagmus
   b. Constricted pupils, drowsiness, attention deficit
   c. Lip-licking, nausea and vomiting, dyskinesia
   d. Coughing, dyspnea, watery eyes

7. A client is admitted to the inpatient unit with a diagnosis of chronic alcohol use disorder and Wernicke–Korsakoff syndrome. Which intervention would the nurse include in the client's plan of care?
   a. Methadone maintenance program
   b. Client teaching in stress management
   c. Thiamine and niacin vitamin supplements
   d. Fifteen-minute–interval suicide precautions

8. A client is receiving treatment for methamphetamine dependence. Which activity would be most helpful for the client in remaining drug-free after discharge?
   a. Understanding how the drug is affecting them
   b. Admission that they have a drug problem
   c. Moving to a new geographic location
   d. Becoming involved in a community activity center

9. A client is in the emergency department after first responders prevented them from attempting to jump from a 10-story building. The urine sample tests positive for LSD. What is the client experiencing?
   a. Illusion
   b. Temporary insanity
   c. Perceptual changes
   d. Delirium tremens

10. The nurse is collecting data on the client who has been admitted for substance use detoxification. What statements made by the client would support this admission? *(Select all that apply)*
    a. "I don't need to be here. I don't have a drug problem."
    b. "Sometimes when I drink I wake up the next morning and don't remember what happened."
    c. "I have perfect attendance at my job."
    d. "This is the fourth time in the past 2 years I've been admitted for this."
    e. "My parents are both alcoholics."

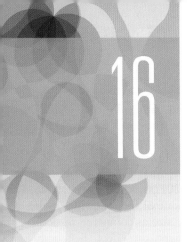

16 Eating Disorders

Introduction

In all cultures, food is customary at events and family gatherings. Changing family structures, norms, and busy schedules have made fast food a multibillion-dollar industry. While food is essential for the body, emotions and expectations can also be tied to eating in some families. Social media and advertising emphasize different body styles that are promoted as "ideal." "Body shaming" is a tactic used in online bullying. Numerous dieting approaches are advertised and sold as quick-fix remedies to curb an increasing trend in obesity. The perceived need to conform to a specific body size or weight can overshadow sensible and nutritionally safe food intake. All of these factors can lead some individuals to have a difficult time distinguishing between realistic ways of healthy eating, controlling weight and body image, and what constitutes a severe disturbance and often dangerous pattern of eating behaviors.

> **Just the Facts** Although obesity is considered a medical condition, and has varying causative factors, it is not considered a mental disorder.

The three most common eating disorders are anorexia nervosa, bulimia nervosa, and binge-eating disorder. Binge-eating disorder is the most common of the eating disorders accounting for almost half of the cases while 12% of the cases are diagnosed as bulimia nervosa and 3% are diagnosed as anorexia nervosa (National Eating Disorders Collaboration, 2022a).

The exact cause of eating disorders is unclear. Genetic, social, and psychological components impact the individual's risk for developing an eating disorder. Individuals with eating disorders often have an underlying misperception that their self-worth is related to shape and weight and the ability to control them. Other symptoms tend to evolve out of this irrational thinking and the individual's coping strategies. It is important to recognize the relationship or significance food has to the person and their sense of self. This helps the understanding about how food can become a negative and menacing threat to their life.

> **Just the Facts** Eating disorders are more common in the Western countries than in other countries.

Anorexia Nervosa

Anorexia nervosa is an eating disorder characterized by an individual who loses weight, either by restricting calories or excessive exercise, has an inappropriate weight for their age and stature, and has a distorted body image (National Eating Disorders Association, 2022a). The distorted body image includes at least one of the following: their actual weight and body size as compared to their perception of their weight, the effect their body size has on their self-worth, or denial of the seriousness of their low body weight.

Although the term "anorexia" means a loss of appetite, the absence of appetite is not used to describe this disorder. When the disorder develops during childhood or adolescence, the symptom may be a failure to maintain a growth pattern instead of weight loss. These criteria, however, must be viewed with the individual's body build and that of other family members in mind. Genetic tendencies for a smaller body frame and bone structure need to be considered.

> **Just the Facts** Anorexia nervosa is characterized by an extreme fear of gaining weight that results in an ongoing and focused quest for thinness and calorie restriction to maintain or lose weight.

Signs and Symptoms

The individual with anorexia nervosa has an extreme fear of gaining weight. However, the fear of weight gain is not relieved as the individual experiences weight loss. This fear may even intensify as weight loss accumulates. When the individual reaches a weight that is below the standard for age and stature, they continue to mentally visualize themselves as overweight and continue their quest to lose more weight. The behaviors the individual uses to achieve weight loss categorize anorexia nervosa into one of two subtypes: restricting or binge-eating/purging.

The restricting type includes those whose weight loss is achieved through dieting, starvation, or excessive exercise. Weight loss is often accomplished by reducing total food intake to only a few foods, with a drastic exclusion of both overall caloric intake and essential nutrients or food groups. The individual may avoid food or meals, weigh their food, or methodically count all calories in their food. In addition, they may

"Wendy"

Wendy Chu, 16 years old, is brought to the health care provider's office after she passed out during her physical education (P.E.) class. She is accompanied by her grandmother who is her primary caregiver. During the nurse's data collection, Wendy reports her menstrual periods are irregular and she can't remember when her last one was. Her grandmother states, "She always does well in school and she's taking extra classes this year to graduate early. Her mother graduated from high school early too. She's probably tired from the extra classes."

The nurse's data collection reveals that Wendy is a thin, small-framed teenaged female with excess body hair and amenorrhea who complains that the exam room is "freezing cold" and asks for a blanket.

Digging Deeper

1. *Amenorrhea is common in individuals with eating disorders, due to low hormone levels, but what other causes should also be investigated?*

2. *When collecting data on clients with eating disorders, why is it important to collect data on the family and recent life events in addition to physical data?*

3. *While these are typical findings in a female client with anorexia nervosa, what other causes of these findings should also be considered?*

CASE STUDY 16.1

---

attempt increased weight loss through purging or increased compulsive exercise.

Individuals with the binge-eating/purging type restrict their food intake as described above but also regularly indulge in binge-eating, purging, or both. **Binge-eating**, or binging, is eating an unusually large amount of food, usually within a 2-hour time frame, that is more than most people would eat in a similar circumstance. **Purging** is the eliminating of consumed food through self-induced vomiting or with excessive use of laxatives or diuretics. Most individuals with anorexia who engage in binge-eating also follow these episodes with purging methods.

> **Just the Facts** Anorexia nervosa may cause the individual's hair and nails to become brittle, fragile, and easily broken resulting from the lack of essential nutrients needed for body maintenance.

The individual with anorexia nervosa exhibits a distorted view of body weight and size with the actual reality of their body proportions. The actual image of what they see in the mirror does not match the image they have in their mind of themselves (Fig. 16.1). Some may see their entire body as being "fat," whereas others may realize

they are thin but see certain body areas such as the buttocks, arms, abdomen, or thighs as too large. They may use methods such as repeated weighing, measuring of body parts, or viewing themselves in a mirror to reinforce their self-image. The individual's self-esteem is dependent on their body shape and size. Weight loss is seen as a major accomplishment of self-control, whereas weight gain is viewed as a failure. Distorted thinking is also seen in the repeated denial of the dangerous medical implications of their disorder. The starvation and malnutrition that are seen in

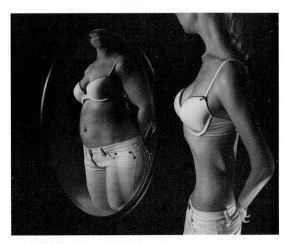

Figure 16.1 Distorted body image seen in anorexia nervosa.

Medical Conditions Caused by Anorexia Nervosa

- Anemia
- Cardiac arrest and death
- Electrolyte imbalances
- Hypothyroidism
- Impaired kidney function
- Malnutrition
- Metabolic disturbances
- Osteoporosis

Physical Findings Associated With Anorexia Nervosa

- Amenorrhea
- Arrhythmias including bradycardia
- Calluses on dorsal hand surface from inducing vomiting (Russell sign)
- Constipation
- Decrease in white blood cell (WBC) count
- Dehydration
- Dental erosion
- Dizziness
- Dry skin
- Elevated liver enzymes
- Fainting
- Fatigue
- Hypotension
- Lanugo on trunk, face, upper arms, and shoulders
- Low levels of sex hormones (estrogen/testosterone)
- Swollen salivary glands
- Subnormal body temperature or sensitivity to cold

anorexia nervosa can cause serious medical conditions, some life-threatening. Medical conditions that are caused by anorexia nervosa are described in Box 16.1.

Just the Facts

An indicator of physiologic dysfunction in the patient assigned female at birth with anorexia nervosa (who has already reached menarche—that is, their first menstrual period—and is otherwise physically capable of menstruation) is decreased levels of the pituitary hormones follicle-stimulating hormone (FSH) and luteinizing hormone (LH) and ovarian estrogen secretion, which results in amenorrhea, or the absence of menstrual periods.

Other symptoms or physical findings include a depressed mood, social withdrawal, irritability, insomnia, swollen joints, a decreased libido, and loss of bone mass (Box 16.2). Symptoms of depression may be secondary to the effects of starvation and lack of nutrition to body cells. Vital signs and electrolytes can become imbalanced, sometimes leading to cardiac arrest and death. Most of the physical conditions can be reversed as weight returns to normal.

Individuals with anorexia nervosa also exhibit an obsessive preoccupation with thoughts related to food. They may hoard food items or collect magazines and recipes related to food. Many actually prepare flavorful meals for their families but do not actually consume any portion of the food themselves. Behaviors seen as part of food avoidance or weight loss are listed in Box 16.3.

Incidence and Etiology

Anorexia nervosa is usually first seen between the ages of 13 and 18. It occurs in about 0.6%

of the United States adult population. It is seen three times more often in females than males in the general population. However, in clinical settings the ratio of females to males is even higher, ranging from 10:1 to 20:1 (Yager, 2022a). Neurotransmitter, psychosocial, and genetic factors are thought to be related to the cause of anorexia nervosa.

In anorexia nervosa, neurotransmitter imbalances are seen in low dopamine and serotonin functioning. Dopamine is thought to be responsible

Behaviors Seen in Anorexia Nervosa

- Concern about eating in public
- Wants to isolate to eat
- Excuses to miss mealtimes
- Compulsive exercise
- Obsessive preoccupation with food
- Leaving table immediately after meal (to purge)
- Wearing layers of clothing to keep warm or to hide body size
- Self-esteem dependent on body shape and size
- Weight loss seen as accomplishment
- Denial of potential medical problems
- Repeatedly weighing themselves
- Social withdrawal
- Smoking
- Alcohol or drug use

for an individual's eating, motivation, and reward behaviors while serotonin is thought to be responsible for the impulse control and obsessive behavior (Yager, 2022a).

Symptoms commonly follow stressful life events, such as starting high school, moving to a new location, experiencing sexual abuse, or having traumatic family relationships. Individuals with this disorder are typically in high school, or high school graduates, and have middle- to upper-income families. These families at first seem to be loving and cohesive, with model compliant, obedient, and perfectionist children who aim to please parents and teachers. However, further evidence usually reveals unresolved family conflicts with inconsistent patterns of overprotective and rigid parenting in which the child remains in a dependent state. The eating disorder may be a desperate attempt by the adolescent to separate from the family system, in particular from a dominant and overcritical parent.

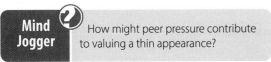

Mind Jogger Considering both the distorted view of self and compulsive need for perfection, in what type(s) of occupations might the individual with anorexia nervosa be employed?

Individuals with anorexia nervosa are often shy, quiet, orderly, and oversensitive to rejection with heightened feelings of inferiority, self-imposed guilt, and unreasonable expectations for perfection. These personality characteristics of excessive self-criticism and sensitivity commonly lead to emotion-focused problem solving. They believe the only way to overcome their lack of self-worth and value and gain control of their lives is by exercising control over their body.

A sense of worth and value becomes intertwined with the ability to lose weight. Their need for autonomy and control of self is demonstrated by controlling what they eat, which is ultimately their body image. They have a distorted view of their body and perceive weight gain as a lack of control over themselves and failure to meet their unrealistic self-standards.

Mind Jogger How might peer pressure contribute to valuing a thin appearance?

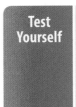

Test Yourself
✔ How does anorexia nervosa differ from the medical term anorexia?
✔ Describe the two subtypes of anorexia nervosa.
✔ List four medical conditions and four physical findings that can be seen in the individual with anorexia nervosa.

Bulimia Nervosa

In **bulimia nervosa,** the individual either binge-eats or regularly overeats and then uses self-induced methods, such as vomiting or the use of laxatives, to counteract the food consumed. Individuals with bulimia nervosa often report a "feeling of being out of control" during the episode of binge-eating or overeating. Those with bulimia nervosa typically do not have the distorted body image that is seen with anorexia nervosa. In fact, those with bulimia nervosa often recognize that their eating is abnormal and report feelings of guilt, anxiety, or shame regarding their eating and or the food consumed. However, the binge-eating and purging that is seen in bulimia nervosa can be seen in a subtype of anorexia nervosa. The individual with bulimia nervosa is typically within a normal weight range for height and age which is different from the individual with anorexia nervosa.

Signs and Symptoms

The components of bulimia nervosa include both binge-eating episodes and the use of compensatory methods to prevent weight gain. **Compensatory methods** are laxatives, diuretics, or enemas used to counteract the amount of food consumed. Typically, the episodes occur on average once a week. There is a lack of control or inability to stop eating during a binge episode. The type of food consumed varies, but typically is an indulged craving for high-calorie, sweet, or carbohydrate foods such as pastry, ice cream, cake, or pizza. Rapid hidden consumption of food is typical, with continued eating despite an uncomfortable feeling of fullness. The individual with bulimia nervosa usually consumes more calories during a binge episode than those without the disorder consume in an entire meal. Individuals are usually ashamed of their eating problem and attempt to hide their behaviors.

Binging usually occurs after a depressed mood state, individual stressors, periods of strict dieting, or negative self-talk about body image. The binge

BOX 16.4

Signs and Symptoms of Bulimia Nervosa

- Binging with inability to stop eating
- Craving for high-calorie or sweet foods
- Consumption of many calories in a binge
- Shame about eating problem
- Attempting to hide food consumption
- Depression
- Negative self-image
- Repeated use of induced vomiting
- Use of laxatives, diuretics, or enemas
- Normal weight for age and height with little fluctuation
- Outward preoccupation with food
- Stashing of food
- Associated personality and anxiety disorders
- Leaving table frequently during meal, or immediately after (in order to purge)

used method is self-induced vomiting. Purging is used by most individuals who present for treatment of this eating disorder. They may feel a temporary sense of relief after the vomiting, both physically and psychologically. Purging is usually easily induced after repeated stimulation of the gag reflex by inserting fingers or other flat objects into the pharynx. Over time, a callus can develop on the dorsal hand surface from the rubbing of the teeth against the skin during induced vomiting. Individuals with bulimia nervosa may use compensatory methods along with induced vomiting.

Fasting for a period of time may also be used in combination with excessive exercise to alleviate the guilt felt after binging. The individual may engage in exercise during inappropriate times in unusual places. They may secretively stash food or make excuses for spending extended time in the bathroom, usually after consuming a large amount of food.

Physical findings seen in individuals with bulimia nervosa are related to the effects of altered nutrition and the results of the purging methods (Box 16.5). Medical problems related to bulimia nervosa include dehydration, hypokalemia, menstrual irregularities, and electrocardiogram changes (from the hypokalemia). A typical finding seen in an individual who regularly vomits is the erosion of dental enamel from the acidic stomach contents. A dental hygienist may be one of the first people to notice this condition.

may temporarily relieve the dysphoric state; however, increased depression and self-dislike quickly emerge after the episode. A continued pattern of binge-eating results in an impaired ability to refrain from indulging in the binge or to stop it once the eating begins. See Box 16.4 for signs and symptoms associated with bulimia nervosa.

The second primary symptom of bulimia nervosa is the repeated use of purging methods after binge-eating or overeating. The most commonly

CASE STUDY 16.2

"George"

George is a 20-year-old college student who has come to the student health center and is accompanied by his dorm assistant. The dorm assistant was worried that George had the flu after the roommate reported that George had been throwing up several times a day. The data collected shows that George is 5 feet 8 inches and weighs 175 pounds. He has calluses on the back of his knuckles. He states the vomiting usually occurs after his hardest class and occasionally gets constipated and needs to use a laxative. After developing trust with the client, the nurse asks questions about his vomiting episodes. George admits that he binge-eats after his hardest class and then self induces vomiting because he "feels disgusted" with himself. The health care provider at student health center refers George to a mental health provider for outpatient therapy.

Digging Deeper

1. The individual with bulimia nervosa is often within normal weight for their height and age. What other data should be collected in a client that would indicate an eating disorder?

2. What means does an individual with bulimia nervosa use to prevent weight gain or deal with the excess food consumed?

3. What potential insights could George gain through outpatient therapy?

Physical Findings Associated With Bulimia Nervosa

- Loss of dental enamel—teeth appear ragged and "moth-eaten"
- Increased dental caries
- Swollen salivary glands
- Calluses or scars on dorsal surface of hand
- Menstrual irregularities
- Constipation
- Rectal prolapse
- Tears in esophageal or gastric mucosa
- Electrolyte imbalances
- Metabolic alkalosis (due to loss of stomach acid) or metabolic acidosis (due to frequent diarrhea)
- Gastric distress or bleeding
- Kidney failure

Incidence and Etiology

Bulimia nervosa is typically first seen around the age of 18. It occurs in about 1% of the U.S. adult population; however, this number is an estimate, as eating disorders are often hidden from others, including health care professionals. It is seen three times more often in females than males. However, in the clinical setting the ratio of females to males is even higher at 13:1 (Yager, 2022a).

Many individuals with bulimia nervosa have symptoms of depression, anxiety, panic disorder, or post-traumatic stress syndrome. Substance use is also common. Social and coping skills are inadequate and interpersonal relationships usually suffer from the lying and hidden behaviors.

Just the Facts ① Individuals with bulimia nervosa are more aware of their own eating disorder and more distressed by the symptoms than those with anorexia nervosa. Even after clinical recovery, many continue to experience considerably more body image problems and psychosomatic symptoms than those who have never had bulimia nervosa.

Mind Jogger ② It is said that the individual with bulimia nervosa replaces anxiety felt before the binge with guilt following the binge. How might this lead to other self-abusive behaviors?

Test Yourself
- ✔ Describe the two main symptoms seen in bulimia nervosa.
- ✔ Describe compensatory methods and why they are used.
- ✔ How does body weight differ between anorexia nervosa and bulimia nervosa?

Binge-Eating Disorder

Binge-eating disorder involves recurrent binge-eating episodes during which the individual loses control over the eating compulsion, like that seen in bulimia nervosa. These episodes, however, are not followed by purging, use of compensatory methods, or excessive exercise. Individuals with binge-eating disorder report similar behaviors, feelings, and thoughts regarding their eating episodes as those with bulimia nervosa. Some common feelings include a lack of control over the eating (either being able to stop or the amount of food consumed), eating alone as they are embarrassed by the amount of food consumed, or feeling disgusted with themselves or guilt after overeating. The severity of the disorder is determined by the number of episodes of binge-eating the individual has in a week (Box 16.6).

Signs and Symptoms

The individual with binge-eating disorder tends to be overweight or obese as a result of the binge-eating. The binge-eating episode may occur from stress, anger, or loneliness, and the eating is used as a coping mechanism to avoid the emotional distress. They usually feel guilt and shame about their eating, which can initiate another binge to help cope with the feelings experienced. Food consumption is usually accomplished quickly and often alone in secret. The amount eaten is usually in excess of 10,000 calories at one time. The fact that the individual feels full does not stop the binging. Restricting food in between binges also seems to trigger more binging. Box 16.7 lists signs and

Severity of Binge-Eating Disorder

Mild: 1–3 binge episodes per week
Moderate: 4–7 binge episodes per week
Severe: 8–13 binge episodes per week
Extreme: 14 or more binge episodes per week

symptoms associated with binge-eating disorder. The individual is at a higher risk for experiencing chronic pain and developing diabetes mellitus or hypertension.

Incidence and Etiology

Binge-eating disorder typically first develops in the late teenage years to early 20s. It occurs in about 1.2% of the U.S. adult population. It is seen twice as often in females than males. Approximately 75% of individuals with binge-eating disorder have at least one or more mental disorders including specific phobias, social anxiety disorder, depression, post-traumatic stress disorder (PTSD), attention deficit hyperactivity disorder, or substance use or dependence, usually with alcohol. Personality disorders are seen in about 30% of individuals with binge-eating disorder.

Although it is not known exactly what causes the binge-eating, most individuals with the disorder tend to have a low self-image and impulsive behaviors. A family history of an eating disorder increases the risk for an individual to develop binge-eating disorder. Media emphasis on weight and appearance is considered an underlying stigma that adds to the self-criticism, shame, and guilt.

Treatment of Eating Disorders

Treatment for eating disorders involves psychotherapy (usually cognitive-behavioral therapy) in addition to individual and family therapy. Treatment also includes nutritional support and sometimes antianxiety or antidepressant medications. Topics covered during treatment include the individual's ability to recognize the relationship between food, eating patterns, and the complications of the disorder.

For individuals with anorexia nervosa, goals of treatment revolve around reversal of the restrictive or maladaptive patterns of eating and thinking about food and their perceived body image. Individual planning is also centered on the reestablishment of healthy eating habits. Weight gain is considered the goal of treatment. Physical problems often correct themselves as weight is regained and normal nutritional intake is consistent.

The client must confront dysfunctional thoughts and irrational beliefs about self-image and food and replace them in realistic terms. Behavior therapy may involve a reward contract in which privileges are exchanged for increased food intake. Gradual increase in caloric intake may also be used to help the client overcome the fearful avoidance of food. Antidepressant medications including fluoxetine, nortriptyline, olanzapine, and mirtazapine may be used in combination with psychotherapy. In some cases, antianxiety medications such as lorazepam or chlorpromazine may be useful for short-term relief of anxiety.

Treatment of the individual with bulimia nervosa includes relinquishing the behaviors of binging and purging as normal eating patterns are restored. In the individual with bulimia nervosa, therapy is designed to help them take a self-inventory of eating, binging, and purging behaviors along with the events and feelings that precede the maladaptive eating behaviors. Encouraging them to keep a food and emotional diary will help them to see the relation between their feelings and behaviors. Education is provided about healthy nutritional habits along with efforts to reorganize the maladaptive thinking related to food, body image, and personal achievement.

Behavioral methods include a means of exposing the individual to situations that invite binging, but the action is prevented. With repeated exposures, they gradually become less fearful of the circumstances that previously initiated the compulsive behavior. Anxiety-reducing relaxation techniques are used to decrease the need for compensatory action and introduce preventative strategies. Antidepressant medications have been used successfully for clients with bulimia nervosa when combined with psychotherapy. Fluoxetine and desipramine are commonly used with careful monitoring for side effects.

The method of treatment program varies with the needs of the individual. Care is often provided in outpatient therapy utilizing a multidisciplinary approach involving a psychotherapist, physician, and registered dietitian. Inpatient programs are more intense and more structured than

BOX 16.8

Information Sources on Eating Disorders

- National Institute of Mental Health (NIMH)
  https://www.nimh.nih.gov/health/topics/eating-disorders
- National Eating Disorders Association
  https://www.nationaleatingdisorders.org
- National Association of Anorexia Nervosa and Associated Disorders
  https://anad.org

outpatient treatment can provide. Hospitalization may be necessary in severe cases that involve medical complications. Follow-up counseling and referrals to support groups are helpful to reinforce treatment outcomes and prevent a return to maladaptive eating habits. National websites offer information about eating disorders and treatment (Box 16.8).

Test Yourself

✔ How does binge-eating disorder differ from bulimia nervosa?
✔ List three behaviors exhibited in binge-eating disorder.
✔ Describe the treatment for eating disorders.

Nursing Process and Care Plan *for the Client With an Eating Disorder*

Because eating disorders are often hidden from others, the client may be reluctant to share specifics related to their behaviors and feelings. The nurse must use an accepting, caring, and nonjudgmental approach in order to establish a therapeutic relationship with the client who has an eating disorder. Nursing interventions and plan of care to stabilize the client should be viewed as safety interventions and take priority over psychosocial nursing interventions when the client is admitted.

Assessment (Data Collection)

Many individuals with eating disorders deny their problem and maintain their maladaptive eating patterns for several years before treatment is sought, often by concerned family members or during a medical crisis episode such as loss of consciousness from hypotension or electrolyte imbalance. Behaviors such as binging and purging are done in secret and may not be detected until more objective symptoms are noted.

The nurse's attitude and approach when interacting with the client, whether in an emergency room or other clinical situation, is essential to earning the trust of the client. Many individuals with eating disorders are ashamed of their behaviors and may want to divulge the magnitude of their problem but may refrain because of negative or blocking statements made by the nurse or if the client perceives the nurse is uncaring or judgmental. It is important for the nurse to self-examine their own feelings about food, dieting, and body image to maintain an objective view of the client's situation. A nonconfrontational and nonjudgmental approach without an authoritative attitude is important to convey caring, compassion, and willingness to understand the extent of the client's feelings and behaviors towards eating.

Information about dietary intake and eating patterns should be gathered with caution to avoid questions that may imply that the client has an eating disorder. In the client's mind, they may not see themselves as having a problem. Questions that ask how often the client induces vomiting after eating or inquire about feelings after binge-eating would imply that a problem exists. Because they are usually supersensitive to criticism, it is best to avoid asking clients questions that can be misinterpreted in this context. Use of active listening and open-ended techniques will aid in encouraging the client to communicate freely. Questions such as, "Tell me how you feel about your body." "How do you feel after eating?" or "What happens after you eat?" will help the nurse gain more insight to the client's relationship with eating. This approach also allows the client to provide data that they may not provide with direct questions.

Objective data to be collected includes the client's vital signs (look for hypotension and bradycardia), height and weight, body stature, and body mass index (BMI). A blood glucose level should be done to check for hypo or hyperglycemia. Observe the body for general signs of inadequate nutrition including turgor; nail, skin, and hair status for brittleness and dryness; and erosion of tooth enamel. Look for abrasions or calluses on the back of the hands related to induced purging. Examine the client's body for increased hair growth (lanugo). An electrocardiogram may be ordered to look for arrhythmias. Laboratory data that might be ordered includes a complete blood count (to check for anemia and leukopenia), a metabolic profile (to check electrolytes and kidney function), cholesterol levels, liver enzymes, protein, albumin, and thyroid levels. A urinalysis would be done to check for color, specific gravity, and presence of ketones or glucose. An A1C test may be done to gauge the client's average blood glucose over the past 6 weeks. The client should also have a pregnancy test since they may have irregular to absent periods and may be pregnant without knowing it.

Inquire about the date of last menstrual period (LMP). Obtain date of last bowel movement and typical elimination pattern. Determine patterns in bowel elimination. Gather information about insomnia, fatigue, and intolerance or sensitivity to cold temperatures. Determine if the client is taking any prescribed medications or herbal supplements. Collect data on any smoking, alcohol, or substance use.

Inquire about family and client history of any mental disorders including depression, specific phobias, social anxiety disorder, and death by suicide or suicide attempts. Have the client describe any recent stressors such as starting a new school or job, family conflicts, or any relationships that ended.

Nursing Care Focus

The effects of eating disorders may affect several body systems and create safety issues in addition to the mental health focus of nursing care. The focus of nursing care for the client with an eating disorder initially is on stabilization of medical issues related to the eating disorder and can include Altered Tissue Perfusion, Dehydration, Diarrhea, Electrolyte Imbalance, Hypotension, Hypovolemia, and Vomiting.

After medical stabilization, the focus of nursing care for the client with an eating disorder can include: Anxiety, Activity Intolerance, Altered Body Image Perception, Chronic Low Self-Esteem, Constipation Risk, Feeding ADL Deficit, Injury Risk, Malnutrition Risk, Overweight, Situational Low Self-Esteem, or Vomiting.

Outcome Identification and Planning

After medical stabilization, the anticipated outcomes for the client with an eating disorder are focused on having the client identify situations that lead to avoidance of food or binging, stabilizing the weight loss pattern, and normalizing eating patterns. Box 16.9 lists common desired outcomes for the client with an eating disorder.

BOX 16.9

Common Desired Outcomes for a Client With an Eating Disorder

The client:
- Verbalizes decreased fear and anxiety related to weight gain and inability to maintain control
- Consumes adequate nutritional intake to meet body requirements for height and age
- Demonstrates appropriate eating behaviors
- Verbalizes events or thoughts that precipitate anxiety
- Does not engage in binge-eating or purging
- Participates in activity level appropriate for health maintenance
- Verbalizes realistic view of body image
- Expresses understanding of relationship between feelings and eating behaviors
- Identifies ways to maintain a healthy means of weight control
- Identifies strengths and makes positive self-statements
- Demonstrates improved interpersonal skills in social setting

---

Nursing Care Focus

- Ineffective health maintenance, related to decreased food intake and weight loss

Goal

- The client will demonstrate regular, independent, nutritional eating habits.

(Note: this is an example of a goal for a client who is not severely nutritionally compromised and does not require total parental nutrition or nasogastric tube feedings.)

Implementations for Improving Food Intake and Weight Gain

When working with the client who has an eating disorder, one intervention that can help the client feel a sense of control is the initiation of a contract that details goals and expectations of both the client and the treatment team. This also helps the client with their sense of self responsibility. However, if the client does not agree or is not part of setting the contract, it will not be effective.

Nursing interventions should reflect normalized behaviors that the client can follow after discharge. These include weighing, eating, mealtimes, food choices, and physical activity. The nurse's reactions can model to the client a neutral reaction regarding being weighed. Avoid weighing the client daily as this puts an emphasis on the weight and not the healthy eating. Once a week, weights should be done on the same scale, prior to breakfast but after voiding, with the client wearing a hospital gown. Some clients try to increase their weight with a full bladder or by hiding objects in pockets or wearing weights. The nurse should not tell the client the weight or let the client see the number. The nurse should use a matter-of-fact attitude that does not convey approval or disapproval of the weight gain or loss, as this helps to separate emotions from the client's food consumption.

The nurse should keep a record of the client's food consumption, but the records should not be visible to the client or kept in the client's room to prevent them from focusing on the details of their eating. The nurse should be unobtrusive and neutral when monitoring the client's intake. This also helps to separate emotions from food consumption. The client should not be the one to fill out their diet intake as they may record a false amount.

The unit should have boundaries to mealtimes that include what time meals occur, length of mealtime, where the client can eat, who can be present during meals, and visiting the bathroom or unsupervised activity should not be allowed after mealtime. Expectations can include that the client will eat in the dining room at a table at the scheduled time. Mealtimes should not be allowed to be missed for any reason and cannot be done alone in their room without a staff member present. A set schedule and expectations to mealtimes that is followed by all staff in a neutral manner avoids a power struggle with the client. Visitors or other clients may provide unhealthy feedback to the client for avoiding eating. The nurse should avoid bribing or coaxing the client to eat as this places a focus on the food and attaches emotions to eating. After the limit of time has been met for the meal (usually mealtimes limited to 30 minutes), the client's food should be removed. While this seems counteractive to getting a client to increase their food intake, it actually minimizes the secondary gains the client could receive from not eating. Secondary gains could include the extra attention staff give to the client, such as coaxing them to eat or observing them eating, or not eating. To help the client refrain from purging behaviors or disposing of food they have hidden instead of eaten, the client should not be left unsupervised after mealtimes. A typical plan is for 90 minutes of supervision initially and then gradually decrease the supervised time. This helps the client to transition to being responsible for self-control of refraining from purging. As the client's food intake increases and weight is gained, the client should be allowed increasing choices of foods for their meals. All of these interventions help the client recognize and follow normal eating patterns that they can independently repeat at home. This is important to helping increase food consumed and subsequent weight gain.

Activity should also be monitored in the client with an eating disorder. Many individuals with an eating disorder use activity or exercise to "burn off" calories from food consumed. Activity should be monitored and documented for length, type, and location. Some clients may try to do "hidden exercise" such as in the shower or in bed. However, the client should not be restricted from doing all exercise, as maintaining a healthy lifestyle does require some form of moderate exercise. For some clients, preventing them from doing exercise may increase their anxiety which can in turn cause a return to the unhealthy eating behaviors.

The nurse should recognize that mealtimes can be a stressful event for the client with an eating disorder. The environment for mealtimes should be free from excess stimuli and distractions. Mealtime should be pleasant and not a setting for power struggles or control by the nurse. After mealtime the client may experience negative emotions regarding their eating. The nurse should help the client with relaxation techniques or a quiet activity during this stressful time period.

Evaluation of Goal/Desired Outcome

The client:

- consumes a minimum of 50% of three meals a day.
- gains at least 2 pounds within 7 days of admission.
- eats three meals a day in the dining room.
- does not engage in purging behavior after meals.

Nursing Care Focus

- Coping Impairment, evidenced by unhealthy eating behaviors

Goal

- The client will demonstrate coping mechanisms that are not related to food.

Implementations for Improving Coping

To effectively use healthy coping strategies, the client must refrain from using manipulative behaviors. Some clients may not recognize they are being manipulative. Actions should be taken to minimize manipulation. Most important is that the staff works together as a team and gives the same information to all the clients. The staff must follow the unit policies consistently and adhere to the client's plan of care. To do this effectively, there should be one staff member per shift who is identified as the treatment lead and has the decision-making role but with staff input. This helps staff from being manipulated by a client and helps to ensure treatment plans are followed. When the staff do not follow the unit policies or randomly change the rules for select clients, it gives the clients opportunity to manipulate the staff. Also, to help minimize manipulation and maintain consistency, a limited number of staff should be assigned to the client's care upon admission. As the client adheres to the treatment plan and avoids manipulative tactics, the staff can begin to vary and increase in number. This helps to model postdischarge interpersonal interactions.

Clients with an eating disorder are at an increased risk for suicide attempt. Due to their ineffective coping and impulsive behaviors, they should be observed closely for any suicidal ideation or behaviors that may indicate they are planning a suicide attempt. Nursing interventions related to safety issues are a priority.

Food should only be offered at scheduled meal and snack times. The nurse should never use food as a reward for the client exhibiting desired behaviors. The nurse should avoid actions that connect feelings with eating or place a focus on food. This includes not having discussions with the client that surround food and weight. The exception to this is when the nurse reinforces teaching regarding meals, food preparation, and nutritional value of foods. This reinforcing of teaching must not be done during a mealtime.

Encourage the client to verbalize their feelings and give them positive feedback for doing so. This reinforces to the client that verbalization of feelings is preferred. However, do not allow this verbalization to occur during mealtime. Efforts should be made to separate mealtimes and discussion of feelings. If the client starts to verbalize feelings during mealtime, remind them of this guideline. Reinforce to the client that post discharge it is important to adhere to this guideline as well. Their family members may not recognize the importance of separating mealtimes and emotional discussions and may need education regarding this point. This is a vital postdischarge goal for the client's continued recovery.

The nurse should help the client identify ways to express their feelings that are not food related. One method is to have the client keep a journal of their feelings that are felt before, during, and after eating. Some other times they should journal their feelings includes when they are having the urge to binge or purge, after an emotional conflict, after a positive encounter, when successfully achieving a goal, or after a therapy session. Many clients find it easier to write about their feelings than discuss them verbally. Other nonfood methods for expressing their feelings include art and role-playing.

In addition to expressing feelings, the client should have activities that are nonfood related and provide an opportunity for relaxation, pleasure, or success. This usually involves a multidisciplinary approach with recreational, occupational, and music therapies. These activities have the benefit of encouraging emotions that are distinctly separated from food and can help to relieve or decrease anxiety. Give the client honest praise for their participation and growth with these therapies but do not use false praise or flattery. Clients are able to perceive when staff are being insincere. Compliment the client for observed successes such as helping another client or completing a goal. These successes, no matter how small, should be acknowledged as this helps the client build self-esteem. During the acknowledgement, the nurse should also point out a strength the client exhibited. The nurse's verbalizing the success and strength helps the client place an emphasis on a nonfood behavior. If the client counters with a feeling of inadequacy, have them recall the success and the feelings they have associated with that event.

Have the client write a list of their identified strengths and skills. Do not tell the client what their strengths and skills are, as this is nontherapeutic. The client needs to use their insight for this exercise to be effective. The nurse, however, may need to help to guide the client in recalling events and recognizing the strengths they exhibited. Have the client identify potential situations where they can utilize their identified strengths and how they can use their strengths to benefit their coping.

The nurse should reinforce teaching regarding the problem-solving process. To do this, have the client identify a problem (it can be as simple as how to do their laundry when the machines are already in use) and then come up with several solutions to that problem. Have them list the pros and cons for each potential solution and decide upon one to try. Then have them describe the steps they will take and how to see if their plan was effective. Using this approach helps the client gain self-confidence in their problem-solving abilities.

The nurse should self-examine their own behavior when working with the client. It is possible for the nurse to reinforce the sick role and unintentionally provide the client with a secondary gain. For example, the client is still in school and states they are unable to complete an assignment and asks the nurse to write an excuse note for their teacher. If the nurse writes the note and the teacher offers sympathy to the client, they have received a secondary gain for their eating disorder. The nurse should also expect age-appropriate behavior from the client. Ignoring inappropriate behavior or excusing it because of their hospitalization only reinforces to the client that their eating disorder gives them an excuse to misbehave instead of accepting responsibility for their behavior. The nurse should use a neutral matter-of-fact approach and point out the behavior to the client and state that it is unacceptable. Do not allow the client to isolate in their room; instead, have them be present in the unit activities.

Evaluation of Goal/Desired Outcome

The client:

- does not use manipulation.
- does not harm themselves during hospitalization.
- identifies three coping strategies they can use.
- practices using the problem-solving process.

"Cassidy"

Aleksey Mnogosmyslov/
Shutterstock

Cassidy is a recently married 23-year-old college graduate. She has been brought to the outpatient clinic after being found unresponsive at her home. Cassidy is 5 feet 8 inches tall and weighs 101 pounds. Her spouse states they knew she was on a crash diet during the months prior to their wedding but had no idea that her weight loss was a serious problem. Prior to her wedding she often found ways to avoid eating and would spend countless hours working out in the university gym. Cassidy has often described herself as "fat," even though she seemed to get thinner. Her college roommate felt Cassidy wasn't eating right, but thought it was just the stress of finishing school. She is the oldest of three children from a single-parent family. Her parent worked many hours and left Cassidy to manage her two younger brothers. She would state that her family "needed" her but did not care about her.

Cassidy is pale, thin, and somewhat emaciated, with sunken cheeks and dry mucous membranes. She hesitates to open her mouth, which when examined reveals numerous dental caries and brownish stained enamel. Cassidy states that she started self-induced vomiting when she was 13 years old. She had started getting "pudgy" and her mother told her she was going to be fat if she didn't stop eating. She also states that her friends told her she could keep herself from gaining weight by making herself vomit after she ate. Cassidy says she binges on things like pie, chocolate, and banana splits, after which she purges with vomiting and laxatives. She admits to taking as many as 8 to 10 laxative pills at a time to feel relief from the guilt she feels over her food intake and to ensure weight loss after the binge. She works out for as much as 4 hours daily at the gym to compensate for the food she eats. Cassidy relates a feeling of shame for her eating problem and is embarrassed that everyone now knows the secrets she has tried so hard to conceal.

Digging Deeper

1. What factors put Cassidy at risk for an eating disorder?

2. What data was collected that indicates Cassidy has an eating disorder?

3. Cassidy expresses sadness because she wants to have a baby, but she is afraid that her behavior will hurt her chances of having a healthy pregnancy. What factors related to an eating disorder may affect the issue of pregnancy?

4. How can the nurse help Cassidy to view her self-image in a positive way excluding body appearance and weight?

CASE STUDY 16.3

Cultural Considerations

Culture and Ideal Body Size

In the United States, pressure from social media and advertising gives a subtle message about what an ideal body size looks like. Some platforms and advertising campaigns have recently taken an opposite stand and are spreading the message about the importance of accepting all different body types, and that healthy eating is more important than a specific weight or body size.

In some cultures around the world, an overweight or large body size historically was desirable. In these cultures, overweight or larger bodies were seen as a symbol of wealth, power, or fertility. Societies that historically have viewed a larger body size as attractive include: Tahiti, Nauru, Fiji, Jamaica, and some Arab countries. With the spread of industrialization and social media, these ideals and the practices that led to cultural-specific weight gain are changing.

However, there are still those who continue to hold the historical belief and view of the ideal body size.

Source: Bradley University. (2022). *The Body Project: Cross-cultural perspectives.* https://www.bradley.edu/sites/bodyproject/perspectives/#

SUMMARY

- Research indicates that genetics, psychosocial influences, environment, and neurotransmitters are factors in the development of an eating disorder. The exact cause is not known.
- Anorexia nervosa is characterized by an individual restricting calories and nutrients to maintain a subnormal body weight for height and age. There is an accompanying disturbance in the individual's perception of their body shape and self-image, and an intense fear of becoming overweight.
- There are two subtypes of anorexia nervosa. The restrictive subtype is characterized by weight loss accomplished through dieting, starvation, or excessive exercise. The second subtype involves binge-eating and/or purging.
- Binge-eating, or binging, is eating an unusually large amount of food, usually within a 2-hour time frame, which is more than most people would eat in a similar circumstance. Purging is the eliminating of consumed food through self-induced vomiting or with excessive use of laxatives or diuretics.
- Research demonstrates that many individuals with anorexia nervosa come from families with unresolved conflicts of parent–child relationships, often with an overindulgent and controlling parent. A sense of worth becomes entwined in the ability to lose weight.
- Bulimia nervosa is characterized by binge-eating. Despite an uncomfortable feeling of fullness, the individual is unable to stop eating. After the binge, there is usually a feeling of shame and effort to hide the symptoms.
- The individual with anorexia nervosa is underweight for height, age, and stature while the individual with bulimia nervosa is typically within a normal weight range for height and age.
- In binge-eating disorder, the episodes of binge-eating relate to the ingestion of an amount of food in a limited time period of 2 hours or less that is larger than the ordinary person would consume in the same time period under the same circumstances. Individuals lose control over their eating but do not follow with purging or other compensatory methods such as laxative or diuretic use. Individuals with this disorder often are overweight or obese.
- Treatment methods for individuals with eating disorders focus on reversing the restrictive or maladaptive patterns of eating and thinking about food and reestablishing healthy eating habits. Psychotherapy may employ education about healthy nutritional habits, behavioral methods and contracting, group therapy, and cognitive therapy to reorganize the maladaptive thinking related to food, body image, and personal achievement.
- The attitude and approach of the nurse are paramount to establishing a trusting relationship in which the client is willing to participate in treatment. To gain insight into the problem, it is important to hear the symptoms and perception of the illness from the individual's perspective and to remain nonjudgmental.

BIBLIOGRAPHY

Bradley University. (2022). *The Body Project: Cross-cultural perspectives.* https://www.bradley.edu/sites/bodyproject/perspectives/#

Engel, S., Steffen, K., & Mitchell, J. E. (2021). Bulimia nervosa in adults: Clinical features, course of illness, assessment, and diagnosis. *UpToDate.* Retrieved July 8, 2022, from https://www.uptodate.com/contents/bulimia-nervosa-in-adults-clinical-features-course-of-illness-assessment-and-diagnosis

Klein, D., & Attia, E. (2021). Anorexia nervosa in adults: Clinical features, course of illness, assessment, and diagnosis. *UpToDate.* Retrieved July 8, 2022, from https://www.uptodate.com/contents/anorexia-nervosa-in-adults-clinical-features-course-of-illness-assessment-and-diagnosis

Maguire, S., Li, A., Cunich, M., & Maloney, D. (2019). Evaluating the effectiveness of an evidence-based online training program for health professionals in eating disorders. *Journal of Eating Disorders, 7*(14). https://doi.org/10.1186/s40337-019-0243-5

Mehler, P. (2021). Anorexia nervosa in adults and adolescents: Medical complications and their management. *UpToDate.* Retrieved July 8, 2022, from https://www.uptodate.com/contents/anorexia-nervosa-in-adults-and-adolescents-medical-complications-and-their-management

National Eating Disorders Association. (2022a). *Anorexia nervosa.* https://www.nationaleatingdisorders.org/learn/by-eating-disorder/anorexia

National Eating Disorders Association. (2022b). *Substance use and eating disorders.* https://www.nationaleatingdisorders.org/substance-use-and-eating-disorders

National Eating Disorders Collaboration. (2022a). *Anorexia nervosa.* https://nedc.com.au/eating-disorders/eating-disorders-explained/types/anorexia-nervosa/

National Eating Disorders Collaboration. (2022b). *The care team.* https://nedc.com.au/eating-disorders/treatment-and-recovery/the-care/

National Institute of Mental Health. (2021). *Eating disorders: About more than food.* U.S. Department of Health and Human Services, National Institutes of Health. NIH Publication No. 21-MH-490. https://www.nimh.nih.gov/health/publications/eating-disorders

U.S. Department of Health & Human Services. (2022). *Bulimia.* https://www.mentalhealth.gov/what-to-look-for/eating-disorders/bulimia

US Preventive Services Task Force (2022). Screening for eating disorders in adolescents and adults: US Preventive Services Task Force recommendation statement. *JAMA, 327*(11), 1061–1067. https://jamanetwork.com/journals/jama/fullarticle/2789963

Wu, W. L., & Chen, S. L. (2021). Nurses' perceptions on and experiences in conflict situations when caring for adolescents with anorexia nervosa: A qualitative study. *International Journal of Mental Health Nursing, 30*(S1), 1386–1394. https://doi.org/10.1111/inm.12886

Yager, J. (2022a). Eating disorders: Overview of epidemiology, clinical features, and diagnosis. *UpToDate.* Retrieved July 8, 2022, from https://www.uptodate.com/contents/eating-disorders-overview-of-epidemiology-clinical-features-and-diagnosis

Yager, J. (2022b). Eating disorders: Overview of prevention and treatment. *UpToDate.* Retrieved July 8, 2022, from https://www.uptodate.com/contents/eating-disorders-overview-of-prevention-and-treatment

Fill in the Blank

Fill in the blank with the correct answer.

1. The individual with anorexia nervosa demonstrates a disturbance in the _____ of the shape and size of their body.
2. The anorexic client sees weight loss as a major accomplishment of _____ _____, whereas weight gain is seen as _____.
3. The search for autonomy is often seen in the adolescent with anorexia who makes a desperate attempt to separate from a(n) _____ parent.
4. _____ is used by most individuals with bulimia to achieve a temporary sense of relief after a binge.
5. The individual with bulimia nervosa is typically within a normal _____ for height and age.
6. When caring for the client with an eating disorder, the nurse restricts meal time to _____ minutes to reduce the focus on food and eating.

Matching

Match the following terms to the most appropriate phrase.

1. _____ Purging
2. _____ Binging
3. _____ Reward contract
4. _____ Amenorrhea
5. _____ Compensatory methods

a. Absence of menstrual periods
b. Privileges are exchanged for increased food intake
c. Self-induced vomiting or use of laxatives
d. Use of laxatives, diuretics, or enemas to prevent weight gain
e. Eating a large amount of food in a short time with inability to stop

Multiple Choice

Select the best answer from the multiple-choice items.

1. What would most likely be present during data collection on a client being evaluated for anorexia nervosa?
   a. Periodic patterns of weight gain and loss over the past year
   b. Refusal to talk about the subject of food and nutritional planning
   c. Extreme weight loss from self-imposed restricted food and nutrient intake
   d. Periods of overeating and self-induced vomiting with no change in weight pattern

2. What nursing intervention would be important to include for the client with anorexia nervosa?
   a. Provide opportunities for independent decision making.
   b. Confront the client with the severity of their distorted thinking.
   c. Use an approach that conveys a sense of concern and sympathy.
   d. Encourage the client to talk about the caloric value of various food items.

3. Treatment for bulimia nervosa includes psychotherapy and which medication?
   a. Antithyroid
   b. Antidepressant
   c. Anticholinergic
   d. Beta-adrenergic blockers

4. A client has been self-admitted for treatment of bulimia nervosa. What would be the best initial approach by the nurse?
   a. "Why would you want to lose weight when you look so good already?"
   b. "I just don't understand why you make yourself vomit after you eat."
   c. "Tell me about the last time you did binge-eating and what you did afterward."
   d. "Most people go on a weight-reduction diet instead of binging."

5. The nurse is collecting data on a young client in the emergency department with an electrolyte imbalance. The nurse notes poor oral condition and calluses on the index and middle fingers of the client's right hand. What are these findings characteristic of?
   a. Purging behavior
   b. Starvation
   c. Binge-eating
   d. Excessive stress

6. Which finding would be consistent with an individual diagnosed with bulimia nervosa? *(Select all that apply)*
   a. Excessive craving for high-calorie, sweet, or high-carbohydrate foods
   b. Continued eating despite feeling full
   c. Frequent mirror-viewing and measuring of body parts
   d. Stashing of food with hidden food consumption
   e. Collecting recipes and cooking gourmet meals for their family

7. The care plan for the client with an eating disorder would include which intervention?
   a. Weighing the client every morning
   b. Providing privacy during mealtime
   c. Making a strict diet plan for the client to follow
   d. Having the client document their feelings in a journal after each meal

8. The nurse is caring for a client with an eating disorder who is underweight, performs excessive exercise, and is experiencing intolerance to cold temperatures. Which of the following are appropriate statements for the nurse say to the client? *(Select all that apply)*
   a. "Keeping a food journal that lists all of your food choices and your daily calorie intake helps track your progress."
   b. "We will weigh you every day so you can see the treatment plan is working."
   c. "We do not allow clients to eat alone in their room."
   d. "As your weight increases you will start to feel less cold."
   e. "Keeping an emotion and food journal will help you understand why you throw up after eating."

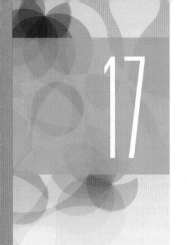

17

Mental Health Issues Related to Gender and Sexuality

Sexual Health and Related Mental Health Concerns

The goal for sexual health is for the client to have a healthy self-image and satisfactory adult sexual desires that respect the rights of others. Some individuals may not desire a sexually intimate relationship. Some may not have any sexual partners or may have more than one.

Discussing Sexuality With Clients

An important part of the client's health history includes their sexual health. In order to gather this data accurately, the nurse first needs to examine their own feelings and opinions related to sexual and gender issues and if their personal views would bias the nursing care they provide. Box 17.1 lists some sample questions for the nurse to begin their self-assessment regarding sexuality.

Prior to gathering client data, it is important to ensure a private environment. Questions of a sensitive nature, including those related to issues of sexuality, should not occur in common areas, or where others could overhear the conversation. Remember that curtains between client beds still allow for conversations to be overheard and should not be considered as ensuring privacy and confidentiality. Communication techniques that aid data collection regarding sexuality are listed in Box 17.2.

The Center for Disease Control (CDC, 2022) gives guidelines for taking a sexual history and refers to these as the "5 Ps." The 5Ps stand for *Partners, Practices, Past History of STI(s), Protection, and Pregnancy.* The National Coalition for Sexual Health (2021) recommends another category, *Plus,* which includes questions regarding pleasure, problems, and pride (questions related to sexual orientation or gender identity). Box 17.3 lists examples of topics that should be covered in each category.

It is important to remember that not all clients are comfortable talking about sexual topics.

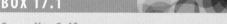

BOX 17.1

Sexuality Self-assessment

These are examples of statements the nurse can ask themselves related to sexuality. Typical responses would be "Never," "Sometimes/Occasionally," "Fairly Often/Pretty Well," or "Always/Very Well." This is not a test, rather questions for the nurse to help them think about their views on sexuality.

- I have examined my own personal sexual history.
- I have explored my own attitudes about sexuality.
- I am aware of my feelings when I encounter differences in sexual orientation.
- I have listened to different attitudes of others about sexuality.
- I interact with people of all genders in respectful and appropriate ways.
- I affirm my own sexual orientation and respect the sexual orientation of others.
- I am aware of the stereotypes I hold and have developed personal strategies to manage them.
- I recognize and affirm family diversity.
- I seek ongoing opportunities for education and information regarding sexuality.
- I recognize and respect my own personal limitations and boundaries for handling issues related to sexuality.
- I accept that there can be situations discussing sexuality that I might feel uncomfortable with.
- I recognize that people have intersecting multiple identities drawn from race, gender identity, sexual orientation, religion, ethnicity, etc., that vary from person to person.

Questions complied from: Cultural Competence Self-Assessment Checklist from https://www.avma.org/sites/default/files/2022-02/DiversityCulturalCompetence Checklist.pdf

---

BOX 17.2

Communication Techniques for Gathering Data Related to Sexuality

- Avoid making assumptions based upon age, gender, marital status, ethnicity, or any other factor.
- During the first encounter with the client gather basic information including preferred name, pronouns, and gender identity.
- Use neutral terms such as "partner" or "spouse".
- Establish rapport before asking any questions.
- Obtain permission to continue the conversation if other persons are present.
- Begin conversation by asking permission to discuss sensitive issues.
- State that you ask all clients these questions.
- Be nonjudgmental.
- Let client know they can stop the conversation if they want to.
- Be sensitive to client preferences regarding gender or age of health care provider.
- Don't assume the client has the same definition of terms as the nurse (example, "sex" may only mean to the client penile–vaginal intercourse and not include anal or oral sex). Tactfully ask for clarification.

Sample Sexual History Topics

- Partners: current or past partners, any unwelcomed sexual activity
- Practices: type of sexual activity, use of drugs or alcohol with sex
- Past History of STIs: which type and treatment
- Protection: type of protection used, vaccinations (HPV, Hepatitis A or B)
- Pregnancy: desire to have children, birth control used in past and currently
- Plus: satisfaction with current sexual life, difficulties with sex and sex drive, support from family or friends regarding sexual orientation or gender identity

This may be due to their culture, upbringing, personal views, or a history of trauma or sexual abuse. Let the client know that they have the right not to answer any question and can request that the conversation stop. This allows the client to feel in control.

A majority of clients want to talk about their sexual concerns but prefer for the health care provider to bring up the topic; however, most health care providers rely on the client to initiate the conversation on sexual health. Studies show that sexuality is the least commonly discussed health topic. The most common barriers adult clients report for not discussing sexual concerns include embarrassment, nervousness, and concern about their information being kept confidential, while younger clients identify embarrassment and concern regarding discrimination/being treated poorly as barriers. This nurse can initiate this subject with a question such as, "Are there any topics that you would like to discuss or discuss with the health care provider including sexuality topics?" or "We have clients that have questions regarding sexuality or sexual concerns. Do you have any questions like this for the health care provider?" The second format lets the client know that the practice is open to questions and that the client is not "alone" in their questions.

Ethical Nursing Care

A component of ethical nursing care is to provide unbiased, nonjudgmental, and equal care to all clients. It is important for the nurse to develop a self-awareness of their attitudes and beliefs toward any issue, including sexuality, which may hinder providing effective care of any client. When caring for the client with a sexual concern, self-awareness allows the nurse to provide ethical and unbiased nursing care, be a client advocate, present factual information about sexual development, and promote an understanding of this human need for all age groups.

The nurse should be prepared to care for a client with a sexual issue regardless of the setting

CASE STUDY 17.1

Monkey Business Images/Shutterstock

"Did I just see that?"

You are working in the emergency department when a client is brought in by paramedics and accompanied by law enforcement. The client has several large cuts that are bleeding, large reddened areas over their lower back, and a black eye. The report you receive is that the client was arrested while raping a young child. As the newest member of the team, you are assigned to observe and be available to help as needed. While observing, you notice one of team members use excessive pressure while turning the client and starting an IV. You haven't seen this nurse use excessive pressure before. You even enjoy working with this nurse as you both have children the same age. Afterward you overhear them say, "Maybe now they'll remember not to do that again."

Digging Deeper

1. What are your initial feelings regarding the client?

2. After caring for the client, what would be your next action?

3. Who would you identify to help you debrief from this client encounter?

4. How would you react if the client had been accused of shoplifting instead of raping a child?

they practice in. However, there are some settings in which the nurse is more likely to encounter clients with concerns related to sexuality than other settings. For example, the nurse working in an emergency department or a correctional facility may encounter a client who is charged with rape or solicitation. Other client examples might be a resident of an extended care facility that has a paraphilia in which they desire to engage (see later section on Paraphilia) in or a pediatric client who is questioning their sexual orientation. The nurse needs to recognize their feelings regarding the sexual behavior of the client and evaluate their ability to provide competent and unbiased care. The nurse who feels that they cannot treat the client in an ethical an unbiased manner and provide the same level of care that is provided to other clients must seek guidance from their charge nurse.

Test Yourself	✔ List four things that can aid in gathering data related to sexuality. ✔ Name six sexual history topics.

Sexuality and Gender Identity

When discussing sexuality and gender identity, it is important to understand that historically only binary terminology (e.g., "man or woman") was used to define gender and that "homosexuality" was diagnosed as a disorder through much of the 1900s. Additionally, sexuality and discussing sexual matters were historically taboo topics. In the later 1900s and early 2000s, these viewpoints began to shift. However, stigma is still often attached to sexual orientation and gender identity. Therefore, the nurse needs to be aware of potential concerns surrounding gender identity, sexuality, and sexual disorders that may impact a client's mental health.

It is vital to recognize that a person's sexuality or gender identity is just one part of their personality, not a totality. The LPN/LVN will not see clients for mental health issues related to sexuality and gender unless the client is experiencing distress because of them. This could include when an individual feels unaccepted for their gender or sexual orientation, if they are experiencing issues related to sexual intimacy, or if these issues are causing them to harm or be at risk of harming themselves or others. The nurse should let the client take the lead on explaining to the nurse what their concerns are or are not. The nurse should

never assume that the client's viewpoints are the same as their own.

While sexuality was introduced in the different developmental theories that were discussed in Chapter 3, it is important in this chapter to define terms regarding sexuality, sex, and gender. The term sex refers to an individual's biologic make-up whereas gender is a social construct. At birth, infants are typically assigned as female or male based on their external genitalia. All individuals have a **gender identity**, which is the innate sense of feeling male, female, neither, or a combination of both, or something else. It is important to recognize that all people have a gender identity (American Psychological Association [APA], 2021). An individual's **sexual orientation** is their gendered pattern of attraction to others. Sexual orientation for some includes attraction to one gender, while others are attracted to multiple genders, and others do not experience sexual attraction. The individual's gender identity is not the same as their sexual orientation (APA, 2021).

Gender Identity

As discussed, all people have a gender identity, and gender identities are not mental health conditions. However, until recently, certain gender identities were not only stigmatized but were considered to be mental disorders. Significant work has been done to change society's and health care professionals' understanding of these identities as variations of human identity and experience, rather than mental health disorders that require treatment. People with different gender identities often *do* experience mental health issues, but it is important to emphasize that these mental health concerns are often caused by societal views and internalized stigma, and not by the identities themselves (Robles et al., 2021).

Definitions of Gender Identities

A person's gender identity is a personal experience, and there are many ways someone might identify. The nurse should never assume that someone identifies a certain way and may encounter different terms than those used in this chapter. Still, it is helpful to understand the definitions of some terms people commonly use to describe gender identity. Someone who is cisgender feels that the sex they were assigned at birth aligns with their experience of their gender. **Transgender** (sometimes abbreviated as trans) is an adjective that describes an individual whose gender identity is different from the sex they were assigned at birth. Some transgender people may be men or women, while some might identify outside the conventional gender binary and may describe themselves as nonbinary, meaning they do not identify as male or female; they may be (to name a few possibilities) neither, both, a third gender, or have a fluid sense of their gender. People who are nonbinary may or may not consider themselves to be transgender (APA, 2022). In this chapter, however, the term transgender is used in alignment with the APA's (2022) use as an umbrella term that describes "persons whose gender identity, expression, and/or role does not conform to what is culturally associated with their sex assigned at birth."

Transgender individuals may choose to transition as part of their gender affirmation process. It is important to recognize that not all individuals have the same personal goals for transition. Some may choose only to make social or legal changes to affirm their gender (clothing, name, medical and legal records changed) while others may choose to have medical transition (which can include hormone therapy) and/or surgical transition. Not all transgender individuals choose to have all or any therapies or surgeries, but the incidence of gender-affirming surgery is increasing as it becomes more mainstream and more care health care providers are trained in providing transgender care (Ferrando & Thomas, 2022).

For all clients, the nurse should note the client's preferred name and pronouns, if listed, on the intake form before meeting the client. Some clients are apprehensive about listing information they expect they may feel judged for. The nurse can use a nonjudgmental statement such as, "The reason we ask these questions is to learn about the organs that are present in your body so we can ask the right questions to appropriately treat the health concerns you have." The nurse could further ask, "Have you had any organs removed from your body or are there any organs that are causing you concern?"

Mental Health Concerns Related to Gender Identity

Some transgender individuals will experience **gender dysphoria,** which is psychological distress due to a sense of incongruence between sex assigned at birth and gender identity (American Psychiatric Association, 2023). Not all transgender people experience this distress, and therefore, transgender or nonbinary identity does not automatically equate to gender dysphoria.

Other mental health issues transgender individuals report include depression, suicidality, substance use disorders, eating disorders, and stress (Paceley et al., 2021). Rates and causes of death for transgender individuals are similar to those in the U.S. population except for suicide, which is higher in the transgender population. Eighty-two percent of transgender individuals have considered suicide and 40% have attempted suicide, with suicidality highest among transgender youth (Austin et al., 2022). Depression and suicidality are decreased by 40% if a transgender or gender-diverse youth has at least one supportive adult in their life (Paceley et al., 2021). It is important to note that suicidality is not an inherent part of being transgender; rather, the higher rates of suicide for transgender individuals are due to contributing factors including gender-based victimization, discrimination, bullying, feeling excluded by peers, emotional neglect by family, internalized self-stigma, and ill treatment within health care systems.

A transgender individual's family, friends, peers, and social groups can be sources of support or stress. Many transgender individuals report rejection by their family and/or community, harassment, discrimination, and social stigma or isolation. Mental health concerns include anxiety, depression, and sadness. Psychological distress related to harassment, bullying, and physical attacks is reported by almost half of transgender individuals (Paceley et al., 2021).

As the LPN/LVN is one of the first professionals to help collect data and create a rapport with the client, it is essential for the nurse to be nonjudgmental and accepting of the client. This helps to reinforce respect for the client as an individual and their concerns. Respect for the client and an accepting approach are vital for the client to share their concerns with the nurse and other medical professionals. In addition to collecting data related to the client's gender identity or sexuality, it is important to collect data on all clients regarding any concerns related to their safety in regards to bullying, depression, and suicidality.

Test Yourself
- ✔ Describe the difference between gender identity and sexual orientation.
- ✔ Define gender dysphoria.
- ✔ Identify potential mental health concerns for transgender individuals.

"Blake"

The nurse is working in the health clinic. A client, Blake, arrives and states they are here for "a regular check-up." The nurse takes the client to the exam room. As the information intake begins, the nurse notes the client is tapping their foot and wiping their palms on their pants.

Digging Deeper

1. How should the nurse proceed with the data collection?

2. What could the nurse do in response to the nonverbal behavior observed?

3. What is the best way to address a patient whose preferred name doesn't match the name on their intake form?

Noting from Blake's nonverbal cues that Blake seems nervous, the nurse asks, "Is there anything causing you distress you'd like to talk about?" Blake responds, "I've been thinking about my gender identity for a long time, and recently, I've been wondering about hormone treatment."

Digging Deeper

1. What thoughts or biases might the nurse need to consider after hearing Blake's response?

2. How might the way the nurse proceeds be different if Blake was an adolescent versus an older adult?

3. How can the nurse proceed if they incorrectly use the wrong pronoun or name for the client?

CASE STUDY 17.2

Sexual Function

It is helpful for the nurse to recognize phases of the sexual response cycle so that they can better understand any differences in sexual response the client is experiencing that may be causing them mental distress (Box 17.4). The initial phase consists of the individual's desire to have sexual activity which is also known as their libido. This is followed by the arousal phase which includes physiologic changes throughout the body and erection of the penis or nipples. This is followed by the orgasmic stage with orgasm being the peak of the sexual response cycle. After orgasm, the resolution phase begins which includes vital signs

returning to baseline and can include fatigue or relaxation and contentment.

It is important to note that the sexual response cycle, which definitions of sexual dysfunction are based on, can be considered ethnocentric and not applicable to all cultures and therefore not all cultures share the same definition of sexual dysfunction. In some cultures, the topic of sexual activity is taboo and statistical data may not be fully representative.

Just the Facts It is important to recognize that the sexual response cycle is not always relevant when discussing sexual orientation and it is not related to gender identity.

Not experiencing a phase, such as arousal, is not considered a dysfunction on its own and may not cause mental distress to the individual. It is only a concern if the lack of, or difficulty with, a phase causes the individual distress. Some individuals are asexual and would not

BOX 17.4

Phases of the Sexual Response Cycle

- Desire (libido)
- Arousal/Excitement
- Orgasm
- Resolution/Recovery

identify with the phases of the sexual response cycle and are comfortable with that. The nurse should rely on the person, not the health care team, to be the one to identify if part of the sexual response cycle applies to them or not. The nurse *should not* indicate the client is experiencing sexual dysfunction solely because the client does not experience any, or all, phases of the sexual response cycle.

Sexual Dysfunction

Sexual dysfunction is a condition that the client identifies as causing them distress that occurs during any phase of the sexual response cycle or interferes with sexual function. Sexual dysfunction can also include pain associated with sexual intercourse. Issues with sexual function can cause marked discomfort and anxiety and can interfere with interpersonal relationships. For these reasons, sexual dysfunction is discussed as a mental health issue.

Treatment for sexual dysfunction often is sought first from a medical health care provider; however, mental health care providers also treat sexual dysfunctions. Some clients may first utilize cultural remedies or receive treatment from a cultural healer. To receive treatment the individual must first report the dysfunction to the health care provider. Some individuals may deny the need for treatment of sexual dysfunctions or are unaware that treatment may be available. Others may avoid or deny the issue which can add to any internal conflict or disrupted sexual relationships. The nurse needs to recognize that the client may be reluctant to discuss sexual problems with health care workers or that such discussions may be culturally prohibited. Other contributing factors could be a lack of understanding about anatomic functioning and effective sexual stimulation techniques. Because sexual desire is a mind and body process, an individual's past experiences may impact their current views regarding their sexual function and, in some individuals, may contribute to sexual dysfunction.

The dysfunction may be seen in sexual interest or arousal, ineffective orgasms (absent or premature), erectile disorder, and pain with penetration (see Box 17.5 for examples). Remember that what one individual considers a sexual concern and is labeled as a dysfunction may not be considered a dysfunction in another individual.

BOX 17.5

Examples of Sexual Dysfunction

- Decreased sexual desire
- Dislike and avoidance of sexual activity
- Lack of desired sexual arousal
- Inability to achieve or maintain erection
- Inability to achieve orgasm during intercourse
- Premature ejaculation
- Pain during intercourse
- Involuntary perineal muscle contractions preventing vaginal penetration
- Medical conditions or medications that interfere with sexual functioning
- Sexual inhibition related to use of substances

Note: These are sexual dysfunctions that are identified by the American Psychological Association. The presence, or absence, of the examples does not automatically indicate a dysfunction for all individuals. For example, the individual who identifies as asexual and is not distressed by a decreased sexual desire is not considered to have a sexual dysfunction.

Again, this distinction is based on whether or not the client experiences distress. For example, while one person may be very distressed about not having an orgasm, another individual may be unconcerned with not having an orgasm.

Causes of Sexual Dysfunction

Sexual dysfunction can have origins in a mental health issue, related to a mental health or medical-surgical condition, or as a side effect from a medication. Table 17.1 summarizes some of these conditions. The dysfunction may be related to a particular set of circumstances or a problem that exists with some or all types of stimulation, situations, or partners. The level of distress indicated by the individual regarding the dysfunction and the impact on their life is a determining factor in the level of medical attention sought and the level of mental health involvement. The problem may be present over the individual's lifetime or may be acquired after a period of normal functioning and response.

The individual's culture is important to take into consideration when discussing sexual dysfunction and sexual norms. For example, in some cultures masturbation may be considered a sign of a sexual problem and contribute to relationship difficulties (Bhavsar & Bhugra, 2018). Cultural norms for sexual activity should be considered. For example, adherence to cultural gender roles

TABLE 17.1	Common Causes of Sexual Dysfunction
Origin	**Examples**
Mental Health Issue	• Anxiety • Depression • Emotionally traumatic event: rape, post-traumatic stress disorder
Related to a Mental Health Condition	• Anhedonia related to depression • Anxiety
Related to a Medical-Surgical Condition	• Cardiovascular disease • Diabetes mellitus • Female genital mutilation • Genital injury or infections • Hypertension • Mastectomy • Multiple sclerosis • Neuropathy • Oophorectomy without hormone replacement therapy • Prostatectomy • Spinal cord injury • Treatments: chemotherapy and radiation • Uterine prolapse • Vaginitis
Side Effect from a Medication	• Alcohol • Anticonvulsants: carbamazepine, valproic acid, phenytoin • Antidepressants: SSRIs • Antihypertensives: clonidine, methyldopa, beta blockers • Antipsychotics: haloperidol, risperidone • Benzodiazepines: alprazolam, lorazepam, diazepam • Beta blockers • Digoxin • Diuretics: spironolactone, hydrochlorothiazide • H2 blockers: cimetidine and famotidine • Hormone replacement therapy • Lithium (especially when combined with benzodiazepines) • Marijuana • Methadone • Methamphetamine • Parkinson medications: benztropine, bromocriptine, levodopa

Note: These are not comprehensive lists.

or sexual activity for older adults may contribute to the individual's positive view or dissatisfaction with their sexual activity.

Mind Jogger What situation or circumstances within a relationship might lead to a sexual dysfunction?

Mental Health Issues Related to Sexual Dysfunction

There are sexual conditions that may cause some individuals distress while others may have the same experience and not be concerned, distressed, or interested in the condition. Again, the nurse should let the client be the judge of what is normal, or right, for them.

Conditions that involve sexual interest or arousal include a hypoactive sexual desire (also referred to as decreased libido), absent or reduced pleasure during sexual activity, a lack of arousal from physical or visual stimulation, and recurring episodes of difficulty attaining or maintaining acceptable excitement response (such as decreased lubrication or erectile dysfunction) to complete sexual activity. For some individuals, the condition may cause painful intercourse or avoidance of sexual encounters. Substance use and medications can contribute to, or cause, hypoactive sexual desire. In some, sexual or physical abuse may be a causative factor. Causative factors for erectile dysfunction are age, alcohol, medications, and prostatic hypertrophy. Medical issues that involve vascular or neurologic function may also cause erectile dysfunction. Examples of these conditions would be cardiovascular disease, multiple sclerosis, prostatectomy, and diabetes mellitus. Mental health issues encountered by individuals with hypoactive sexual desire may include decreased self-esteem or self-worth, relationship difficulties, or depression.

Just the Facts Medications such as antihypertensives, antipsychotics, antidepressants, anxiolytics, and anticonvulsants can cause hypoactive sexual desire.

Conditions that involve orgasms may include a reoccurring delay or absence of orgasm following sexual activity. Contributing factors to orgasmic issues can include alcohol, age, or the type of sexual stimulation provided, especially if it is not the individual's desired partner or type of stimulation. Orgasmic conditions can lead to mental health issues of anxiety, self-esteem, a sense of lacking in sexuality, negative body-image, or satisfaction in sexual relationships.

Dyspareunia, genital–pelvic pain occurring prior, during, or after sexual intercourse, can impair an individual's sexual functioning. Causes may include penetration, lubrication, injury, female

Laurin Rinder/
Shutterstock

CASE STUDY 17.3

"Juan Carlos"

Juan Carlos is seeing the health care provider for an annual physical and a prescription renewal. He was diagnosed 5 years ago with diabetes mellitus and hypertension. His medications include glipizide 5 mg by mouth once a day and lisinopril 10 mg/hydrochlorothiazide 12.5 mg by mouth once a day.

Digging Deeper

1. What questions would be important to ask Juan Carlos regarding his sexual health in regards to his history?

2. What nonverbal behaviors would indicate that Juan Carlos was uncomfortable with the discussion?

3. What would be an appropriate response by the nurse at this point?

---

genital mutilation (also called female circumcision; see Cultural Considerations box), inflammation, spasms of vaginal walls (vaginismus), history of sexual abuse, or side effects of testosterone on the genital area. Dyspareunia can lead to mental health issues related to self-image, self-esteem, satisfaction in sexual relationships, depression, anxiety, or hypervigilance to pain.

> **Test Yourself**
> ✔ Describe three groups of sexual dysfunctions.
> ✔ Identify four causes of sexual issues and name two examples for each one.

Paraphilia

A **paraphilia** is often defined as a sexual interest that falls outside what is generally considered "typical" within a certain culture. A paraphilia may involve an erotic activity, or it may be focused on specific objects or people. For some individuals, these activities are required for erotic arousal and are consistently included in each sexual encounter.

Paraphilic Disorders

Most people with paraphilia do not have a mental disorder. A paraphilia is only classified as a paraphilic disorder if the individual acts on their urges on nonconsenting individuals and/or if the urges or the behaviors cause the person clinically

significant distress or impairment. In paraphilic disorders, the paraphilia may impose anxiety or problems to the individual's functioning in social or occupational roles or within their personal relationships. If the paraphilic act takes place on nonconsenting individuals and is illegal, as in the case of pedophilia or exhibitionism, the individual may be arrested and incarcerated. Paraphilic disorders are not often seen in the clinical setting, nor do people typically seek treatment for them.

Table 17.2 outlines some examples of paraphilias, but not all people describe these behaviors using these terms and not all people who experience these sexual urges identify this way. These paraphilias would be considered paraphilic disorders if the individual acts on the urge or fantasy in a way that causes harm to a nonconsenting individual or causes the person with the paraphilia distress.

Nursing Process and Care Plan *for the Client With a Sexual Concern*

Sexuality is a normal part of human development. Most clients prefer that the health care team initiate discussion regarding sexual health. In order to gather data related to the client's sexual health, the nurse needs to first self-reflect on their own values and beliefs regarding sexuality and address any bias they may have. This is necessary to provide ethical nursing care to all clients. When discussing sensitive topics, such as sexual history and

TABLE 17.2	Example of Paraphilias
Paraphilia	**Description**
Exhibitionism	Exposure of genitals to a stranger with or without masturbation. There is often no further attempt at sexual activity with the stranger.
Fetishism	Sexual activity involving an inanimate object (fetish). Contact with or view of the item is usually required for orgasm.
Frotteurism	Touching or rubbing of the genitals against a stranger while fantasizing intimacy with them. Often performed in an area where a crowd or dim lighting will obscure the activity.
Pedophilia	Sexual activity with a prepubescent child. Victims can be of any gender.
Voyeurism	Sexual arousal from the visual observation of a stranger undressing, naked, or engaging in sexual behavior without the stranger's knowledge. Generally, no further sexual contact is pursued.

concerns, it is important for the nurse to initiate a therapeutic rapport with the client using an empathetic and nonjudgmental attitude. The nurse should encourage the client to verbalize feelings and perception of the sexual problem and clarify any ambiguous terms the client uses such as "down there." The nurse should utilize therapeutic communication techniques to encourage the client to discuss sexual concerns. At all times the nurse must ensure the client's privacy and confidentiality during disclosure and treatment.

Assessment (Data Collection)

The nurse can assist in gathering data related to a concern the client may be experiencing with sexual functioning. Questions should be asked in regards to the CDC's 5 P's (Partners, Practices, Past History of STI(s), Protection, and Pregnancy) as well as questions related to pleasure, problems, and pride. This will help to determine the particular areas that may be involved. All efforts should be made to ensure confidentiality and to respect the private content of the issues being discussed. The client should be encouraged to share feelings and concerns so that appropriate information and treatment can be provided. A complete sexual and social history should be taken. Information regarding the client's sexual and gender identity should be noted in the client's record.

Nursing Care Focus

Once data has been collected, the client's main nursing care focus regarding their sexual health

can be determined. Some clients may not express concern over their sexual health, even when the data collected otherwise indicates a possible dysfunction. For this reason, it is important to validate with the client what their concern or need is. For some clients the focus of nursing care is an anticipatory need that might arise. An example of this might be Acute Anxiety for the client with a new diagnosis of HIV. Others that might apply to the client with a sexual concern include: Altered Body Image Perception, Chronic Low Self-Esteem, Depression, Fear, Knowledge Deficiency, Psychosocial Needs, Risky Health Behavior, Self-Harm Risk, Suicide Attempt Risk, and Violence Risk.

Outcome Identification and Planning

Anticipated outcomes for the client with a sexual concern are often long term in nature. The nurse should include this in the reinforcement of teaching. Letting the client know that these concerns may take some time to resolve helps the client to have realistic expectations about their plan of care. Box 17.6 lists common anticipated outcomes for the client with a sexual concern.

Nursing Care Focus

- Knowledge deficiency related to sexual performance

Goal

- The client will restate factual information related to sexual performance.

BOX 17.6

Common Desired Outcomes for a Client With a Sexual Concern

The client:
- Describes the side effects of medications or disease process on sexual functioning.
- Expresses techniques to maintain and/or sustain arousal.
- Expresses ability to be intimate and satisfaction during sexual encounters.
- Develops an insight into the feelings of their partner related to sexual concern.
- Engages in healthy sexual relationships.
- Acknowledges their sexuality.
- Expresses comfort with their sexual identity.

Implementations for Improving Knowledge Regarding Sexual Performance

Inquire how the client likes to learn best. Determine their preferred vocabulary for genitals and sexual acts. Provide information in a matter-of-fact tone. Acknowledge sexuality is a sensitive subject and embarrassment is a common feeling when discussing sex. Provide the client with information utilizing learning methods the client prefers. Information can be pamphlets, online resources, wall charts, or drawings. Use terminology the client is familiar with. Have the client repeat the information back to you to determine client's understanding of information.

Evaluation of Goal/Desired Outcome

The client is able to describe sexual performance with factual information.

Nursing Care Focus

- Acute Anxiety related to sexual dysfunction

Goal

- The client will report reduced anxiety during sexual activity.

Implementations for Reducing Anxiety

Have client state what physical and emotional symptoms they have when they are anxious during sexual activity. Have the client state what situations during sex cause them anxiety. Assure the client that these are normal reactions, even among individuals who do not report a sexual dysfunction. Have the client identify methods they use in other anxiety provoking situations. Let the client know these anxiety reducing techniques can be useful during sexual activity. The techniques should be practiced when the client is not anxious and prior to sexual activity. Let the client know that some practices may decrease sexual performance such as alcohol and smoking.

Evaluation of Goal/Desired Outcome

The client:

- reports anxiety is reduced during sexual activity.
- reports satisfaction with sexual activity.

Cultural Considerations

Female Genital Mutilation

Female genital mutilation (FGM), also known as female circumcision, is the practice of removing all or part of the female genitalia. It can involve partial or total removal of the clitoris and/or the clitoral hood, or removing the labia minora and/or the labia majora with or without removal of the clitoris. In some cases it also involves narrowing of the vaginal opening (medically this is referred to as infibulation) by cutting and repositioning the labia minora or labia majora. Female genital mutilation (FGM) typically occurs before the child is 15 years old and can occur as young as in infancy or 5 years of age.

There are no health benefits or medical reasons for female genital mutilation (FGM) and it is not supported by any religion. It is recognized as a violation of human rights, and the World Health Organization (WHO) is opposed to female genital mutilation (FGM). It is a common practice in certain countries of Africa, the Middle East and Asia including Egypt, Ethiopia, Indonesia, Kenya, Sierra Leone, Somalia, Sudan, and Yemen (UNICEF,

2020). It is estimated that there are over 200 million girls and women alive today that have undergone this practice and a rate of about 3 million procedures done annually (WHO, 2023). Reasons given for this practice are that it is a cultural tradition, that it is preparation for adulthood and marriage, or it promotes premarital virginity and prevents adultery. It is usually done because of a social norm and the fear that the girl will later be rejected by the community or shunned by peers.

Female genital mutilation (FGM), in any form, has the risk of health complications. Immediate complications include pain, hemorrhage, infection, and urinary problems. Long-term complications include urinary problems, menstrual problems, painful intercourse (dyspareunia), decreased sexual satisfaction, and also an increase in complications during childbirth. In addition to these health complications, mental health issues reported by those who have been subjected to female genital mutilation (FGM) include depression, anxiety, post-traumatic stress disorder and low self-esteem.

Reference: World Health Organization. (2023). *Female genital mutilation.* https://www.who.int/news-room/fact-sheets/detail/female-genital-mutilation; UNICEF. (2020). *Female genital mutilation country profiles.* https://data.unicef.org/resources/fgm-country-profiles/

SUMMARY

- An important part of the client's health history includes their sexual health.
- The nurse needs to examine their own feelings and opinions related to sexual and gender issues and if their personal views would bias the nursing care they provide.
- The 5 Ps of a sexual history are Partners, Practices, Past History of STI(s), Protection, and Pregnancy. A sixth category has been included which is termed "Plus" and covers topics of pleasure, problems, and pride (questions related to sexual orientation or gender identity).
- Clients prefer the health care provide initiate the topic of sexual health however, most health care providers wait for the client to start the discussion.
- The way a person views their sexuality is part of their personality, not a totality.
- The term sex refers to an individual's sex assigned at birth based on external genitalia, while gender is a social construct.
- All individuals have a gender identity which is the innate sense of feeling male, female, neither, a combination of both, or something else. Gender identity applies to all individuals.
- An individual's sexual orientation is their gendered pattern of attraction to others and is not the same as their gender identity.
- Not all clients are comfortable discussing sexual matters. The nurse should let the client know that they can stop the conversation at any time and also choose not to answer any questions that they are uncomfortable with.
- The goal for sexual health is a healthy self-image and satisfactory adult sexual desires that respect the rights of others. A sexually intimate relationship is not desired for some individuals or may not include a partner.
- Mental health issues related to gender identity include depression, suicidality, substance use disorder, eating disorders, and stress. Transgender individuals are at a higher risk for suicide than the overall population risk.
- The sexual response cycle consists of four phases: desire (libido), arousal/excitement, orgasm, resolution/recovery. Not experiencing a phase, such as arousal, is not considered a dysfunction on its own and may not cause mental distress to the individual. Some individuals identify as asexual and would not identify with the phases of the sexual response cycle and are comfortable with that.
- Sexual dysfunction would include a condition that the client identifies as causing them distress that occurs during any phase of the sexual response cycle or interferes with sexual function.
- Sexual dysfunctions include disturbances in sexual interest or arousal, ineffective orgasms (absent or premature), erectile disorder, and pain with penetration.
- Sexual dysfunction can have origins in a mental health issue, related to a mental health or medical-surgical condition, or as a side effect from a medication.
- A paraphilia is often defined as a sexual interest that falls outside what is generally considered "typical" within a certain culture. Most people with paraphilia do not have a mental disorder. Examples of paraphilia include exhibitionism, fetishism, frotteurism, pedophilia, and voyeurism.

BIBLIOGRAPHY

Agronin, M. (2021). Sexual dysfunction in older adults. *UpToDate*. Retrieved September 28, 2022, from https://www.uptodate.com/contents/sexual-dysfunction-in-older-adults

American Psychological Association. (2021). *Equity, diversity, and inclusion: Inclusive language guidelines*. https://www.apa.org/about/apa/equity-diversity-inclusion/language-guidelines.pdf

American Psychiatric Association. (2023). *What is gender dysphoria?* https://www.psychiatry.org/patients-families/gender-dysphoria/what-is-gender-dysphoria

Austin, A., Craig, S. L., D'Souza, S., & McInroy, L. B. (2022). Suicidality among transgender youth: Elucidating the role of interpersonal risk factors. *Journal of Interpersonal Violence, 37*(5–6), NP2696–NP2718. https://doi.org/10.1177/0886260520915554

Bhavsar, V., & Bhugra, D. (2018). Cultural factors and sexual dysfunction in clinical practice. *Advances in Psychiatric Treatment, 19*(2), 144–152. https://www.cambridge.org/core/journals/advances-in-psychiatric-treatment/article/cultural-factors-and-sexual-dysfunction-in-clinical-practice/1315F95D-78451DE2438D85C245A621BC

Bradford, A. (2021). Female orgasmic disorder: Epidemiology, pathogenesis, clinical manifestations, course, assessment, and diagnosis. *UpToDate*. Retrieved September 28, 2022, from https://www.uptodate.

com/contents/female-orgasmic-disorder-epidemi-ology-pathogenesis-clinical-manifestations-course-assessment-and-diagnosis

Brown, G. R. (2022). *Overview of paraphilic disorders (Paraphilias)*. Merck Manual Professional Version. https://www.merckmanuals.com/professional/psychiatric-disorders/paraphilic-disorders/overview-of-paraphilic-disorders

Centers for Disease Control and Prevention. (2022). *Discussing sexual health with your patients*. Division of HIV Prevention, National Center for HIV, Viral Hepatitis, STD, and TB Prevention. https://www.cdc.gov/hiv/clinicians/screening/sexual-health.html#

Feldman, J., & Deutsch, M. B. (2021). Primary care of transgender individuals. *UpToDate*. Retrieved October 21, 2022, from https://www.uptodate.com/contents/primary-care-of-transgender-individuals

Ferrando, C., & Thomas, T. N. (2022). Gender-affirming surgery: Male to female. *UpToDate*. Retrieved September 28, 2022, from https://www.uptodate.com/contents/gender-affirming-surgery-male-to-female

Ferrando, C., Zhao, L. C., & Nikolavsky, D. (2022). Gender-affirming surgery: Female to male. *UpToDate*. Retrieved September 28, 2022, from https://www.uptodate.com/contents/gender-affirming-surgery-female-to-male

Hirsch, M., & Birnbaum, R. J. (2022). Sexual dysfunction caused by selective serotonin reuptake inhibitors (SSRIs): Management. *UpToDate*. Retrieved September 28, 2022, from https://www.uptodate.com/contents/sexual-dysfunction-caused-by-selective-serotonin-reuptake-inhibitors-ssris-management

Martin, S. F., & Levine, S. B. (2021). Fetishistic disorder. *UpToDate*. Retrieved September 28, 2022, from https://www.uptodate.com/contents/fetishistic-disorder

National Coalition on Sexual Health (2021). *Asking essential sexual health questions*. https://nationalcoalitionforsexualhealth.org/tools/for-health-care-providers/asset/AskingEssentialSexualHealthQuestions_2021.pdf

Paceley, M. S., Ananda, J., Thomas, M. M. C., Sanders, I., Hiegert, D., & Monley, T. D. (2021). "I have nowhere to go": A multiple-case study of transgender and gender diverse youth, their families, and healthcare experiences. *Int J Environ Res Public Health*, *18*(17), 9219. https://www.ncbi.nlm.nih.gov/pmc/articles/PMC8431416/

Robles, R., Real, T., & Reed, G. (2021). Depathologizing sexual orientation and transgender identities in psychiatric classifications. *Consortium Psychiatricum*, *2*(2), 45–53. https://doi.org/10.17816/CP61

Rosen, R. C., & Khera, M. (2022). Epidemiology and etiologies of male sexual dysfunction. *UpToDate*. Retrieved September 28, 2022, from https://www.uptodate.com/contents/epidemiology-and-etiologies-of-male-sexual-dysfunction

Savoy, M., O'Gurek, D., & Brown-James, A. (2020). Sexual health history: Techniques and tips. *American Family Physician*. https://www.aafp.org/dam/AAFP/documents/journals/afp/Savoy.pdf

Schifren, J. L. (2022a). Overview of sexual dysfunction in females: Epidemiology, risk factors, and evaluation. *UpToDate*. Retrieved September 28, 2022, from https://www.uptodate.com/contents/overview-of-sexual-dysfunction-in-females-epidemiology-risk-factors-and-evaluation

Schifren, J. L. (2022b). Overview of sexual dysfunction in women: Management. *UpToDate*. Retrieved September 28, 2022, from https://www.uptodate.com/contents/overview-of-sexual-dysfunction-in-women-management

Tangpricha, V., & Safer, J. D. (2020). Transgender men: Evaluation and management. *UpToDate*. Retrieved September 28, 2022, from https://www.uptodate.com/contents/transgender-men-evaluation-and-management

Tangpricha, V., & Safer, J. D. (2021). Transgender women: Evaluation and management. *UpToDate*. Retrieved September 28, 2022, from https://www.uptodate.com/contents/transgender-women-evaluation-and-management

Fill in the Blank

Fill in the blank with the correct answer.

1. _____ _____ is an individual's gendered pattern of attraction to others.
2. The nurse does a sexuality _____-_____ when they examine their own feelings and opinions related to sexual and gender issues and if their personal views would bias the nursing care they provide.
3. Transgender individuals are at a higher risk for _____.
4. The phases of the sexual response cycle include desire, _____, orgasm, and recovery.
5. Antihypertensive medications are known to cause the sexual dysfunction of _____ _____.

Matching

Match the following terms to the most appropriate phrase.

1. _____ Exhibitionism
2. _____ Fetishism
3. _____ Gender identity
4. _____ Pedophilia
5. _____ Transgender

a. Sexual activity with a prepubescent child
b. The innate sense of feeling male, female, neither, or a combination of both, or something else
c. Intentional exposure of one's genitals in public
d. Adjective that describes an individual whose gender identity is different from the sex they were assigned at birth
e. Sexual arousal using inanimate objects

Multiple Choice

Select the best answer from the multiple-choice items.

1. The nurse is reinforcing teaching for a 45-year-old male client newly diagnosed with diabetes mellitus. The client states, "I really don't want to talk about my sexual life. That is my business." What is the best response by the nurse?
   a. "That is fine if you prefer not to discuss this issue. I will make a note to that effect on your record."
   b. "I understand. I would not want to tell someone about that part of my life either."
   c. "I know it must be difficult for you to talk with a stranger about such a private matter. We can discuss it at a later time."
   d. "We can't help you if you choose not to give us information. There are lots of people with your condition who have problems."

2. The nurse is talking with a client who is experiencing pain during sexual intercourse. Tearfully, the client states their spouse "expects me to have sex even though it hurts." What is the best response for the nurse to make at this time?
   a. "We will be glad to refer you to a counselor who works with people who have experienced sexual assault."
   b. "Tell me more about what happens when you have sexual intercourse."
   c. "After the health care provider does a physical exam, we will try to help you with your problem."
   d. "I don't know how you put up with that. It must be very difficult."

3. The nurse is admitting a client with a diagnosis of poly-substance use disorder to the emergency department. The client is also a registered sex offender. Which nursing intervention is most important for the nurse to implement?
   a. Gathering information about their sexual behaviors
   b. Warning other clients about their sexual behavior
   c. Taking them into an exam room and shutting the door to take a sexual history
   d. Using a nonjudgmental approach

4. A client is being followed in an outpatient clinic for treatment of depression and anxiety. Which statement by the client would indicate a possible sexual dysfunction related to medication side effects?
   a. "I really want to respond to my spouse, but the feeling just isn't there."
   b. "Nothing seems to matter anymore. I don't even want talk to anyone."
   c. "I know I am not the best company, but my spouse is supportive."
   d. "It takes all my energy just to get out of bed in the morning."

5. Which of the following statements would be asked when taking a sexual history? *(Select all that apply)*
   a. "Who do you have sex with?"
   b. "How often do you use alcohol?"
   c. "In what situations, or with whom, do you avoid condoms?"
   d. "Have you told your current partner you were treated for gonorrhea in the past?"
   e. "What are your current plans or desires regarding pregnancy?"

Unit V | Age-Specific Disorders and Issues

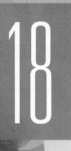

18

Disorders and Issues of Children and Adolescents

LEARNING OBJECTIVES

After learning the content in this chapter, the student will be able to:

1. Describe why the conditions discussed are considered mental health issues.

2. Identify common signs and symptoms of the mental health issues seen in children and adolescents.

3. Identify common causes for intellectual and/or developmental disability.

4. Discuss treatment options for the child or adolescent with a mental health issue.

5. Identify coexisting conditions that may be seen in the child or adolescent with a mental health issue.

6. Describe the nursing process for the child or adolescent with a mental health issue.

KEY TERMS

copropraxia

dyslexia

echopraxia

enuresis

intellectual and/or developmental disability

pica

stuttering

tic

Mental Health Issues in Children and Adolescents

In Chapter 1, it was discussed that mental health includes a balance between the individual's cognitive, behavioral, and emotional states as well as the individual's ability to handle stress, relate and communicate with others, and emote (express) their feelings. The issues discussed in this chapter may not seem like they are mental health in nature, however, they directly impact the individual's mental health. Many of these issues will exist for the individual's lifetime. Some of the issues may resolve prior to adulthood but the individual may have residual emotions as an adult. An example of this would be the child who experienced nocturnal enuresis (repeated episodes of urine incontinence during the night after being toilet trained, the lay term is "bed wetting"), was bullied, and then as an adult is diagnosed with depression related to the persistent bullying.

There are mental health disorders that are seen in childhood and adolescence, as well as adulthood. Some of these may not be diagnosed until the individual is an adult, but with a detailed history, it may be discovered that they existed to some extent when the individual was younger. Examples of these mental health diagnoses include anxiety, panic, depression, post-traumatic stress disorder (PTSD), and substance use disorder. Although the mental health issues discussed in this chapter are typically first diagnosed, or occur, during childhood and adolescence, there is no defined age limit that distinguishes between childhood and adult mental health issues. The mental health issues discussed in this chapter are divided as being either neurodevelopmental or behavioral in nature.

Neurodevelopmental Disorders

The neurodevelopmental disorders include those conditions in which the child demonstrates deficits or symptoms during the normal periods of development. Typically, the deficits are seen early in the child's development prior to school age. These disorders are characterized by performance testing of mentality, skills, coordination, or activity that is substantially below that anticipated for the child's chronologic age and education level. The identified deficits impact the child's functioning in their personal, social, academic, or occupational areas. Neurodevelopmental disorders include language and communication disorders, intellectual and/or developmental disability, autism spectrum disorder, and attention deficit hyperactivity disorder (ADHD).

Language and Communication Disorders

These disorders cause impairment with some component of speech and/or language. Children with this type of disorder have difficulty acquiring and using language due to deficits in comprehension or production of vocabulary, sentences, and speech. The language difficulty interferes with the child's performance in school and social functioning.

The child with language disorder may have limited speech and vocabulary with difficulty learning new words or applying grammar concepts. Children with an expressive disorder have a difficult time expressing themselves through language and may use gestures or verbal sounds to express themselves. These children usually begin talking later than usual and progress at a slower rate than that which is considered age appropriate. Children with a receptive disorder have difficulty understanding the message that is being sent to them verbally. The child with a mixed language disorder also has a problem in understanding words and sentences and also difficulty expressing themselves. The inability to comprehend may be less apparent than the ability to speak effectively. The lack of comprehension is often seen when the child does not follow commands correctly or respond appropriately to questions. The ability to complete a thought process or follow rules of a game may also indicate the lack of understanding. Box 18.1 lists other signs and symptoms of a language disorder.

BOX 18.1

Signs and Symptoms of Language Disorder

- Limited speech and vocabulary
- Difficulty learning new words
- Difficulty applying grammar concepts
- Delayed talking
- Slow progress in speech
- Difficulty in understanding words and sentences that require complex thinking
- Decreased ability to process incoming sounds
- Difficulty associating and organizing words and sentences
- Inability to speak effectively
- Lack of comprehension
- Failure to follow commands
- Inappropriate responses to questions
- Inability to follow rules of a game

Stuttering

Stuttering is characterized by repetitive or prolonged sounds or syllables that include pauses and monosyllable broken words. It causes considerable discomfort for the child in both academic and social situations, but may be absent when they are singing or reading aloud. There may be accompanying motor movement such as jerking, twitching, or tremors. Increased levels of anxiety and stress will often initiate the problem, which leads to further anxiety, frustration, and low self-esteem. Box 18.2 lists other signs and symptoms of stuttering. The development of stuttering is typically seen before 6 years of age and frequently resolves itself. The child should be checked for a hearing impairment that can contribute to the speech problem.

Dyslexia

Dyslexia is a type of learning disorder characterized by difficulty in the visual reading domain. In this disorder, there is a difference between the child's intellectual ability and their success in reading and spelling. Even though these children are of average or higher intelligence, they may be behind in the level of reading expected for their grade level. The problem seems to stem from an inability to process incoming sensory stimuli with the correct interpretation. Dyslexia can affect social interactions in school, such as the child may be teased or bullied because of their reading and writing ability, moved to a remedial class, or not advanced to the next grade level.

The child with dyslexia usually does not read for pleasure. Spelling and writing by hand may be difficult, with a consistent pattern of letter confusion. Letter reversal is common; for example, "p" may be used for "g," or "b" used for "d." The child often sees

words from right to left with failure to see similar or different characteristics of words. For instance, instead of seeing "cat" the child sees "tac." There may also be a problem with sounding out words phonetically. Individuals who have difficulty learning may exhibit accompanying signs of discouragement, low self-esteem, and inadequate social skills. Signs and symptoms for dyslexia are found in Box 18.3.

Dyslexia is often not discovered until elementary school when reading skills become more complex and increased comprehension is required. Hearing loss or visual impairment must first be ruled out as a primary cause of the disorder. The quality and number of educational opportunities that are available to the child may be a factor in the child's reading ability.

Just the Facts The way children think about their successes or failures determines what effects these will have on their motivation and attitude toward learning. Children who attribute their failures to a lack of effort may try harder the next time, whereas those who attribute them to a lack of ability often quit trying.

Tics and Tourette Syndrome

A **tic** is a sudden, brief, repetitive, arrhythmic, stereotyped motor movement or sound. Tics occur before the age of 18 years. In a tic disorder, there is never a symptom-free period of more than 3 months. Tourette syndrome is a type of tic disorder where the individual has experienced tics for at least 1 year. Most people with tics meet the criteria for Tourette syndrome.

Simple tics may involve such movements as blinking of the eye, wrinkling of the nose, jerking of the neck or shoulder, or grimacing. More complex movements may include hand gestures, contortions of the face, or physical actions such as jumping, retracing steps, hopping, and skipping over lines. Occasionally, the person may assume unusual positions or posturing. Vocal tics are meaningless recurrent sounds such as sniffing, snorting, and throat clearing. More complex behaviors include verbal outbursts of words or phrases, speech blocking, or meaningless changes in tone or volume of speech. **Echopraxia** is mimicking the movements of another person without a reason. While echopraxia is a symptom that is also seen in psychosis, in children, it is more evident of a tic and not psychosis. **Copropraxia**, or a sudden tic-like obscene gesture, along with repetitive movements, can also occur, but usually in a small number of individuals with a tic disorder.

The person with a tic disorder usually experiences an irresistible urge to perform the tic and feels relief once the behavior has occurred. Tics tend to occur in spells that may last from seconds to hours. The severity or frequency of the spells usually changes during the course of the day or as environmental location changes. Some children may be able to suppress tics during a school session but return to the behavior during recess. Tics generally tend to decrease during sleep or during concentrated activity such as reading or playing the piano. The incidence may increase during periods of stress, illness, or when the individual is tired. The emotional discomfort, shame, and self-consciousness caused by the behavior may lead to social isolation or personality changes. Tic disorders tend to be genetic and often the individual outgrows them. If the symptoms cause the individual distress, medications and cognitive behavioral therapy may be helpful.

Selective Mutism

In some cases, the child repeatedly does not speak during situations where they are expected to, such as in school. This is called selective mutism. For this to be considered a mental health issue, it needs to occur for at least a month and interfere with the individual's schooling or social interactions. Selective mutism does not include instances when the child does not know the language, such as a recent immigrant, and is not comfortable speaking the new language, or in cases where there is an existing communication disorder. Behavioral therapy is the most common treatment for selective mutism. Antianxiety medications may also be used.

Test Yourself
- ✔ How does stuttering differ from a tic?
- ✔ Would a 3-year-old be diagnosed with dyslexia? Describe why or why not.
- ✔ What other mental health disorder is echopraxia a symptom of?

Intellectual and/or Developmental Disability

Intellectual and/or developmental disability is a broad term that covers a variety of conditions that cause significant limitations in intellectual functioning, social interactions, and practical living skills. The disability almost always is evident before adolescence. Table 18.1 lists some common causes and examples of intellectual and/or developmental disability. In many individuals, there is no clear cause that can be determined. The limitations are seen in the individual's inability to meet expected standards of personal growth, independence, and social adaptation in all areas of daily functioning.

Just the Facts The term mental retardation carries with it a negative stigma and is considered offensive. Therefore, it should not be used by the nurse.

The impact of the disability is classified as mild, moderate, severe, or profound. These levels are not based upon IQ but by evaluating the individual's ability to perform day-to-day life skills,

Mind Jogger How is the support of the family important in helping the child with a communication disorder?

TABLE 18.1	Causes of Intellectual and/or Developmental Disability
Category	**Example(s)**
Chromosomal/Genetics	Down syndrome (Trisomy 21)
	Fragile X syndrome
Birth related issues	Prematurity
	Cerebral Palsy
Prenatal damage	Toxins (heavy metal ingestion)
	Maternal alcohol intake (fetal alcohol syndrome)
	Maternal substance use (cocaine, methamphetamine)
	Infection (cytomegalovirus)
Metabolic	Untreated phenylketonuria
Childhood injury	Head injury
	Stroke
	Illness (meningitis)

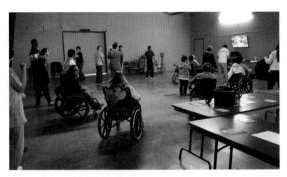

Figure 18.1 Group exercise activity at Mental Health Day-hab Center for individuals of all ages with Intellectual and/or Developmental Disability.

activities, developmental milestones, and cognitive processes (such as communicating and learning capabilities), as this is what determines how much support the individual needs. The majority of persons with an intellectual and/or developmental disability fall into the mild disability category and a small percentage in the severe and profound categories. Children usually are brought in by their family caregivers for evaluation when the child does not meet developmental milestones appropriate for their age such as rolling over, walking, or speaking. Although the intellectual and/or developmental disability usually remains unchanged, interventions can provide some improvement of functional life skills in most cases of mild to moderate disability (Fig. 18.1). Treatment is individualized based upon the individual's strengths, needs, and medical needs. No treatment will completely remove the disability. The goal is to help the individual live at their highest level of functioning, as well as be as independent as possible in any activities they can perform.

Signs and Symptoms

The individual with an intellectual disability typically has intellectual functioning that is significantly below average, an IQ score of around 70 to 75 or lower, which is usually accompanied by deficits in conceptual, social, and practical skills. Cognitive impairment is seen in the delay of the individual's skills in areas such as language, reading, time, numbers, money, and self-care skills. There is usually impairment at some level in reasoning, problem solving, judgment, or comprehension.

Practical daily skills may be difficult or neglected and include skills related to personal hygiene and care, attending to health care needs, transportation, daily routines, and schedules. Some

individuals may be unable to use communication devices such as a telephone. Interpersonal skills necessary for social interactions and relationships are also affected. Impairments in interpersonal skills and a tendency to being gullible or naïve predispose the individual with an intellectual and/or developmental disability to safety issues and vulnerable to experiencing physical and/or sexual abuse.

Temperament varies in individuals with an intellectual and/or developmental disability. Some individuals are passive, serene, and compliant, whereas others may be more aggressive and impulsive in their actions. The aggressive tendencies may stem from the inability to communicate in a meaningful way, which leads to frustration.

Issues Concurrent With Intellectual and/or Developmental Disability

One of the purposes of establishing a diagnosis of intellectual and/or developmental disability is to assist the individual and family caregivers with individualized services such as therapy (physical, speech, or occupational), education, skills training, home- and community-based waiver services, and government Social Security Administration and health care benefits.

Research has been trying to establish the incidence of coexisting mental health issues in individuals with an intellectual and/or developmental disability. Difficulty with limited communication and cognition can make the coexisting diagnosis difficult, so objective symptoms such as depressed mood, irritability, anorexia, or insomnia may be the basis for determining that an additional problem exists. Biologic and psychological factors contribute to this disparity. Biologic factors include genetic abnormalities or brain injury and psychological factors include stigmatization and impaired social interactions.

Mind Jogger How might the presence of a child with an intellectual and/or developmental disability affect home life? What possible impact could this diagnosis have upon their siblings? What adjustments in the family might be necessary as the individual reaches adulthood?

Mind Jogger What nursing interventions might the nurse need to implement, or change, when caring for a client with difficulty in comprehension and expression?

Autism Spectrum Disorder

Autism spectrum disorder refers to a range of complex neurodevelopmental disorders that involve differences in the development of various basic skills, including communication and socializing with others. It is considered a spectrum as there is a variety in the types of symptoms seen in the individual. The behaviors seen in one individual may not be the same in another. The term Asperger syndrome is no longer used as the symptoms seen are part of autism spectrum disorder.

The child with autism spectrum disorder has difficulty processing and understanding input from the world around them. The child may have specific areas in which problems exist and other areas of daily functioning. This disorder is characterized by differences in development of the ability to socially interact and communicate with others. Symptoms usually appear before 3 years of age. Children with this disorder often are withdrawn and inwardly focused with little interest in their environment, exhibit repetitive behaviors or interests, have magnified emotional responses, and are routine driven.

Behaviors Seen in Autism Spectrum Disorder

Early language delays that might indicate autism spectrum disorder may exist include a lack of babbling by 1 year of age, no single words by 16 months, or no two-word phrases by 2 years of age, and a lack of response when being addressed by name. Nonverbal behaviors such as eye contact, facial expression, and gestures used to communicate are not used as frequently in children with autism spectrum disorder as in their peers. The child often does not develop age-appropriate peer relationships. This may be from lack of interest in or enjoyment from peer relationships and play activities with other children or from a lack of communication skills. The child may have different ways of playing with toys and other objects than their peers, such as arranging their toys in a certain way or repetitious banging of an object. Time is occupied with an inflexible and consistent routine of nonpurposeful behaviors and rituals. Children with autism spectrum disorder can have accompanying intellectual disability ranging from mild to profound. Verbal skills and the ability to comprehend written words are usually below the level appropriate for the child's age.

Other behaviors may be exhibited such as hyperactivity, impulsivity, aggressiveness, and inattention to the world around them. The child

---

> ## BOX 18.4
>
> ### Signs and Symptoms for Autism Spectrum Disorder
>
> - Lack of responsiveness to others
> - Unusual play behavior with toys
> - Temper tantrums
> - Severe difficulty with communication
> - Repetitive routines
> - Does not like to be touched or held
> - Withdrawal from social contact
> - Heightened responses to environmental stimuli (e.g., head banging, hand flapping, rocking, clinging to inanimate objects)

may demonstrate heightened responses to sensory stimuli, such as screaming when touched, or exhibit a lack of anticipated response to painful stimuli. The child may be very sensitive to some noises, but ignore others. Some children exhibit a fascination with certain colors, objects, or music. Eating patterns may be stereotyped, such as repeatedly eating the same food. The child may awaken during sleep and engage in rocking movements, head banging, or other self-stimulating behaviors. Mood instability often occurs with sudden outbursts of laughing or crying. Adolescents with autism spectrum disorder may experience depression. Box 18.4 lists signs and symptoms for autism spectrum disorder. Autism spectrum disorder is lifelong, and affects not only the individual, but family and those around them (Box 18.5).

Incidence, Causes, and Concerns

The symptoms of autism spectrum disorder may be difficult to distinguish in the child under the age of 2 years, because social and communication skills are in an early stage of development. Some family caregivers indicate seeing early signs of developmental delays, whereas others report no obvious indicators of a problem. The incidence of this disorder is rising in the United States with 1 in 44 children are identified with autism spectrum disorder (CDC, 2021). Males are affected more often than females and there is an increased incidence in siblings of individuals with the disorder. Most individuals identified with autism spectrum disorder were not diagnosed prior to the age of 4, although it can be diagnosed as early as age 2. There is no definite cause of autism spectrum disorder. Research studies show that genetics and environmental influences may be partly responsible. Studies have also looked at the reasons for

BOX 18.5

Malachi—Autism Early Diagnosis: From a Mother's Perspective

"Malachi's early development seemed normal. He crawled and walked at the usual milestones; he was even trying to talk. But when he was 18 months old, he stopped talking, he stopped looking at me when I talked to him, and wouldn't respond to me or to other children. At the encouragement of family members, he was taken to a clinic that specialized in autism and behavior issues with children, where at the age of 3 years he was diagnosed with autism. He attended special classes for autistic and intellectually disabled children and was given speech therapy. His teacher took a special interest in Malachi and worked tirelessly to engage him in social interaction and play with other children. She still calls to see how he is doing.

His special education teachers have been so helpful in working with him and teaching me as his mother how to handle his behaviors and to help him adjust to the world around him. At times, his behavior has been violent. This is usually at times when he cannot handle his emotions—the most recent was when his maternal grandmother died. He was very close to his grandmother and called her frequently. He couldn't handle the sadness and grief which led to destructive behaviors and admission to a behavioral inpatient unit for stabilization. Most of the time, he does very well. He rocks and paces constantly, always in some sort of motion. He loves his camera and his pictures downloaded on the computer. He has hundreds of pictures that he loves to show to anyone who will look at them."

Malachi is now 16 years old, lives with his mother and is a happy young man who loves to take pictures and have his picture taken. He has a very special and bonded relationship with his mother. He is in the Big Brother–Little Brother program, likes to participate in athletics at his school, and attends church regularly with his mother.

the increasing incidence seen which may include more awareness of symptoms and broader determination criteria which can lead to more diagnoses being made.

Concurrent health issues that are commonly seen in autism spectrum disorder include epilepsy, depression, obesity, and anxiety. Drowning, accidents, and bullying are commonly seen in individuals with autism spectrum disorder. The individual may age out of autism services that are school based when they turn 18 years old. This may impact the family as many individuals with autism spectrum disorder face unemployment or difficulty with postsecondary education or skills training. Health care issues and poverty are also concerns for families with adult members with autism spectrum disorder. Family members who act as case managers or advocates for the individual may not be able to hold full-time jobs, which can impact the family's income.

"Martin"

Dubova/Shutterstock

Martin, a 6-year-old, is admitted to the hospital's pediatric unit with asthmatic bronchitis. In addition to their medical condition, Martin has autism spectrum disorder. Martin does not seem aware of the nurse's presence in the room but is intensely staring out the window. The nurse is preparing to administer scheduled oral medications. Martin's family caregiver is present in the room.

Digging Deeper

1. *What approach would help the nurse to establish a trusting relationship with Martin?*

2. *How will Martin likely use eye contact in communicating with the nurse?*

3. *What other behaviors might the nurse anticipate as Martin attempts to deal with the unfamiliar surroundings and activities?*

CASE STUDY 18.1

Treatment

Treatment for autism spectrum disorder is focused upon the individual's specific needs. Occupational therapy for daily tasks such as brushing teeth, using buttons and zippers, utilizing public transportation, or grocery shopping may be indicated. Therapy for enhancing social skills, anger management, or speech skills may be necessary for some individuals. Medications may be prescribed for associated conditions such as anxiety or depression. Agitation and irritability that is associated with autism spectrum disorder may be treated with risperidone or aripiprazole.

Attention Deficit Hyperactivity Disorder

In attention deficit hyperactivity disorder (ADHD), a persistent pattern of inattention, hyperactivity, or impulsive behaviors is more frequently exhibited than in a child of comparable age and developmental level. Some display of these symptoms must be present before the age of 12 years, often appearing between ages of 3 and 6. Many children are diagnosed after the behaviors have been present for some time.

Just the Facts Attention involves the filtering of incoming sensory stimuli to screen out most information. This allows only a select few stimuli to pass into conscious awareness.

Signs and Symptoms

Primary symptoms of inattention, hyperactivity, and impulsive actions are the key behaviors seen in children with attention deficit hyperactivity disorder (ADHD). The behavior causes significant difficulty for the individual in home, school, or social settings. There is usually an obvious pattern of disruption and inappropriate functioning as a result of the behavior. To be diagnosed with attention deficit hyperactivity disorder (ADHD), the symptoms must be present for a period of 6 months or longer.

The symptoms of hyperactivity may not be the same at all developmental age levels. Toddlers and preschool children with attention deficit hyperactivity disorder (ADHD) usually exhibit more exaggerated activity than other children of the same age. Continual and often destructive physical activity is seen, along with an inability to remain seated for activities such as a television show or story-telling session. In school-age children, these behaviors may be minimized in intensity although fidgeting, noise-making, and other restless behaviors increase. The child often gets up from the table during meals or seated activities in the classroom. Although symptoms of the disorder often diminish in late adolescence or adulthood, many continue to exhibit restlessness and difficulty with activities requiring quiet attentiveness or concentration. This results in an unorganized approach to schoolwork and work-related activities with minimal ability to follow through on task-oriented projects. Risk-taking behaviors are common, with little regard for the potential consequences of these actions. Impulsivity, which can occur in any age group, is demonstrated by impatience, the inability to refrain from interrupting, and discourteously intruding on the rights of others. Children with attention deficit hyperactivity disorder (ADHD) lack the self-control to delay their responses. The impulsive and fearless nature of physical activity often leads to accidental injury and destruction of property. Because children have different personalities and temperaments, and mature at varying rates, it is important that the child's behavior is observed during different situations and activities.

Additional symptoms may include a low tolerance or frustration with accompanying temper tantrums, mood changes, low self-esteem, stubbornness, demanding behavior, and poor caregiver–child and peer relationships (Box 18.6). These behaviors tend to be labeled as willful, leading to conflict within the family and school systems. Family maladjustment and poor caregiver–child interaction are usually present. These relationships may improve with successful intervention and therapy. The intelligence level of individuals with this disorder ranges from lower than average to gifted.

Attention deficit hyperactivity disorder (ADHD) is more commonly seen in children who have a first-generation biologic relative with the disorder. Children born to families with members who have substance use disorders or other mental health issues have higher incidence of attention deficit hyperactivity disorder (ADHD). It is most commonly diagnosed in school-age children, with a higher incidence seen in boys. With research and increased awareness of the symptoms, adults are also being diagnosed with attention deficit

Signs and Symptoms of Attention Deficit Hyperactivity Disorder (ADHD)

- Inattention to close detail or errors in homework or assigned tasks
- Inability to maintain focus on a task or play activity
- Often seems preoccupied and inattentive to the person who is speaking
- Repeatedly moves focus from one activity to another, failing to follow directions
- Failure to follow a task to completion
- Dislikes tasks that require maintained mental concentration and effort (e.g., reading, mathematics, mental games), often avoiding them
- Marked disorganization and inattentive handling or loss of materials necessary to perform a task or complete homework
- Easily distracted by irrelevant external stimuli such as a lawn mower or car honking
- Fidgety and frequent squirming with inability to remain seated when asked to do so
- Difficulty following instructions or taking turns in games or classroom activities
- Excessive and spontaneous talking and interruptions of others at inappropriate times
- Difficulty in playing quietly; perpetually in motion
- May engage in potentially dangerous or destructive activity, oblivious of the possible consequences
- Impaired relationships (caregiver–child and also peers)
- Low tolerance to frustration
- Temper tantrums, low self-esteem, stubbornness, demanding

hyperactivity disorder (ADHD) more frequently. In adults, a historical review of symptoms often reveals that the behaviors were present early in childhood but a diagnosis was never made. In addition to genetics, other possible links to attention deficit hyperactivity disorder (ADHD) include brain injury, environmental exposure, premature birth, low-birth weight, nutrition, or substance use during pregnancy.

Treatment

Attention deficit hyperactivity disorder (ADHD) can be successfully managed using a combination of medication and behavior therapy. Medication can be used to better control behavior challenges. While no one particular medication works successfully for every individual, it is important to find one that works best. Stimulants are the most commonly used treatment with most children

responding favorably to their effects. The benefits of these medications result in improved attention, less hyperactive or restless behaviors, and improved peer relationships. Improvements in the child's academic functioning are also seen. Most children do not experience side effects in response to these medications. However, some may experience insomnia, stomach aches and anorexia, headaches, drowsiness, irritability, or nervousness. Some nonstimulant medications are available for treating attention deficit hyperactivity disorder (ADHD) with fewer reported side effects. Family caregivers should be taught not to alter the established dose regimen or abruptly discontinue the medication. Withdrawal symptoms can be induced with sudden interruption in the medication levels. Common stimulant and nonstimulant medications used in children with attention deficit hyperactivity disorder (ADHD) are listed in Box 18.7.

In addition to medication, behavioral therapy is a vital part of the treatment program. The interventions are designed to help the child create a structured routine that centers on behavior modification, goals and rewards, and discipline using consequences for inappropriate conduct. Family caregivers are educated in child-rearing skills to maintain consistency in the approach to behavior change. A large percentage of children continue to demonstrate at least one of the essential symptoms into adulthood.

Medications Used in Treatment of Attention Deficit Hyperactivity Disorder (ADHD)

STIMULANTS (Some are approved for use in children over 3, others approved for children over 6 years of age)

- methylphenidate
- amphetamine sulfate
- dextroamphetamine sulfate
- pemoline
- dexmethylphenidate

NONSTIMULANTS

- atomoxetine
- guanfacine (extended release, for children/teens between ages 6 and 17)

ANTIDEPRESSANTS

- desipramine
- bupropion
- venlafaxine

Behavioral Disorders

Behavioral disorders include conditions that involve problems in the self-control of emotions, behaviors that violate the rights of others, or behaviors that bring the child or adolescent into conflict with the norms of society or authority figures.

Oppositional Defiant Disorder

Oppositional defiant disorder is a repetitive pattern of angry mood, negative/defiant, and hostile behavior toward authority figures typically beginning in the home. Children with oppositional defiant disorder demonstrate the tendency to argue incessantly with adults, lose their temper, and actively defy or refuse to comply with rules and requests imposed upon them. There is a pattern of deliberately acting in a way that annoys others, while blaming others for the behavior. Children with this disorder are usually vindictive, spiteful, and resentful in their interpersonal relationships and usually exhibit resistance to compromise or negotiation with peers or adults. The problematic behaviors may lead to suspension or expulsion from school and frequent encounters with law enforcement officials. There is an increased incidence of sexually transmitted diseases and teenage pregnancy reported in these clients. The tendency for suicidal ideation and suicide attempts increases and may be the factor in seeking treatment. Warning signs for suicidal risk in children and adolescents are listed in Box 18.8.

Parental rejection and neglect with harsh and abusive physical punishment or sexual abuse are often cited as predisposing factors for this disorder. The child may have been removed to a foster or group home situation with a frequent shift in caregivers. Rejection by peers may lead the child

BOX 18.8

Warning Signs for Suicide Risk in Children and Adolescents

- Verbal threats or behavioral hints about suicide
- Decline in quality of schoolwork
- Truancy from school or running away from home
- Sudden withdrawal from friends or family
- Withdrawal from previously enjoyed activities
- Drug or alcohol use
- Giving away prized possessions
- Excessive fatigue or physical symptoms
- Prolonged expression of sadness or uselessness
- Lack of response to praise and rewards
- Neglect of personal appearance or hygiene
- Unusually rebellious behaviors

to an association with those who engage in delinquent antisocial behaviors, violence, and drug-related activity (see Box 18.9). These children have a low tolerance for frustration with frequent angry outbursts and conflict with family members and teachers. It is usually evident before the age of 8 years but no later than early adolescence. A familial pattern of psychiatric problems is often preexistent in the child. It is also seen more often in families where there is serious marital conflict between spouses. A thorough evaluation of the child is important, because many of the behaviors seen in this disorder may normally be seen occasionally in children of preschool age through adolescence in milder outbursts.

Intermittent Explosive Disorder

Intermittent explosive disorder is characterized by angry, aggressive outbursts that have a rapid onset, typically lasting less than 30 minutes. These

BOX 18.9

Signs and Symptoms of Oppositional Defiant Disorder

- Arguing without compromise
- Willful defiance of rules
- Hostility and anger
- Low tolerance to frustration
- Argumentative, angry, irritable mood
- Use of drugs or alcohol
- Physical violence
- Violation of curfews
- Spiteful or vindictive acts

"Anthony"

Csaba Peterdi/
Shutterstock

Anthony is a 14-year-old client who has been admitted to the adolescent psychiatric center after repeated incidents of suspension from school for disruptive and defiant behaviors toward his teachers and peers. He is an only child from a single-parent family. His father died when he was 3 years old, leaving his mother with minimal employment skills to support her young son. Anthony has had recurrent episodes of nocturnal and diurnal enuresis since he was 5.

His mother relates that Anthony was always a hyperactive child. When he started school, the teachers were calling several times a week to tell her that they could not manage him in their classroom. He was given time-out suspensions from class in addition to receiving many failing grades in his academic learning. Anthony was placed in an alternate class situation for children with learning disabilities. In addition to being easily distracted, Anthony cannot sit still nor concentrate on any one task long enough for its completion.

Anthony's mother says that she is afraid he is going to end up in jail if something isn't done. She says, "He has been a hassle for me ever since he was born. Sometimes I really wish he had never been born. Maybe he would be better off in jail—then I wouldn't have to deal with him."

He is given a diagnosis of attention deficit hyperactivity disorder (ADHD) with oppositional defiant disorder. It is also determined that Anthony has an intelligence level in the gifted range.

CASE STUDY 18.2

Digging Deeper

1. What psychological factors may be underlying Anthony's disruptive behavior?

2. What may have contributed to his performance in the school setting?

3. What feelings may Anthony be having related to his mother's attitude toward him?

4. What approach might be used to help Anthony's mother to deal with her son's illness?

---

outbursts are usually in response to a minor situation and may involve damage and/or physical aggression toward another person, animal, or property.

Onset of intermittent explosive disorder is typically during late childhood or adolescent years, and accounts for many incidents of school-based violence. The impulsive, aggressive response is significantly out of proportion to the psychosocial stressor that seemingly triggers the behavior. The impulsive aggressive behavior (see Box 18.10) typically occurs in recurrent episodes that follow a chronic pattern over the individual's lifetime. The outbursts are usually unplanned and do not have ulterior motives attached (e.g., money, power, or property). Intermittent explosive disorder is more prevalent in younger individuals and occurs more frequently in males. The disorder appears to be more common in individuals with family history of mood disorders or substance use disorders. The onset of the disorder is frequently unexpected with no warning period of behaviors leading up to the time of diagnosis.

Conduct Disorder

Conduct disorder is defined as a pattern of repetitive and continuous behavior that either infringes on the basic rights of others or defies the rules of society that would be appropriate for the child's age level. This behavior may have an onset prior to the age of 10 years, with many also having a history of other disruptive disorders. Individuals with adolescent-onset type tend to demonstrate conduct problems in group situations, although their behaviors may be less aggressive.

BOX 18.10

Behaviors Seen in Intermittent Explosive Disorder

- Recurrent verbal or physical aggression that involves damage or destruction of property
- Physical violence that causes harm to animals or another person
- Impulsive assaultive behavioral outbursts
- Feeling of relief from the tension immediately after the explosive behavior
- Assaultive behavior is out of proportion to the precipitating stressor
- Tends to see the motives of others as malicious and directly targeting them personally
- Blames others for provoking their violence
- May experience racing thoughts or heightened emotions during an assault

Children with this disorder demonstrate aggressive actions that result in or threaten harm to other people or animals. They tend to initiate hostile and bullying-type behavior, using threats and fighting with or without weapons that can inflict serious physical injury. They may steal, rape, mug, assault other people, or seriously abuse animals. It is common for these children to lie and "con" by asking personal favors with no intention of repayment. Other behaviors may cause damage or loss of property, such as setting fires or vandalism. The behaviors usually exist in several situations such as the home, school, or community setting. There is usually a pattern starting before the age of 13 years. Defiance of home and family rules and curfews with a pattern of "running away" from home overnight or truancy from school is common.

Preschool children with conduct disorder usually exhibit aggressive behaviors in their home situation and toward other children. They often deliberately destroy other people's property. School-age children continue the deliberate aggressive behaviors, both physical and verbal. In the adolescent, there may also be an early onset of sexual promiscuity, substance use, and physical violence that accompany the earlier behavioral pattern. Conduct disorder may be associated with other risk-taking behaviors, school problems, substance use, and bullying (Box 18.11). Conduct disorder is influenced by both genetics and environmental factors, with the risk increased in children with a first-degree biologic relative with the disorder or families with a history of substance use and other mental health issues.

Test Yourself

✔ Describe the difference between oppositional defiant disorder and intermittent explosive disorder.
✔ What would be a priority nursing intervention when a client with conduct disorder is admitted to a nursing unit?

Separation Anxiety Disorder

During early childhood development, it is expected that the child will experience anxiety in response to encounters with unfamiliar objects or people or when leaving a trusted caregiver. This is seen in infants starting as early as 8 months and is seen until about 4 years of age. In comparison, the child with separation anxiety disorder experiences excessive anxiety related to separation from home or attachment figures. The disturbance must occur before the age of 18 years and cause significant distress or impairment in functioning for a period of at least 1 month. Symptoms may become evident following a stressful period in the child's life such as starting school, parental divorce, a neighborhood move, or death of a pet or close relative.

The child with separation anxiety disorder is uncomfortable to the point of misery when separated from the person with whom a love attachment is formed. When the separation is necessary, as in attending school, the child may feel the need to stay in constant touch with the person or be preoccupied with the need to return home. The child may experience somatic symptoms such as abdominal pain, nausea and vomiting, or headaches during or before the separation. Excessive worry about the event or of losing the loved ones during a separation may become persistent. There may be a fear of going to sleep without the loved one present or worry that something terrible is going to happen to that person. The degree of anxiety can range from uneasiness to panic and depression. Depending on the age of the child, fears and concerns may vary. The younger child may have fears of the dark, monsters, burglars, fires, water, or other situations that could pose a danger to the family or self. Apathy, sadness, depression, and feelings of being unloved or unwanted are common. These children are often described as demanding of attention, leading to frustration and resentment within the family circle.

BOX 18.11

Signs and Symptoms of Conduct Disorder

- Repeated disruptive and destructive behaviors
- Willful defiance of family rules
- Violation of age-appropriate and societal norms
- Aggressive behavior
- Truancy from school or running away from home
- Sexual promiscuity
- Substance use and misuse
- Vandalism and physical violence
- Cruelty toward animals
- Bullies and initiates physical fights
- Deliberate destruction of property belonging to others
- Intentional setting of fire with property damage
- Lying and deceit

Treatment is aimed at reducing the anxiety and reinforcing a sense of security in both the child and the family during periods of separation. Cognitive-behavioral therapy and group therapy are utilized in addition to antianxiety medications to help the child or adolescent to cope with their fears and uncertainties. Family caregivers, or the whole family, may be included in the therapy sessions to assist them in understanding the nature of the disorder and how to support their child.

Although some children are successful in accomplishing these goals, others go on to develop a chronic anxiety disorder, panic disorder, or depression. This disorder is more common in children whose family caregivers have anxiety, panic disorders, or who are overprotective. The symptoms tend to decrease as the child reaches adolescence (Box 18.12).

Enuresis

Enuresis (involuntary urination) may be related to physiologic or psychological causes. Physiologic causes include a urinary tract infection or a delay in development that may resolve over time. The child with nocturnal enuresis has repeated episodes of urine incontinence during the night. The symptoms must occur at least twice a week for at least 3 months to be categorized as a disorder. An isolated event such as the child becoming incontinent at school while playing or delaying urination is not considered a mental health issue. The child must be at least 5 years of age or have control over urination (in other words, already have been toilet trained). The symptoms may occur only during the day (called diurnal enuresis) or night, or both. Most children with enuresis tend to feel ashamed and embarrassed to the point of social isolation, and they avoid any activities, such as sleepovers or going away to camp, that would predispose them to the embarrassment.

Most children tend to outgrow enuresis. A thorough medical exam is first done to rule out any physical cause. Once it is determined that the disorder is from a psychological standpoint, various behavioral approaches can be utilized. These methods gradually train the brain to respond to elimination signals during sleep or at controllable intervals.

> **Just the Facts**
>
> Physiologic factors for incontinence include psychosocial stress (such as being on stage during a school play), physical urinary tract abnormalities, medication side effects, increased fluid intake, or a urinary tract infection.

Pica

Pica is the repetitive eating (ingestion) of nonfood substances that lasts more than 1 month. It is considered a mental health issue when it occurs after 3 years of age (when normal oral sensory learning stops) and occurs outside of a cultural norm. Pica can also occur during pregnancy and the postpartum period and usually self-resolves.

Some people refer to it as "dirt-eating" since dirt is a common substance ingested in pica. Other common substances include clay, starch, ice, and crayons. Children may imitate a pet by eating the pet's food. Most children outgrow pica. The incidence is higher in individuals with intellectual and/or developmental disability. Pica can be a side effect of some medications such as risperidone, olanzapine, and tramadol (Leung & Hon, 2019). Children with pica have a higher incidence of anemia than in peers of their same age. Individuals with pica are at an increased risk for ingesting a harmful substance such as lead-based paint chips.

> **Test Yourself**
>
> ✔ Describe the difference between an 18-month old with nocturnal enuresis as compared to an 8-year old with the same condition.
> ✔ What is the major issue that a child with nocturnal enuresis faces?
> ✔ Describe pica.

Nursing Process and Care Plan *for the Child or Adolescent With a Neurodevelopmental Mental Health Issue*

The developmental level of the child or adolescent must be taken into account when working with a child or adolescent with a neurodevelopmental metal health issue. If the nurse only considers the chronologic age of the child, safety issues might be overlooked, and nursing interventions may be inappropriate. The family, including any caregivers, should be included in the plan of care in addition to the child or adolescent.

General nursing approaches for any mental health nursing care focus include: Establish a trusting relationship, do not immediately provide the child with tactile stimuli such as touch or hugs as these may be offensive or overstimulating, plan activities that provide a chance for the child to succeed, provide a distraction-free environment for task-oriented activity, maintain a safe, physical environment, and identify any suicide risk, ideation, or actions.

Assessment (Data Collection)

The child or adolescent with a mental health issue is referred for evaluation by family caregivers, teachers, other health care professionals, or the judicial system. Family caregivers are often concerned and frustrated with the child's actions and inability to adapt to daily living. To assess all factors that may contribute to the child's behavior, data is collected regarding the child, family, and related environmental factors. The data assists the health care team to determine, if there are any relevant issues. It is important that family members be included in both identifying areas of concern and contributing to the treatment plan.

Family caregivers, teachers, and other social contacts of the child are the usual sources of information regarding the child's behavior of concern. A history should include the time at which the problematic behaviors began and any other significant information such as treatment of pets, disruptions at school, and also the discipline style and pattern used by family caregivers. A thorough physical and emotional assessment is completed by the health care provider. The child's ability to communicate and interact with others is observed using play activities. Thorough data collection is done for the child's feelings, self-image, distorted thinking, or other subjective symptoms such as abuse, depression, or suicidal ideation. It is not unusual for the child to reveal problems related to familial relationships, such as abuse, that are not divulged or known by others within the family circle. In addition, it is important to observe communication and interaction patterns between all family members and to collect data on the degree to which the child's behavior and actions are disrupting the family functioning or other social settings in which the child participates.

Nursing Care Focus

Selecting an appropriate nursing focus of care can be difficult because the child is in a period of constant growth and development with behavior that is influenced by both genetics and environmental factors. Because many of these disorders may overlap and coexist in the same child, the data collection may identify multiple problem areas. Common nursing diagnoses that can be applied to children and adolescents with neurodevelopmental mental health issues include: Acute Anxiety, Activities of Daily Living Deficit, Caregiver Fatigue, Communication Impairment, Coping Impairment, Depression, Fear Injury Risk, Knowledge Deficiency, Psychosocial needs, Safety, Self-Harm Risk, Situational Low Self-Esteem, and Sleep deprivation.

Outcome Identification and Planning

Once an appropriate focus of nursing care has been selected, planning includes determining anticipated outcomes. These outcomes should be structured so that the child or adolescent can see successes, even small ones. Realistic time frames will depend on the individual's capabilities and level of cognition. Box 18.13 lists common desired outcomes for a child or adolescent with a neurodevelopmental mental health disorder.

Nursing Care Focus

- Injury Risk

Goal

- The client will be free from injury.

Implementations for Preventing Injury

When planning nursing interventions for preventing injury in a child or adolescent, it is most

Common Desired Outcomes for a Child or Adolescent With a Neurodevelopmental Mental Health Disorder

The client:

- Remains free of self-harm and does not harm others
- Establishes effective alternative communication
- Chooses and initiates appropriate social interactions with peers
- Demonstrates consistent progress in development toward maximum potential
- Demonstrates increased autonomy and reliance on self
- Remains free from injury
- Exhibits ability to control impulsivity
- Expresses positive feelings about self
- Tolerates overnight separation periods from attachment figure
- Verbalizes decreased anxiety during separation from parent or caregiver
- Exhibits decreased reports of somatic symptoms
- Identifies possible coping strategies for different situations
- Applies improved alternative coping strategies

Expected outcomes for family caregivers may include the following:

- Identify strengths and weaknesses of the child
- Participate in planning and implementation of behavior improvement program
- Establish and maintain consistency in boundaries for acceptable behavior
- Describe appropriate ways to express feelings of frustration regarding child's inappropriate behaviors
- Develop appropriate ways to cope with feelings toward the child's inappropriate behaviors

important to consider the developmental level of the individual. A child who uses a wheelchair has different needs than the child who bolts out of any open door and tends to wander. Provide supervision as appropriate for the client. Some individuals may need assistance with eating while others need assistance with mobility. Anticipatory guidance is necessary for the individual with intellectual and/or developmental disability. Keep sharp or hazardous items out of reach or in a locked area. Be alert for potential hazards that are left unsecured such as cleaning supplies, or caps from syringes that could be ingested. Even though the nurse may not see these items as something to eat, they may be tested orally by an individual with an intellectual and/or developmental disability.

Use headgear such as a helmet or hand coverings to prevent self-inflicted injury during behaviors such as head banging, scratching, or hair pulling. Intervene to prevent injury from aggression or acting-out behaviors. Determine precipitating factors that lead to agitated and self-injurious behavior. Provide adequate supervision and limits for the child's activity.

Evaluation of Goal/Desired Outcome

The client will:

- not ingest nonfood substances.
- not sustain an injury during mobility or transfers.
- not wander off unit.
- not injure self during self-stimulating behaviors.

Nursing Care Focus

- Communication Impairment

Goal

- The client's needs will be made known to the nursing staff.

Implementations for Improving Communication

The child or adolescent with a communication impairment is at risk for their wants and needs being unmet. The parent or caregiver who interacts with the client on a daily basis is the best source for assisting with communication techniques. However, communicate to the child or adolescent directly—not only to the parent or caregiver. Call the client by name. Avoid using generic endearing terms such as "Honey," "Sweetie," or calling them a "big boy" or "big girl." Make eye contact, as appropriate, with the client and avoid staring at them. Direct your questions to the client, not the family. Even if the client is unable to respond, they deserve to be talked to—not talked over, or ignored. The nurse should not assume the client desires to be touched. Take cues from their nonverbal behavior, if they are comfortable with a handshake, "fist-bump," or "high-five."

Make a poster or write on a white board, if the client has a specific word, gesture, or sound for a need, food, toy, or television show. When communicating with a client who has limited communication, be alert to nonverbal responses. Some of these may be subtle. Allow the client time to respond. Talk to the client as you would to all other clients. Avoid unnecessary chatter. Do not use baby talk.

Remember that intelligence is not based upon the client's ability to verbally communicate.

Observe for signs of overstimulation. Decrease stimuli in the client's room as appropriate.

Evaluation of Goal/Desired Outcome

• The client's needs are expressed.

Cultural Considerations

More Than Just Dirt

Pica is seen world-wide. The substance consumed tends to vary in different cultures, but the most common substance is dirt, soil, or clay, the consumption of which is termed geophagia. Starch eating during pregnancy seems to help with morning sickness. In some parts of Africa, eating clay is thought to increase sexual power. In North India, some people believe that the pregnant person's pica cravings are related to the sex of the unborn child. In the South of the United States, kaolin (aluminum silicate hydroxide), a chalky white substance, is available to purchase. This substance helps with diarrhea and was the original source for some antidiarrheal medications. Pica is also part of some religious ceremonies. For example, the soil from El Santuario de Chimayo in New Mexico is said to have healing properties and pilgrims will mix some of the soil with water to drink or make a mud to apply to skin.

Reference: Bhatia, S., & Kaur, J. (2014). Pica as a culture bound syndrome. *Delhi Psychiatry Journal, 17*(1), 144–147. https://static1.squarespace.com/static/575f16758259b52cea318166/t/5b61fe68575d1fdc0a3987c5/1533148812826/Pica+article.pdf

---

SUMMARY

• The most prevalent factor that may contribute to the incidence of a mental health issue in the child or adolescent is a familial history of mental health issues.

• Delays or deficits seen in intellectual and/or developmental disability may exist in various developmental areas including neurodevelopmental and intellectual level, interactive and communicative skills, and coordination or activity. Impairment may range from mild to profound, and may interfere with the child's ability to adjust and interact with the world around them. The level of severity is not based upon IQ.

• Children and adolescents with autism spectrum disorder have challenges with social skills and may not appear interested in their environment in the same way that their peers are. The rate of their mental or social development is often different from others in their age group or education level.

• Inattention, hyperactivity, and impulsive actions are the key behaviors seen in children with attention deficit hyperactivity disorder (ADHD). This disorder does not affect intelligence and is more often diagnosed in boys. The symptoms must be present for a period of 6 months or longer for a diagnosis to be made and can be successfully managed using a combination of medication and behavior therapy.

• Learning disorders and language impairment interfere with the individual's performance both socially and academically. The frustration experienced often leads to decreased motivation and premature exit from the school system.

• Because both social and academic advancement require basic skills in reading, mathematics, writing, and communicative language, it is difficult for children and adolescents with learning and communication disorders to adjust and function as they grow older.

• Early intervention and treatment can help the child with a learning or communication disorder to adapt to and accommodate the symptoms of the disorder.

• A difficult situation for family caregivers is caring for the child or adolescent with a disruptive, impulse-control, or conduct disorder. Because of the disruptive and destructive nature of the behaviors, these children often become entangled with law enforcement officials early in their lives. The child is unable to understand or control the erratic episodes of behavior, which leads to frustration and ambivalent feelings in family members, teachers, and others who come in contact with the child.

• Family maladjustment and poor caregiver–child interaction are common among children and adolescents with disruptive, impulse-control, or conduct disorders. If the individual's conduct is aggressive or hostile in nature, the likelihood increases that the behavior will lead to arrest and disciplinary action by the judicial system. There is often a familial pattern of psychiatric problems in children and adolescents who are diagnosed with conduct or defiant disorders of this level.

- Other mental health issues in children are often the result of stress-related symptoms that manifest themselves in the form of anxiety, repetitive tic movements, or inappropriate elimination.
- Children and adolescents with mental health issues may also have concurrent issues related to stigma, self-esteem, and poor school performance.
- Therapeutic interventions include developing a trusting relationship and helping the child to understand the relationship between the psychological symptoms and the condition.

- Many of the mental health issues seen in children and adolescents continue to manifest symptoms into the adult years. Some are not diagnosed until adulthood but may have been present since childhood, while others are not symptomatic until adolescence and beyond.
- Early intervention is necessary to assist both the child and family to develop skills that promote functioning to the highest level possible.

BIBLIOGRAPHY

Al Nasser, Y., Muco, E., & Alsaad, A. J. (2022). Pica. In: *StatPearls [Internet]*. StatPearls. https://www.ncbi.nlm.nih.gov/books/NBK532242/

American Association on Intellectual and Developmental Disabilities. (2022). *Defining criteria for intellectual disability*. https://www.aaidd.org/intellectual-disability/definition#.WdsHNIWcEt0

Augustyn, M., & von Hahn, L. E. (2021). Autism spectrum disorder: Clinical features. *UpToDate*. Retrieved August 10, 2022, from https://www.uptodate.com/contents/autism-spectrum-disorder-clinical-features

Bennett, S., & Walkup, J. T. (2022). Anxiety disorders in children and adolescents: Assessment and diagnosis. *UpToDate*. Retrieved August 11, 2022, from https://www.uptodate.com/contents/anxiety-disorders-in-children-and-adolescents-assessment-and-diagnosis

Bhatia, M. S., & Kaur, J. (2014). Pica as a culture bound syndrome. *Delhi Psychiatry Journal*, *17*(1), 144–147. https://static1.squarespace.com/static/575f1675-8259b52cea318166/t/5b61fe68575d1fdc0a3987c5/1533148812826/Pica+article.pdf

Centers for Disease Control and Prevention. (2022). *Attention-Deficit/Hyperactivity Disorder (ADHD): Data & statistics about ADHD*. National Center on Birth Defects and Developmental Disabilities. https://www.cdc.gov/ncbddd/adhd/data.html

Centers for Disease Control and Prevention. (2022). *Autism Spectrum Disorder (ASD)*. National Center on Birth Defects and Developmental Disabilities. https://www.cdc.gov/ncbddd/autism/index.html

Centers for Disease Control and Prevention. (2022c). *Children's mental disorders*. https://www.cdc.gov/childrensmentalhealth/symptoms.html

Krull, K. R. (2022). Attention deficit hyperactivity disorder in children and adolescents: Overview of treatment and prognosis. *UpToDate*. Retrieved August 10, 2022, from https://www.uptodate.com/contents/attention-deficit-hyperactivity-disorder-in-children-and-adolescents-overview-of-treatment-and-prognosis

Leung, A. K. C., & Hon, K. L. (2019). Pica: A common condition that is commonly missed–An update review. *Current Pediatric Reviews*, *15*(3), 164–169. https://doi.org/10.2174/1573396315666190313163530

Maenner, M. J., Shaw, K. A., Bakian, A. V., Bilder, D. A., Durkin, M. S., Esler, A., Furnier, S. M., Hallas, L., Hall-Lande, J., Hudson, A., Hughes, M. M., Patrick, M., Pierce, K., Poynter, J. N., Salinas, A., Shenouda, J., Vehorn, A., Warren, Z ... Cogswell, M. E. (2021). Prevalence and characteristics of autism spectrum disorder among children aged 8 years—Autism and Developmental Disabilities Monitoring Network, 11 sites, United States, 2018. *Morbidity and Mortality Weekly Report, Surveillance Summaries*, *70*(11), 1–16. https://www.cdc.gov/mmwr/volumes/70/ss/ss7011a1.htm

Pivalizza, P. (2022). Intellectual disability (ID) in children: Clinical features, evaluation, and diagnosis. *UpToDate*. Retrieved August 10, 2022, from https://www.uptodate.com/contents/intellectual-disability-id-in-children-clinical-features-evaluation-and-diagnosis

Weissman, L. (2019). Autism spectrum disorder in children and adolescents: Overview of management. *UpToDate*. Retrieved August 10, 2022, from https://www.uptodate.com/contents/autism-spectrum-disorder-in-children-and-adolescents-overview-of-management

Fill in the Blank

Fill in the blank with the correct answer.

1. _____ is the most common underlying contributor to the probability of a mental health issue in children.
2. _____ is the most common type of learning disorder.
3. Levels of severity in intellectual and/or developmental disability are not based upon _____ but by evaluating the individual's ability to perform day-to-day life skills and activities.
4. Speech that is characterized by repetitive or prolonged sounds or syllables that include pauses and monosyllable broken words is _____.
5. The filtering of sensory input to allow a select few to pass through into conscious awareness is termed _____.
6. Eye blinking, jerking of the neck or shoulder, or grimacing are examples of simple _____.

Matching

Match the following terms to the most appropriate phrase.

1. _____ Attention deficit hyperactivity disorder (ADHD)
2. _____ Enuresis
3. _____ Conduct disorder
4. _____ Intellectual and/or developmental disability
5. _____ Oppositional defiant disorder
6. _____ Autism spectrum disorder

a. Repetitive and continuous behavior that infringes on the rights of others or defies rules of society appropriate for age level
b. Deficits in general mental abilities, problem solving, and learning from experience
c. Repeated episodes of urine incontinence
d. Persistent patterns of inattention, hyperactivity, or impulsive behaviors, more frequent than those seen in the average child
e. Repetitive pattern of negative, defiant, disobedient, and hostile behavior toward authority figures
f. Differences in the development of various basic skills, including communication and socializing with others

Multiple Choice

Select the best answer from the multiple-choice items.

1. Which of the following are seen in treatment plans for a child with attention deficit hyperactivity disorder (ADHD)? *(Select all that apply)*
   a. Stimulant medications
   b. Nonstimulant medications
   c. Antibiotic medications
   d. Behavioral therapy
   e. Electroconvulsive therapy

2. A 7-year-old child is having difficulty with reading and writing assignments in school. The teacher has suggested testing for which disorder?
   a. Stuttering
   b. Dyslexia
   c. Attention deficit hyperactivity
   d. Tic

3. A 6-year-old whose parents divorced 6 months ago begins to cry and vomits each time their parent brings them to school. The parent is asked to take them home each day. Which disorder is this behavior seen in?
   a. Conduct
   b. Separation anxiety
   c. Oppositional defiant
   d. Pervasive developmental

4. A 14-year-old has been admitted to the adolescent behavioral health unit. Behaviors the adolescent has done in the past 2 years include being truant from school four times in the past month, setting fire to the grandmother's garage, assaulting a parent when asked to clean their room, and suspension from school for writing graphic language on the school sidewalk with spray paint. Which of the following nursing interventions should receive priority?
   a. Supervise the client during all interactions with other clients.
   b. Ask the client how they feel about being admitted.
   c. Have the client journal their feelings about their parent.
   d. Set up a contract regarding expected behavior.

5. A 16-year-old has been admitted to the psychiatric unit with severe depression and placed on suicide precautions. Which of the following signs might be suggestive of suicidal behavior?
   a. Chooses to limit their visitor list to four people
   b. Asks the nurse for shampoo when taking a shower
   c. Sleeps during the day in between therapy sessions
   d. Gives their favorite novel to their best friend

6. The child with a language and communication disorder would most likely have a problem with which task?
   a. Following rules for a game
   b. Being touched or held by another person
   c. Staying overnight with a relative
   d. Compromising during an argument

7. A 5-year-old has difficulty articulating syllables in a way that their speech can be understood. They often have repetitive or prolonged sounds separated by pauses that make them anxious and upset. Which of the following describes the speech problem?
   a. Syntax
   b. Copropraxia
   c. Stuttering
   d. Echopraxia

8. A 7-year-old who exhibits characteristic signs of severe intellectual and/or developmental disability. Which of the following would be a realistic outcome for the child?
   a. Institutional care to provide adequate supervision
   b. Independent living with ability to provide own income
   c. Simple job with supervised independent living
   d. Self-care needs of feeding and toileting

9. A 7-year-old is being evaluated for a learning disorder. The nurse collects the following data. Which factor most likely indicates a contributing factor to the child's performance?
   a. Turns up the TV to volume that is uncomfortable for others
   b. Likes to play on swings and gym equipment at school
   c. Tends to pick on younger siblings
   d. Is afraid of the neighbor's dog

10. A 15-year-old is verbally aggressive toward the principal of their school after being reprimanded for breaking a school rule stating loudly, "You don't own me. Nobody owns me. I don't have to follow your silly rules." This type of behavior is characteristic in which disorder?
    a. Intellectual and/or developmental disability
    b. Oppositional defiant disorder
    c. Separation anxiety disorder
    d. Tic disorder

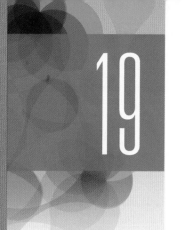

19

Disorders and Issues of the Older Adult

LEARNING OBJECTIVES

After learning the content in this chapter, the student will be able to:

1. Describe characteristics of older adults.
2. Describe psychosocial issues relating to the mental health of the older adult.
3. Differentiate between delirium and dementia.
4. Describe the signs and symptoms seen in the three types of dementia.
5. Describe the different stages seen in Alzheimer disease.
6. Discuss treatment for the client with dementia.
7. Describe causative factors and symptoms of depression in the client with dementia.
8. Describe the nursing process for clients with delirium and dementia.

KEY TERMS

ageism	confabulation
aging	delirium
agnosia	dementia
Alzheimer disease	disorientation
anomia	Lewy bodies
aphasia	primary aging
apraxia	secondary aging
catastrophic reaction	sundowning syndrome

Mental Health Care for Older Adults

Aging is defined as the changes that occur in a continuous and progressive manner during the adult years. The older adult population typically exhibits physical symptoms of aging such as graying of hair, a decrease in subcutaneous supportive tissue resulting in wrinkling of the skin, and presbyopia (decline in the ability to focus on close-up objects). It is important to recognize the flexible nature of health and functioning among those older than 65 years. There are effects of **primary aging**, or those changes that occur as a result of genetics or natural factors, and those of **secondary aging**, which are influenced by the environment. A pattern of coping with environmental stressors is often established as a result of social learning early in life. Successful adaptation to the process of aging is encouraged by the ability to give meaning and perspective to life experiences. This is reflected in findings that most older adults, despite coexisting chronic medical conditions (Box 19.1), rate their physical or mental health as good or excellent. Although the changes that accompany aging are inevitable, it is recognized that older adults who can adapt to these changes with relative acceptance experience the highest level of satisfaction with their lives. It is important for the nurse to know, and communicate to their clients, that depression *is not* a normal or expected part of the aging process.

Mind Jogger ② In what way do childhood experiences influence how an individual adapts to the aging process?

BOX 19.1

Chronic Medical Conditions Most Common in People 65 Years and Older

- Arthritis
- Visual disturbances
- Hypertension
- Peripheral vascular disease
- Congestive heart failure
- Urinary dysfunction
- Parkinson disease
- Hearing loss
- Stroke
- Chronic obstructive pulmonary disease (COPD)
- Thyroid disease
- Diabetes mellitus

BOX 19.2

Potential Changes That Older Adults Face

- Health
- Employment
- Spouse or loved ones (health issues or death)
- Income
- Status
- Friends (dying or moving away)
- Cognitive decline
- Home
- Independence
- Roles
- Purpose

Issues Faced by Older Adults

Older adults face changes in employment, finances, and family structure. They also may have concerns related to chronic disease, potential memory impairment, deaths of close friends or relatives, and changes in independence (Box 19.2). The potential for these concerns to become actual issues typically increases with age. Social and behavioral aspects of life and the concerns related to growing older can have a great influence on an individual's mental status and the prevalence of mental health issues in later life.

Psychosocial Issues Related to Aging

Ageism is a prejudice based on age (in this chapter, referring to older age), driven by the common misconception that deterioration, senility, and mental health issues are a part of the normal aging process. Ageism stereotypes and minimizes the worth of the older adult by assuming they are incompetent and somehow an inferior population of society. Unfortunately, many older adults also believe that with growing older they have to accept for themselves these mental health issues as well as physical and mental decline. Many symptoms are unreported by those who may see these changes as a sign of weakness, loss of control, or inevitable. There is also added fear of institutionalization, which is being "placed in a nursing home." The individual may have been raised in a manner or a culture where discussion of feelings or emotions was not typical or was looked down on. This can prevent recognition of the problem. The cost of mental health care may also be a prohibitive factor due to limited or restricted finances. Limited income and existing medical and pharmacologic health care costs may also decrease the likelihood that mental health issues will be addressed.

Care of the older adult with mental health issues has received some federal government attention with legislative regulation of both psychiatric treatment facilities and nursing homes. Mental health disorders are often seen among the residents of long-term care facilities. Specialized units and programs to address the needs of these residents in long-term care facilities have seen tremendous growth, related to an increased focus on escalating inpatient hospital costs. Cost containment by private and national funding sources as well as national legislation have brought about the emergence of supportive community care.

> **Test Yourself**
> ✔ What is the difference between primary and secondary aging?
> ✔ Name five chronic medical conditions that may be present in an older adult.
> ✔ Name five changes the older adult may experience.
> ✔ Define ageism.

Cognitive Functioning

The subtle memory changes attributed to the normal aging process are seldom evident in the day-to-day functioning of the older adult. Minor memory lapses such as misplacing an item, forgetting someone's name, or forgetting an appointment are considered typical as one ages. Changes may become more evident when there is an increase in anxiety produced by the need to perform under pressure. There is much variance among older adults and most continue to function at a very high level. Some individuals compensate with written reminders and lists. The greatest mental changes with aging are seen in the areas of learning and retaining information. Some older adults experience a change in their ability to do abstract reasoning and complex problem-solving.

In contrast, cognitive impairment is a more defined problem centered on memory loss. There may be a significant loss in the ability to remember the content of what is read or descriptive details of what is seen or heard. Important events may be repeatedly forgotten. This degree of impairment is quite different from that seen in normal aging. Memory is the basis for thinking processes. The loss of memory leaves the individual unable to remember past experiences, which are used to make current decisions and judgments. They experience a state of confusion, unable to understand present experiences.

The term *cognitive disorders* has replaced the previously used terms of "organic brain disease." In cognitive disorders, there is a noticeable change in cognition as compared to a former level of functioning. Underlying these disorders is a cause for the altered cognitive state. Causes of cognitive disorders include medical conditions, infections, medications, depression, or imbalances such as metabolic or endocrine.

Delirium

Delirium is characterized by a disturbance of the consciousness and a change in cognition that develops over a short time, such as within hours to a few days. Delirium presents with a disturbance in the level of awareness and cognitive functioning but may have different etiologies. The most common underlying causes of delirium in older adults are listed in Table 19.1. Once the cause is determined and treated, the condition is usually reversed and improvement in the mental state is seen.

Signs and Symptoms

In delirium, the deterioration in the level of consciousness and cognitive functioning is evident in the individual's behavior and inability to carry out previously routine activities of daily living (ADLs). Delirium develops rapidly, with symptoms that may fluctuate depending on the time of day. There is a change in the level of consciousness with impaired thinking, concentration, attention, and awareness of the surrounding environment. Speech and motor coordination or activity rapidly change from the individual's baseline. Speech may become slurred or the individual may forget a word they had recently used without difficulty. The individual may become unstable and need assistance walking whereas they had no difficulty with balance or independent walking just days or hours prior to the onset of the delirium. The individual may experience hallucinations and delusional thought processes. Appetite and sleep are disturbed as the mental changes occur. Behavior

TABLE 19.1	Common Causes of Delirium in Older Adults	
	Causes	**Examples**
Medical conditions	Infection	Urinary tract infection (UTI)
		Sepsis
	Metabolic imbalance	Hypoglycemia
		Hyperthermia
	Endocrine imbalance	Hypothyroidism
	Fluid and electrolyte imbalance	Dehydration
		Hyponatremia
	Hepatic or kidney disease	High level of ammonia or uric acid
Medications	Prescriptions	Medication toxicity
		Polypharmacy with interactions
	Medications with anticholinergic activity	Benzodiazepines
		Third-generation cephalosporins
		Diuretics
		Digitalis
		Tramadol
		Corticosteroids
		Tricyclic antidepressants
	Narcotics	Morphine
		Codeine
		Narcotics in high doses
	Medications known to adversely affect older adults	Diphenhydramine HCl
		Metoclopramide HCl
Substances	Usage	Alcohol
		Sedatives, hypnotics, or anxiolytics
	Withdrawal	Abrupt discontinuation of any substance

can be categorized as either agitation or psychomotor stupor ("sluggishness"). Box 19.3 lists the common signs and symptoms of delirium.

BOX 19.3

Signs and Symptoms of Delirium

- Rapid onset (hours to days)
- Fluctuating course with more confusion in late afternoon/early evening
- Intermittent memory loss
- Changes in level of consciousness
- Decreased awareness of surroundings
- Inability to maintain attention or focus
- Impaired cognition (concentration, judgment, communication, perception)
- Changes in speech
- Increase or decrease in psychomotor activity
- Hallucinations (usually visual) and illusions
- Fleeting, poorly organized thoughts
- Involuntary tremors or movements
- Appetite and sleep disturbances

Just the Facts Perceptual disturbance may include hallucinations (e.g., seeing and talking to a dead parent), illusions (e.g., seeing intravenous tubing as a rope), or delusions (e.g., may see injection as a threat of harm).

Risk and Treatment

As noted previously, symptoms of delirium may be caused by different factors. Older adults are more at risk for delirium because of their higher incidence of chronic illness and their use of multiple medications to manage those disorders. The increased chance of hospitalization for acute infections, and exacerbations of chronic illnesses, such as congestive heart failure, adds to the risk. The combined use of both prescription and over-the-counter medications can contribute to the development of delirium. Significant risk factors for delirium are the body's decreased ability to metabolize and excrete medications as the body ages, dosages not being tailored to meet the metabolism needs of the older adult, and sensitivity to adverse medication reactions. In addition, other factors such as sensory deprivation, an altered sleep–wake cycle, and nutritional or fluid deficiencies can contribute to the onset of delirium.

Treatment for delirium is the correction of the causative factor. If the causative factor is a medication, the individual's cognitive functioning returns to baseline as the medication wears off. For acute infections, once antibiotics have been started, the delirium usually begins to resolve. Some individuals with delirium who have hyperactive delirium or are agitated and aggressive may be prescribed a medication to help with the temporary symptoms. Medications given to counteract these symptoms should not be used in an ongoing or routine basis.

Test Yourself
- ✔ Describe the onset of delirium.
- ✔ List three causes of delirium.
- ✔ Identify three prescribed medications that can cause delirium.
- ✔ How is delirium treated?

Dementia

Dementia is characterized by irreversible, progressive deterioration in cognitive functioning, including a loss of memory, awareness, judgment, and reasoning ability. This deterioration in

"Bertha"

Bertha is an 86-year-old resident of the assisted living center. She eats her meals in the dining room with other residents and likes to spend her time outdoors in the center's garden or visiting with others in the living area. When she does not come to the dining hall for breakfast the nurse checks in on Bertha. The nurse notes that Bertha's speech consists of irrational sentence fragments unrelated to any conversation directed to her. Bertha is crying and restless, going aimlessly from room to room in her apartment. Her temperature is 99°F (37.2°C) and she is shaking. The nurse notes a strong urine odor to Bertha's clothes. Bertha is unable to describe the location of any discomfort.

Digging Deeper

1. What might the changes in Bertha's behavior indicate?

2. How might her behavior be related to other symptoms?

3. What action should the nurse take?

CASE STUDY 19.1

Berna Namoglu/
Shutterstock

intellectual functioning is severe enough to interfere with an individual's normal daily activities and ability to communicate or interact with others. Although not a specific disease in itself, dementia is a set of symptoms caused by a number of different disorders that affect the brain. Primary dementia does not result from any other disease, while secondary dementia occurs as a result of another condition. Most familiar is the progressive type of dementia, in which cognitive ability gradually worsens over a period of time. Box 19.4 lists the characteristics of dementia.

There are several different types of progressive dementia, with Alzheimer disease being the most common. In addition, vascular disease and Lewy body disease fall into this category and will be discussed. Other conditions that may have symptoms similar to dementia are listed in Box 19.5.

Because memory impairment is common to both delirium and dementia, it is necessary to recognize that an individual with delirium can also have a pre-existing dementia. One way that may help distinguish between them is that, except in late dementia, most individuals with dementia alone are usually alert to the environment, whereas those with delirium also have a disturbance in consciousness. This means that the

---

BOX 19.4

Characteristics of Dementia

- Irreversible
- Progressive
- Loss of memory
- Loss of awareness
- Loss of judgment
- Loss of reasoning

BOX 19.5

Conditions With Symptoms Similar to Dementia

- Frontotemporal lobar degeneration
- HIV infection
- Untreated syphilis
- Substance/medication use
- Traumatic brain injury
- Huntington disease
- Creutzfeldt–Jakob disease
- Parkinson disease
- Multiple sclerosis
- Amyotrophic lateral sclerosis (ALS)
- Nutritional or vitamin deficiencies
- Chronic alcohol use disorder
- Infections
- Brain tumors
- Anoxia
- Chronic lung or heart disease
- Normal pressure hydrocephalus
- Depression
- Thyroid imbalance

individual who is alert but disoriented and confused because of dementia may develop a deteriorating level of consciousness as a result of an acute state of delirium.

Dementia Due to Alzheimer Disease

Alois Alzheimer, a German physician, first identified what became known as Alzheimer disease in the early 20th century. A female client in her 50s was described as having the signs of what appeared to be a mental illness. Following her death, an autopsy revealed this woman had dense deposits, or neuritic plaques, outside and around the nerve cells in her brain. Inside the cells were twisted strands of fiber, or neurofibrillary tangles. Today, a definite diagnosis of Alzheimer disease is still only possible when an autopsy shows these classic signs of the disease.

Alzheimer disease primarily affects the cerebral cortex, which is involved in conscious thought and language, the production of acetylcholine (a neurotransmitter involved in memory and learning), and the hippocampus, essential to memory storage. In the areas of the brain affected by this disease, the neurons degenerate and lose their synaptic connections to other neurons. The positron emission tomography (PET) scan in Figure 19.1 shows the reduced brain activity in the brain of a person with Alzheimer disease versus a brain without.

Signs and Symptoms

As the neurons of the hippocampus degenerate, short-term memory fails. The ability to perform routine tasks begins to diminish. Once the disease progresses to the cerebral cortex, the individual loses language skills and judgment is impaired. This leads to impulsive emotional outbursts and behaviors such as the wandering and agitation that are commonly seen in Alzheimer dementia. As the disease progresses, remote memory loss leaves the individual with the inability to recognize even close family members or to communicate in any meaningful way. In addition, there is a progressive, irreversible loss of memory that affects temporal and spatial orientation, abstract thinking, ability to carry out mathematical calculations, and capacity to learn new things or concepts. Personality changes lead to a diminished and lost sense of self as memory fades and with it the mental pictures that give meaning to one's life. Memories erode into small pieces that gradually disappear and are lost beyond recall.

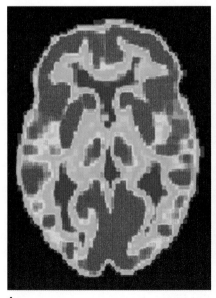
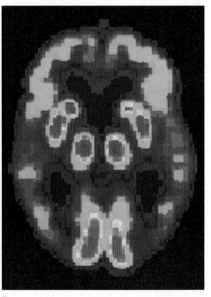

A   **B**

Figure 19.1 A. PET scan of brain of a healthy person. **B.** PET scan of a brain of a person with Alzheimer disease. The blue areas indicate reduced brain activity. (Images courtesy of the Alzheimer's Disease Education and Referral Center, a service of the National Institute on Aging.)

Initially, the individual may write down what they want to remember, and then forget to check the written reminder. There is difficulty encoding material to be recalled or an inability to make a connection between the meaning of the spoken word and words to be remembered. Early in the course of the disease, individuals are usually aware of their memory deficit and try to compensate for their losses by using **confabulation**, filling in the gaps with fictitious statements. As memory deficits increase, the individual may become frightened and anxious and get discouraged. As the disease progresses, they lose insight into their memory loss and are no longer aware of it.

Additionally, there is an inability to acquire and process new information—for example, a new house or address may not be recognized and they show up at a previous address. Language difficulties become more marked as the disease progresses and are listed in Box 19.6.

The problems related to language include the following:

- **Anomia**—inability to find the right word. For example, when shown a watch, the person may refer to it as a "timepiece," or referring to someone who has died, may say that the person is at the "resting place" or "sleeping place" instead of the cemetery.
- **Agnosia**—inability to identify an object. For example, the person may try to eat soup with a knife, eat the paper wrapper on a piece of candy, or attempt to shave with a toothbrush and toothpaste. This can also be sensory, such as the inability to identify hot temperature (e.g., they may not realize their bath water is too hot and may burn themselves) or recognize the meaning of traffic lights. Agnosia can also be seen when the individual does not recognize themselves in the mirror but instead thinks there is an intruder in the room.
- **Aphasia**—impairment in the significance or meaning of language that prevents the individual from understanding what is heard, following instructions, and communicating needs, for example, the need to use the toilet or to communicate pain.

As Alzheimer dementia continues to progress, visual and spatial skills deteriorate, and the individual may get lost while driving a car or walking. They develop **apraxia**, or an inability to carry out purposeful movements and actions despite intact motor and sensory functioning. The individual may try to water plants with a hose but is unable to connect the hose to the water faucet or is unable to transfer food from plate to mouth with silverware when trying to eat. The ability to use correct judgment or to make logical decisions is lost. Usually, the first noticeable sign of this is a difficulty in managing finances and is often the symptom that leads families to seek medical attention. They may pay bills twice or not pay bills, buy unnecessary items, make large charitable donations, or be unable to balance a bank account.

Amnesia, the loss of memories, is the symptom most people associate with dementia. The amnesia first starts with forgetting recent events, such as what they ate for the previous meal or the month or year, while still being able to recall long-term memories such as their wedding or songs from their youth. Then the amnesia progresses to the loss of long-term memories, often their children's names or what they did for an occupation. See Figure 19.2.

In addition, there is evidence of declining self-awareness, as they show a lack of attention to appearance and dress. Layering of clothing and an

BOX 19.6

Language Deterioration in Dementia Due to Alzheimer Disease

- Sentence fragments used instead of conversational speech
- Repeating words and questions (echolalia)
- Repeating one word (paralalia)
- Repeating one syllable (logoclonia)
- Unintelligible and repetitive babbling
- Mutism

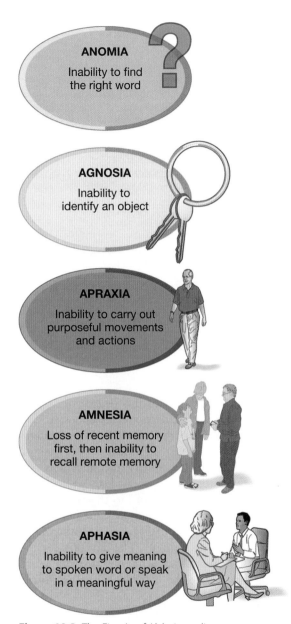

ANOMIA
Inability to find the right word

AGNOSIA
Inability to identify an object

APRAXIA
Inability to carry out purposeful movements and actions

AMNESIA
Loss of recent memory first, then inability to recall remote memory

APHASIA
Inability to give meaning to spoken word or speak in a meaningful way

Figure 19.2 The Five As of Alzheimer disease.

unkempt appearance in one who was previously neat and well-groomed is typical. Personality and mood changes are noticeable as well as a loss of interest and energy for doing previously enjoyed activities. Depression is common, with decreasing interaction and social withdrawal. As the disease progresses, catastrophic reactions may occur. **Catastrophic reactions** include agitation and verbal and/or physical responses of fear and panic (such as crying, shouting, or laughing uncontrollably or inappropriately) with a potential of harm to self and others. Catastrophic reactions are often precipitated by frustration and a perceived threat or

BOX 19.7

Interventions to Help Decrease Incidence of a Catastrophic Reaction

- Maintain a consistent schedule
- Avoid rushing the individual
- Remove stimuli including television and radio
- Remain calm and avoid arguing or yelling with the individual
- Do not blame or scold the individual for their behavior
- Cover mirrors to minimize the illusion that an intruder is in the room, because the client may no longer recognize self in a mirror

fear, often trivial in nature such as a change in routine or environment. Box 19.7 gives tips to decrease incidence of a catastrophic reaction.

Test Yourself
✔ Describe a situation that might cause a catastrophic reaction.

Behavior problems such as stubbornness, resistance to care, abusive language, acting out in response to hallucinations or delusions, or urinating in inappropriate places may occur. Older adults with Alzheimer dementia tend to hide their belongings and develop a suspicion of others, thinking misplaced things have been stolen when the items cannot be found. There may also be increased restlessness that leads to rummaging, wandering, aimless walking (pacing), and interruption of the sleep–wake cycle. This behavior puts the individual at risk for injury. Some exhibit a peak period of agitation and acting-out behavior during the evening hours, which is sometimes referred to as **sundowning syndrome**. Signs and symptoms of dementia due to Alzheimer disease are listed in Box 19.8.

Test Yourself
✔ Describe an example of confabulation.
✔ Describe three problems related to language seen in dementia.
✔ List 10 signs or symptoms seen in Alzheimer disease

In advanced dementia from Alzheimer disease, the individual may be totally unaware of their surroundings and require total and constant supervision

CASE STUDY 19.2

Ground Picture/
Shutterstock

"Annie"

Annie is a retired teacher who helps out with delivering sack lunches to homebound senior citizens in her town. One day Annie walks into the school where she taught for 30 years and hands the secretary a sack lunch and states, "I don't know where I need to go with this food." When the center is advised of the situation, the supervisor remembers that several people on Annie's route have reported that they have not been receiving their lunches. However, when she asks Annie about this, Annie states she must "have left them at another house by mistake." Realizing that there is a problem, the supervisor notifies Annie's daughter, Katy, of the situation. When Katy visits her mother's house, she finds piles of unopened mail and bills with notices of nonpayment. There are spoiled food items in the refrigerator and soiled laundry is piled in a corner of the bathroom. Katy realizes something is very wrong with her mother and brings her to the clinic for evaluation.

Digging Deeper

1. Katy feels that her mother can no longer continue to live independently and chooses to admit Annie to a nursing home. Annie does not understand why she has to be there, crying and saying she needs to go and "I have to feed the hungry people." What would be the best nursing approach to Annie at this time? How did Annie exhibit confabulation?

2. Annie begins to take food items from the plates of other clients, stating they have stolen "her food." She becomes physically aggressive if the food is taken away from her. What nursing approach would be most appropriate when Annie is removing the food? How can distraction and redirection be used when Annie becomes agitated?

BOX 19.8

Signs and Symptoms of Dementia Due to Alzheimer Disease

- Confabulation
- Short-term memory loss occurs first—then long-term memory loss occurs
- Decreasing ability to perform routine tasks
- Hiding objects with inability to relocate them
- Suspiciousness
- Restlessness, rummaging, wandering, and pacing
- Interruption of sleep–wake cycle
- Language deterioration (anomia, aphasia)
- Impaired judgment
- Inability to cognitively be independent in daily activities (money management, paying bills, taking medications)
- Impulsive emotional outbursts (catastrophic reactions)
- Inability to recognize family or friends
- Inability to recognize familiar objects (agnosia)
- Loss of spatial and temporal orientation
- Loss of abstract thinking and mathematical concepts
- Inability to learn anything new or encode incoming information
- Personality changes
- Inability to carry out purposeful movements (apraxia)
- Stubbornness
- Abusive language
- Hallucinations and delusions
- Eliminating in inappropriate places
- Sundowning syndrome

---

and care. Individuals with this degree of impairment are at risk for accidents and infectious diseases that often lead to death. The three most common causes of death for the individual with Alzheimer disease are pneumonia, urinary tract infections, and infected pressure injuries. Individuals with Alzheimer disease live an average of 4 to 10 years after the onset of the disease, although in some individuals, the duration from time of diagnosis to death may be as many as 20 years or more. The final phase of the disease may last from a few months to several years, during which time the individual becomes totally disabled. The clinical stages of Alzheimer disease are identified in Table 19.2.

Mind Jogger What environmental stimuli might cause behaviors to accelerate with evening hours?

Incidence and Etiology

There is a familiar pattern with some forms of Alzheimer disease. Some families exhibit an inherited pattern that suggests possible genetic transmission. There are studies that indicate that younger-onset cases (those diagnosed before the age of 65 years) are more likely to be familial than late-onset cases. The majority of individuals with dementia are over the age of 75 with women being

TABLE 19.2	Stages of Alzheimer Disease
Stage	**Characteristics**
Mild	Poor short-term memory
	Unable to acquire new information (may have difficulty balancing a bank account, preparing a complex meal, or remembering medication schedules)
	Mild anomia
	Personality changes
	Disorientation—may get lost
	Some decrease in judgment
Moderate	Significant memory loss
	Impaired judgment (difficulty with simple food preparation, housework or yard work, may require assistance with activities of daily living [ADLs])
	Increased cognitive loss
	Anxiety, suspiciousness
	Agitation, depression
	Problems with sleeping
	Wandering or pacing
	Difficulty recognizing family or friends
Severe	Severe cognitive impairment
	Physical unsteadiness and loss of mobility (requires considerable assistance with personal care and activities of daily living [ADLs]; often chair- or bed-bound and dependent on others for care)
	Total loss of speech
	Loss of appetite, weight loss
	Incontinence

affected more than men. Alzheimer disease is the most common form of dementia. It is estimated that as many as 6.5 million Americans are living with Alzheimer disease. Alzheimer disease is the seventh leading cause of death in the United States (Alzheimer's Association, 2022a).

Mind Jogger How will this increase in the incidence of Alzheimer dementia impact nursing as the over-65 segment of the population increases?

Dementia Due to Vascular Disorder

Dementia due to vascular disease is caused by the effects of one or more strokes (cerebrovascular accidents) or from the effects of hypertension. It is characterized by an abrupt onset and follows a step-like pattern of cerebrovascular disease and symptoms. The pattern of deficit is related to the portion of the brain that has been affected by the stroke. Some functions are affected while others may remain intact. Each step is accompanied by a decrease in cognitive functioning.

BOX 19.9

Signs and Symptoms of Dementia Due to Vascular Disease

- Series of strokes (cerebrovascular accidents [CVAs])
- History of hypertension or cerebrovascular disease
- Hemiplegia or weakness of extremities
- Gait disturbances
- Step-like cognitive decline
- Exaggerated reflexes
- Foot drop
- Aphasia
- Apraxia
- Agnosia
- Decreased thought processing

Signs and Symptoms

Slow thoughts and an inability to make decisions are usually some of the early symptoms seen in dementia related to vascular disease. Personality and insight tend to remain unchanged as compared to the person with Alzheimer dementia. Depression is common as the condition advances. Neurologic symptoms such as hemiplegia, abnormal reflexes, slow gait, and poor balance are seen. The parts of the brain as well as the number and size of the infarcts determine the symptoms seen. There may be cognitive deficits such as aphasia, apraxia, agnosia, and the inability to organize thought processes. Box 19.9 lists signs and symptoms of dementia due to vascular disease.

Just the Facts Vascular changes that start with a decreased blood supply to certain brain areas important in storing and retrieving information may cause memory loss very similar to Alzheimer disease.

Incidence and Etiology

The onset of vascular dementia may occur any time in the older adult but is less common after age 75. The initial onset is typically earlier than the onset of Alzheimer disease. The two types of dementia can coexist in the same person. Vascular dementia tends to be more common in men than in women. The incidence of this form of dementia is much lower than that of the Alzheimer type.

Dementia Due to Lewy Body Disease

Lewy body disease is a form of progressive dementia in which abnormal deposits of proteins develop in nerve cells in the cortex of the brain, and these deposits are called **Lewy bodies**. Since the protein deposits are in the cortex of the brain it causes cognitive symptoms related to planning, navigating, and memory. The proteins associated with this disorder are also associated with Parkinson disease. However, in Parkinson disease, the Lewy bodies are often found in the midbrain portion of the brainstem, which causes the symptoms of tremors and stiffness.

Signs and Symptoms

Initially the individual with dementia caused by Lewy body disease has sleep disturbances and visual hallucinations of colors, people or animals, paranoia, or delusional thinking. Mental alertness is intermittent with the individual seemingly lucid one day, and confused, lethargic, distracted, and semiresponsive to the environment the next. Apathy, agitation, and anxiety are other symptoms common to Lewy body dementia. Parkinson-like symptoms of slow, rigid movements and shuffling gait are also seen. Later symptoms seen in this form of dementia are similar to those of Alzheimer disease. Box 19.10 lists signs and symptoms of dementia due to Lewy body disease.

Incidence and Etiology

Lewy body dementia is usually seen in those over 65 years of age, and is more common in men than in women. Because of its similarity to Alzheimer disease and Parkinson disease, it is difficult for health care providers to give a definitive diagnosis. Findings suggest that Lewy body disease and Alzheimer disease usually occur together and only about 5% of cases of dementia are caused solely by Lewy body disease.

BOX 19.10

Signs and Symptoms of Dementia Due to Lewy Body Disease

- Sleep disturbances
- Recurring detailed visual hallucinations
- Fluctuating mental alertness and cognition
- Shuffling gait, stiff or rigid movements
- Depression
- Mild tremors
- Cognitive deficits interfere with independence in daily activities (e.g., paying bills, managing medications)
- Cognitive deficits that interfere independence in activities of daily living (ADLs)

Test Yourself
- ✔ Describe the three stages of Alzheimer disease.
- ✔ Describe the difference in dementia due to vascular disease and Lewy body disease.

Depression

Although not categorized as a cognitive disorder, depression is a mood disorder (see Chapter 10) that can occur in any age group. Depression often accompanies the early stages of dementia, particularly in Alzheimer disease. The individual still has the mental ability to understand that something is happening, that memory lapses are occurring, and that they are unable to do things that previously were easily accomplished. These disturbing changes may lead the individual to feelings of loss, decreased self-worth, hopelessness, and depression. These feelings can lead them to thoughts that life is not worth living. Depression can actually intensify the symptoms of dementia. It is important to recognize these feelings in the early stages of dementia when the individual still may have the ability to carry out a plan for suicide.

As many of the symptoms found in depression are also characteristic of dementia, it may easily go unrecognized. Changes in appetite, changes in sleep patterns, and loss of energy and initiative are common to both disorders. The individual may demonstrate other symptoms such as withdrawal from others, self-neglect, and feelings of failure, inadequacy, helplessness, and powerlessness. The diagnostic work-up for all dementia of the Alzheimer disease type includes testing for depression. Usually when asked questions, the depressed individual will answer with, "I don't know," indicating a lack of energy to formulate an answer, whereas the individual with dementia will attempt to answer, demonstrating the existing mental deficits.

Risk factors for the development of depression in the early stages of dementia include a previous depressive episode or a very achievement-oriented lifestyle. Difficult family situations or financial strain may also precipitate depressive symptoms such as sadness and emptiness, which may be reinforced by a coexisting dementia. If the existence of depression is determined, it is important that treatment be initiated, because this can lead to improvement in the individual's overall functioning.

In addition to the individual with dementia, it is common for family caregivers to experience signs of depression. The constant demands of the unpredictable behaviors in the individual with dementia take their toll on the caregiver. The burden increases as an attempt is made to balance this schedule with other family responsibilities. Communication with family and friends may become strained or minimal as the caregiver becomes increasingly protective and isolated. Programs such as support groups can allow the caregiver to express feelings that are shared by others in the group. These groups can also provide information and suggestions for dealing with the problem behaviors and the frustration or fear that may accompany them. Box 19.11 lists some websites that provide information on dementia.

Treatment of Neurocognitive Disorders in the Older Adult

Currently, there is no cure for dementia due to Alzheimer or Lewy body disease. Treatment is focused on symptoms. Management is aimed at controlling the cognitive and behavioral symptoms that result from the progressive decline in the dementias. In Lewy body disease, there is also treatment geared toward controlling the motor movements or Parkinson-like symptoms. Various therapies are combined with medications to reduce the effects of these mental diseases. Support groups may be of help to spouses and family members who take care of the victims of this disease (Box 19.11).

There are currently several medications available that can sometimes delay the progression of the disease and symptoms. These may differ depending on the type of dementia being treated. The cholinesterase inhibitors are useful in increasing the levels of neurotransmitters or chemical messengers to the portions of the brain affected by Alzheimer disease. They can improve mental alertness and cognition, along with reducing the behavioral problems. The cholinesterase inhibitors can delay worsening of symptoms for 6 to 12 months for some who take them. Another neurotransmitter, glutamate, is needed for memory and learning processes in the brain. Research shows that an excess of glutamate may lead to destruction of brain cells in the individual with Alzheimer disease. A medication, memantine, is a glutamate receptor antagonist that has demonstrated effectiveness in the later stages of the disease. Antipsychotic medications may be useful in decreasing verbal and physical aggressiveness in individuals with Alzheimer dementia, and may improve delusional thinking or hallucinations. Individuals with Lewy body dementia, however, often are very sensitive to these medications related to the Parkinson-like symptoms and may have an increase in the psychotic symptoms. Parkinson disease medications may be used to reduce the movement symptoms in the individual with Lewy body dementia. Medications used in the treatment of dementia are found in Table 19.3.

TABLE 19.3   Medications Used in Treatment of Dementia

Medication Classification	Medications	Common Side Effects	Comments
Cholinesterase inhibitors	Galantamine Donepezil Rivastigmine	Nausea, vomiting, anorexia, diarrhea, abdominal pain, headache, dizziness, rash, urinary frequency, insomnia, blurred vision, muscle cramps	Most effective when treatment begun in early stages. Tacrine is rarely prescribed today due to serious side effects and possible liver damage
(*N*-methyl-D-aspartate) NMDA receptor antagonist	Memantine	Fatigue, dizziness, headache, insomnia, constipation, nausea, vomiting, anorexia, diarrhea, muscle aches, coughing, rash, frequent urination	Treatment of moderate to severe Alzheimer disease
Antipsychotics	Risperidone Haloperidol	Orthostatic hypotension, sedation, drowsiness, headache, insomnia, agitation, anxiety, extrapyramidal symptoms, dry mouth, dyspepsia, nausea, vomiting, diarrhea, constipation, hyperglycemia, cough, photosensitivity, urinary retention, decreased libido	May be used to decrease verbal and physical aggressiveness

CASE STUDY 19.3

Dragana Gordic/ Shutterstock

"Frank"

Frank is a 67-year-old resident of a special dementia unit of a long-term care facility. His family admitted him following an incident in which he drove a neighbor's car to the interstate and proceeded to enter an exit access going the wrong direction. Several vehicles were forced into the median to avoid an accident. He was eventually stopped by police officers who informed his wife, Ruth that arrangements would have to be made for his safety.

Frank owns a construction business and told the police officers he was "going to work," although he had been unable to work for the past 3 years because of diagnosed early-onset Alzheimer dementia. Since admission to the nursing home facility, Frank paces the halls, pulling on hand rails, doorknobs, and window casings. He repeatedly runs his hands over all door hinges and latches, kicks the wall and doors, and moves furniture around in the rooms. Frank wears a sock on his left foot, but refuses to wear shoes. He becomes agitated and strikes out with a fisted hand if any attempt is made to put a sock or shoe on the right foot. Frank will only take a bath if Ruth is present. He becomes physically aggressive when nursing staff try to attend to his hygiene needs unless she is talking to him. The staff has placed pictures of Ruth on several doors in his room and in the shower room hoping to give him a feeling of security with her perceived presence. Ruth comes to the facility several times each day to help with her husband's care.

Digging Deeper

1. What may be the precipitating factor in Frank's aggressive behavior?

2. What methods can the nurse use to address the behavior?

3. What purpose do the pictures serve for Frank?

4. It is noted that Frank is limping with limited weight bearing on his right foot. An order is received for an x-ray that reveals a comminuted fracture of the third metatarsal. Calcification surrounding the fracture indicates the injury occurred several weeks ago, and it is decided to allow calcification to continue and not to intervene surgically at this point. How is this injury affecting Frank's behavior?

5. What approach can the nurse use to help Frank with the pain he does not understand?

6. What nursing approaches may be used to relieve some of the caregiver strain for Ruth?

The most effective treatment in the older adult with depression is a combination of antidepressant medication and various psychotherapeutic approaches. Nursing observations related to antidepressant therapy should take into consideration the age-related physiologic changes that slow the body's response and the elimination of medications in older adults. It is also important to monitor for the many side effects caused by these medications and to report and document any adverse effects. Older adults may experience negative effects that may worsen other existing conditions.

Test Yourself

✔ Describe how depression can impact dementia.
✔ Name five medications used in the treatment of dementia and the expected effect for each one.

Nursing Process and Care Plan *for the Client With Delirium*

The client with delirium is often already in the hospital or is taken to the hospital for stabilization. While some symptoms, nursing care focuses, and nursing interventions overlap between delirium and dementia, the nursing care plan needs to be tailored to the individual's situation. The client with delirium is most likely agitated or frightened. It is important for the nurse to remain calm and reorient the client frequently. Most individuals with delirium will have a full recovery. Many older adults develop delirium during a hospital stay because of existing medical conditions that increase their risk of complications. There is an increase in the morbidity rate associated with this risk.

Assessment (Data Collection)

It is crucial to determine the cause of the mental decline and any disorientation. Disorientation is the inability to be knowledgeable of time (such as time of day, month or year), place or location, and person. Disorientation in older adults can be caused by sensory loss such as hearing loss, an unfamiliar environment such as the hospital, a coexisting mental disorder such as dementia, or an underlying physical or medical condition. When sensory factors are noted to be an issue, a simple adjustment of lighting or checking the battery in a hearing aid may be all that is needed to resolve the problem. In the case of physical causes, prompt detection and treatment is imperative to restoring mental function.

Data collection will include a complete history and physical examination. Nurses play a major role in collecting data. If the client is unable to provide information, it may be acquired from family members or others who may be aware of the client's health history and circumstances leading up to the current episode.

A detailed description of the client's behaviors that indicate a change from their normal baseline should be documented. Obtain a list of the client's current medications and dosages so that the possibility of medication toxicity or interactions can be determined and note if any changes were recently made. Over the counter, herbal remedies, and PRN (as needed) medications also need to be investigated. Treatment and nursing interventions will depend on the precipitating factors causing the delirium. Data collected should also be considered in comparison to the client's baseline physical condition and previous level of functioning. Monitor level of consciousness for further deterioration or improvement.

Nursing Care Focus

Although each situation of delirium may differ, commonalities exist in caring for the client with an acute change in mental state. When selecting the nursing care focus for the client with delirium it is important to determine if the client is agitated or stuporous. Nursing care focus for the client with delirium may include: Acute Anxiety, Acute Confusion, Electrolyte Imbalance, Fear, Injury Risk, Memory Impairment, Polypharmacy, Safety, Sleep Deprivation, or Violence Risk.

BOX 19.12

Outcomes for the Client With Delirium

Outcomes may include the following:
- Remains safe from harm or injury
- Accurately states time, place, person, situation
- Meets basic needs and independently performs activities of daily living (ADLs)
- Responds appropriately to incoming stimuli
- Identifies the fear and focuses on eliminating or reducing the source
- Is free of signs of sleep deprivation
- Regains or maintains ideal body weight for height and age
- Demonstrates understanding of current health problems

Outcome Identification and Planning

Realistic outcomes for a client with delirium will depend on the cause, the client's psychomotor state (agitation or stupor), and if the client also has dementia or not (Box 19.12).

Nursing Care Focus

- Acute Confusion

Goal

- The client will return to their baseline mental and cognitive status.

Implementations for Managing Confusion

Most clients with delirium will be cared for in the acute care setting. In providing nursing care for the client, the nurse must carry out all interventions to ensure that permanent brain damage or death is avoided. Because the course of delirium is short and critical, plans of care and goals are short term, and the focus of the medical and nursing teams should be directed toward correcting the underlying problem. Nursing interventions for managing confusion will be directed toward the acute phase of the illness.

Delirium is a frightening experience for the individual and those who witness it. Nursing care for the client with delirium includes ensuring the client's safety which may require constant observation. Reorient the client frequently to date, time, and place and restate who you are. Avoid lengthy explanations. Give short, direct directions. Let them know this is not a permanent experience.

To assist with reorienting the client, provide glasses or hearing aids to facilitate orientation and place family photographs or favorite objects within view. Explain all procedures and what is happening to the client. Initiate safety precautions.

Important nursing interventions involve decreasing environmental stimuli. Decrease lights but do not make them too dim; doing so could increase the risk of visual illusions. Decrease auditory stimulation (reduce noise) by keeping television or radios off. Closing the client's door to make the room quiet should only be done if someone is with them for observation. If possible, decrease volume on alarms and silence phones. Avoid restricting the client's movement unless there is a safety issue.

The client who is in a state of delirium may not recognize the need for toileting. Provide frequent opportunities for the client to visit the bathroom and remind them that they need to void. Along with not recognizing the urge to void or defecate, they may not recognize hunger or thirst cues. Provide assistance with eating as needed, and observe for swallowing and any potential choking. Offer water on a regular basis.

Evaluation of Goal/Desired Outcome

The client will:

- not experience further confusion.
- be oriented date, time, and place.

Nursing Care Focus

- Safety

Goal

- The client will remain safe and free from injury.

Implementations for Promoting Safety

Implementations for promoting safety are closely aligned with those for managing confusion. Reorient the client, provide enough light for the client to move about (to the toilet for example) without tripping, maintain the bed in lowest position or use a floor bed, provide constant observation of the client, and ensure the client has glasses or hearing aids as needed. Avoid having any tripping hazards on the floor. Use bed alarms as needed. Keep side rails to a minimum as appropriate and avoid restraining the client. Provide frequent opportunities for toileting needs. Provide nonskid socks as needed. Minimize IV lines and use wireless monitoring if needed.

Evaluation of Goal/Desired Outcome

- The client does not experience injury while in state of delirium.

CASE STUDY 19.4

"Patty"

Dusan Petkovic/Shutterstock

Patty is a 74-year-old woman who is a resident of the dementia unit of a nursing care facility. Prior to her retirement she worked as a hotel custodian. She is constantly pacing the hallway with a broom, sweeping the floor as she goes. Patty has lost 14 pounds in the 3 months since her admission to the nursing home. She is unable to sit at the table long enough to eat her meals and resumes her constant walking after eating only a few bites.

Digging Deeper

1. How would the nurse document Patty's behavior?

2. What nursing interventions could be used to assist Patty with eating?

3. What nursing interventions could be used to help with her constant motion?

4. What other health conditions could Patty be at risk for?

Nursing Process and Care Plan *for the Client With Dementia*

The nursing care plan for the client with dementia can change within days or weeks and for some clients it may remain unchanged for years. As the client may not be a reliable historian for data, the nurse must use their strong observation skills and obtain data from a variety of sources. Support of family caregivers should be included in the nursing care plan of the client with dementia.

Assessment (Data Collection)

Data collection for the client with dementia should include a past health and medication history. Asking the client questions or reviewing the current level of functioning with family members may help the nurse to obtain data concerning recent and remote memory loss. Other information to obtain is listed in Box 19.13.

Identify the primary caregiver, support systems, and the knowledge base of the family members. The role of caregiver to an individual with dementia is a difficult, stressful, and time-consuming task. A spouse or adult child most often assumes this role. It is important for the nurse to actively listen to the feelings and concerns of the family members. An individual with dementia is dependent on the caregiver and often will be reassured and calmed by their presence. However, caregivers often feel overwhelmed by the responsibility imposed by the disease as it progresses and may be increasingly isolated as the individual's cognition and physical health continue to decline. The nurse can assist the caregivers in locating support groups and respite care (programs to temporarily relieve the burden of primary caregiving) alternatives for the family.

Nursing Care Focus

The needs of the client with dementia are varied and change over time. Each individual must be viewed from the perspective of their own particular situation and the losses that are evident and continuous in their decline. Nursing care focus for the client with dementia may include: Acute Anxiety, Activities of Daily Living (ADLs) Deficit, Bowel Incontinence, Caregiver Fatigue, Chronic Confusion, Deconditioning, Dehydration, Depression, Fall Risk, Fear, Injury Risk, Malnutrition Risk, Safety, Suicide Attempt Risk, and Violence Risk.

Outcome Identification and Planning

Outcomes for the client with dementia are based upon their current level of functioning. As dementia progresses and the client's abilities deteriorate, outcomes will need to be revisited. Outcomes will depend on the individual problems identified (Box 19.14).

BOX 19.13

Data Collection for the Client With Dementia

- Disorientation
- Mood changes, feelings of hopelessness
- Fear and frustration level—develops as the individual is unable to give meaning to incoming sensory messages and leads to agitation and catastrophic reactions
- Inability to concentrate—leads to pacing behaviors
- Suspiciousness, agitation, or aggressive behaviors
- Self-care deficit
- Inappropriate social behavior—public disrobing or sexual behaviors such as masturbation
- Level of mobility, wandering, or pacing behaviors
- Judgment ability—safety becomes a major concern
- Sleep disturbance—sleeps more often for shorter periods of time
- Speech or language impairment
- Hallucinations, illusions, or delusions
- Bowel and bladder incontinence
- Apathy (flatness of gestures, tone of voice, facial expression)
- Recognition of family members, child, or spouse (may have difficulty deciding to whom feelings should be directed)
- Any decline in nutritional status
- Sensory needs and limitations

BOX 19.14

Outcomes for the Client With Dementia

Outcomes may include the following:
- Demonstrates decreased anxiety levels
- Remains safe and free from injury
- Does not harm self or others
- Experiences minimal catastrophic reactions
- Participation in self-care activities as able
- Remains oriented at level of ability
- Follows scheduled routine of activity and rest
- Feels valued and accepted

An additional outcome is that the caregiver and family will identify and utilize community support systems.

Outcomes for an individual with dementia must be considered on a day-to-day and moment-to-moment basis, because their behavior is a response to the immediate world around them. The most important thing that caregivers can do is provide a safe environment and protection from injury. The nursing interventions listed below allow clients to participate in self-care to the extent of their ability. With the assistance of caregivers and nursing staff in controlling the environment, the individual is helped to control the impulsive aggressive actions precipitated by frustration and confusion. Reassurance and calm are encouraged by consistency and simple, routine day-to-day activities. The nurse's reflection and observation of what works and what does not work with each client will promote individualized care and aid with the achievement of outcomes planned. In addition, caregivers will need understanding of the disease process and be able to demonstrate adaptive coping strategies in dealing with the stress of the caregiver role.

Nursing Care Focus

- Impaired Communication

Goal

- The client will understand staff and have their own needs understood by staff.

Implementations for Improving Communication

One of the most important aspects of caring for the individual with dementia is communication. Both verbal and nonverbal approaches must be adapted to the limited ability they have to understand what is being said or the intended meaning.

When a catastrophic reaction is occurring, distraction and redirection are the most useful interventions. It is important for the nurse not to overreact, as this may increase the intensity of the situation. Remember, the individual with dementia is unable to control the behavior but will quickly forget the incident if allowed time to do so. It is important to intervene to prevent injury to the individual or others. Nursing observations should be made as to *who* is involved in the incident (do certain persons tend to trigger the behavior?), *what* is going on in the environment at the time of the incident, *where* the incidents tend to occur (does one location precipitate the behavior

> ## BOX 19.15
>
> ## Interventions to Facilitate Communication
>
> - Use touch, eye contact, unhurried movements, a smile, or a pleasant affect.
> - Speak clearly, softly, and slowly using short, simple words and sentences—a raised voice will trigger agitation.
> - Identify yourself and call the individual by name at each meeting.
> - Avoid questions that challenge memory—instead of asking the individual who a relative is, tell them the relative's name and the relationship to them.
> - Focus on one piece of information at a time.
> - Use gestures or cues to accompany speech or commands.
> - Use face-to-face contact.
> - Repeat questions or commands exactly as they were first stated—saying them another way adds another challenge.
> - Validate at the client's level of functioning—this helps the client to cope with feelings of loss.
> - Ask questions and make comments that allow the client to remember or reminisce on subjects that have emotional meaning for the client. Do not argue or disagree with what the client is saying. When the client is delusional, acknowledge their feelings and reinforce reality or divert attention to another issue.
> - Recognize the client's feelings and redirect attention to another subject that is pleasant if a client becomes verbally aggressive.
> - Minimize excess sounds or background noise when talking to the client. Misleading stimuli, such as excess noise or television, can produce agitation—as the sounds are often too confusing or move too fast.

more than others?), *when* the individual tends to become more agitated (is there a particular time of day when the incidents reoccur?), and *why* the individual might be responding with agitation (e.g., pain, infection, uncomfortable clothing, incontinence). Interventions to enhance communication are listed in Box 19.15.

Evaluation of Goal/Desired Outcome

The client will:

- understand staff.
- have their own needs understood by staff.

Nursing Care Focus

- Activities of Daily Living (ADLs) Deficit

Goal

- The client will perform Activities of Daily Living (ADLs) as independently as possible.

Implementations for Assisting the Client With Activities of Daily Living (ADLs) Needs

As dementia advances, the ability to independently carry out the steps of self-care is diminished. Nursing interventions that may support the client's self-care needs are listed in Box 19.16.

Most clients with dementia will have weight loss. Nursing interventions related to maintaining adequate nutritional intake include monitoring intake of food and fluids. As clients with dementia are often moving and not able to sit for long periods, provide finger foods that can be eaten while pacing—make sandwiches out of meat, vegetables, or fruit. Too many choices may be overwhelming and result in refusal to eat. Set one item or bowl of food in front of the client at a time. Face the individual if assisting with eating. Alzheimer disease tends to decrease peripheral vision and a side approach may frighten the client. Prevent the client from eating nonfood items such as napkins, food wrappers, or plants. Offer between-meal snacks. Consider a mechanical alteration in food consistency as the disease progresses, because swallowing may be impaired.

As dementia progresses, the ability to locate the bathroom and follow through with the steps of toileting is lost. The individual may become incontinent with little recognition that urination or defecation has occurred. The nurse can best assist the client with dementia by labeling the bathroom door with a picture or large-print wording to identify the purpose of the room. Simplify clothing (e.g., using pants with an elastic waist, slip-on shoes instead of shoes with laces). Use toileting schedules. Watch the client for nonverbal messages such as fidgeting with pants, increased pacing, or going in and out of doors.

BOX 19.16

Nursing Interventions That Support Activities of Daily Living (ADL) Needs in the Client With Dementia

- Allow client time to perform those tasks they are able to do.
- Assist with dressing—minimize the choices by selecting items of clothing. Different color items help the client to separate socks from pants, for example. Avoid tight clothing or complicated zippers and fasteners—Velcro fasteners decrease frustration with laces and buttons.
- Use simple step-by-step instructions, providing cues as needed.
- Try again later if client resists care—they may forget the issue in a few minutes.
- Maintain a consistent routine or schedule with the same caregivers as much as possible. This will promote calmness and decrease agitation.
- Use tub baths—many clients with dementia are frightened by the falling water of a shower on their skin.
- Use a same-sex staff member to bathe the client, which is sometimes accepted better by the client.
- Bathe the client at the time the client is accustomed to bathing (day vs. evening).
- Provide rest periods between activities—fatigue produces negative behaviors.
- Use a bed closer to the floor to prevent serious injury when ataxia is present.

Evaluation of Goal/Desired Outcome

- The client's Activities of Daily Living (ADLs) needs are met.

Just the Facts Key areas of concern in the care of the individual with dementia include communication, self-care deficit, nutrition, safety, fatigue, and confusion.

Cultural Considerations

Dementia in Language, Literature, and Common Beliefs

Words for dementia in some languages have dual meanings. For example, the Chinese term *chi dai zheng*, used in China, Hong Kong, and Singapore for dementia, also implies "stupidity." Meanings for the Arabic word *khabal* include "dementia" and "lunacy" (Low & Purwaningrum, 2022). Shakespeare portrayed dementia in his tragedy *King Lear*. During the Middle Ages, dementia was thought to be a sign of sin or being "demon-possessed." Then, and as recently as 2010, dementia has been associated with witchcraft.

Dementia continues to have a negative stigma and is often combined with the term "suffer," as in, "He suffers from dementia." Rarely is dementia shown as a positive. Individuals with dementia are portrayed as frail and incapacitated. Terms or phrases used to describe an individual with dementia may be very dehumanizing such as "living dead."

It is important for the nurse to recognize the individual—*not* the diagnosis or the symptoms. The nurse must be aware of their own bias and terminology so the individual with dementia, or their family, is not dehumanized or minimized.

Reference: Low, L.F., Purwaningrum, F. (2020). Negative stereotypes, fear and social distance: a systematic review of depictions of dementia in popular culture in the context of stigma. *BMC Geriatrics, 20*, 477. https://bmcgeriatr.biomedcentral.com/articles/10.1186/s12877-020-01754-x

SUMMARY

- Aging is an inevitable part of life in which changes occur that may have natural causes or be imposed by environmental and/or societal factors. Many older adults continue to live active and viable lives beyond the retirement age, whereas others are restricted by decreased income and limitations imposed by chronic illness.
- With age comes changes that may present the older adult with an emotional issue to work through. Although many older adults have adequate coping skills to adapt to these changes, others may encounter difficulty in meeting these emotional demands.
- The aging adult is often unaware of the signs that indicate a need for professional help in dealing with cognitive changes. A lack of resources further discourages some older adults from seeking help.
- Although some cognitive decline is probable as a person ages, it is subtle and causes few complications for them. In contrast, cognitive impairment leads to a significant memory loss and a decline in the ability to perform activities of daily living (ADLs).
- The two most common causes of cognitive impairment in the older adult are delirium and dementia.
- Delirium is marked by a sudden onset of a disturbance of consciousness and follows a short and critical course. In most cases, with treatment of the underlying cause, this disorder is reversible. Treatment is dependent on the cause, with the goal being to restore the client to the previous level of functioning. Many older adults develop delirium as a complication of an existing medical problem, which leads to a decrease in the likelihood of a full recovery.
- In contrast, dementia is characterized by a deterioration in cognitive functioning that is irreversible and progressive, leaving the individual with vague memories of past experiences.

- The most common types of progressive dementias are Alzheimer disease (most common), vascular disorder, and Lewy body disease.
- Alzheimer disease develops slowly with its deteriorating process leaving the individual with an inability to recognize once familiar objects, functions, and people.
- Personality and mood changes accompany a loss of interest and energy in previously enjoyed activities. Behavior problems arise out of the fear and confusion the individual is faced with as they attempt to cope with stimuli that are not understood. Impulse control is also impaired.
- In advanced dementia, the individual may be totally unaware of the environment and require constant care.
- Nursing interventions should be directed at providing for the safety and basic needs of the individual. Use of simple one-step commands in a stable and consistent environment provides a milieu that offers security and comfort to the individual with dementia and promotes an optimal response.
- Excessive or misunderstood stimuli lead to fear, which in turn may result in outbursts or catastrophic reactions. These are best managed by a calm approach, using redirection and refocusing of the individual's attention.
- The symptoms of depression can also be evident in the individual with dementia. However, it is important to recognize the existence of depression in older adults who do not have dementia.
- Because depression and dementia have similar symptoms, a diagnostic work-up is essential to distinguish between the two conditions. Treatment of depression usually leads to improvement in the cognitive level and overall functioning of the individual.
- Nursing interventions are directed at maximizing the functional ability of the person with cognitive impairment and to improve the quality of the individual's life and that of family members.

BIBLIOGRAPHY

Alzheimer's Association. (2022a). *2023 Alzheimer's disease facts and figures.* https://www.alz.org/media/Documents/alzheimers-facts-and-figures.pdf

Alzheimer's Association. (2022b). *Medications for memory, cognition and dementia-related behaviors.* https://www.alz.org/alzheimers-dementia/treatments/medications-for-memory

Alzheimer's Association. (2022c). *Dementia vs. Alzheimer's disease: What is the difference?* https://www.alz.org/alzheimers-dementia/difference-between-dementia-and-alzheimer-s

Deshaies, S. (2022). *Caring for patients with dementia and Alzheimer's: Tips & resources for nurses.* Nurse-Journal.org. https://nursejournal.org/resources/nursing-care-patients-with-alzheimers-dementia/

Francis, J. (2019). Delirium and acute confusional states: Prevention, treatment, and prognosis. *UpToDate.* Retrieved September 2, 2022, from https://www.uptodate.com/contents/delirium-and-acute-confusional-states-prevention-treatment-and-prognosis

Francis, J., & Young, G. B. (2022). Diagnosis of delirium and confusional states. *UpToDate.* Retrieved September 2, 2022, from https://www.uptodate.com/contents/diagnosis-of-delirium-and-confusional-states

Goodarzi, Z., & Ismail, Z. (2019). Neuropsychiatric aspects of Alzheimer's disease. *Practical Neurology.* https://practicalneurology.com/articles/2019-june/neuropsychiatric-aspects-of-alzheimers-disease

Koch, J., Amos, J. G., Beattie, E., Lautenschlager, N. T., Doyle, C., Anstey, K. J., & Mortby, M. E. (2022). Non-pharmacological interventions for neuropsychiatric symptoms of dementia in residential aged care settings: An umbrella review. *International Journal of Nursing Studies, 128,* Article 104187. https://doi.org/10.1016/j.ijnurstu.2022.104187

Kułak-Bejda, A., Bejda G., & Waszkiewicz, N. (2021). Mental disorders, cognitive impairment and the risk of suicide in older adults. *Frontiers in Psychiatry, 12.* https://doi.org/10.3389/fpsyt.2021.695286

Lauretani, F., Bellelli, G., Pelà, G., Morganti, S., Tagliaferri, S., & Maggio, M. (2020). Treatment of delirium in older persons: What we should not do! *International Journal of Molecular Science, 21*(7). https://www.ncbi.nlm.nih.gov/pmc/articles/PMC7177924

National Institute on Aging. (2021). *How is Alzheimer's disease treated?* National Institutes of Health. https://www.nia.nih.gov/health/how-alzheimers-disease-treated

National Institute on Aging. (2021). *Depression and older adults.* National Institutes of Health. https://www.nia.nih.gov/health/depression-and-older-adults

Press, D. (2022). Management of neuropsychiatric symptoms of dementia. *UpToDate.* Retrieved September 2, 2022, from https://www.uptodate.com/contents/management-of-neuropsychiatric-symptoms-of-dementia

Yakimicki, M. L., Edwards, N. E., Richards, E., & Beck, A. M. (2019). Animal-assisted intervention and dementia: A systematic review. *Clinical Nursing Research, 28*(1), 9–29. https://doi.org/10.1177/1054773818756987

STUDENT WORKSHEET

Fill in the Blank

Fill in the blank with the correct answer.

1. The most common causes of cognitive impairment are _____ and _____.
2. Delirium is characterized by a change in _____ and a change in cognition that occur in a _____ period of time.
3. An altered response to the effects of medication is seen in older adults because of the decreased ability of the body to _____ and _____ the medication.
4. Dementia is characterized by mental decline that is _____ and _____.
5. The three most common causes of death in the individual with Alzheimer dementia are _____, _____, and _____.
6. Periods of agitation in the person with Alzheimer disease are referred to as _____ reactions.

Matching

Match the following terms to the most appropriate phrase.

1. _____ Confabulation
2. _____ Paralalia
3. _____ Anomia
4. _____ Echolalia
5. _____ Apraxia
6. _____ Logoclonia
7. _____ Agnosia
8. _____ Aphasia

a. Inability to carry out purposeful movement
b. Repetitive verbalization of one word
c. Inability to understand what is heard
d. Filling in the gaps with fictitious statements
e. Inability to find the right word
f. Repeating words or questions
g. Inability to identify an object
h. Repeating one syllable

Multiple Choice

Select the best answer from the multiple-choice items.

1. A client goes into the bathroom and leaves. After leaving the bathroom they wander into the dayroom and urinate in the trash can. This is an example of:
   a. Amnesia
   b. Anomia
   c. Agnosia
   d. Apraxia

2. What is the reason a client with dementia may urinate in the trashcan instead of the toilet? *(Select all that apply)*
   a. Anxiety created by an illusion that someone else is in the bathroom
   b. Inability to remember why they are in the bathroom
   c. Failure to recognize the purpose of the commode
   d. Difficulty in managing clothing to facilitate using the bathroom
   e. Following the voices in their head that tell them to

3. The nurse is caring for a client who is diagnosed with delirium related to urosepsis. Which of the following would correctly describe the course of this cognitive disorder?
   a. Progressive
   b. Insidious onset
   c. Reversible
   d. Long term

4. A client is telling their family about a trip to the doctor yesterday afternoon. The client is unable to recall the reason for the visit and states they just needed some papers filled out. Which of the following describes the client's behavior?
   a. Anomia
   b. Confabulation
   c. Sundowning
   d. Logoclonia

5. A client says, "I don't want it, I don't want it, I don't want it." The term referring to this level of spoken language is:
   a. Babbling
   b. Paralalia
   c. Logoclonia
   d. Echolalia

6. The nurse prepares to administer oral medication to an older client with dementia. As the nurse attempts to put the tablets in their mouth, the client curses and strikes the nurse's hand. The nurse's best choice of action at this time would be to:
   a. explain to the client that the medications are to help them get better.
   b. leave the client alone and give the medication at a later time.
   c. omit the dose and document the medication as refused.
   d. call the health care provider and report the incident.

7. The nurse asks a client with dementia to sit down so their shoestrings can be retied. The client looks blankly at the nurse and continues to pace. What is the nurse's best action to help the client understand this command?
   a. Repeat the command using different words to explain what is meant.
   b. Explain why it is important to keep the shoestrings tied.
   c. Guide the client to a chair and point to the chair seat while telling the client to sit.
   d. Allow the client to pace and retie the shoestring when the client sits down on their own.

8. A client has sustained several lacerations and bruises from falling while getting out of bed and attempting to ambulate to the bathroom. The client does not remember verbal reminders to call for help to go to the bathroom. Which of the following nursing interventions would be the best approach to provide for the client's safety?
   a. Provide a bed closer to the floor.
   b. Provide a bedside commode.
   c. Place full side rails on the bed.
   d. Ask the doctor for a sedative at bedtime.

9. A client with dementia is given a breakfast tray with multiple items on it. The client proceeds to get up and wander away from the table. The appropriate nursing action is to:
   a. Save the tray and allow the client to eat at a later time.
   b. Redirect client back to table and provide one food item at a time.
   c. Accept actions to indicate client is not hungry.
   d. Verbally tell the client their breakfast is ready.

10. The family member of a client with dementia approaches the nurse and says, "Mom doesn't recognize me. She thinks her son is a little boy. How can I make her understand who I am?" What is the nurse's best response?
    a. "Remind her you are grown and that she does not have a little boy anymore."
    b. "Give her current pictures of you to remind her you are grown."
    c. "Ask her each time if she knows who you are before you tell her."
    d. "Tell her who you are each time and have her reminisce about your childhood."

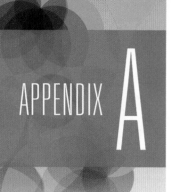

Patient Health Questionnaire-9 (PHQ-9)

The PHQ-9 is a multipurpose instrument for screening, diagnosing, monitoring, and measuring the severity of depression. The client answers the following nine questions.

Over the **last 2 weeks**, how often have you been bothered by the following problems?	Not at All	Several Days	More Than Half the Days	Nearly Every Day
1. Little interest or pleasure in doing things	0	1	2	3
2. Feeling down, depressed, or hopeless	0	1	2	3
3. Trouble falling asleep, staying asleep, or sleeping too much	0	1	2	3
4. Feeling tired or having little energy	0	1	2	3
5. Poor appetite or overeating	0	1	2	3
6. Feeling bad about yourself—or that you're a failure or have let yourself or your family down	0	1	2	3
7. Trouble concentrating on things, such as reading the newspaper or watching television	0	1	2	3
8. Moving or speaking so slowly that other people could have noticed. Or, the opposite—being so fidgety or restless that you have been moving around a lot more than usual	0	1	2	3
9. Thoughts that you would be better off dead or of hurting yourself in some way	0	1	2	3
For Office Coding PHQ-9 score is total score obtained from answers from all 9 questions.	0 +	____ +	____ +	____ = Total Score _____

If you checked off any problems, how difficult have these problems made it for you to do your work, take care of things at home, or get along with other people?

Not Difficult at All	Somewhat Difficult	Very Difficult	Extremely Difficult
☐	☐	☐	☐

PHQ-9 score and depression severity:

0–4	None–minimal
5–9	Mild
10–14	Moderate
15–19	Moderately Severe
20–27	Severe

(Developed by Drs. Robert L. Spitzer, Janet B.W. Williams, Kurt Kroenke, and colleagues, with an educational grant from Pfizer Inc. No permission required to reproduce, translate, display or distribute.)

Notes:
a. *Question 9 is a single screening question on suicide risk. A patient who answers yes (either a 1, 2, or 3 score for that question) to question 9 needs further assessment for suicide risk by an individual who is competent to assess this risk.*
b. *Clients who report a score that correlates to the "Severe" category should have immediate attention.*

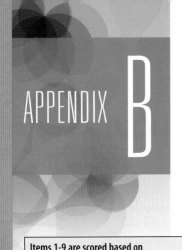
Abnormal Involuntary Movement Scale (AIMS)

Items 1-9 are scored based on					
Abnormal movements are not observed (0)					
Minimal or infrequent movements difficult to detect (1)					
Mild infrequent, but easy to detect (2)					
Moderate, frequent, easy to detect (3)					
Severe, almost continuously (4)					
Facial and Oral Movements					
1. Muscles of facial expression (frowning, blinking, smiling, grimacing)	0	1	2	3	4
2. Lips and periorbital area (puckering, pouting, smacking)	0	1	2	3	4
3. Jaw (biting, clenching, chewing, mouth opening, lateral movements)	0	1	2	3	4
4. Tongue (thrusting, tremors, athetoid movements)	0	1	2	3	4
Extremity Movements					
5. Upper (include choreic or rapid, objectively purposeless, irregular, spontaneous movements; athetoid or slow, irregular, complex, serpentine movements); Does NOT include tremors (repetitive, regular, and rhythmic)	0	1	2	3	4
6. Lower (lateral knee movement, foot tapping, heel dropping, foot squirming, inversion, and eversion of foot)	0	1	2	3	4
Trunk Movements					
7. Neck, shoulders, hips (rocking, twisting, squirming, pelvic gyrations)	0	1	2	3	4
Global Judgment					
8. Severity of abnormal movements	0	1	2	3	4
9. Incapacitation due to abnormal movements	0	1	2	3	4
10. Client's awareness of abnormal movements No awareness (0); Aware, no distress (1); Aware, mild distress (2); Aware, moderate distress (3); Aware, severe distress (4)	0	1	2	3	4
Dental Status					
11. Current problems with teeth or dentures? None (0), Partial (1), Full (2)	0	1	2		
12. Does the client usually wear dentures? None (0), Partial (1), Full (2)	0	1	2		
13. Level of cooperation. None (0), Partial (1), Full (2)	0	1	2		

AIMS Examination Procedure

Observe the client unobtrusively at rest. The chair to be used in the examination should be hard, firm, and without arms.

1. Ask client, whether there is anything in mouth (i.e., gum, candy) and if there is, to remove it.
2. Ask client about current condition of their teeth. Ask if client wears dentures. Do teeth or dentures bother client now?
3. Ask whether client notices any movement in mouth, face, hands, or feet. If yes, ask to describe and to what extent they currently bother client or interfere with activities.
4. Have client sit in chair with hands or knees, legs slightly apart, and feet flat on floor. (Look at entire body for movement while in this position.)

5. Ask client to sit with hand hanging unsupported. If male, between legs, if female and wearing a dress, hanging over knees. (Observe hands and other body areas.)
6. Ask client to open mouth. (Observe tongue at rest within mouth.) Do this twice.
7. Ask client to protrude tongue. (Observe abnormalities of tongue movement.) Do this twice.
8. Ask client to tap thumb, with each finger, as rapidly as possible for 10 to 15 seconds, separately with right hand, then with left hand. (Observe facial and leg movements.)
9. Flex and extend client's left and right arms (one at a time). Note any rigidity separately.
10. Ask client to stand up (observe in profile). Observe all body areas again (hips included). Ask client to extend both arms outstretched in front with palms down. (Observe trunk, legs, and mouth.)
11. Have client walk a few paces, turn, and walk back to chair. (Observe hands and gait.) Do this twice.

Public Health Service
Alcohol, Drug Abuse, and Mental Health Administration, National Institute of Mental Health

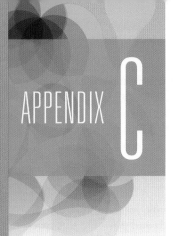
Answers to Student Worksheet

Chapter 1

Fill in the Blank

1. Balance
2. Fight, flight
3. Overwhelming, behavior
4. Unpredictability
5. Empty clichés

Matching

1. C
2. E
3. H
4. D
5. I
6. B
7. A
8. F
9. G

Multiple Choice

1. **Correct Answer: B, E,** Indicate feeling of isolation and anhedonia. A: Shows active interaction with others. C: Indicates person is comfortable being alone. D: Indicates adaptive coping.
2. **Correct Answer: C,** Mental disorders often interfere with interpersonal relationships. A, B, D: Indicators of a healthy mental state.
3. **Correct Answer: C,** Description indicated overall exhaustion and apathy toward work which is indicative of burnout. A: Is a response to a threat or challenge, description does not indicate a threat. B: Disorganization of mental state not evident. D: Requires the individual to adjust or adapt to the environment.
4. **Correct Answer: A,** Recognizes individual strengths and weaknesses. B: Unrealistic view of one's abilities. C: Indicates negative view of self. D: Self-defeat through negative view of self.
5. **Correct Answer: B,** Temporarily relieves the anxiety but problem still exists. A: With adaptive coping, the problem would be resolved. C: Maladaptive would mean unsuccessful methods are used to reduce anxiety. D: Dysfunctional would indicate no attempt is made to reduce anxiety.

6. **Correct Answer: B, D,** Offers opportunity for client to talk about present feelings. A: Closes the conversation and minimizes client's feelings. C: Belittles client's statement and feelings. E: "Why" puts client on the defensive to respond.
7. **Correct Answer: C,** Avoiding reality of the situation. A: Bargaining cannot occur until reality of inevitable is acknowledged. B: There is no evidence of feelings of anger. D: Depression indicates a loss of hope and mourning for that which is gone.
8. **Correct Answer: D,** Seen in those who are facing a major loss in the near future. A: Seen when grief process is incomplete. B: Grief experienced following a loss. C: Failure to complete the grief process and successful coping not evident.
9. **Correct Answer: C,** Client is demonstrating symptoms of severe anxiety. A: Client would be restless but have good concentration. B: Physical symptoms described are more intense than seen in moderate anxiety. D: Symptoms of panic include the individual being incoherent, withdrawn, and having unintelligible speech.

Chapter 2

Fill in the Blank

1. Psychotropic/antipsychotic
2. Seclusion, restraint(s)
3. Ethics
4. Informed consent
5. Confidentiality
6. Involuntary commitment

Matching

1. C
2. D
3. F
4. B
5. E
6. A

Multiple Choice

1. **Correct Answer: D,** The nurse used the word "crazy" which has a negative association. A, B, and C are questions used to evaluate or eliminate barriers to care.

2. **Correct Answer: C,** Evidence of mental state posing an immediate threat to self or others is required to have an order of protective custody granted by a court official. A, B, D: Do not indicate an immediate threat to client safety or that of others and would not be reason for involuntary commitment.

3. **Correct Answer: A,** Coping abilities both past and present would be included in data collection. B, C, D: All would be included in the planning phase of the client care plan for this client.

4. **Correct Answer: A, C, D,** An inmate who voices current suicidal ideation, has had previous treatment for depression, or has a history of intervention for prior suicide attempts will need referral to be further evaluated for any current symptoms and treatment. B, E: Are common responses of incarcerated individuals.

5. **Correct Answer: D,** Outpatient care offers client treatment without admission to a mental health inpatient unit. A: Referral does not include accepting or refusing treatment. B: The question is asking about the health care provider's action of referral and does not mention the provider's qualifications. C: Treatment plan is discussed at the time of admission.

6. **Correct Answer: B,** Intent to commit a crime is a legal reason for disclosure. A: Information cannot be given to spouse unless client has given consent. C: Only personnel directly involved in client care legally have access to the information. D: Disclosure to the media would violate HIPAA policies.

7. **Correct Answer: C,** The initial action should be to try to de-escalate the behavior by a calm and nonthreatening approach and to protect the safety of all clients. This will allow the client a chance to regain control of their behavior without the use of restraint. A: Sedation may be necessary if behavior becomes unmanageable by nonrestraining methods. B: Threat of seclusion or restraint is inappropriate. D: Allowing the confrontation to continue could pose a threat to all involved.

8. **Correct Answer: A,** Chemical restraint is the least restrictive of the options listed. B: Seclusion should only be used if behavior cannot be controlled by other means and requires a timeframe. C: Seclusion would only be used if sedation was not effective in behavior management; they should not be used together. D: Physical restraint is the most restrictive and only used in an emergency situation.

9. **Correct Answer: C,** Seclusion is never appropriate when a client is suicidal. A, B, D: All indicate inappropriate social behaviors for which seclusion may be used until client regains control or seclusion is determined to be ineffective.

10. **Correct Answer: C,** Since competency of the client may be questionable at the point of admission, it would be advisable to include a family member or guardian to verify information was received. A: If present psychologic state of the client is irrational, it will not help to go over the information again. B: It is important that information on client rights and unit policies is explained at the time of admission. D: A coworker cannot legally provide a signed statement of understanding from the client or family.

Chapter 3

Fill in the Blank

1. Personality
2. Basic needs
3. Temperament
4. Defense mechanisms
5. Industry, inferiority
6. Nurse–client
7. Solid self

Matching

1. C
2. G
3. B
4. D
5. H
6. A
7. F
8. E

Multiple Choice

1. **Correct Answer: C,** Demonstrates a lack of fulfillment and satisfaction with life choices in age group over 65 years. A, B, D: All relate to earlier life stages of development.

2. **Correct Answer: B,** Having hypothermia indicates the individual was exposed to the elements. A and C, while they are basic needs, are not indicated to be unmet in the question. D is a higher-level need, not a basic need. Basic needs must be met before higher-level needs can be addressed. Additionally, being homeless does not automatically indicate security needs are not met.

3. **Correct Answer: B,** Egocentric view where child is unable to see another point of view except their own. A: Involves growth of abilities related to five senses and motor function. C: Cognitive connections based on actual events. D: Stage of abstract thought process and problem-solving.

4. **Correct Answer: C,** Choice based on the number of people who would be affected and hurt by telling their friend the truth. A: No indication that there is personal gain from the choice. B: Does not show influence either by society or the

law. D: There is no law of society that is involved in this decision.

5. **Correct Answer: D**, Observed and learned behavior with reinforcement of punishment and aggression. A, B: Behaviorism implies that thinking and feeling are irrelevant. C: Assault does not relate to an environmental threat to survival.

6. **Correct Answer: A,** Actions based on observation and imitation of others for approval. B: Behaviors are result of conscious choice, not conditioning which is automatic. C: Freudian focus on adolescent sexuality is not an issue in this situation. D: Feelings and peer relationships would be irrelevant in behaviorism.

7. **Correct Answer: B**, Awareness that behaviors are the result of own choices with option for change. A: Reflects Freudian theory of personality development. C: Does not indicate behavior is influenced by external forces. D: Freudian theory.

8. **Correct Answer: C,** Client unable to see the truth because the trauma of the rape is too painful at this time. A: No blame is being attributed by the client. B: No physical symptoms are present as a result of emotional conflict. D: Client is not offering justification for a behavior.

9. **Correct Answer: A,** Client exhibits suspicion and inability to believe in the credibility of company policies. B: Feelings not based on fear of independence. C: Does not indicate the client has a feeling of inadequacy.
D: Does not indicate a fear of failure or feeling of unworthiness.

10. **Correct Answer: C,** The child took some time to interact with the nurse which is seen in a slow-to-warm-up temperament.

Chapter 4

Fill in the Blank

1. Safe, structured
2. Treatment team
3. Unbiased, nonjudgmental
4. Psychotherapy
5. Psychotropic
6. Lipid solubility
7. Protein, more

Matching

1. F
2. E
3. D
4. C
5. A
6. B
7. G

Multiple Choice

1. **Correct Answer: C,** Observation of behavior and response to treatment is a responsibility of the nurse. A, B: Role of the psychologist, psychiatrist, or therapist. D: This is the responsibility of the social worker.

2. **Correct Answer: A,** Modeling is an effective method of reinforcing socially appropriate behavior. B: Is a therapeutic communication response by the nurse. C: Reprimands are not therapeutic and demean the client. D: Does not involve client interaction.

3. **Correct Answer: D,** Social worker works with community agencies to secure continued support and care for the client. A: Works with direct day-to-day care of the client. B: May be involved with psychotherapy. C: Securing placement is not a nursing function.

4. **Correct Answer: B,** As a client advocate, the nurse functions to protect the rights of the client through acceptance, respect, and support of the client's perspective and decisions. A: As educator, the nurse provides and reinforces information. C: In the role of counselor, the nurse provides active listening and therapeutic communication. D: As caregiver, the nurse implements nursing interventions.

5. **Correct Answer: A,** Observation of response to treatment and assessment are part of the caregiver role. B: Therapeutic interaction with the client. C: Patient teaching. D: Protecting patient rights.

6. **Correct Answer: C,** Modeling assists the client with learning communication skills and social interaction. A: Ignoring the behavior does not provide guidance or supportive intervention. B: Isolating the client will not support improved social skills. D: Punitive methods are not therapeutic.

7. **Correct Answer: B,** Psychotropic agents used in combination with therapy will reduce the disabling symptoms and promote functional levels of living. A: Medications by themselves cannot help the client with the behaviors imposed by the illness. Therapy helps the client to understand the symptoms and manage them. C: Medications can reduce the symptoms, but there is no guarantee they will ever be totally free of them. D: Psychotropic agents are not curative.

8. **Correct Answer: A,** Slowed metabolic rate and renal excretion time allow the medication to remain in the body longer. B: There is a higher fat composition of tissue in the older adult. C, D: There is less serum albumin and protein to bind with the medication, which allows more of the free medication to circulate in the blood.

9. **Correct Answer: A, C,** Taking all medicine in the morning could indicate dosages are not taken as prescribed, and feeling worse after taking medicine could indicate possible side effects. Nurse

should ask more questions to clarify the statements. B, D: Nurse can respond with explanation and note the request for the provider. E: Client is taking medication correctly to assist with difficulty swallowing.

10. **Correct Answer: D,** Dry skin with decreased fluid intake could indicate dehydration, which increases the concentration of the medication in the body. A: Indicates safety issue related to side effects. B: Increased drowsiness is a side effect of antidepressant medication. C: Usual symptoms of depressed state.

Chapter 5

Fill in the Blank

1. Empathy
2. Self-awareness
3. Situation, needs
4. Independence
5. Boundaries
6. Anxiety

Matching

1. C
2. D
3. F
4. B
5. A
6. E

Multiple Choice

1. **Correct Answer: A, E,** Trust is dependent on the nonjudgmental approach, honesty, and integrity of the nurse. B: Sympathy can cause the nurse to overidentify with the client's problem and is nontherapeutic. C: Clients are accepted regardless of their background. D: It is the quality, not quantity, of that time spent with the client that is important.
2. **Correct Answer: D,** Client is attempting to manipulate the nurse by complaining about others and showing favoritism. A: Statement does not indicate client is evading a topic. B: The client is interacting with the nurse, not withdrawing. C: There are no ambivalent statements expressed by the client in this scenario.
3. **Correct Answer: A,** Acknowledging the behavior helps the client to recognize their behavior. B: Threatens the client and is nontherapeutic and unethical. C: Distance should be maintained— touching an aggressive client is unsafe. D: Does not attempt to understand meaning behind the behavior.
4. **Correct Answer: A, D, E,** Awareness of the nurse's own thinking and behavior allows the nurse to be aware of any unrecognized feelings or biases which can affect client's care. Observing a client after limits are imposed can help the nurse notice

if the client's behavior changes; limit-setting can increase the risk for violence in a client. Avoiding all oncoming staff changing at the same times decreases risk of unsupervision of clients. B, C: These actions put the nurse in an unsafe position by either preventing a means of leaving a room or causing them to be unable to see what is happening in the group behind them.

5. **Correct Answer: A,** Explanations of rules and boundaries are explained at the beginning of the relationship to establish a baseline for the next phase. B: Working phase involves planning and goals to improve client's behavior. C: Termination phase occurs when the client is able to practice learned skills. D: Not a phase of the relationship; is part of the nursing process.
6. **Correct Answer: B,** Nurse should encourage the client to be independent and promote reliance on their own ability to deal with problems. This prevents dependence of the client on the nurse. A: Time spent with client is continued until discharge. C: The nurse–client relationship must not extend beyond the client's discharge. D: This is a focus in the working phase.
7. **Correct Answer: C,** Any contact by phone, mail, e-mail, or socialization with any client following discharge is in clear violation of professional ethics. A, B, D: All within acceptable roles of the nurse.
8. **Correct Answer: D,** Focuses on the client's problem and feelings without responding to the attempted personal reference. A: Encourages further isolated contact and overinvolvement with the client. B: Demeans client without recognizing the feelings behind the statement. C: Focuses on the nurse and is risking overinvolvement.
9. **Correct Answer: A,** Accepting a client's gift is overinvolvement and violates professional limits for behavior. B, C, D: All are acceptable within the nurse–client relationship.

Chapter 6

Fill in the Blank

1. Trait anger
2. Stalking
3. Bullying
4. Intimate partner violence
5. Risk, protective
6. Assertion

Matching

1. D
2. F
3. E
4. G
5. C
6. B
7. A

Multiple Choice

1. **Correct Answer: C,** Gathering data on how the client has coped in the past helps the nurse with understanding how the client may cope with the current situation. A, B, D: These statements do not gather information on the client's coping. B and D are inappropriate questions at this time.
2. **Correct Answer: C,** Suicidal gesture indicates the person has defined their plan and may be about ready to carry out the plan. A: Suicidal erosion is the accumulation of negative experiences that may lead to suicidal thoughts. B: Suicidal ideation indicates a verbalized thought or idea that includes the person's desire to do self-harm or destruction. D: A suicidal attempt means the person has actually carried out the suicide plan.
3. **Correct Answer: A,** Situational crisis related to a series of unpredictable events in one's life that leave one void of coping skills. B: Maturational crisis refers to a predictable period of development in life stages when the person may be unable to adjust and move to next phase. C: Developmental crisis refers to the same as maturational crisis. D: Identity crisis would be applicable to adolescent developmental stage.
4. **Correct Answer: A, B, D,** All factors that are warning signs for violence. C: Action-packed movies can be enjoyed without related violent behavior. E: Numerous relationships do not indicate violence.
5. **Correct Answer: C,** Indicates bullying, as it is occurring daily, verbally, and is frightening to the individual. A: Situational and not necessarily daily. B: Adult is present and the behavior is not necessarily occurring daily. D: Isolated social media incident.

Chapter 7

Fill in the Blank

1. Congruent
2. Intermittent
3. Blocking
4. Neologism
5. Loose association
6. Nonverbal communication
7. Arm's length

Matching

1. E
2. C
3. A
4. D
5. B

Multiple Choice

1. **Correct Answer: B,** Reinforces reality while acknowledging and validates the symptoms are real and frightening to the client. A: Minimizes client's feelings. C: Belittling statement. D: Puts client on the defensive.
2. **Correct Answer: D,** Clarification to verify perceived meaning of client statement. A: Minimizes client's feelings. B: False reassurance with superficial attitude. C: Minimizing or belittling and devalues the client's feelings.
3. **Correct Answer: A,** Client behavior indicates anxiety about the topic. Silence will allow client to continue talking when able. B: Client has not stated feelings about the situation. C: Client's nonverbal behavior indicates the nurse should wait rather than restating at this time. D: Concentrating not an issue at this point.
4. **Correct Answer: B,** Open-ended statement that allows the client to talk freely about the issue. A: Could be used later in the interaction. C: Statement belittles client's feelings and is a closed-ended question. D: Clarification statement would be better used later in the interaction.
5. **Correct Answer: A,** Validates nurse's perception of client's feelings and offers the client an opportunity to talk about them. B: Minimizes the client's fears and anxiety. C, D: False reassurance.
6. **Correct Answer: D,** Client's statement indicates a feeling of being controlled by others. A: "Why" puts client on defensive. B: Belittling comment. C: Statement is offering the nurse's opinion of the situation.
7. **Correct Answer: A,** Open-ended statement allows client to discuss feelings freely. B: "Why" puts client on the defensive. C: Closed-ended question that could be answered in one word. D: Minimizes client feelings.
8. **Correct Answer: B, E,** Focusing helps the client concentrate on a specific issue that may be uncomfortable to talk about. A, D: Closed-ended questions that could be answered in one word. C: Puts client on defensive and demands an answer.

Chapter 8

Fill in the Blank

1. Nursing process
2. Subjective
3. Objective
4. Problem, data
5. Outcomes

Matching

1. C
2. D
3. A
4. E
5. F
6. B

Multiple Choice

1. **Correct Answer: A,** Subjective data is best documented using exact words as stated by the client to avoid attempts at interpreting the intended meaning. B: This can validate subjective data but cannot provide client perspective. C: Objective data, which does not offer client's perspective. D: Nurse's perspective may differ from intended meaning.

2. **Correct Answer: D,** An accepting and nonjudgmental attitude by the nurse fosters a trusting environment. A: Cooperation of the client is a result of the trusting relationship. B: Provides an environment that is therapeutic but does not establish trust on its own. C: Client's perception does not create a trusting environment.

3. **Correct Answer: B,** Mood and affect are components of the mental status assessment. A, C: Do not relate directly to mental status. D: Established from collected data.

4. **Correct Answer: A, B, C, E,** Descriptions of attitude. D: Used to reference slowed motor activity or mood .

5. **Correct Answer: D,** The components of a nursing care focus. A: A nursing care focus can be actual or risk problems. B: A nursing care focus is never based on a medical diagnosis. C: The nursing care focus can be updated or resolved during the admission based upon a continuous process of evaluation and reassessment. E: The health care provider determines the therapies; the nursing plan of care reflects the therapies in the nursing interventions component.

6. **Correct Answer: B,** The outcome is not specific and is therefore not complete. A: Can measure if the client verbalizes thoughts or not. C: Time listed is "by discharge." D: Verbalizing thoughts by discharge is realistic.

7. **Correct Answer: D,** The nurse is clarifying, or evaluating, the client's understanding about the medication. A: Occurs prior to implementation of planned interventions. B: Identifies the problem. C: Question describes the nursing intervention that has occurred.

8. **Correct Answer: D,** Evaluation is where reassessment, additional planning, and updating nursing interventions occurs. A, B, C: All are steps that occur in the nursing process and the process cannot be validated until evaluation has occurred.

Chapter 9

Fill in the Blank

1. Connect, stimulus
2. Automatic relief behaviors
3. Specific phobia
4. Agoraphobia

5. Obsessions
6. Reduced

Matching

1. F
2. G
3. B
4. H
5. D
6. C
7. E
8. A

Multiple Choice

1. **Correct Answer: C,** Reassurance and calm relays a sense of security to client in panic. A: Medications are not an initial intervention with this level of anxiety and medications do not provide reassurance. B: Client in panic is unable to listen to any explanation. D: Touching or approaching can pose additional threat or invade personal space and can increase anxiety.

2. **Correct Answer: D, E,** Linking the behavior to a particular situation can help client develop an awareness of feelings that precede anxiety attacks. A: False reassurance that minimizes client's feelings. B: Providing medication does not help the client identify causative factors to their anxiety. C: Giving the client extra attention when they have anxiety symptoms provides secondary gain for the client and does not help them address the anxiety.

3. **Correct Answer: B,** Feelings of suffocation are triggered by sympathetic nervous system responses that usually accompany a state of panic. A, C: Not typically displayed in panic state. D: Person in panic attack cannot think logically.

4. **Correct Answer: D,** Anticipatory anxiety comes well in advance of a particular situation leading to thoughts of dread and actions to avoid the situation. A: In free-floating anxiety the client cannot attach a stimulus to the anxiety; here the client is reacting to the public speaking. B: Automatic relief behaviors are subtle unconscious behaviors that are aimed at relieving the anxiety. C: In an uncued panic attack the client cannot identify a stimulus to the panic attack.

5. **Correct Answer: C,** Demonstrates progress of client in coping with fear of being in public place. A: Relates to person with social phobia. B: Does not relate to agoraphobia. D: Would show progress in a client with obsessive-compulsive disorder.

6. **Correct Answer: D,** Recognizes the client's need to perform rituals to deal with acute anxiety created by the obsessive thoughts. This is an initial reaction but not a long-term intervention. A: Invalidates the client's underlying anxiety from the obsession and compulsions. B: Intervention is inappropriate and punitive. C: Conforming to

a schedule would lead to extreme anxiety for the client.

7. **Correct Answer: A,** Smoking decreases the sedative and antianxiety effects of benzodiazepine medications. B, C, D: Benzodiazepines not affected by caffeine, jogging, or working.

8. **Correct Answer: C,** Antianxiety medications are contraindicated during pregnancy and lactation. The client is asking for medication so the fact that the client is breast-feeding should be reported. A, B, D: Are all common symptoms of panic attack.

9. **Correct Answer: B,** Antianxiety medications should not be combined with alcohol or other CNS depressants. A: The most common side effect of antianxiety medications is drowsiness which tends to improve as adjustment to the medication occurs. C: Clients may experience several weeks' time before onset of therapy and reduction of symptoms is experienced. D: Most antianxiety medications are taken short term.

10. **Correct Answer: B, C, E,** are different classifications of medications that have shown to relieve anxiety. A, D: These medication classifications do not have an effect on anxiety and are not prescribed for anxiety.

Chapter 10

Fill in the Blank

1. Affect
2. Cyclothymic
3. Dysthymia
4. Persecution
5. Lithium carbonate
6. Electroconvulsant
7. Lethality

Matching

1. J
2. F
3. D
4. G
5. A
6. B
7. H
8. I
9. E
10. C

Multiple Choice

1. **Correct Answer: C,** It is important to provide nutrition for the increased energy level when the client is unable to sit long enough to eat. These foods can be eaten while standing or walking. A: Client in manic state will go for long periods without eating if no intervention is provided and may not remember to ask for food. B: Does not address the problem created by the continuous

activity. D: Client is not able to receive teaching while in manic state.

2. **Correct Answer: C, D,** Atypical speech patterns can be seen during manic attacks, Loss of inhibitions can lead client to dress in a manner that is excessive and atypical for the client. A: Flashbacks are seen in PTSD, not mania. B: Is a normal sleep amount. In mania, sleep is fragmented or not present. E: Is a normal finding. In mania the client may not eat or may take few bites as they are unable to sit and focus on eating.

3. **Correct Answer: D,** Client has loss of inhibitions during manic episodes and needs reminders of appropriate behavior. A: Implies disapproval of the client's behavior and is punitive. In a manic episode the client may not be able to control impulsivity. B: Allowing continuance of delusional thought processes is nontherapeutic. C: Clients can pace for extended periods without breaks. This would distract the nurse from other clients and is nontherapeutic for the client as they are responding to internal stimulation and not feedback from the nurse.

4. **Correct Answer: B,** Nursing plan of care should provide structured activities that offer opportunity for positive and encouraging experiences. A: Client may not have physical energy to exercise and may not have emotional energy to socialize. C: Supports the client's feeling of worthlessness and withdrawal. D: May be too demanding for client or set client up for self-defeating thoughts.

5. **Correct Answer: C,** Therapeutic lithium serum levels are 0.6 to 1.2 mEq/L. Giving additional doses could push levels to a toxic level. A: Not indicated as level too high, not too low. B: Level indicates a reduction is needed rather than increase. D: Medication dosage adjustment may be all that is needed to maintain therapeutic response.

6. **Correct Answer: D,** Photosensitivity is a side effect of tricyclic antidepressant medications. A: A side effect of tricyclic antidepressants is cardiac arrhythmias and therefore stimulants, including caffeine, should be avoided. B: Medication must be tapered and should not be discontinued unless supervised by the health care provider. C: Therapeutic levels of the chemical neurotransmitters must be maintained in order for effective response of the drug.

7. **Correct Answer: A, B, E,** These contain tyramine and should be avoided when taking an MAOI. C, D: No interactions with these foods.

8. **Correct Answer: A,** Anhedonia is a lack of pleasure in things the individual previously enjoyed. B: Anergia relates to a decrease in energy level. C: Euphoria is an excessive feeling of happiness. D: Negativism is a learned sense of helplessness or a negative view of situations.

9. **Correct Answer: D,** Validating the client's feelings of worthlessness and hopelessness begins to establish a trusting relationship with the client. A: "Why" questions put the client on the defensive and are nontherapeutic. B: This statement is a non-reassuring cliché that closes the interaction to further response. C: It is more therapeutic to access the client's feelings than reasoning behind the words.

10. **Correct Answer: B,** Client in state of depression may need assistance with hygiene, elimination, and nutrition needs. A, C: These will be addressed as treatment progresses. D: Depression alone does not indicate relationship problems.

Chapter 11

Fill in the Blank

1. Anticholinergic, extrapyramidal
2. AIMS
3. Illusions
4. Water-intoxication
5. Grandeur
6. Blunted or flat

Matching

1. C
2. G
3. E
4. B
5. D
6. A
7. F

Multiple Choice

1. **Correct Answer: B,** Client believes others are telling them to harm themselves. A: Hallucinations are perceptual disturbances rather than disorganized thinking. C: Would be expressed as thoughts of individual doing a grandiose act or believing they are more powerful than they really are. D: Loose associations are speech patterns where unrelated concepts are spoken as though they are complete thoughts.

2. **Correct Answer: D,** Poverty of speech indicates a decreasing quality of speaking in which the person may speak very slowly, not answer questions, or stop in the middle of thoughts. A: Describes word salad. B: Rhyming is referred to as clang associations. C: Describes thought insertion.

3. **Correct Answer: A,** Acknowledges the feelings produced by the perceptual alteration, while reinforcing reality of it as nonexistent to others is most therapeutic. B: Encourages the client to continue the perceptual alteration. C, D: Belittling the distorted reality and the discomfort it is causing the client is nontherapeutic.

4. **Correct Answer: A,** Protrusion of the tongue and pill-rolling of the fingers are both late-appearing and irreversible movements indicating the extrapyramidal side effect of tardive dyskinesia. B: Tardive dyskinesia is common after long-term use but is not a normal response. C: These symptoms are definitely related to the medication and not part of the illness. D: Indication that reduced, not increased, dosage is needed or medication to counteract these effects is also needed.

5. **Correct Answer: C,** Risperidone can cause the side effect of photosensitivity. The client should be advised to wear sunscreen and protective clothing to avoid any negative consequences from being in the sun. A: Medication should be taken with food to avoid gastric irritation, so this is a correct statement. B: Medication can actually take several days to weeks to achieve full benefit, so this is a correct statement. D: Orthostatic hypotension can occur as a side effect of this drug, so this is a correct statement.

6. **Correct Answer: D,** Benztropine is an anticholinergic drug for counteracting the extrapyramidal side effects of tardive dyskinesia as a result on antipsychotic drugs. Protruding tongue movements would indicate symptoms of tardive dyskinesia. A: Antipsychotic medication haloperidol should diminish the delusional thinking. B: Not an indication for benztropine administration. C: These are expected negative symptoms of schizophrenia and benztropine is not indicated for these symptoms.

7. **Correct Answer: B, D,** Perceptual disturbances and disorganized thinking appear early in the disease and are considered positive symptoms. Positive symptoms are those that are typically associated with psychosis. A, C, E: Are all negative symptoms which are the absence or deficits of typical behaviors and affect.

8. **Correct Answer: B,** Dry mouth is one of the anticholinergic side effects of antipsychotic medications. A: This is an intervention for clients taking lithium carbonate. C: Haloperidol is not known to affect oral cavity or cause secondary infection in the mouth, so this intervention is not indicated. D: Unrelated to haloperidol.

9. **Correct Answer: D,** Clients with paranoia often misinterpret things and sounds in the environment as endangering them and will act defensively in response. A: Most clients with paranoia are very alert to environmental changes. B: Clients with schizophrenia have very little insight into the illogical nature of their symptoms. C: Recognition of the distortions in thinking is lacking in most cases of schizophrenia.

10. **Correct Answer: A,** A firm, matter-of-fact approach reassures the client of reality and the need for medication to treat the illness. B, C: Reinforce the distorted thinking and paranoid delusion. D: Delay will cause an increase in symptoms.

Chapter 12

Fill in the Blank

1. Personality traits
2. Schizotypal
3. Medications
4. Entitlement
5. Self-mutilation
6. Antisocial

Matching

1. F
2. E
3. I
4. G
5. A
6. D
7. H
8. B
9. C

Multiple Choice

1. **Correct Answer: B,** Self-injury is an outward focus of control over inner pain and a chronic sense of emptiness and self-hate. A: Arrogance is not typical in the person who self-mutilates. C: Suspicion is more common in paranoid disorder. D: Not a component of self-mutilation.
2. **Correct Answer: D,** With little insight into their behavior, those with personality disorders need limits with consequences that require taking responsibility for the behavior. A: Puts client on the defensive and invokes negative response. B: Behavior modification is more effective in these disorders than medications. C: This should be used only in the event the client poses an actual threat to self or others and only if least-restrictive measures are not effective.
3. **Correct Answer: B,** The individual tends to be self-indulgent, arrogant, and demanding. Treatment is ineffective because of the person's denial or inability to identify the problem in their inflexible and maladaptive behavior. A: Most persons with these disorders are unable to identify the problem. C: Most are oblivious to the problem with their behaviors and when aware, most have no desire to change their behavior patterns. D: They tend to be unaware of how their behavior is seen by others. E: Medications have almost no effect on their behavior and are used only for symptoms that are present due to other reasons such as anxiety.
4. **Correct Answer: B,** Persons who become involved in repeated abusive or destructive relationships are actually reinforcing and feeding a type of self-hate and redirected self-injury. A: Avoidance tends to be done as a self-defense mechanism not self-destruction. C: Would be seen as atypical behavior but not self-destructive. D: Sense of importance is the opposite of self-destructive.
5. **Correct Answer: C,** Demonstrates a grandiose sense of self-importance and claim that others owe them because of this superiority. A: Projection is blaming others for one's own problem. B: Splitting is seeing the world in "all or none" terms. D: Conflicting views of a situation is sign of ambivalence.
6. **Correct Answer: C,** The client is showing awareness of the problem and its impact on subsequent behavior. A: Client is focusing on cutting and not identifying the causative feelings or situations prior to cutting. B: Client can do this and not identify the problem in their own behavior. D: This might place the client in a situation where they choose to cut in private.
7. **Correct Answer: B,** Clients should be given one individual to refer to so staff do not follow different expectations or rules. A: This feeds into the personality disorder by addressing the requests but not the behavior. C: Imposing limits can increase risk for violence. D: Persons with personality disorders have little insight into their behavior.
8. **Correct Answer: B,** The person with a histrionic personality displays a pattern of egocentric and excessive emotion in a demanding manner to gain personal attention, and are uncomfortable in situations where they are not the center of attention. A, C, D: Do not typically exhibit this type of behavior.
9. **Correct Answer: D,** Narcissistic personality disorder indicates a continued need for self-indulgent attention and admiration with little regard for the feelings of others. A: Describes a dependent personality. B: Descriptive of an obsessive-compulsive personality. C: Commonly seen in schizotypal personality disorder.
10. **Correct Answer: A,** All personality disorders incorporate deeply ingrained, persistent, inflexible, and maladaptive patterns of behavior that are in conflict with a cultural norm. B: Seen in paranoid, schizoid, and schizotypal personality disorders but not all personality disorders. C: Seen in paranoid personality disorder. D: Seen in schizotypal personality disorder.

Chapter 13

Fill in the Blank

1. Somatization
2. Secondary gain
3. Primary gain
4. *La belle*
5. Psychogenic

Matching

1. E
2. D

3. A
4. B
5. C

Multiple Choice

1. **Correct Answer: C,** A person with illness anxiety disorder would have excessive fear that they have a serious illness despite medical testing and reassurance the disease does not exist. A, B, D: Common statements made by individuals with somatization disorder.

2. **Correct Answer: B,** Focus on the symptoms provides attention and concern for the client by physicians and family. The primary gain is achieved as the anxiety is relieved by diverting the focus to a physical problem. A: In somatic disorders is there is no medical evidence to support the symptoms. C: Client is usually unaware of the psychological basis for the symptoms. D: In conversion disorder there an attitude of indifference or little concern over the implication of the symptoms.

3. **Correct Answer: A, D,** Helps the client to focus on using energy for positive outcomes; observations may demonstrate psychological nature of complaint. B: The focus should be on reducing the need for a perceived dependency which provides secondary gain. C: Since the client is unaware of the underlying psychological conflict, confrontation should be avoided. E: Clients are encouraged to express feelings of anxiety and recent emotional events but not to focus on the physical symptoms.

4. **Correct Answer: A, B,** In somatic disorders the discomfort is real to the individual. It is therapeutic to acknowledge this. Redirecting the client's focus to other concerns, not the somatic ones, helps the client to begin to recognize causative factors to their physical ones. C: Confronting the client will cause their anxiety to increase. Focusing on their physical symptoms helps decrease the anxiety. D: Focusing on the pain does not help the client begin to recognize the connection to their feelings and the pain they are experiencing. E: Having the client keep a detailed log of pain does not address the underlying cause.

5. **Correct Answer: C,** Clients with factitious disorder are not concerned with lengthy hospital stays or multiple tests. A: Normal response to extended hospitalizations or tests. B: This would be seen by a client who is displaying drug-seeking behaviors; they are trying to gain from the system. D: Would be seen in somatic disorder.

6. **Correct Answer: C,** The somatic symptoms provide a psychologic or primary gain as the anxiety is relieved and focus is diverted to the physical problem. A: The client using somatization is unaware of the psychologic factors. B: Using somatization relieves but does not effectively resolve the psychologic discomfort. D: In some instances, the person may acknowledge the disease does not exist, but the fear and distress over the symptoms continue.

7. **Correct Answer: B,** Chronic pain poses a significant risk factor for depression, regardless of the cause of the pain. Depression from chronic pain can lead to suicide. A: Sleep disturbances are common with chronic pain but are not the most significant health risk. C: This occurs in conversion disorder where little concern is shown over the symptoms. D: The person with chronic pain is more likely to receive increased attention as primary and secondary gain is achieved.

8. **Correct Answer: A,** Inadvertent movement of the limb when attention is directed away can be a clue to the conversion nature of the symptoms. B: Concern of a spouse over the symptoms is not unusual and does not indicate conversion disorder. C: Functional use of unaffected limb would be expected. D: This statement would be seen in illness anxiety disorder, not conversion disorder.

Chapter 14

Fill in the Blank

1. Dissociation
2. Repressed
3. Host
4. Switching
5. Depersonalization

Matching

1. D
2. A
3. E
4. B
5. C

Multiple Choice

1. **Correct Answer: C,** The person with dissociative fugue has an inability to recall some or all of their past identity and may be accompanied by a sudden and unexpected travel away from home where a new identity may be assumed. A: Feeling of detachment while illogical nature of the feelings is recognized. B: Intentional dissociation to avoid a legal, financial, or unwanted personal situation. C: Feeling of being detached from mental thoughts of body but disorientation does not occur.

2. **Correct Answer: B,** Focus on the primary personality with reassurance for positive outcome. A: Places focus on dissociated identity. C: The nurse is exhibiting avoidance with this response, which is nontherapeutic. D: Response should emphasize a trusting environment. "Why" statements put the client on the defense and are not therapeutic.

3. **Correct Answer: A,** Provides increased perception and insight into present symptoms and problems.

B: Outcome for depersonalization. C: Outcome for dissociative identity disorder. D: Would not be an outcome as question does not mention client has any self-care deficits.

4. **Correct Answer: C,** Flooding the client with details of past traumatic events may cause the client to regress further into the dissociative state that is serving as protection from the emotional pain. To help prevent flooding, the nurse should look for signs that the client is ready to revisit the memory of the traumatic incident. A, B: In these two options, the focus is on current stressors and orientation. The question asked about "past memory deficits. Flooding does not occur when discussing current feelings. D: Introducing details on the first session will likely be too overwhelming for the client and cause further regression.

5. **Correct Answer: C,** Describes clarification of events the client is describing to the nurse. Having the client restate facts can help them to recognize the situation or what might have led up to the amnesia. A: There is no indication from the client to convey a message of anger. B: Minimizes the client's difficulty with the amnesia and the word "overreact" is a judgment. D: Demeaning statement that will likely block communication efforts.

6. **Correct Answer: B,** Although she can remember portions of her life, the client does not remember the painful details of the death of her child. A, B, D: All describe other types of amnesia.

7. **Correct Answer: D,** Host or primary personality usually is submissive, depressed, and the one that seeks treatment. A, B: True of alternate personality states that assume persona to deal with feelings and emotions that are overwhelming to the primary personality. C: Host personality is usually unaware of the other personality states.

8. **Correct Answer: B,** Clients with depersonalization disorder have persistent and repetitious feelings of being detached from their thoughts or body without the presence of disorientation. A: Seen in dissociative identity disorder. C: Seen in fugue not depersonalization disorder. D: Seen in dissociative identity disorder.

9. **Correct Answer: A, B, C, D,** Descriptive of derealization. E: In derealization the client knows who they are.

Chapter 15

Fill in the Blank

1. Substance
2. Enabling
3. Addiction
4. Detoxification
5. Delirium tremens
6. Wernicke–Korsakoff syndrome

Matching

1. B
2. J
3. H
4. E
5. G
6. F
7. D
8. I
9. A
10. C

Multiple Choice

1. **Correct Answer: D,** It is important for the nurse to notify the health care provider of changes in vital signs that could indicate complications during withdrawal. A: Fluids are not increased during withdrawal—the client has been usually been consuming fluids through drinking for a period of time. B: Fall precautions are not indicated with the symptoms identified in the question. C: Irrelevant to the situation.

2. **Correct Answer: A,** Blood alcohol level, slurred speech, and staggering gait are symptoms of alcohol intoxication. B, C, D: Symptoms listed do not define any of these situations.

3. **Correct Answer: A,** Client is denying responsibility for their actions by saying "I can handle it," and that they do not have an alcohol use disorder, despite their drinking pattern. B: Projection would be seen by shifting blame to another person and is not indicated by the client statement. C: Client is not transferring feelings to another person. D: Client is not substituting false reasoning for their behavior.

4. **Correct Answer: D,** Acknowledges and demonstrates respect for the client as a person with a problem who needs treatment. A: Minimizes the client's feelings. B: Puts client on the defensive—"why" questions block communication. C: Client has not admitted they have a problem.

5. **Correct Answer: B,** Agreeing accepts their excuses for the behavior and does not help them to take responsibility for their own actions and problems. A: Assists the client to identify differences between causes of problem and behaviors expressed. C: Acknowledging that their behavior has consequences is part of the recovery process. D: Participating in a support group is part of recovery treatment.

6. **Correct Answer: D,** Watery eyes and other respiratory symptoms are symptoms of recent substance inhalation. A, B, C: Indicate symptoms of other types of drug intoxication.

7. **Correct Answer: C,** People who engage in chronic alcohol use are usually deficient in thiamine and niacin. A: Methadone is not used for alcohol treatment. B: Stress management is not

a priority at this point in treatment. D: Client safety would be more related to psychosis or confusion that is seen with this disorder—not suicide.

8. **Correct Answer: B,** Client must first acknowledge that they have a problem in order to be committed toward abstinence. A, C, D: All may be necessary once the client has taken the initial step toward recovery.

9. **Correct Answer: C,** Hallucinogenic drugs alter the perception causing distortions of reality, such as distance or height. A, B: Symptoms would not be defined in these terms. D: Seen in chronic alcohol use, not LSD.

10. **Correct Answer: A, B, D, E,** Denial (A) is one of the common defense mechanisms used by people with substance use disorders. Blackouts (B) are seen with substance use and can be a reason for seeking treatment; readmission for treatment (D) is seen in substance use and substance use is seen more frequently in children of people with substance use disorders (E). C: With substance use, frequent call-ins or tardiness to work is seen as well as job loss—not perfect attendance.

Chapter 16

Fill in the Blank

1. Perception
2. Self-control, failure
3. Controlling/overprotective
4. Purging
5. Weight
6. 30

Matching

1. C
2. E
3. B
4. A
5. D

Multiple Choice

1. **Correct Answer: C,** Extreme weight loss from self-imposed restricted food and nutrient intake is characteristic of anorexia. A, D: Weight gain and overeating are not seen in the pattern of anorexia. B: Usually talks about and prepares food for others but does not consume any.

2. **Correct Answer: A,** Provide opportunities for independent decision-making. Fosters a sense of control for the client. B: Further depletes the client's sense of value and self-worth. C: A firm supportive approach should be used rather than one of sympathy which enables behaviors to continue. D: Discussions that focus on food are nontherapeutic.

3. **Correct Answer: B,** Antidepressant medications combined with psychotherapy have been used successfully to combat feelings of worthlessness.

A, C, D: Medications not used in treating the eating disorders.

4. **Correct Answer: C,** "Tell me about the last time you did binge eating and what you did afterward." Open-ended statement to encourage communication and acquire information. A: Puts client on defensive and minimizes their underlying psychological problem and feelings. B: Demeaning and critical of the client. D: Does not show understanding of the underlying issues in eating disorder. Nurse is also offering their opinion.

5. **Correct Answer: A,** Electrolyte imbalance, teeth enamel erosion, and calluses of the fingers and hands are common signs of purging behaviors. B: Starvation would be evident by a body weight less than the client's expected range. C: Binge-eating would not result in these symptoms. D: Excessive stress may result in weight loss but would not cause the symptoms seen.

6. **Correct Answer: A, B, D,** Seen in bulimia nervosa. C: Frequent mirror-viewing and measuring of body parts is seen in anorexia nervosa. Viewing oneself in the mirror and measuring of body parts are an attempt to reinforce their perceived self-image which is dependent on body shape and size. E: Clients with anorexia nervosa often make meals for family members or collect recipes but do not consume the food.

7. **Correct Answer: D,** Journaling can help the client tie their feelings with their behavior. A: Weighing the client each day emphasizes the weight. Focus should not be on weight but on healthy eating habits and feelings. B: Clients with an eating disorder who are left alone may hide or dispose of food in order to seem like they have eaten. Goal is to normalize eating habits. C: Clients prefer strict plans as it gives them control over their food. Normal eating habits should be emphasized, not strict plans.

8. **Correct Answer: C, D, E,** Having the client eat in a public area normalizes eating habits. Clients with an eating disorder will often hide or throw away food when left alone. Feelings of being cold are due to low muscle mass and body fat. As the client gains weight and replaces these tissues the client should feel less cold. Clients with an eating disorder focus on food and calories and not on their feelings or how they react to an emotional situation; an emotional journal would be an appropriate suggestion. A: Keeping a food and calorie journal is inappropriate as it keeps the client's focus on food. Clients with an eating disorder focus on food and calories and not on their feelings or how they react to an emotional situation. An emotional journal would be an appropriate suggestion instead. B: Daily weights are inappropriate as this helps the client focus on weight and not their feelings or emotional reactions to situations.

Chapter 17

Fill in the Blank

1. Sexual orientation
2. Self-assessment
3. Suicide
4. Arousal
5. Erectile dysfunction

Matching

1. C
2. E
3. B
4. A
5. D

Multiple Choice

1. **Correct Answer: C,** "I know it must be difficult for you to talk with a stranger about such a private matter. We can discuss it at a later time." The nurse would use an empathetic approach that acknowledges the client's right to choose when to discuss sexual functioning, but also offers to listen when the client is ready to do so. A: Blocks further communication with the client about any problem they may be experiencing related to their sex life. B: Sympathetic response that agrees with the client and closes communication. D: Attempts to force client to talk about an uncomfortable subject.
2. **Correct answer: B,** "Tell me more about what happens when you have sexual intercourse." Open-ended statement that encourages the client to continue talking about the problem. A: Client's statement does not mention sexual assault, making response inappropriate. C: Delaying when client is ready to talk discourages communication. D: Statement makes judgmental assumption.
3. **Correct answer: D,** Using a nonjudgmental approach. Nurse would appropriately use an empathetic approach that acknowledges the client has a substance use disorder but does not judge the client based on their history. A: Incorrect because information about the client's sexual behaviors is not important for the situation in the emergency department. They were admitted for polysubstance use disorder and in the emergency department time is limited. B: This action is a violation of HIPAA. C: This action puts the nurse in a potentially unsafe situation. The client with polysubstance use disorder can be unpredictable and violent. In addition, due to the client's history of being a sex offender it is inappropriate and unsafe to be alone with the client in a closed room.
4. **Correct Answer: A,** "I really want to respond to my spouse, but the feeling just isn't there." Client statement indicates a possible sexual desire or arousal disorder related to effects of antidepressant medication. Most clients with depression experience some decrease in libido. B, C, D: Usual symptoms of a depressive state.
5. **Correct answers: A, C, E,** These questions relate to topics of partners, practices, and pregnancy. B: Only asks about alcohol use; however, it is important to ask in a sexual history if the client uses alcohol along with sexual activity. D: Does refer to a sexually transmitted infection (STI) but response refers to a treated past infection. While a history of STIs is important to ask in a sexual history, asking if the client has revealed a prior treated infection to their partner is not asked.

Chapter 18

Fill in the Blank

1. Genetics
2. Dyslexia
3. IQ
4. Stuttering
5. Attention
6. Tics

Matching

1. D
2. C
3. A
4. B
5. E
6. F

Multiple Choice

1. **Correct Answer: A, B, D,** These are medications and therapy used in ADHD. C, ADHD is not an infection and antibiotics are not used in the ADHD treatment plan. E: Electroconvulsive therapy is used in the treatment of depression and bipolar disorders not ADHD.
2. **Correct Answer: B,** The child with dyslexia has difficulty in the reading and spelling domains of cognitive skills. A: Stuttering is a speech disorder. C: Would involve more than difficulty in school; would also involve behavioral symptoms such as fidgeting or inability to focus. D: Is an involuntary movement or speech and is not related to reading and writing.
3. **Correct Answer: B,** The child with separation anxiety experiences excessive anxiety related to separation from home or attachment figures. A, C, D: Not applicable to the symptoms in the question.
4. **Correct Answer: A,** Client's history shows a pattern of violent and aggressive behaviors that have resulted in or threatened harm to other people. The potential for serious injury to other clients or personnel would receive a priority. B, C, D: All may be applicable at some point in the treatment plan but safety is priority.

5. **Correct Answer: D,** Giving away prized possessions is a warning sign for suicide risk. A, B, C: Not indicative of suicidal behavior.

6. **Correct Answer: A,** The child with a language and communication disorder has difficulty understanding words and sentences or associating and organizing incoming information. This would make it difficult for the child to follow rules of a game. B: More common in autism spectrum disorder. C: Indicative of separation anxiety disorder. D: Symptom of behavioral disorder.

7. **Correct Answer: C,** Repetitive or prolonged sounds separated by pauses describe a stuttering disorder. A: Syntax refers to the structural area of language. B: Copropraxia is a sudden tic-like obscene gesture. D: Echopraxia is repetitive movements and may or may not involve speech.

8. **Correct Answer: C,** A child with severe intellectual and/or developmental disability could work at simple jobs and have independent supervised living in adulthood. A: Institutional care would be more indicated at the profound level if no caregiver could provide constant supervision. B: At the severe level, the individual could not be capable of independent living or providing own income. D: Would be seen at mild level of intellectual and/or developmental disability.

9. **Correct Answer: A,** Turning up the volume indicates child may have a hearing problem that would contribute to the learning disorder. B, C, D: Irrelevant data for learning disorder.

10. **Correct Answer: B,** Child with oppositional-defiant disorder has a repetitive pattern of negative, defiant, disobedient, and hostile behavior toward authority figures. A, C, D: Not relevant to the behavior described.

Chapter 19

Fill in the Blank

1. Delirium, dementia
2. Consciousness, short
3. Metabolize, excrete
4. Irreversible, progressive
5. Pneumonia, urinary tract infections (UTIs), infected pressure sores
6. Catastrophic

Matching

1. D
2. B
3. E
4. F
5. A
6. H
7. G
8. C

Multiple Choice

1. **Correct Answer: C,** Inability to recognize the purpose of an object is symptomatic of agnosia, or loss of comprehensive ability to recognize objects or individuals. A: Amnesia is forgetting memories. B: Anomia relates to words. D: Apraxia relates to the inability to carry out a purposeful movement.

2. **Correct Answer: A, B, C, D,** Because of the inability to recognize themselves in the mirror, they may believe someone else is in the bathroom. This may trigger anxiety that there is something wrong and cause them to retreat to another location to eliminate. Not remembering the purpose of the toilet, why they were in the bathroom, or difficulty with clothing may create a situation where urinating in a trashcan may occur. E: Hearing voices is not a symptom of dementia.

3. **Correct Answer: C,** The symptoms can usually be reversed once the cause is determined. A: Delirium is not progressive. B: The cause is urosepsis—which is not gradual or subtle (insidious). D: Delirium is short term—not long term.

4. **Correct Answer: B,** Filling in the gaps when memory falters (confabulation) is common in the early stages of dementia. A, C, D: Do not describe the example in the question.

5. **Correct Answer: D,** Repeating words or sentences describes echolalia. A: Babbling would be unintelligible sounds. B: Repetition of one word. C: Repeating one syllable.

6. **Correct Answer: B,** Clients with dementia may misinterpret the nurse's action, and trying again later will usually allow the client to forget the issue. A: Client would be unable to comprehend the explanation. C: Client is not cognitively able to refuse the medication. D: This action is indicated only if repeated efforts to give the medication are unsuccessful.

7. **Correct Answer: C,** Client may be unable to understand the spoken verbal message. Cueing will assist the client to follow through with the requested action. A: Saying the words another way adds another challenge. B: Client unable to comprehend or reason. C: It would be unsafe for client to continue ambulating with loose shoestrings.

8. **Correct Answer: A,** Placing them on a lower bed would provide the safest means of avoiding a fall. B: Bedside commode may not be understood as appropriate by the client and would add clutter to the environment. C: The client will likely attempt to get out, over, or through side rails, which poses a safety hazard. D: A sedative increases the likelihood of the client being confused and/or unstable and falling, which poses a safety threat.

9. **Correct Answer: B,** Client is most likely overwhelmed and confused by the variety of items on the tray. Reduce choices by setting one item

or bowl of food in front of the client at a time. A: Keeping a regular schedule adds structure and reduces confusion about mealtime and sleep–wake cycles. C: Actions demonstrate confusion, not lack of appetite. D: Client most likely unable to interpret verbal command.

10. **Correct Answer: D,** The person with dementia loses the ability to recognize the present and will likely remember grown children as they were when they were young, and often will think grandchildren or children not related to them are their own children. Helping family members to understand this and encouraging reminiscence about the past may help the client with the confusion. A: Arguing or correcting the mother may induce negative behavior in response. B: Pictures from the past are a better approach for reminiscence since current time period is not remembered. C: Asking for information reminds client of their memory impairment and can intensify feelings related to the impairment such as anger or sadness.

Glossary

Abuser: inflicts harmful or offensive conflict, the abuse, on their partner; gains power and control over their partner through violence that causes the partner to be fearful and intimidated. The violence can take the form of threats or emotional, physical, economic, or sexual abuse.

Acceptance: when the person begins to experience peace and serenity. This is the time of letting go and allowing life to provide new experiences and relationships.

Acetylcholine: neurotransmitter found in various organs and tissues of the body, thought to play an important role in the transmission of nerve impulses at synapses and myoneural junctions. It is quickly destroyed by an enzyme, cholinesterase.

Active listening: a learned skill that includes observing nonverbal behaviors, giving critical attention to verbal comments, listening for inconsistencies that may need clarification, and attempting to understand the client's perception of the situation.

Adaptation: successful management of stress or anxiety.

Adaptive coping: use of a rational and productive way of resolving a problem to reduce stress or anxiety.

Addiction: a physiologic and psychological dependence on a substance to the extent that withdrawal symptoms are experienced when the substance is discontinued.

Affect: describes the facial expression an individual displays in association with the mood, for example, smiling when happy, grimacing when angry.

Ageism: a prejudice based on age (in this text, referring to older age), driven by the common misconception that deterioration, senility, and mental health issues are a part of the normal aging process.

Aggression: behavior that may result in both physical and psychological harm to oneself or another verbally or nonverbally.

Aging: the changes that occur in a continuous and progressive manner during the adult years.

Agnosia: inability to identify an object.

Agoraphobia: an avoidance of certain places or situations where escape is impossible.

Akathisia: motor restlessness, inability to sit still.

Alogia: decrease in amount or speed of speech where the individual may not answer questions or stop talking in the middle of a thought (see also, poverty of speech).

Alzheimer disease: type of dementia that primarily affects the cerebral cortex, which is involved in conscious thought and language, the production of acetylcholine (a neurotransmitter involved in memory and learning), and the hippocampus, essential to memory storage.

Amnesia: loss of memories applied to episodes during which individuals forget their identity, though they conduct themselves properly and following which no memory of the period exists.

Anal stage: Freudian stage from 2 to 4 years during which pleasure is achieved from an awareness and control of urination and defecation.

Anergia: marked decrease in energy level; may make the individual depend on others for even basic needs.

Anger: emotion triggered in response to threats, insulting situations, or anything that seriously hampers the intended actions of an individual.

Anhedonia: little interest in things an individual previously enjoyed.

Anomia: inability to find the right word.

Anorexia nervosa: an eating disorder characterized by an individual who loses weight, either by restricting calories or excessive exercise, has an inappropriate weight for their age and stature, and has a distorted body image (National Eating Disorders Association, 2022a).

Anticipatory anxiety: anxiety that occurs in advance of a feared situation, such as a public speech or social event).

Anticipatory grief: grief experienced when the person is expecting a major loss in the near future.

Antidepressant: medication used in the treatment of depression to elevate mood, increase physical activity and mental alertness, improve appetite and sleep, and restore interest or pleasure in usual activities and things previously enjoyed.

Antimanic: mood-stabilizing agent used to treat manic episodes associated with bipolar disorder or to diminish future episodes.

Antipsychotic agents: medications, sometimes referred to as neuroleptics, used to treat serious mental illness such as bipolar affective disorder, major depressive disorder, substance-induced psychosis, schizophrenia, and autism spectrum disorder.

Anxiety: a feeling of apprehension, uneasiness, or uncertainty that occurs in response to a real or perceived threat.

Anxiolytic (antianxiety agents): medication used to counteract or diminish anxiety.

Aphasia: impairment in the significance or meaning of language that prevents the individual from understanding what is heard, following instructions, and communicating needs.

Apraxia: inability to carry out purposeful movements and actions despite intact motor and sensory functioning.

Assertion: standing up for one's rights, beliefs, or values in such a way that it does not hurt others in the process.

Assessment: involves the collection of psychosocial, subjective, and objective data about the client, also referred to as data collection.

Automatic relief behaviors: unconscious behaviors aimed at relieving the individual's anxiety.

Avolition: lacking motivation to make decisions or initiate self-care such as hygiene and grooming.

Behavioral therapy: emphasizes the principles of learning with positive or negative reinforcement and observational modeling.

Bereavement: adapting to loss, characterized by reactions of grief and sadness.

Binge-eating: also known as binging; eating an unusually large amount of food, usually within a 2-hour time frame, that is more than most people would eat in a similar circumstance.

Biofeedback: a training program used for specific types of anxiety that is designed to develop the client's ability to control heart rate, muscle tension, and other autonomic or involuntary functions of the nervous system by using monitoring devices during situations that trigger this reaction.

Bipolar disorder: mental illness characterized by atypical and erratic shifts in mood, energy, activity, behavior, sleep, and cognition.

Blackout: a form of amnesia for events that occurred during the drinking period.

Blocking: speech pattern where the client unconsciously blocks out information, which results in loss of thought process and causes the client to stop speaking.

Bulimia nervosa: eating disorder characterized by the individual either binge-eating or regularly overeating and then uses self-induced methods, such as vomiting or the use of laxatives, to counteract the food consumed.

Bullying: psychological harassment or physical confrontation used repeatedly to intentionally bring harm or humiliation to one seen as weak or different.

Catastrophic reactions: include agitation and verbal and/or physical responses of fear and panic (such as crying, shouting, or laughing uncontrollably or inappropriately) with a potential of harm to self and others. Catastrophic reactions are often precipitated by frustration and a perceived threat or fear, often trivial in nature such as a change in routine or environment.

Catalepsy: extreme form of posturing for extended periods of time.

Catatonic: behaviors that display a decreased reaction to environmental surroundings with movements that may be severely decreased or absent and accompanied by a stupor.

Chemical restraint: the use of medication to restrict a client's behavior.

Circumstantiality: speech pattern where the client cannot be selective when speaking and describes in lengthy, great detail.

Clang associations: speech pattern where words are strung together in rhyming phrases or that have no connected meaning such as "Hair is bare and bear is a scare, scare is a fair, fair is there, you are a pear…" or "The sky is blue, so are you… two plus two, much to do so to fear, far and near, let's have a beer…"

Clinical psychologist: mental health professional who administers and interprets psychological testing used in the diagnostic process, and provides various types of therapy to assist in resolution of mental health issues.

Codependent: individual who feels a responsibility for the person with a substance use disorder's problem and internalizes a form of guilt for the behavior of that person. As a result, the codependent individual continues to do everything possible to sustain the relationship and is unable to recognize the detrimental effects of the codependency on their own physical and mental health.

Cognitive behavioral therapy: based on the cognitive model that focuses on identifying and correcting distorted thinking patterns that can lead to emotional distress and problem behavior.

Compensatory methods: laxatives, diuretics, or enemas used to counteract the amount of food consumed.

Compulsions: the repetitive behaviors or rituals the person engages in to reduce their anxiety.

Concrete mental operations: stage of cognitive development in Piaget's theory of development, in which the individual engages in mental manipulations of internal images of tangible objects.

Confabulation: behavioral reaction to memory loss in which the individual fills in memory gaps with fictitious statements.

Confidentiality: client's right to prevent written or verbal communications from being disclosed to outside parties without authorization.

Conscious: Freudian stage of the psyche relating to present awareness; being aware and having perception of the environment; having the ability to filter that information through the mind with the awareness of doing so.

Continuous amnesia: encompasses a period up to and including the present that is lost from conscious recollection.

Contracting: a behavioral technique in which the client and therapist draw up a contract to which both parties are obligated.

Conventional grief: feelings of sadness experienced following a loss.

Conversion disorder: when an individual exhibits symptoms that indicate a sensory or neurologic impairment; however, the impairment is not supported by results of diagnostic testing (sometimes called functional neurologic symptom disorder).

Copropraxia: sudden tic-like obscene gesture.

Countertransference: the response that is elicited in the person receiving the transferred feelings or communications.

Craving: a strong desire to use a substance for the reward of the intense feelings the substance produces.

Cued: a panic attack where an identified trigger can be associated with the attack.

Cultural identity: binding force between members of a group that may include a common language, family structure, customs, country of origin, religious and political beliefs, food, dress/clothing, traditions, and holidays.

Defense mechanism: automatic, psychological processes that are used to protect the person from anxiety and the awareness of internal or external stressors.

Delirium: state of mental confusion characterized by a disturbance of the consciousness and a change in cognition that develops over a short time, such as within hours to a few days.

Delirium tremens: a state of profound confusion and delusions along with all of the usual symptoms of alcohol withdrawal.

Delusion: fixed, false ideas or beliefs without appropriate external stimuli that are inconsistent with reality and that cannot be changed by reasoning.

Delusions of grandeur: false or outrageous beliefs about oneself.

Delusions of persecution: when an individual fully believes someone is planning to harm them or are conspiring against them.

Delusions of reference: false beliefs by an individual that the behavior of others in the environment is directed at them personally.

Dementia: characterized by irreversible, progressive deterioration in cognitive functioning, including a loss of memory, awareness, judgment, and reasoning ability. This deterioration in intellectual functioning is severe enough to interfere with an individual's normal daily activities and ability to communicate or interact with others.

Depersonalization: a persistent and repetitious feeling of being detached from one's mental thoughts or body.

Depression: a persistent and prolonged mood of sadness that extends beyond 2 weeks' duration or longer.

Derailment: inability to organize and connect ideas; with sudden changes in thought processes that are vague, unfocused, and illogical. The thoughts or ideas frequently jump from one topic to another that are unrelated (see also, loose associations).

Derealization: the person perceives the external environment as unreal or changing.

Detoxification: the first phase of dependency treatment and consists of immediate withdrawal from the physical and psychological effects of the drug that usually last from 3 to 5 days.

Developmental crisis: occurs at a predictable time period in an individual's life related to maturational stages and changes.

Disorientation: the inability to be knowledgeable of time (such as time of day, month, or year), place or location, and person.

Dissociation: the mechanism that allows an individual's mind to separate certain memories, most often of unpleasant situations or traumatic events, from conscious awareness.

Dissociative amnesia: characterized by an inability to remember important personal information that is usually of a traumatic or stressful nature.

Dissociative fugue: inability to recall some or all of a person's past or identity, accompanied by the sudden and unexpected travel of the person away from home or place of employment.

Dissociative identity disorder: two or more distinct identities or personalities present in the same person that alternate in assuming control of the person's behavior (formerly known as multiple personality disorder).

Distress: negative stress in response to a threat or challenge that is actually harmful to one's health.

Dopamine: catecholamine neurotransmitter; a precursor in the synthesis of norepinephrine important in understanding the pathology of schizophrenia and parkinsonism.

Drug-induced parkinsonism: symptoms that mimic parkinsonism such as tremors, rigidity, akinesia, or absence of movement with diminished mental state.

Dysfunctional grief: failure to complete the grieving process and cope successfully with a loss.

Dyslexia: a type of learning disorder characterized by difficulty in the visual reading domain.

Dystonia: rigidity in muscles that control posture, gait, or eye movement.

Echolalia: speech pattern where the individual repeats another's speech word for word.

Echopraxia: mimicking the movements of another person without a reason.

Ego: in Freudian theory, the conscious self where sensations, feelings, adjustments, solutions, and defenses are formed.

Electroconvulsive therapy (ECT): a treatment using low-voltage electric shock waves passed through the brain to induce short periods of seizure activity.

Emotional abuse: words or nonverbal language that is used to criticize, demean, or humiliate and inflict psychological trauma on another person.

Emotional numbness: not feeling or expressing emotions.

Empathy: ability to hear what another person is saying, to have temporary access to that person's feelings, and to perceive the situation from that person's perspective.

Enabling: pattern of either consciously or unconsciously helping someone else's maladaptive behavior to continue.

Entitlement: belief seen in narcissistic personality disorder where the individual believes others owe them because of their superiority.

Enuresis: involuntary urination that may be related to physiologic or psychological causes.

Ethics: a set of principles or values that guides behavior, helps determine right or wrong in a situation, and helps determine how activity should be conducted.

Euphoria: an excessive feeling of happiness or elation.

Eustress: positive and motivating stress shown by one's confidence in the ability to master a challenge or stressor.

Evaluation: step of nursing process which determines if the outcome was met, partially met, or not met at all.

External stressors: aspects of the environment that may be adverse to one's well-being.

Extrapyramidal side effects: side effects of antipsychotic medications which include the inability to sit still, involuntary muscle contractions (such as repeated arm jerking), tremors, and involuntary facial movements, also called drug-induced movement disorders.

Factitious disorder: where the individual intentionally falsifies, simulates, or creates medical symptoms as though there is an illness when in fact, there is not one, for the sole purpose of primary gain.

Fight-or-flight response: reaction to an immediate threat in which there is a surge of adrenalin into the bloodstream.

Flight of ideas: speech pattern where the client rapidly shifts between topics that are unrelated to each other.

Focusing: communication technique that helps client concentrate on a specific issue.

Formal operations: stage of cognitive development in Piaget theory where abstract thought processes, problem solving, and systematic purposeful mental relationships develop, beginning at age 11 and older.

Free-floating anxiety: occurs when the individual is unable to connect the anxiety to a stimulus.

Gender dysphoria: psychological distress due to a sense of incongruence between sex assigned at birth and gender identity.

Gender identity: the innate sense of feeling male, female, neither, or a combination of both, or something else.

Generalized amnesia: condition in which the individual is unable to recall any aspect of their life.

Genital stage: Freudian psychosexual stage that occurs as the child enters puberty and adolescence where sexual feelings reemerge and become directed towards establishing a relationship.

Genuineness: attribute of realness and concern that fosters an honest and caring foundation for trust shown by the nurse accepting the client as a person with worth and dignity, who is not judged or labeled by the nurse's standards.

Grandiosity: larger-than-reality self-esteem or feelings (e.g., the individual thinks they have more wealth or intelligence than they really do); this sounds arrogant or boastful to the observer.

Grief: emotional process of coping with a loss.

Group therapy: therapy in which a trained therapist leads a small group of people with similar problems who discuss individual and common issues.

Hallucination: false sensory perceptions that have no relation to reality and are not supported by actual environmental stimuli.

Hierarchy: some needs are more basic or more powerful than others.

Holistic: concept of nursing care that incorporates the entire scope of human needs, addressing the physical, emotional, psychosocial, cultural, and spiritual issues of the client.

Hostility: intense feeling of animosity toward someone or something.

Humanistic therapy: nondirective approach that centers on the client's view of the world and their problems.

Hypomania: a state of mild to moderate mania that lasts for a period of at least 4 days.

Id: One part of the personality according to Freud that operates on the pleasure principle and demands instant gratification of drives, is present at birth and contains the instincts, impulses, and urges for survival.

Ideas of reference: the individual believes that everyday occurrences have a special and significant personal meaning. For example, the individual may think a news headline was written specifically for them.

Illness anxiety disorder: when the individual may or may not have a medical condition, but they do have increased body sensations and are extremely anxious about the possibility of an existing serious undiagnosed illness (previously called hypochondriasis).

Illusions: are experienced when sensory stimuli actually exist but are misinterpreted by the individual. For example, the individual may refer to spots on the floor as insects or to an electric cord as a snake.

Informed consent: when the client gives permission to undergo a specific procedure or treatment <u>after</u> being informed about the procedure, risks, and benefits.

Inhalants: volatile substances such as gasoline and paint, if used for the purpose of intoxication.

Intellectual and/or developmental disability: broad term that covers a variety of conditions that cause significant limitations in intellectual functioning, social interactions, and practical living skills.

Internal stressors: adverse aspects that cause stress that are from within the individual and can be physical or psychological.

Interpersonal: concerning the relations and interactions between persons.

Intimate partner violence (IPV): a pattern of behavior displayed by a current or former intimate partner using physical or sexual violence, psychological intimidation, aggression, or stalking (previously called domestic abuse or domestic violence).

Intoxication: the state where an individual's physical or mental status is affected or diminished due to the consumption of a substance such as alcohol or drugs.

Involuntary commitment: when a person is admitted to a psychiatric unit against their will.

Job-related burnout: condition of mental, physical, and emotional exhaustion with a reduced sense of personal accomplishment and apathy toward one's work.

Labile: rapid shifts in mood in a short period of time, alternating from euphoria to dysphoria and irritability.

La belle indifference: is seen in conversion disorder and is an attitude demonstrating little to no anxiety or concern over the implications of their symptoms.

Latency stage: Freud's psychosexual theory stage during middle childhood in which the sexual desires and feelings remain subdued.

Learned helplessness: individual behaves in helpless manner and overlooks possible solutions.

Lewy bodies: abnormal deposits of proteins develop in nerve cells in the cortex of the brain which cause a type of dementia.

Localized amnesia: usually occurs within a few hours following a traumatic incident such as war combat, natural disasters, or severe trauma. Fragments of the individual's identity are forgotten.

Loose association: inability to organize and connect ideas, with sudden changes in thought processes that are vague, unfocused, and illogical. The thoughts or ideas frequently jump from one topic to another that are unrelated (see also, derailment).

Loss: actual or perceived change in the status of one's relationship to a valued object or person.

Magical thinking: the belief that the individual's thoughts, words, or actions can cause or prevent an occurrence in another person, usually by extraordinary means.

Maladaptive coping: unsuccessful attempts to decrease anxiety without attempting to solve the problem allowing anxiety to continue.

Malingered fugue: type of dissociation occurring in a person who is trying to avoid a legal, financial, or unwanted personal situation.

Malingering: when the individual is intentionally being deceptive regarding their symptoms or an illness to avoid a situation such as work or incarceration or to gain something such as opioids or disability benefits.

Mannerisms: repetitive and goal-directed movements such as saluting or bowing. These behaviors involve excessive motor activity that is triggered by an internal, not external, stimulus.

Mania: a mood characterized by overactivity, extreme euphoria, impulsivity, and lowered inhibitions, and may lead to delusions or hallucinations.

Manipulation: involves behavioral tactics of deceit, devious thinking, or actions used to meet the individual's self-serving needs at the expense of another person.

Mental health: involves the components of emotional, psychological, and social well-being; the balance between the individual's cognitive, behavioral, and emotional states; and the individual's ability to handle stress and adversity, relate to others, emote (express) their feelings, and make healthy choices.

Mental Health Patient Bill of Rights: document set by the US government that covers the rights of the mental health client regarding their treatment.

Mental illness: when the individual demonstrates a change in one or more of the following: emotions (sometimes referred to as mood), thinking, or behavior; these changes are accompanied by problems relating to others in personal, work, or social relationships or an inability to perform activities of daily living (ADLs).

Monoamine oxidase inhibitor (MAOI): a category of antidepressant medications that inhibit monoamine oxidase; monoamine oxidase is an enzyme that metabolizes or inactivates the monoamine neurotransmitters.

Mood: emotion that is prolonged and permeates the individual's entire psychological thinking.

Mood-stabilizing agents: medications indicated for manic episodes associated with bipolar disorder and maintenance therapy to prevent or diminish future episodes.

Narcissism: derived from the Greek, meaning "excessive love and attention given to one's own self-image"; person has continued need for lavish attention and admiration with little regard for the feeling of others.

Neologism: speech pattern where the individual makes up new words and definitions, such as, "The malitars are coming to get me." The neologism has meaning to the individual but not to others.

Neuroleptic malignant syndrome: a potentially fatal reaction most often seen with the high-potency antipsychotic medications causing muscular rigidity, tremors, inability to speak, altered level of consciousness, hyperthermia, hypertension, tachycardia, tachypnea, diaphoresis, and elevated white blood cell count.

Neurotransmitter: the chemical messenger proteins stored in the presynaptic compartment and when released, travel across the synapse to act on the target cell to either inhibit or excite.

Nursing care focus: the identification of a client problem based on an actual or a potential problem that falls within the range of the nursing scope of practice, also referred to as a nursing diagnosis.

Nursing interventions: actions taken by the nurse to assist the client in achieving the anticipated outcome.

Nursing process: scientific and systematic method for providing effective individualized nursing care that serves as an aid in resolving client problems.

Objective data: data the nurse observes or that is provided by additional members of the health care team.

Objectivity: the ability to view facts and events without distortion by personal feelings, prejudices, or judgments.

Obsessions: reoccurrence of persistent unwanted thoughts or images that cause the person intense anxiety.

Opiates: a substance that naturally occurs from opium and are heroin, morphine, and codeine.

Opioids: refers to all natural, synthetic, and semisynthetic forms of opium.

Oral stage: Freud's psychosexual theory stage that occurs during a person's first 2 years where the child seeks pleasure from sucking and oral gratification of hunger.

Orientation phase: introductory phase of the therapeutic relationship that involves meeting and getting to know the client, an explanation of the purpose for the nurse–client interaction; is a means of building trust, establishing roles, and identifying client problems and expectations.

Outcomes: specific, measurable, and realistic goals that include a time frame for when it should be accomplished by.

Palliative coping: coping strategy where the solution temporarily relieves the stress or anxiety but the problem still exists and must be dealt with again at a later time.

Panic attack: intense feeling of fear or terror that occurs suddenly and intermittently without warning.

Paraphilia: a sexual interest that falls outside what is generally considered "typical" within a certain culture. A paraphilia may involve an erotic activity, or it may be focused on specific objects or people.

Passive-aggressive: behaviors, in which the individual indirectly and subtly acts on hostile feelings by displaying a passive and pleasant affect, but acts based on underlying pessimism and bitterness.

Perseverance: continuing to do, or follow through with, something that is difficult or has a delay in the outcome or faced with obstacles.

Personality disorder: deeply ingrained, persistent, inflexible, and maladaptive patterns of behavior that are in conflict with a cultural norm.

Personality traits: persistent ways in which an individual views and relates to other people and to society as a whole including controlling their behavior, emotionally responding to situations, how they think about themselves or others, and how they relate to other people.

Phallic stage: psychosexual theory stage around the age of 4 years in which the child discovers pleasure in genital stimulation while also struggling to accept a sexual identity.

Physical abuse: intentional injury to another person and can include slapping, pinching, choking, scratching, stabbing, shooting, and homicide.

Physical restraint: the use of a method or physical device to restrict movement by the client.

Pica: the repetitive eating (ingestion) of nonfood substances that lasts more than 1 month.

Postsynaptic receptor: a cell component located in the neuron distal to the synapse.

Posturing: person in stupor assumes a rigid posture held against gravity, resisting efforts to be moved for extended periods of time.

Poverty of speech: decrease in amount or speed of speech where the individual may not answer questions or stop talking in the middle of a thought (see also, alogia).

Powerlessness: a state of helplessness felt from the lack of control over the effects imposed by a condition.

Preconscious: also referred to as subconscious; that part of the psyche according to Freud that is below current awareness but easily retrieved.

Preoperational: according to Piaget, second stage of cognitive development, which occurs from 2 to 7 years where the child communicates their thoughts, which are largely egocentric without regard for another point of view.

Presynaptic compartment: storage compartment for neurotransmitters located before the nerve synapse.

Primary aging: changes that occur as a result of genetics or natural factors.

Primary gain: when anxiety is relieved by focus being diverted to the physical problem.

Prioritization: the act of putting first the issue, or individual, based upon the intensity and immediate urgency of the problem.

Prodromal phase: the onset of symptoms of schizophrenia that are insidious (subtle and seemingly harmless), with the individual experiencing them for some time before the first full-blown psychotic episode occurs.

Professional boundaries: limits maintained by the nurse to provide for safe interactions with the client.

Pseudoneurologic: false neurologic disturbances.

Psychiatrist: a licensed physician who specializes in the psychiatric or mental disorders.

Psychodynamic therapy: based on Freudian psychoanalytic theory with the assumption that when a client has insight into early relationships and experiences as the source of their problems, the problems can be resolved.

Psychogenic: type of seizure seen in conversion disorder that is nonepileptic.

Psychological crisis: a state of disorganization and disarray occurring in the individual when usual coping strategies fail or are not available.

Psychopharmacology: study of the changes that occur as a medication interacts with the chemicals in the brain.

Psychosis: refers to a set of symptoms that includes perceptual disturbances, disorganized thinking, and behavior alterations. Psychosis is not an illness.

Psychosocial: related to both psychological and social factors.

Psychotherapy: a dialog between a mental health practitioner and the client with a goal of reducing the symptoms of the emotional disturbance or disorder and improving that individual's personal and social well-being.

Psychotropic agents: medications that have their impact on target sites or receptors of the nervous system to induce changes that affect psychiatric function, behavior, or experience.

Purging: the eliminating of consumed food through self-induced vomiting or with excessive use of laxatives or diuretics.

Rapid-cycling: four or more episodes of mania or depression within a year.

Reflection: communication technique that paraphrases message client has conveyed to nurse.

Reframing: way of restructuring thinking about a stressful event into a way that is less disturbing and over which the individual can have some control.

Relapse: return to using a substance after apparent recovery.

Restating: repeating back to client the content of interaction for the purpose of leading and encouraging further discussion.

Reuptake: the action of neurotransmitters being absorbed back into the presynaptic compartment of the previous neuron.

Schizoaffective disorder: form of schizophrenia in which the person demonstrates symptoms of major depression or mania in addition to the primary symptoms of delusions, hallucinations, and disorganized behaviors of schizophrenia.

Schizophrenia: a form of psychosis in which there are disorganized thoughts, perceptual alterations, inappropriate affect, and decreased emotional response as the connections to reality are broken.

Seclusion: the involuntary placement of a client alone, in a controlled environment.

Secondary aging: changes that are influenced by environmental factors.

Secondary gain: the subsequent attention an individual receives from a health care provider or family member in relation to somatic symptoms.

Selective amnesia: when person retains memory of some portions of the event, but does not remember all details.

Self-awareness: a consciousness of one's own individuality and personality

Self-mutilation: intentional act of inflicting bodily injury to oneself without an intent to die as a result.

Self-stigma: when a person believes that, because of their mental illness, they will be rejected personally or when applying for a job; therefore, they begin to avoid others or stop applying for jobs. Also called internal stigma.

Sensorimotor: first stage of cognitive development in Piaget's theory where the growth of abilities related to the five senses and motor functions occurs.

Serotonin: potent vasoconstrictor thought to be involved in neural mechanisms related to arousal, sleep, dreams, mood, appetite, and sensitivity to pain.

Selective serotonin reuptake inhibitors (SSRIs): a category of antidepressant medication designed to block the reuptake of serotonin.

Sexual abuse: any behavior using forced or unwanted sexual acts that are inflicted on an unwilling participant.

Sexual dysfunction: a condition that the client identifies as causing them distress that occurs during any phase of the sexual response cycle or interferes with sexual function. Sexual dysfunction can also include pain associated with sexual intercourse.

Sexual orientation: gendered pattern of attraction to others. Sexual orientation for some includes attraction to one gender, while others are attracted to multiple genders, and others do not experience sexual attraction.

Silence: communication technique where the nurse remains quiet with an attentive manner; this conveys a willingness to continue listening.

Situational crisis: unpredictable and sudden crisis that occurs without warning such as fatal illness diagnosis, plane crash, natural disaster, or sudden death.

Social phobia: characterized by an excessive fear of any social situation in which embarrassment is possible; also known as social anxiety disorder.

Somatic symptom disorder: characterized by one or more somatic symptoms that do not have a medical cause, are disturbing to the individual, and cause disruption in their daily functioning.

Somatization: when the individual's concerns and physical symptoms are experienced as a result of significant psychological stress (soma = Greek for "body").

Specific phobia: characterized by an excessive and persistent irrational fear of specific objects or situations that pose little threat of danger.

Splitting: extreme view of an all or none relationship with the world. Things are seen as all or none, black or white, love or hate, with no neutral ground.

Stigma: the negative association and/or perception attached to a disorder or situation.

Stress: the condition that results when a threat or challenge to one's well-being requires the person to adjust or adapt to the environment.

Stress reaction: physical response to a stressor that is triggered by an arousal of the autonomic nervous system.

Stalking: type of unwanted behavior that includes activities such as harassing or threatening phone calls, e-mails, texts, voicemails, mail, unwanted appearances at the victim's place of employment, home, or other location, vandalism, or forced entry of the victim's place of residence or vehicle.

Stupor: lack of awareness or orientation.

Stuttering: language pattern characterized by repetitive or prolonged sounds or syllables that include pauses and monosyllable broken words.

Subjective data: data spoken by the client or family.

Substance: any drug, medication, or toxin that has the potential for misuse.

Substance use disorder: a maladaptive pattern of substance use that demonstrates physiologic, cognitive, and behavioral indications that the person continues to use the drug despite the adverse substance-related problems they may be experiencing.

Suicidal erosion: long-term accumulation of negative experiences throughout an individual's lifetime that can lead to suicidal thoughts.

Suicidal gesture: action that indicates a person may be about ready to carry out a plan for suicide.

Suicidal ideation: verbalized thought or idea that indicates a person's desire to do self-harm or destruction.

Suicidal threat: statement of intent usually accompanied by behavior changes that indicate a person has defined their plan to end their life.

Suicide attempt: person carries out their plan with actions to end their life.

Sundowning syndrome: a peak period of agitation and acting-out behavior during the evening hours.

Superego: one part of the personality according to Freud, often referred to as the conscience, that starts developing at about 3 to 4 years of age and controls, inhibits, and regulates those impulses and instinctive urges whose unrestricted expression would be socially unacceptable.

Switching process: changing of one personality to another that occurs very abruptly in dissociative identity disorder.

Synaptic cleft: the space between two neurons.

Tardive dyskinesia: extrapyramidal syndrome with irreversible movements of the mouth and face that include lip-smacking and grinding of teeth, protruding tongue movements, a masklike facial appearance, tremors, shuffling gait, cogwheel rigidity, pill-rolling, and stooped posture.

Telehealth: the use of electronic and telecommunication technology to interact with clients.

Temperament: the inherent way an individual behaves or reacts to stimuli, self-regulates (the ability to manage disruptive stimuli), and the intensity of their emotions and reactions.

Termination phase: last phase of the nurse–client relationship that allows the client to depend on their own strengths while continuing to use their adaptive skills.

Therapeutic milieu: a safe and secure structured setting that facilitates the therapeutic interaction between clients and members of the professional team amidst a supportive network in which there is a sense of common goals.

Therapeutic relationship: a helping bond in which one person assists in the personal growth and improved well-being of the other.

Thought broadcasting: false belief that the individual's thoughts can be heard by others.

Thought insertion: false belief by an individual that thoughts of others can be inserted into their mind.

Thought withdrawal: false belief by an individual that others are robbing thoughts from their brain.

Tic: a sudden, brief, repetitive, arrhythmic, stereotyped motor movement or sound.

Tolerance: develops as the brain and body adapt to repeated doses of the substance with a declining effect as it is taken repetitively over time. This results in the need to use greater amounts of the substance to obtain the same effect.

Trait anger: a general biologic leaning toward a volatile personality that reflects a quick response or irritation and fury or a quick temper.

Transference: unconscious transfer of feelings and attitudes from a person or situation in one's past to a person or situation in the present.

Transgender: an adjective that describes an individual whose gender identity is different from the sex they were assigned at birth.

Tricyclic antidepressants (TCAs): a category of antidepressant medication named for their three-ring chemical structure that work by inhibiting the reuptake of the neurotransmitters back into the presynaptic cells, which leads to higher concentration of the neurotransmitters available.

Unconscious: The largest part of the psyche according to Freud, where past experiences and the related emotions have been completely removed from the conscious level. This level is largely responsible for contributing to the emotional discomfort and disturbances that threaten the individual.

Uncued: panic attack where no particular stimulus can be connected with the panic attack.

Unipolar: individual has depression but does not experience mania or hypomania.

Unresolved grief: situations when the grief process is incomplete and life is burdened with maladaptive symptoms continuing months after the loss has occurred.

Validation: verifying the nurse's perception of the verbal or nonverbal message conveyed by the client.

Violence: an expression of anger or resentment in an attempt to maintain power in a situation or relationship.

Visualization: mentally viewing a place of peaceful solitude to allow the individual a momentary reprieve from the stress

Voluntary commitment: when the client is admitted to the mental health unit based on their own decision for admission.

Water intoxication: a psychosis-induced metabolic state of fluid overload that can lead to cerebral edema and other potentially lethal situations. Seen by an excessive amount of water being consumed, leading to abdominal cramps, dizziness, lethargy, nausea and vomiting, convulsions, and possible coma.

Waxy flexibility: where the individual remains fixed in one position until someone changes it. An arm, leg, or other body part can be moved by another person and the body part will remain in that position until moved again.

Wernicke–Korsakoff syndrome: a nutritional disease of the nervous system found in those with alcohol use disorder, caused primarily by thiamine and niacin deficiency.

Withdrawal: occurs as the blood or tissue concentrations of a substance declines in a person who has developed a tolerance for the substance.

Word salad: speech pattern where the individual expresses random unconnected and disorganized thoughts, which indicates severe impairment.

Working phase: a period in which goals are set and interventions planned for behavior change and to improve the client's well-being.

Index

Page numbers followed by b indicate boxes; those followed by f indicate figures; those followed by t indicate tables.